Canine Sports Medicine and Rehabilitation

Canine Sports Medicine and Rehabilitation

Second Edition

Edited by

Chris Zink, DVM, PhD, DACVP, DACVSMR, CCRT, CVSMT, CVA

Janet B. Van Dyke, DVM, DACVSMR, CCRT

WILEY Blackwell

Registered Office
John Wiley & Sons, Inc., 111 River Street, Hoboken, NJ 07030, USA

Editorial Office
111 River Street, Hoboken, NJ 07030, USA

For details of our global editorial offices, customer services, and more information about Wiley products visit us at
www.wiley.com.

Wiley also publishes its books in a variety of electronic formats and by print-on-demand. Some content that appears
in standard print versions of this book may not be available in other formats.

Library of Congress Cataloging-in-Publication data are available

ISBN: 9781119380382

Cover images: (Top image) Courtesy of Rich Knecht; (Bottom left) Canine bone marrow-derived mesenchymal stem
cells isolated by gradient centrifugation, cultured, stained for actin (green) and matrix metalloproteinase (red), and
visualized with confocal microscopy. Courtesy of W. Brian Saunders, DVM, PhD, DACVS. Assistant Professor,
Orthopedic Surgery, College of Veterinary Medicine & Biomedical Sciences, College Station, Texas, USA. Reproduced
with permission; (Bottom right) Courtesy of Janet B. Van Dyke.
Cover design by Chris Zink.

Set in 9.5/11.5pt Palatino by SPi Global, Pondicherry, India

SKY10074464_050324

Contents

Contributors

Stuart Bliss, DVM, PhD, DACVS, CCRP
Staff Surgeon
Port City Veterinary Referral Hospital
Portsmouth, NH, USA

Jennifer Brown, DVM, DACVS-LA,
DACVSMR, CCRT, CVSMT
K-9 SportsVet
Odessa, FL, USA

Sherman O. Canapp, Jr, DVM, MS, DACVS,
DACVSMR, CCRT
Chief of Staff
Veterinary Orthopedic and Sports Medicine
Group
Annapolis Junction, MD, USA

Brittany Jean Carr, DVM, CCRT
American College of Veterinary
Sports Medicine and Rehabilitation Candidate
Yellow Springs, OH, USA

Jody Chiquoine, MSN, FNP, CCRT
CEO, Fitter Critters
Lee, MA, USA

Joan R. Coates, DVM, MS, DACVIM (Neurology)
Professor, Veterinary Neurology & Neurosurgery
Service Leader, Neurology & Neurosurgery
Department of Veterinary Medicine and Surgery
College of Veterinary Medicine
University of Missouri
Columbia, MO, USA

Judy C. Coates, MEd, MSPT, CCRT
Director of Rehabilitation
Coates Canine Physical Therapy
Hanover, NH, USA

Jonathan Dyce, MA, VetMB, MRCVS, DSAO,
DACVS
Associate Professor
Department of Veterinary Clinical Sciences
The Ohio State University
Columbus, OH, USA

David Dycus, DVM, MS, DACVS, CCRP
Orthopedic Staff Surgeon
Veterinary Orthopedic and Sports Medicine
Group (VOSM)
Annapolis Junction, MD, USA

Mark E. Epstein, DVM, DABVP (C/F), CVPP
Senior Partner, Medical Director
Total Bond Veterinary Hospitals, PC
Carolinas Animal Pain Management
Gastonia and Charlotte, NC, USA

Sasha A. Foster, MSPT, CCRT
Founder, Canine Rehab Shop
Rehabilitation Coordinator
Colorado State University Veterinary Teaching
Hospital
Fort Collins, CO, USA

Samuel P. Franklin, MS, DVM, PhD, DACVS-SA, DACVSMR
Assistant Professor, Small Animal Orthopedic Surgery
University of Georgia
Veterinary Medical Center
Athens, GA, USA

Kimberly E. Henneman, DVM, DACVSMR, DABT, FAAVA, CVA, CVC
Owner
Animal Health VIPs
Park City, UT, USA

Amie Lamoreaux Hesbach, PT, DPT, MS, CCRP, CCRT
EmpowerPhysioPeT
Maynard, MA, USA

David Hummel, DVM, DACVS-SA
Staff Surgeon
Skylos Sports Medicine
Frederick, MD, USA

Christine Jurek, DVM, CCRT, CVA, CVC
Associate Veterinarian
TOPS Veterinary Rehabilitation
Grayslake, IL, USA

Martin Kaufmann, C-Ped, BSBA
Owner and Founder
OrthoPets
Denver, CO, USA

Nina R. Kieves, DVM, DACVS-SA, DACVSMR, CCRT
Assistant Professor, Small Animal Surgery
Chief, Small Animal Physical Rehabilitation Services
The Ohio State University College of Veterinary Medicine
Columbus, OH, USA

Kristin Kirkby Shaw, DVM, MS, PhD, DACVS, DACVSMR, CCRT
Staff Surgeon
Animal Surgical Clinic of Seattle
Seattle, WA, USA

Amy Kramer, PT, DPT, CCRT
Owner and Director
Beach Animal Rehabilitation
Torrance, CA, USA

Rosemary J. LoGiudice, DVM, DACVSMR, CCRT, CVA, CVSMT, FCoAC
Senior Staff Veterinarian
Integrative Pet Care,
Hanover Park, IL, USA
Owner
Animal Rehabilitation & Therapy
Yorkville, IL, USA

Faith M. Lotsikas, DVM, CCRT
Skylos Sports Medicine
Frederick, MD, USA

Peter J. Lotsikas, DVM, DACVS-SA, DACVSMR
Skylos Sports Medicine
Frederick, MD, USA

Ellen Martens, MsPT, MT, CCRT
Director
Het Waterhof Rehabilitation
Velm, Belgium

Laurie McCauley, DVM, DACVSMR, CVC, CVA, CCRT
Chief of Staff
Red Tail Rehabilitation, Inc.
Zirconia, NC, USA

Carolina Medina, DVM, DACVSMR, CVA, CVCH, CCRT
Director of Rehabilitation
Coral Springs Animal Hospital
Coral Springs, FL, USA

Patrice M. Mich, DVM, MS, DABVP, DACVAA, DACVSMR, CCRT
Section Head Sports Medicine, Rehabilitation, and Integrative Pain Management
Wheat Ridge Animal Hospital by Ethos
Wheat Ridge, CO USA
Affiliate Faculty
Department of Clinical Sciences
Colorado State University
Fort Collins, CO, USA

Krista Niebaum, MPT, CCRT
Director of Rehabilitation Therapy
Scout's House Clinic
Menlo Park, CA, USA

Antonio Pozzi, DVM, MS, DECVS, DACVS, DACVSMR
Director, Clinic for Small Animal Surgery
Department for Small Animals
Vetsuisse Faculty Zürich
Zurich, Switzerland

Patrick A. Ridge, BVSc, Cert VR, Cert SAS, MRCVS
Recognised Advanced Practitioner in Small Animal Surgery
Ridge Referrals
Dawlish
Devon, England

Shari Sprague, MPT, CCRT, FP-ME, CCKTP
Owner and Founder
PUP Rehabilitation and Conditioning
Tamarac, FL, USA

Lisa Starr, DVM, CCRP, CVA, CVSMT
Medical Director
Pets In Balance
Chicago, IL, USA

Frank Steffen, DECVN
Head of Section Neurology/Neurosurgery
Vetsuisse Faculty
University of Zürich
Zürich, Switzerland

H. Steven Steinberg, VMD, DACVIM (Neurology), CCRT, CVA
Head of Rehabilitation Services
Veterinary Referral Associates
Gaithersburg, MD, USA

Janet B. Van Dyke, DVM, DACVSMR, CCRT
CEO and Founder
Canine Rehabilitation Institute
Wellington, FL, USA

Joseph J. Wakshlag, DVM, PhD, DACVN, DACVSMR
Associate Professor of Clinical Nutrition
Department of Clinical Sciences
College of Veterinary Medicine
Cornell University
Ithaca, NY, USA

Chris Zink, DVM, PhD, DACVP, DACVSMR, CCRT, CVSMT, CVA
Zink Integrative Sports Medicine
Ellicott City, MD, USA

Foreword

The field of canine sports medicine and rehabilitation has rapidly evolved since acceptance of the American College of Veterinary Sports Medicine and Rehabilitation (ACVSMR) in 2010 by the American Veterinary Medical Association as a veterinary specialty. This field addresses the diagnosis, treatment, and rehabilitation of the complex, often multiple, injuries experienced by large numbers of dogs that participate in sports and those with jobs such as police and assistance dogs. In addition, many dogs lead very athletic lives, playing retrieving games, hiking on the weekends, or running with their owners; these, too, often experience the long-term effects of wear and tear on their bodies.

A significant driver in the evolution of the field of canine sports medicine and rehabilitation has been the cross-pollination of expertise and ideas between veterinary and human medicine for the benefit of canine athletes. This, in turn, has raised the bar in terms of our knowledge of orthopedics, neurology, internal medicine, nutrition/exercise physiology, and rehabilitation for the benefit of all dogs. In the spirit of this highly beneficial veterinary-human

medicine collaboration, Drs Chris Zink and Janet B. Van Dyke have brought together a multi-talented group of veterinarians and allied health professionals who have presented the most up-to-date evidence in this outstanding, easy-to-read, and informative Second Edition.

This Second Edition represents the combined work of 36 authors, including 27 veterinarians, nine allied health professionals, and 15 diplomates of the American College of Veterinary Sports Medicine and Rehabilitation. Every chapter has been extensively revised and expanded resulting in a 20% increase in size over the First Edition. As an integrated whole, it provides a wealth of evidence, expertise, and experience to this complex, interactive discipline for the benefit of every veterinary healthcare team. Presented in full color, with outstanding illustrations and abundant case studies, this text provides readers at all levels of experience with detailed yet practical information that can be applied to canine patients of all ages.

Canine Sports Medicine and Rehabilitation should not be present on the bookshelf of every veterinarian, physical therapist, and veterinary technician who works with active dogs. Instead it should occupy an honored space on their desks, to be referred to again and again for its easily accessible and comprehensive information on all aspects of the health care of active dogs. I commend the editors and all of the authors for their contributions to this outstanding text that is so important for the healing of dogs who share our lives, teach us so many life lessons, and even, in turn, heal us.

Prof. Noel Fitzpatrick, MVB DUniv, CVR, DSAS(Orth), DACVSMR, MRCVS
Director, Fitzpatrick Referrals and Fitzbionics
Professor of Veterinary Orthopaedics
University of Surrey, England

Preface

In this textbook, we have provided state-of-the-art information that addresses the complex issues faced by veterinarians, veterinary technicians, physical therapists, and others interested in helping canine patients recover from injury, especially those returning to work, sport, or active lives. We have gathered the top experts in the fields of veterinary sports medicine and rehabilitation, each of whom has provided their unique, evidence-based knowledge. More than a third of the authors are Diplomates of the American College of Veterinary Sports Medicine and Rehabilitation. Their contributions are complemented by those of a number of highly experienced physical therapists who have contributed their knowledge from years of experience working in the field of canine rehabilitation of sporting and working dogs. We were overwhelmed by the willingness of this highly motivated, but highly overworked group to commit their knowledge and experiences to paper. Their material presented here is broad in scope, and deep in science and experience. It has been an honor to compile their extensive and well-written information to create the definitive text on sports medicine and rehabilitation.

This text provides residents, interns, veterinary students, practicing veterinarians, and physical therapy professionals with a resource for their daily practice as well as a basis for future research. This text addresses the needs of this group in several ways, by providing:

- The basic science of exercise physiology, nutrition, and physical therapy concepts.
- The current veterinary approaches to common canine injuries and developmental disorders.
- The current physical therapist's approach to these injuries and impairments.
- Current and cutting edge science to enable the practice of evidence-based medicine.
- Business concepts essential to running a successful sports medicine/rehabilitation practice.
- Case examples in each chapter to better illustrate the concepts covered.

The evidence base available to us is incomplete, but growing daily. We have compiled the evidence currently available, adding those techniques that have proven successful in the hands of our highly experienced authors. The editors and authors of this textbook firmly believe that applying the currently available science, adapting techniques that show promise in the field, and sharing our findings will help this field to grow to the level expected by our dog-owning clients, and deserved by our canine friends.

Chris Zink
Janet B. Van Dyke

Acknowledgments

You would not be holding this book in your hands if it were not for the foresight of Erica Judisch, our executive editor at Wiley Blackwell, who recognized the need to address and disseminate information on the extensive advancements in the field of canine sports medicine and rehabilitation since the first edition was published. We thank Purvi Patel, our project editor, for helping us to transform the manuscript into a beautiful, easy-to-read resource. Throughout the writing and production process both Erica and Purvi have been patient, constructive, accommodating, and most generous with their time.

We are grateful to Marcia Schlehr, a lifetime student of canine structure and function, for her outstanding, anatomically correct illustrations. Thank you also to the graphic designers at Wiley Blackwell, who acquiesced to our desire for an easy-to-read, full-color book and a cover that appropriately illustrates the outcome of canine sports medicine and rehabilitation—a healthy, active dog.

Mary Ellen Goldberg provided expert technical assistance in graphics and reference management.

Most of all we thank the 36 authors of this book, all of whom agreed to write their chapters on a short timeline, incorporating all of the most recent information, assuring that at the time of publication the information presented would be as current as possible.

While they might not realize how grateful we are, we also thank all of the dogs that have taught the authors so much about canine sports medicine and rehabilitation throughout the years and that have posed interminably for photos and videos.

And finally, to our family members and friends, we thank you for your encouragement and patience during our absences.

Chris Zink
Janet B. Van Dyke

1

What Is a Canine Athlete?

Chris Zink, DVM, PhD, DACVP, DACVSMR, CCRT, CVSMT, CVA, and Brittany Jean Carr, DVM, CCRT

Summary

Canine sports medicine and rehabilitation is one of the newest specialties in veterinary medicine. It encompasses and integrates a variety of fields, including orthopedics, exercise physiology, neurology, cardiology, pulmonology, nutrition, and others. Rehabilitation, which includes regaining and maintaining fitness as well as conditioning targeted toward prevention of future injury, is a critical partner to canine sports medicine. Canine athletes include dogs that compete in performance events as varied as agility trials, obedience trials, and disc dog competitions, as well as working dogs such as police/military dogs, search and rescue dogs, and assistance dogs for the disabled. Principles of canine sports medicine and rehabilitation apply to all active dogs, regardless of whether they train or compete; this comprises a large proportion of the canine population. Canine sports medicine and rehabilitation professionals play a pivotal role in helping canine athletes and working dogs recover after injury or illness. They work to prevent re-injury while moving the patient back to a state of muscular ability, endurance, coordination, balance, and flexibility that optimizes their physical abilities. Understanding the physical activities that are involved in different performance events and the jobs that working dogs perform is critical to devising targeted rehabilitation for sports/working dogs after injury or illness, and for retraining them to perform their specific duties. This is best accomplished by attending athletic/working dog training sessions and competitions.

Introduction to canine sports medicine

Humans and dogs have been partners for at least 33,000 years (Galibert *et al.*, 2011; Ovodov *et al.*, 2011; Thalmann *et al.*, 2013; Shannon *et al.*, 2015; Frantz *et al.*, 2016). As working companions, dogs have assisted in hunting food, guarding family and property, gathering and moving livestock, patrolling with soldiers, detecting drugs and explosives, and searching for lost humans.

With increases in disposable income and a change in attitudes toward work/life balance

---

beginning after World War II, there has been an exponential growth in the number of sporting events devised by people to challenge their abilities to train their dogs for competition. The field of canine sports medicine began with veterinarians working predominantly with racing Greyhounds. Veterinarians now work with dogs that participate in dozens, if not hundreds, of different canine sports and working roles.

Canine sports medicine is the branch of veterinary medicine concerned with injuries sustained by canine athletes, including their prevention, diagnosis, and treatment. The field of canine sports medicine comprises many different aspects of traditional and integrative veterinary medicine as well as nonclinical ancillary roles in canine care such as exercise physiology, athletic training, and others (Box 1.1), and encourages significant collaboration between individuals with different areas of expertise. In addition, canine sports medicine is intimately linked to canine rehabilitation, where veterinarians, physical therapists, and veterinary technicians have an opportunity to work together to return injured canine athletes and working dogs not only to health but to full performance.

There are many advantages for veterinarians and rehabilitation professionals working with canine athletes and working dogs (Box 1.2). The field involves assisting clients who have invested significant time, emotion, effort, and finances into raising, training, and competing/working with their canine partners. These clients want the best care and the best outcomes for their dogs, so there is substantial opportunity

---

Box 1.1   Fields included in canine sports medicine

- Anatomy and biomechanics
- Exercise physiology
- Sports conditioning
- Rehabilitation
- Orthopedics
- Internal medicine
- Pulmonology
- Cardiology
- Neurology
- Gerontology
- Nutrition
- Integrative medicine

Box 1.2   Advantages of working with clients with canine athletes and working dogs

- Opportunity to practice state-of-the-art rehabilitation medicine
- Highly educated clients with significant financial, time and emotional investment in their dogs
- High client compliance
- Healthier dogs than in general practice
- Higher success rate due to dogs' better plane of fitness
- Measurable success returning dog to training and competition
- Abundant research opportunities

---

to practice state-of-the-art sports and rehabilitation medicine.

Human athletes have teams consisting of health professionals with diverse expertise who work on maintaining and regaining the athletes' health and fitness. Canine sports medicine and rehabilitation professionals likewise play a pivotal role in helping the clients with canine athletes and working dogs to keep their dogs in athletic condition, prevent injury, and recover after injury or illness. They help move dogs back to a state of muscular ability, endurance, coordination, balance, and flexibility that allows them to optimize their physical condition.

Clients with canine athletes and working dogs are generally highly compliant. Once given detailed individualized conditioning programs, clients will work with their dogs to perform those exercises diligently. This is a key to success for the canine sports medicine and rehabilitation professional, and brings significant job satisfaction, allowing the professional to develop relationships with clients that last through generations of dogs.

Canine athletes and working dogs often enter the rehabilitation program at a much healthier level and a higher fitness plane than most inactive pet dogs. This provides the canine sports medicine and rehabilitation professional with the advantage and enjoyment of working with health more than with illness.

There is significant opportunity for research in the field of canine sports medicine and rehabilitation. Opportunities abound for retrospective studies of outcomes as well as prospective studies that formulate specific hypotheses and design test and control groups to address those hypotheses. Clients with canine athletes and working dogs are generally enthusiastic about participating in studies that will help provide information that they can use to become more efficient in training and more successful in competition and that will result in greater health and longevity.

As an example of the investments that clients have in their dogs, an average annual cost to campaign a show dog in conformation shows is between $80,000 and $100,000 for a dog that had a single Best in Show win, and $250,000–500,000 for a dog that has won more than 100 Best in Show awards (Dugan & Dugan, 2011). This typically includes the costs of entries, travel to shows, advertising, and fees for professional handlers. Many clients with competitive field trial dogs will spend $25,000–50,000 per year to have professional handlers train and compete with their dogs. Most agility competitors spend less than that because they generally train and compete with their own dogs. However, they do have significant costs for lessons, entries, and traveling, and many avid agility competitors will spend $10,000–25,000 per year on their chosen canine sport (Chris Zink, personal communication). This is concrete evidence of the significant temporal, financial, and emotional investment on the part of clients with canine athletes and working dogs. As a result, they are interested in obtaining the best possible care for their canine teammates. They look to canine sports medicine and rehabilitation professionals to help their dogs recover quickly and completely from injuries and to be able to once again compete to their fullest potential.

To be most effective, canine sports medicine and rehabilitation professionals must become as familiar as possible with the requirements for canine athletes' and working dogs' activities. It is also important that they are familiar with terminology and training techniques used with these dogs. Training and practice methods can significantly contribute to the types of injuries that performance and working dogs experience, sometimes more than competition itself.

In addition, an understanding of the functions of each dog breed is critical to devising targeted rehabilitation for sports/working dogs after injury or illness, and for retraining them to perform their specific duties. This is best accomplished by attending athletic/working dog training sessions and competitions. Local competitions can readily be found by searching the Internet. The sports medicine/rehabilitation professional is strongly encouraged to attend local training and practice sessions for a variety of sports and working functions. Clients' videos and photos of their dogs working or training often capture evidence of potential tissue stresses that can lead to injury.

The ability to communicate effectively with performance and working dog clients cannot be overemphasized. Often, these clients are as driven as their dogs so that both handler and dog might ignore a physical problem, working through it until it becomes a major injury. This can result in critical downtime and even permanent loss of work or performance ability. Clients with canine athletes and working dogs are looking for veterinary and rehabilitation professionals who understand their dogs' activities and who can communicate with them about that work.

Types of canine performance and working activities

Canine sports and pleasure activities

These can be divided into two categories: companion events and performance events. *Companion events* are those in which any breed (usually mixed breeds as well) can participate. These are sports events with rules devised by diverse organizations and are usually meant to be inclusive, with events designed for the participation of as many dogs of different sizes and shapes as possible. Examples include the popular sport of agility, as well as obedience, rally, and tracking.

Performance events are sports that are designed to recapitulate the original purposes of various breeds or groups of breeds, and participation is often limited to those breeds. Examples of these sports include herding competitions for breeds such as Border Collies, Shetland Sheepdogs, and Australian Shepherds, and hunt tests for the retrievers, setters, pointers, and spaniels.

This chapter provides brief information on only a few of the most popular and most physical canine sporting events. However, Table 1.1 provides a comprehensive list of popular companion

Table 1.1 Popular companion and performance events

Sport	Brief description	Website(s) and description
Companion events		
Agility	A popular canine sport in which a handler directs a dog over an obstacle course, running against time	en.wikipedia.org/wiki/Dog_agility www.akc.org/events/agility www.usdaa.com/
Obedience	A sport in which judges instruct handlers to have their dogs perform a number of exercises on command. Dogs are judged on the precision of their responses and teamwork with their handlers	www.akc.org/events/obedience
Rally	A sport in which the dog and handler proceed through a course of 10 to 20 designated stations, each of which has a sign providing instructions regarding a skill to be performed	www.akc.org/events/rally/index.cfm
Conformation	A competition in which purebred dogs are judged on their structure and gait against a written description of the ideal dog of that breed	www.akc.org/index.cfm
Tracking	A test in which a dog follows the scent of a person over a 400- to 800-yard track aged from 1 to 5 hours	www.akc.org/events/tracking
Freestyle	A teamwork sport in which dogs and handlers perform a thematic routine, moving together to music	www.canine-freestyle.org/ www.worldcaninefreestyle.org/
Flyball	A relay race in which teams of four dogs run over four small hurdles 10 ft apart, retrieve a ball that is ejected by pressing a pedal on a box, then return over the hurdles	www.flyball.org/
Disc dog	A sport in which dogs retrieve flying discs while performing various movements, such as leaps and flips	en.wikipedia.org/wiki/Disc_dog http://usddn.com
Dock diving	A game in which dogs compete by jumping for distance from a dock into a body of water	http://northamericadivingdogs.com en.wikipedia.org/wiki/Dock_jumping
Weight pulling	A competition in which dogs pull a loaded sled across the ground for various distances	www.iwpa.net
Canine nosework	A sport in which dogs search rooms, containers, a vehicle, and an outdoor area for a specific scent	www.funnosework.com/ https://www.nacsw.net
Barn hunt	A sport in which dogs hunt and find rats safely concealed in ventilated PVC tubes that are hidden among bales of straw	https://barnhunt.com
Performance events		
Lure coursing	A sport in which dogs chase white plastic bags (to imitate prey) that are moved along the ground by a battery-operated string and pulley system	http://www.akc.org/events/lure-coursing/ www.akc.org/events/lure_coursing/ www.asfa.org/
Greyhound racing	An ancient sport in which Greyhounds chase a lure on an oval track. In many countries, Greyhound racing is purely amateur and conducted for enjoyment. In the United States, Australia, and some other countries, Greyhound racing is part of parimutuel betting	en.wikipedia.org/wiki/Greyhound_racing
Herding	A competition in which herding breeds herd sheep, cattle, or ducks over a specified course and move selected animals into a pen	www.usbcha.com/ www.akc.org/events/herding/

Table 1.1   *(Continued)*

Sport	Brief description	Website(s) and description
Field trials/ hunt tests	Sports in which retrievers, setters, pointers, spaniels, and poodles retrieve upland gamebirds on land and in water	www.akc.org/events/hunting_tests/retrievers www.akc.org/events/hunting-tests/ pointing-breeds www.akc.org/events/hunting_tests/spaniels www.akc.org/events/field_trials/beagles/
Earthdog tests	A test in which terriers and Dachshunds run through underground tunnels to find a caged rat	http://www.akc.org/events/earth-dog/
Coon dog tests	A competition that has many different facets, including bench shows, field trials, night hunts, and water races, providing owners with the opportunity to demonstrate the beauty and natural abilities of coonhounds	www.akccoonhounds.org/
Fox hunting	An activity involving the tracking of a fox by trained Foxhounds or other scent hounds, and a group of unarmed followers who follow the hounds on foot or on horseback	en.wikipedia.org/wiki/Fox_hunting
Schutzhund, French ring sport	Competitions that combine obedience, tracking, and protection work	en.wikipedia.org/wiki/Schutzhund https://www.germanshepherddog.com/ about/schutzhund-training/ http://www.ringsport.org/index. php?pg=ringsport
Mushing	An endurance competition in which dogs pull sleds (or land rigs) over a specified course, which may vary from 1 to 1150 miles	https://en.wikipedia.org/wiki/Mushing
Carting	A sport in which a dog pulls a cart filled with supplies, such as farm goods or firewood, and sometimes people over a specified course	en.wikipedia.org/wiki/Dog_carting

and performance events with websites that provide a wealth of additional information.

Agility

Agility is an international sport in which owner/handlers direct dogs over a course consisting of 15–20 obstacles, including jumps (Figure 1.1), tunnels, weave poles, seesaws, A-frames, dog walks, sometimes tables, and sometimes other obstacles, in a race for both time and accuracy. Dogs run off-leash and the handler cannot touch the dog, but instead guides the dog by voice, movement, and various body signals. This requires exceptional training of the dog and coordination of the handler. Dog–handler teams usually run outdoors on grass or indoors on artificial turf, dirt, or rubberized flooring. The handler can walk the course ahead of time to determine strategies to compensate for differences in his or her own

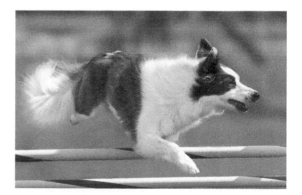

Figure 1.1   Dog jumping during agility competition.

running speed versus that of his or her dog, and for the different physical and training strengths and weaknesses of the handler and the dog. The height that agility dogs are required to jump is determined by their height at the withers (a point just cranial to the highest point

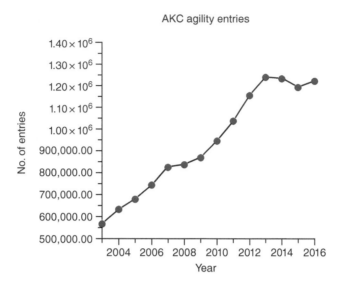

Figure 1.2   The number of entries in American Kennel Club agility trials increased steadily until 2013, when it leveled off, in part due to increased numbers of other organizations holding agility trials and an increasing number of other sports available for dogs. Source: Data from American Kennel Club. Available at: http://www.akc.org/events/agility/statistics/

of the dorsal rim of the scapula). Depending on the organization, dogs can compete in agility as early as 15 months of age, and as a result they begin training at an inappropriately young age.

Agility is a rapidly growing sport worldwide, with over a million entries annually in the last several years in events hosted by the American Kennel Club (AKC) alone (an entry consists of one dog running one course; Figure 1.2). There are dozens of organizations that host agility events internationally, including the AKC, the Canadian Kennel Club, the Kennel Club (United Kingdom), the United States Dog Agility Association, the UK Agility International, the Agility Association of Canada, the United Kennel Club, the Fédération Cynologique Internationale, the North American Dog Agility Council, Canine Performance Events, Teacup Dog Agility Association, Australian Shepherd Club of America, and Dogs on Course North America.

Since the sport of agility involves speed and jumping, agility dogs commonly suffer injuries to the soft tissues, including those to the thoracic limb (especially the shoulder, such as biceps and supraspinatus tendinopathies and medial shoulder syndrome), and to the pelvic limb (particularly the hips and stifles, such as iliopsoas strain and cranial cruciate ligament (CCL) insufficiency) (Levy *et al.*, 2009; Cullen *et al.*, 2013).

Obedience

The sport of obedience started in the 1930s, arising as an adaptation of the work of military dogs. Formal obedience competitions were originally designed to showcase a dog's ability to work with their people and follow specific commands so that together they could go for a walk in a park, have good manners in public, or take a pleasant ride in the car. Obedience competitions are sponsored predominantly by the American Kennel Club in the United States and by many other organizations both nationally and internationally. While obedience trials have competed with agility trials for participants over the last two decades, they still retain a stalwart following.

Basic obedience skills include walking on the handler's left side and staying in place when the handler turns or changes speed (Figure 1.3), sitting when stopped, coming when called, lying down when asked, and staying in position in the presence of other dogs when the handler is about 50 feet away or out of sight. Higher levels of obedience competition include retrieving a dumbbell or a glove when directed, jumping various styles of jumps, selecting a dumbbell with the handler's scent from a group of dumbbells scented by someone else, and

Case Study 1.1   Carpal strain

Signalment: 4-y.o. M/I German Shepherd Dog that works as a detection and apprehension police dog.

History: Dog was chasing a suspect in an apartment complex when it leapt off a balcony 25 feet above the ground and landed on some shrubs. Dog was significantly lame upon standing but the lameness became less severe over the next minute or two if the dog kept moving. However, the lameness was again pronounced when the dog started moving after a period of rest. Handler wanted the dog to be able to continue in his function as a police dog.

Clinical findings: Patient is a large German Shepherd Dog in excellent physical condition, at a correct weight, and well-muscled. On presentation, lameness was scored as 3 on a scale of 6. After 3 minutes of walking, the lameness decreased to a level of 1 to 2. The dog had the typical abundant angulation that is seen in many specimens of this breed. The left carpus was enlarged, with pitting edema present on the cranial aspect. Pain was elicited on palpation and flexion of the left carpus. Radiographs showed no fractures but subcutaneous swelling in a location consistent with the extensor tendons of the thoracic limb.

Diagnosis: Left carpus—strain of the extensor carpi radialis and the lateral and common digital extensor tendons.

Treatment: Room rest for the initial 2 weeks of rehabilitation therapy with bilateral carpal support wraps at all times throughout the rehabilitation period, except when undergoing active rehabilitation exercises. Patient treated with laser therapy, TENS, joint mobilizations, underwater treadmill walking to maintain musculature, and therapeutic exercises twice a week for 4 weeks. Beginning 2 weeks after the initiation of therapy, the dog was walked twice daily with gradually increasing distances and speeds. Handler also performed daily proprioception training including walking slowly forward and backward through a ladder placed flat on the ground as well as on a slight gradation. Carpus iced for 10 minutes after each rehabilitation and exercise period. Four weeks after initiation of therapy, handler began to walk patient slowly over uneven surfaces, up and down low steps, and through deep grass. By 6 weeks post-injury, patient began to work on progressively more difficult surfaces and was trotted for 5 to 10 minutes each day. At this time, patient was also used for detection work that required only moderate exercise. By 8 weeks after the injury, patient went back to work and performed well. Handler chose to have patient wear carpal wraps when not working for the next 3 months.

Comments: Hyperflexion and hyperextension injuries are not uncommon in German Shepherd Dogs. Understanding the unique structure of this breed helped the decision-making process during rehabilitation and was a significant component of the handler's decision to have the dog wear carpal wraps on an ongoing basis.

---

staying in place in the presence of other dogs when the handler is out of sight.

Obedience dogs that are campaigned heavily in the sport most commonly experience chronic strain injuries to the shoulders, such as supraspinatus tendinopathy. This especially affects the left shoulder since more of the dog's weight is borne on the left shoulder when the dog is heeling with its head looking up and to the right toward the handler. Heeling is a major component of obedience at all levels.

Rally

Rally is a sport based on the obedience practice of active warm-up and freestyle exercises. It requires teamwork between dog and handler along with performance skills similar to obedience. However, unlike obedience, instead of waiting for the judge's orders, the competitor proceeds around a course of 10 to 20 designated stations with the dog in heel position. At each station, a sign provides instructions regarding the specific exercise required of the dog. In contrast to obedience competition, in rally trials handlers are allowed to verbally encourage their dogs while on course. Due to the non-concussive nature of this sport, injuries are uncommon.

Conformation

Conformation is a competition in which a judge evaluates individual purebred dogs for how

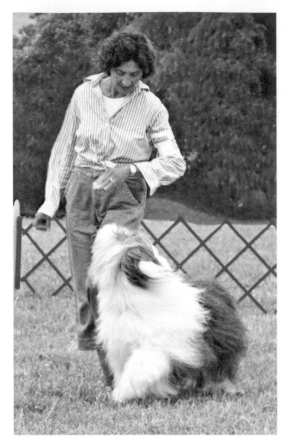

Figure 1.3 Dog heeling during obedience competition. Note the position of the dog's head as it watches the handler, ready to change directions when necessary, always staying in heel position at the handler's left side.

closely the dog conforms to the established standards for its breed. A conformation dog show is not a comparison of one dog with another, but rather a comparison of each dog with the dog's written and illustrated breed standard. The judge evaluates dogs both in a standing position and at a trot. The number of entries annually in this performance event is in the millions.

Flyball

Flyball began as a sport in California in the late 1960s and early 1970s and quickly spread to become an international pastime. In this sport, two teams of four dogs race against each other from a start/finish line, over four jumps placed 10 feet apart to a box that releases a ball to be caught when the dog presses a spring-loaded pad; the dogs then race back over the jumps to their handlers while carrying the ball (Figure 1.4). Two teams run in a heat against each other, with the winning team proceeding to the next heat. The height of the jumps for all dogs is determined by the height at the shoulder of the smallest dog on each team.

Flyball competition involves very high speeds. The world record speed for all four dogs performing a flyball run as of December 2016 was 14.18 seconds. Thus, each dog ran the 102-ft course in an average of 3.545 seconds. This suggests that the dogs are running at over

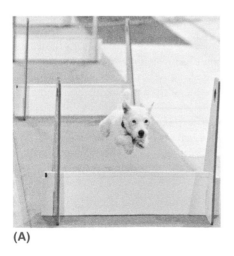

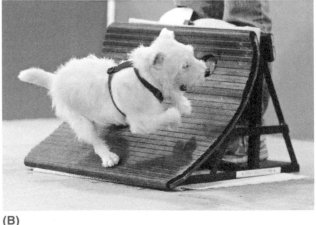

(A)   **(B)**

Figure 1.4   (A) Dog heading over the row of flyball jumps to the box. **(B)** Dog leaving the box with the ball and heading for the jumps. Source: Photos by Steve Surfman.

30 mph when they hit the box. In a typical tournament, dogs might participate in over 25 heats per day.

The injuries that flyball dogs typically experience are associated with chronic repetitive stress and most often occur in the shoulder opposite to and in the coxofemoral joint toward which the dog turns at the flyball box. Typical injuries include carpal desmitis, biceps and/or supraspinatus tendinopathy, medial shoulder syndrome, coxofemoral arthritis, and iliopsoas strain.

Field trials/hunt tests

Field trials and hunt tests require dogs to retrieve upland game birds, such as duck and pheasant, on land and sometimes water, simulating hunting situations where dogs find and retrieve shot birds for hunters (Figure 1.5). Field trials are competitive in that only the dogs placing first through fourth are awarded points, and a certain number of points are required for a championship title. Hunt tests use less complex hunting scenarios and are graded as pass/fail. There are different rules and regulations for field trials and hunt tests for the three different styles of hunting dogs: retrievers, pointing dogs (pointers and setters), and flushing dogs (spaniels).

Dogs that compete in field trials and hunt tests are predisposed to injuries of the feet, carpus, and shoulders, including sesamoiditis, carpal hyperextension/arthritis, and biceps and/or supraspinatus tendinopathy.

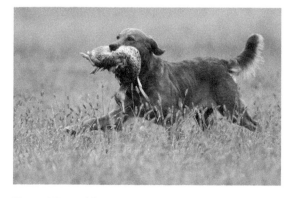

Figure 1.5   Golden Retriever returning to handler after retrieving a duck during a hunt test. Source: Photo by Steve Surfman.

Working dog activities

A vital aspect of canine sports medicine and rehabilitation is working with dogs that perform critical functions for society, including police dogs, detection dogs, search and rescue dogs, and service dogs (Table 1.2). The work these dogs do is critical for the security of national and local communities, the safety of agriculture, and the health and safety of individuals with disabilities. Maintaining the health and full capabilities of these dogs can be a matter of life or death to their handlers.

When dealing with a working dog, it is important for the canine sports medicine and rehabilitation professional to ask the handler to describe the specific activities his or her dog must perform as a part of its duties, since the work that these dogs do varies tremendously

Table 1.2   Working dog activities

Category	Type of work
Search and rescue	Wildland Urban Cadaver Avalanche
Detection	Drugs Explosives Food Cancer Petroleum leaks Mold Insects (termites/bed bugs) Vapor wake (body-worn explosives)
Police, patrol, protection	Police and military patrols Police apprehension Protection and security (secure installations/public gatherings)
Farm dogs	Herding sheep, cattle, ducks, chickens Predator protection Geese police (golf courses)
Service dogs	Dog guides for the blind Hearing dogs Mobility assistance dogs General assistance dogs Seizure/diabetes alert dogs Psychiatric service dogs
Canine actors	Movies Television Print advertisements

between jurisdictions. For example, police dogs may be trained in detection (drugs, weapons, cash, etc.), in suspect apprehension, or both. The canine sports medicine and rehabilitation professional working with these dogs should examine the equipment the dog wears while at work. Some dogs may wear only a collar for their work, while others may wear specialized harnesses that might include additional weight from supplementary equipment. Many harnesses are designed with little consideration of ergonomics for the dog's body (Vanek, 2010).

Working dogs experience injuries and disorders that are often related to overuse (repetitive stress) or trauma because of the intense activities required for their jobs. They also can suffer from conditions more commonly seen in working dog breeds, such as gracilis myopathy, which is seen most often in German Shepherd Dogs (Steiss, 2002). For detailed information on working dogs and their injuries, see Chapter 21.

Noncompetition athletes

Thousands, if not millions of dogs in North America perform athletic activities that do not involve competition. Dogs that run with their owners, romp freely on beaches or on hiking trails, or catch a thrown ball or disc in the yard are all active and athletic and may, in fact, be doing more physical work than some competitive or working canine athletes. Many of them rest all week, and are unprepared for the level of exercise they experience on weekends, making them more susceptible to overuse injuries. These injuries often go unrecognized and untreated for longer periods of time. It is easy to see that the majority of dogs can benefit from the expert problem-solving abilities and skilled care of a canine sports medicine and rehabilitation professional. The training that the canine sports medicine and rehabilitation professional experiences raises the bar for musculoskeletal health for all dogs.

Canine structure and its effects on performance

With each performance and working task come specialized training and activities that create unique physical demands on the canine body. The detailed anatomy of the bones, muscles, tendons, ligaments, innervation, and vasculature of the injured area can be obtained from textbooks (Miller *et al.*, 1979). While all dogs have the same anatomical components, how those components are combined constitutes structure, which is widely varied between breeds. In fact, dogs are the most varied species on Earth. Variation in structure has developed through selective breeding for specific functions, and it is those structure/function relationships that this chapter addresses. Of equal importance to those working with the performance or working dog is an understanding of the ways in which an individual dog uses those structures to perform its particular job. It is also important to be conscious of other anatomical structures that might be affected as the dog compensates for a primary injury.

This prospect is made much more complex by the extreme variation in the structure of different breeds of dogs. Canine sports medicine and rehabilitation professionals can provide a significant service to their clients by helping them understand their individual dog's structural strengths and weaknesses for their chosen activities, how those structural components might comprise an advantage or disadvantage for the dog's activities, and what can be done to mitigate the potential for injuries. For example, a Corgi and a Toy Poodle must navigate the same obstacles on an agility course—jumping the same height jumps and making the same turns, all with the same maximum allowed time—yet the Toy Poodle has a significant biomechanical advantage over the Corgi simply because it weighs one-fifth as much (Figure 1.6). This does not mean that Corgis cannot be successful agility dogs—they are, in fact, very successful—but it does mean that the client who plans to run a Corgi in agility should maintain his or her dog at peak fitness (particularly the core and pelvic limb muscles) and plan to train and compete intelligently, with the dog's heavy-set structure in mind.

Somatotypes

The concept of somatotype (overall body type) in humans was originally popularized by Dupertuis and Sheldon (1947). They described

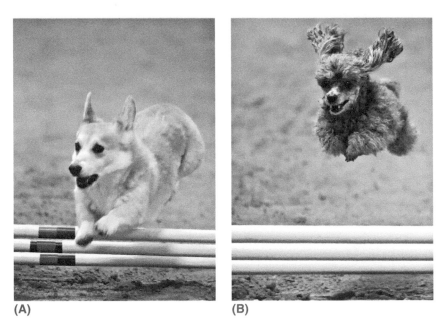

(A)   **(B)**

Figure 1.6 A Corgi (**A**) and a Toy Poodle (**B**) have very different body weights and structures, yet both breeds have the same requirements in agility and obedience. Source: Photos by Steve Surfman.

three body types based on height, leg length, and mass: ectomorphic, endomorphic, and mesomorphic. A similar categorization can be made in dogs. Ectomorphic dogs tend to have a smaller bone structure and be light in mass relative to their height. A key structural feature of these dogs is that the distance between the ground and the olecranon process is greater than the distance from the olecranon process to the dorsal rim of the scapula when the dog is standing with radius and ulna perpendicular to the ground. This added length of the distal limb raises the dog's center of gravity and gives it an advantage by giving it a longer stride length and greater ease in jumping. However, this higher center of gravity also causes these dogs to be less agile at turning, just as a Volkswagen bus has poorer cornering ability than a Corvette. Typical ectomorphic breeds include most of the sighthounds, Weimaraners, German Short-Haired Pointers, Belgian Tervuren and other long-legged, lighter breeds.

At the other extreme, the endomorphic breeds tend to carry more weight on their frame. This group includes all of the chondrodystrophic dwarfs, which have foreshortened limbs, as well as Clumber Spaniels, Newfoundlands, and other heavy-set breeds. The distances

from the ground to the olecranon process and from the olecranon process to the dorsal rim of the scapula are typically equal in these breeds, even in the chondrodystrophic dwarfs. Because of their relatively heavier weight, these dogs have a biomechanical disadvantage in performance events requiring speed and agility.

The mesomorphic breeds lie in between these two extremes and in general are of moderate build with equal distance between the ground and the olecranon and the olecranon and the dorsal rim of the scapula. Most of the highly successful breeds in sports that require speed and agility are mesomorphic. Some typical mesomorphic breeds include Golden Retrievers, Labrador Retrievers, Border Collies, Beagles, and Border Terriers. Their moderate body type means that mesomorphic breeds are often successful in diverse sports.

One way to evaluate the stresses on the musculoskeletal system of a dog is to calculate a dog's weight to height ratio using the following simple formula:

Weight:Height (W : H) ratio = body weight (in pounds) divided by height at the withers (in inches)

This is a useful determinant of the amount of stress on a dog's body during running, jumping, and turning. For example, a typical male Golden Retriever's W:H ratio is $70/24 = 2.9$, while a male Corgi's W:H ratio is $30/11 = 2.7$. This suggests that, despite the obvious size differences in these two breeds, their musculoskeletal systems actually experience similar stresses. Clients with dogs that have a W:H ratio above 2.5 should be advised to train and compete only on surfaces that are nonslip and highly compressible and to frequently train at lower jump heights to reduce the effects of repetitive strain on the musculoskeletal system.

Pelvic limb structure

Different breeds of dogs and individuals within those breeds can have substantial variation in the structure of the pelvic limbs. The most obvious differences in the pelvic limb structure of dogs are the angles at which the long bones meet one another when the dog is standing, a characteristic that is termed pelvic limb angulation, also referred to as *rear angulation* by those who study and evaluate canine structure (Brown, 1986; Elliott, 2009). Pelvic limb angulation is best assessed by having the dog stand with the metatarsals oriented perpendicular to

the ground (Figure 1.7). The distance between a line drawn perpendicular to the ground along the caudal aspect of the metatarsals and the ischial tuberosity provides a rule-of-thumb approximation of the amount of pelvic limb angulation. The longer that line is, the more pelvic limb angulation the dog has. Figure 1.8 shows two dogs of the same breed with substantially different pelvic limb angulation.

There are advantages and disadvantages to having abundant pelvic limb angulation. Dogs with a lot of pelvic limb angulation are able to take longer strides with the pelvic limbs, and thus expend less energy moving from A to B because they take fewer steps. Excessive pelvic limb angulation is often associated with instability, however, since it can require tremendous muscular strength and coordination to stabilize a very angulated rear (Figure 1.9). As a result, dogs with straighter pelvic limbs tend to be more accurate when placing their rear feet and tend to be able to turn more sharply than dogs with very angulated pelvic limbs. For most performance dogs, moderate pelvic limb angulation is the best compromise. Note that an appropriate fitness program is needed to optimize the angulation that each dog was genetically meant to have because appropriate musculature is required to support the dog with the limbs in an angulated conformation.

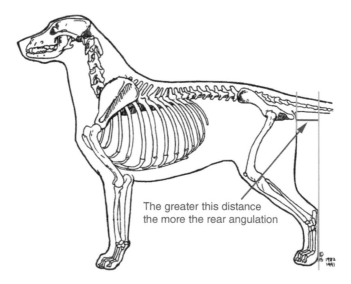

The greater this distance
the more the rear angulation

Figure 1.7   Pelvic limb angulation can be assessed by positioning the dog with its metatarsal bones perpendicular to the ground then drawing a line perpendicular to the ground along the caudal aspect of the metatarsals. The longer the distance between that line and the ischiatic tuberosity of the pelvis, the more pelvic limb angulation the dog has. Source: Illustration by Marcia Schlehr.

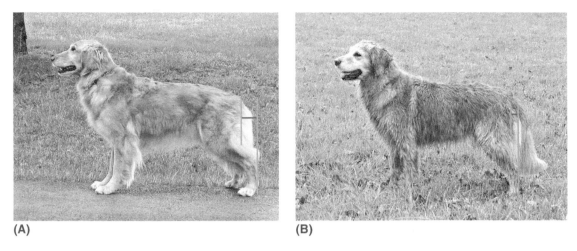

Figure 1.8   Two Golden Retrievers – one with abundant pelvic limb angulation (**A**) and one with minimal pelvic limb angulation (**B**).

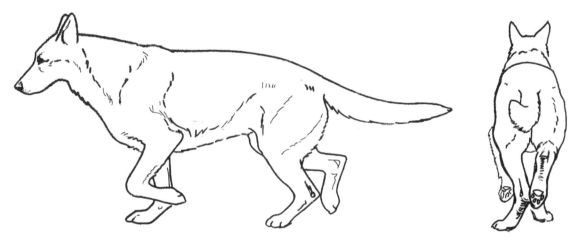

Figure 1.9   Dogs with very angulated pelvic limbs sometimes lack stability in the rear. Source: Illustration by Marcia Schlehr.

Some breeds of dogs have been bred for extreme pelvic limb angulation. One of these is the German Shepherd Dog of which many specimens have such extreme angulation that they must be placed for examination in conformation shows with one pelvic limb in the standing position with the metatarsals perpendicular to the ground but the other pelvic limb placed under the body so that the feet are placed in a tripod configuration for better support. This extreme pelvic limb angulation causes the pelvis to be placed closer to the ground, so that the dog's vertebral column is extremely sloped from cranial to caudal. This extreme angulation often cannot be compensated for by muscular strength, leaving these dogs to swing their

tarsi lateral to medial each time the feet are planted. To the best of our knowledge, this extreme angulation provides no advantages in function. Any potential advantage in function is offset by instability. This breed tends to have laxity in many joints, which may reflect an inadvertent genetic drift toward increased extensibility of the tendons and ligaments.

At the other extreme are breeds with very straight pelvic limb angulation. These tend to be breeds derived from dogs whose original purpose was guarding, such as the Shar-Pei and Chow Chow. Biomechanically, having an angle at the stifle that is closer to 180 degrees when the dog is bearing weight on the pelvic limb tends to increase the potential torque along

Case Study 1.2   Subclinical soft tissue shoulder injury

Signalment: 9 y.o. F/S (spayed at 5 years of age) Golden Retriever competing in agility, obedience, and hunt tests.

History: Patient had been competing in AKC agility at the excellent level approximately one to two weekends per month for the past several years. During the last 4 years, patient would frequently refuse to enter weave poles. When client restarted weave poles, patient would complete them. This happened only during competition, and never when training at home or in training facilities. Client requests complete examination to determine whether any orthopedic problems exist that might result in this change in performance.

Clinical findings: Patient in excellent physical condition, at a correct weight, and generally well-muscled. Pain elicited on flexion of right shoulder. Patient also shows sensitivity on palpation of the psoas musculature and at the insertion of the iliopsoas muscles on the lesser trochanters of both femurs. Musculoskeletal ultrasound shows alterations of echogenicity at the musculotendinous junction of the right supraspinatus tendon and both iliopsoas tendons.

Diagnosis: Right thoracic limb supraspinatus tendinopathy. Bilateral iliopsoas strain.

Treatment: Client advised to cease agility competitions and keep patient in a large pen or room during the day. Rehabilitation therapy, including laser, ultrasound, underwater treadmill work, and therapeutic exercises beginning with gentle stretching, then progressing to isometric, then concentric contraction, then eccentric contraction, instituted twice per week for 4 weeks, then once per week for 4 weeks. Patient then gradually reintroduced to agility by working on short sequences of low jumps with minimal turns, gradually increasing the length of sequences, height of jumps, and tightness of turns over an 8-week period. Weave poles not added to retraining program until 8 weeks after agility retraining initiated. Patient competing successfully in agility 6 months after the diagnosis.

Comments: This case is typical of agility dogs in a number of ways:

(1)   The presenting complaint frequently involves a decline in performance of an obstacle, particularly the weave poles and/or a reduction in the yards per second at which the dog runs during competition. Knowing the requirement for changes in lead legs while performing the weave poles helped direct the veterinarian toward a thoracic limb injury. This dog likely only had problems during competition because she was trained on grass but competed on relatively slippery surfaces; this was noted on video.
(2)   Agility dogs frequently have subclinical abnormalities that do not present as overt lameness.
(3)   Agility dogs frequently have more than one musculoskeletal injury.

the axis of the limb; this may result in an increased risk of cranial cruciate ligament rupture.

In most breeds when viewing the pelvic limbs from the rear, the limbs should extend from the greater trochanter perpendicular to the ground and be parallel to each other. The exception to this is in breeds whose functions require the dog to make quick turns, such as herding dogs, most notably the Border Collie. In these breeds the stifle is externally rotated, such that the tarsi are positioned medial relative to the feet. This limb adaptation provides greater stability as the dog is required to frequently lie down and stand up to reduce or increase, respectively, pressure on the sheep. Further, this pelvic limb conformation provides better contact of the toes with the ground when the dog needs to push off one pelvic limb when turning in response to the sheep's movements.

Thoracic limb structure

There are two different structural features to evaluate when assessing the angulation of the canine thoracic limb: the angle at which the scapula lies from vertical and the length of humerus (Brown, 1986; Elliott, 2009). Each of these components appears to be inherited separately, and together they determine the efficiency with which the thoracic limb functions in the athletic dog.

Angle of the scapula

To evaluate either the angulation of the scapula or the length of the humerus, the dog should be positioned with the radius and ulna perpendicular to the ground, with the head up and the nose pointing forward (Figure 1.10). The thoracic limb is highly mobile due to a lack of bony attachment to the trunk; by positioning the dog in this manner, the location of the thoracic limb relative to the spine is standardized for evaluation of thoracic limb angulation.

The angulation at which the scapula lies from vertical is determined by measuring the angle between a line drawn perpendicular to the ground through the cranial aspect of the greater tubercle of the humerus and another line drawn from the cranial aspect of the greater tubercle of the humerus to the highest point of the dorsal rim of the scapula, as in Figure 1.10. Cineradiographic images have determined this angle should ideally be 30 degrees (Elliott, 2009).

In contrast to pelvic limb angulation, there are no disadvantages to a dog having greater angle of the scapula. Dogs with greater scapular angle are able to take longer steps with each thoracic limb, thus expending less energy going from A to B. In addition, they tend to have more muscle development, particularly of the supraspinatus, infraspinatus and triceps muscles, and less concussion on the shoulder joint, particularly when landing with the limb in extension because the shoulder can better withstand eccentric contraction and absorb the shock (Figure 1.11).

Length of humerus

A second structural variable of the canine thoracic limb is the length of the humerus. Ideally, the humerus should be long enough to place

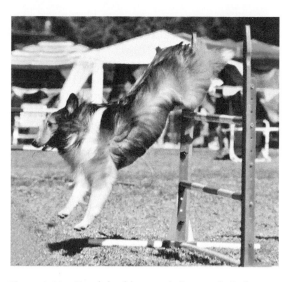

Figure 1.11 Good shoulder angulation results in less concussion when a dog is landing with the forelimb in extension.

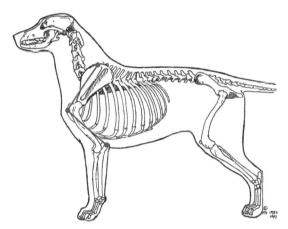

Figure 1.12 If a dog has a correct length humerus, a line from the highest point of the scapula to the greater tubercle of the humerus should be equal in length to a line drawn from the greater tubercle of the humerus to the top of the olecranon process. Source: Illustration by Marcia Schlehr.

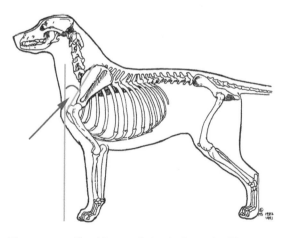

Figure 1.10 Shoulder angulation is determined by measuring the number of degrees from vertical at which the scapula lies. Ideally this angle should be 30 degrees (arrow). Source: Illustration by Marcia Schlehr.

the dog's radius and ulna well under the body when the dog is standing with the radius and ulna perpendicular to the ground. If a dog's humerus is the optimal length, a line from the dorsal rim of the scapula to the cranial aspect of the greater tubercle of the humerus should be equal in length to a line drawn from the cranial aspect of the greater tubercle of the humerus to the olecranon process (Figure 1.12).

A simpler way of evaluating humeral length is to draw a vertical line through the center of the radius and ulna. This line should intersect with the dog's topline at the junction of the neck and the back. When a dog has a short humerus, the entire distal limb is positioned more cranially, resulting in a line that intersects further cranially along the neck (Figure 1.13).

Dogs with a humerus of the optimal length have less concussion, particularly on the elbow joint, and tend to have more well-developed biceps and triceps muscles. To the extent that both scapular angle and humeral length deviate from ideal, thoracic limb function will be compromised. Two dogs with contrasting thoracic limb structure can be seen in Figure 1.14.

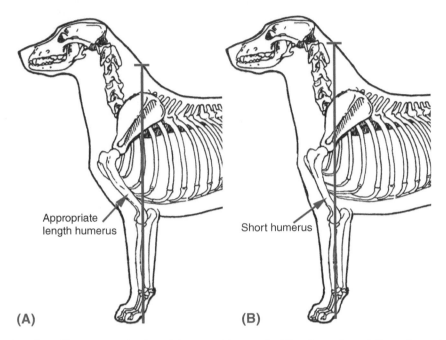

Figure 1.13   In a dog with an appropriate length humerus (**A**), a vertical line drawn through the radius and ulna intersects with the dog's topline near the highest point of the scapula. In a dog with a short humerus (**B**), that line intersects with the topline further cranially, along the neck. Source: Illustrations by Marcia Schlehr.

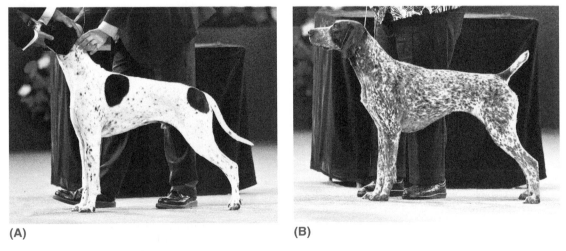

Figure 1.14   Two dogs with contrasting humeral length: a Pointer with a short humerus (**A**) and a German Short-Haired Pointer with appropriate length of humerus (**B**). Source: Photos by Steve Surfman.

Limb angulation is not a static feature of dogs; angulation can change in response to injury and level of fitness. Dogs with injuries to the thoracic limb or pelvic limb generally tend to straighten the limbs, letting the bones and ligaments take over more of the function of supporting the limbs. In addition, dogs that are not optimally conditioned will have reduced angles in the thoracic limbs and/or pelvic limbs because they do not have the muscular strength to fully support the limb in the optimally angled position. One way to monitor progress in rehabilitation after an injury is to observe the improvement in angulation of the limbs when the dog is standing.

As is evident from the previous discussions, there are both advantages and disadvantages to most of the different structural variations in dogs. A summary of the effects of different structural extremes on the function of active dogs is provided in Table 1.3.

The feet

There are two broad categories for shapes of dogs' feet depending on their original function. A dog whose original function was to move over rocky or uneven ground tends to have what is termed *cat feet* in which the toes are all of equal length and form an arch around the central pad (Figure 1.15). These feet could be considered analogous to the knobby tires of an ATV, which have improved grip on uneven surfaces both when moving forward and turning. In contrast, dogs whose function was to run in straight lines tend to have *hare feet*, in which the third and fourth digits are longer than the second and the fifth. This type of foot provides an advantage when running straight and is analogous to the slick tires of a race car. The sports medicine and rehabilitation professional should be aware of the variation of foot shape and

Table 1.3 Canine structure-function correlates

	Advantages	Disadvantages
Body type		
Ectomorphic	Easier to jump Longer stride length (faster)	Harder to turn (high center of gravity) Harder to balance on narrow surfaces (high center of gravity)
Mesomorphic	Ability to participate well in many different sports	None
Endomorphic	Easier to balance on narrow surfaces (low center of gravity)	Harder to jump Harder to accelerate/decelerate Harder to run fast Harder to turn More repetitive stress injuries
Thoracic limb		
Upright scapula	Head held higher in conformation	Shorter stride length, so more steps to cover ground (slower) Increased concussion Harder to jump high More repetitive stress injuries to shoulder
Short humerus	None	Shorter stride length (slower) Increased concussion
Pelvic limb		
Minimal rear angulation	Able to turn faster	More torque on the stifle
Excessive rear angulation	Longer stride lengths, so fewer steps to cover ground	Slower turns Less accurate foot placement due to pelvic limb instability More torque on the coxofemoral joint More hyperextension injuries

should not assume that dogs with hare feet, which are less common, have an abnormality. Due to the insertion of the superficial digital flexor tendon on the distal second phalanx the dog's toes are sprung, allowing for absorption of impact. Chronic stretch of the superficial digital flexor tendon of one or more toes can

change the overall shape of the foot, often flattening the position of the phalanges, resulting in increased concussion.

The dewclaws

Many dogs have their front dewclaws removed at 3 to 5 days of age in the belief that dewclaws are nonfunctional digits and out of concern that they might become injured in active dogs. Breeders who compete in conformation often believe that the removal of these digits makes the legs appear straighter when viewed from the front.

The front dewclaws appear to be nonfunctional when the dog is in a standing position because they are not in contact with the ground. However, the dewclaws do contact the ground when dogs are cantering or galloping and bearing weight on their thoracic limbs (Figure 1.16). At that point, the dewclaw is available to dig into the ground to help stabilize the thoracic limb and reduce torque to the carpus and proximal limb when the dog is turning. Examination of structures associated with the front dewclaws substantiates that they do have function. There are four to five tendons that connect the dewclaw to the muscles of the limb (Figure 1.17) demonstrating that this digit does in fact have a function.

The dewclaws can actually function to save a dog's life. When dogs slip through the ice of a pond (or intentionally go swimming in freezing

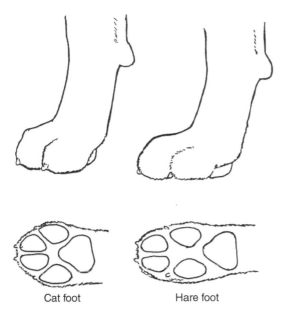

Cat foot   Hare foot

Figure 1.15   Cat foot (left) in which the toes are all of equal length and form an arch around the central pad, and hare foot (right) in which the third and fourth digits are longer than the second and the fifth. Source: Illustrations by Marcia Schlehr.

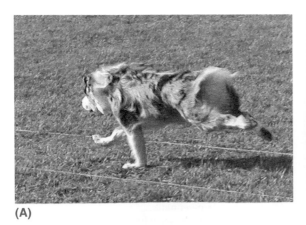

(A)

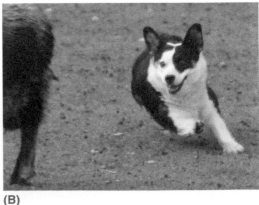

(B)

Figure 1.16   When a dog's legs are on the ground during the gallop or canter, the dewclaw is in contact with the ground and acts to stabilize the carpus if the dog turns (**A**). A Corgi's dewclaw can be clearly seen touching the ground while turning during herding activity (**B**). Source: (**A**) The Dog Camp. (**B**) Jessica Viera.

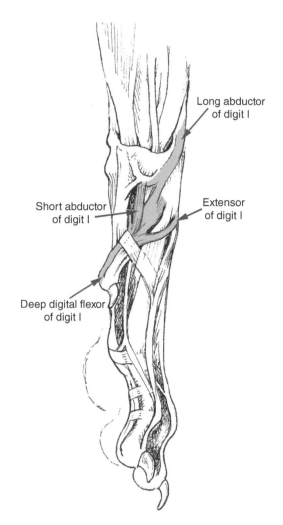

Figure 1.17   Anatomic diagram of the medial side of a dog's left forelimb demonstrating the tendons that attach to the dewclaw. These tendons, with their associated muscles confirm that the dewclaw is a functioning digit. Source: Illustration by Marcia Schlehr.

Long abductor of digit I

Short abductor of digit I

Extensor of digit I

Deep digital flexor of digit I

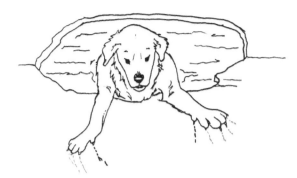

Figure 1.18   The dew claws help a dog lift itself out of water onto ice. By rotating the legs medially, the dewclaws act as little ice picks to grip the ice and pull the dog out of the water. Source: Illustration by Marcia Schlehr.

water), they cannot lift themselves out of the water and onto the ice without the use of the dewclaws acting as little ice picks on the medial side of each leg (Figure 1.18).

Finally, virtually all wild carnivores have front dewclaws, providing further evolutionary proof that they must have a function. Note, however, that dewclaws on the pelvic limb are almost always vestigial and should be removed within a few days of birth, except in those breeds such as the Great Pyrenees, Beauceron, Icelandic Sheepdog, Briard and perhaps a few others whose breed standards specify the presence of rear dewclaws.

The tail

The tail provides a counterbalance for dogs when they turn, either when running on land or swimming in water. It also helps raise the dog's rear after the apex of the trajectory of a jump, thus rotating the dog's front end downward, so that the dog will land on its front feet. Dogs use whatever length of tail they have for a counterbalance. The shorter the tail is docked, the more acute the angle at which the tail is bent laterally on turning. Dogs that have completely docked tails, such as Rottweilers and Australian Shepherds, angle their bodies sideways when turning, banking into turns like a racecar (Figure 1.19). The potential long-term physical effects of this accommodation on the limbs and vertebral column are not known.

History-taking for the canine athlete and working dog

Because of the variety of activities in which canine athletes and working dogs participate, canine sports medicine veterinarians and rehabilitation professionals should query the client in detail about specific aspects of the patient's training and competition for the sports in which the patient participates. The following are some items of additional information that

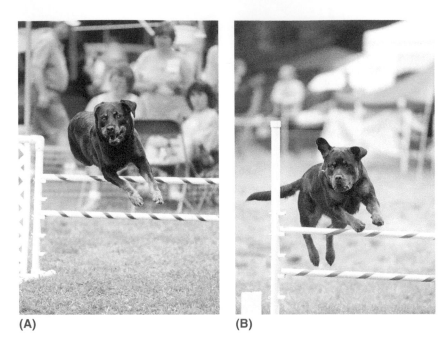

(A)   **(B)**

Figure 1.19   Differences in the way that dogs without a tail (**A**), and with a tail (**B**), angle their bodies when turning. Source: Photos by SpotShots.

should be gathered when taking the history of a canine athlete.

- **Age at which training started.** It is important that the bodies of young puppies not be stressed inappropriately with high or repetitive impact stress. Chapter 10 provides guidelines for age-appropriate training.
- **Gonadectomy status.** Several orthopedic conditions have been shown to be more prevalent in gonadectomized dogs, sometimes regardless of the age of gonadectomy. These include osteosarcoma (Priester and McKay, 1980; Ru *et al.*, 1998; Cooley *et al.*, 2002), CCL insufficiency (Whitehair *et al.*, 1993; Duval *et al.*, 1999; Slauterbeck *et al.*, 2004; Duerr *et al.*, 2007; Hart *et al.*, 2014), hip dysplasia (Spain *et al.*, 2004; van Hagen *et al.*, 2005; Hart *et al.*, 2014), and patellar luxation (Vidoni *et al.*, 2005).
- **Age at which the dog was neutered.** Dogs that are gonadectomized before puberty grow to be taller (Salmeri *et al.*, 1991). This growth can be disproportionate given that the growth plates close at different ages, potentially predisposing the prepubertally gonadectomized dog to orthopedic injuries.

- **All athletic/working events in which the dog participates.** This provides information on the specific types of physical actions that the patient undertakes during training, competition, and just for fun.
- **Number of events in which the dog competes, highest titles achieved in athletic events, level at which the dog is currently competing.** This reveals how much training and competition the dog has experienced and provides information on the total amount of work the dog has performed at its age.
- **Organizations under which the dog competes.** Different organizations can have widely varying athletic requirements. Knowing the organization under which the dog competes provides information on the intensity of the dog's physical activities.
- **Difficulties in performance events.** This can provide information about the specific problem that the dog is experiencing, which might not be obvious during a physical examination. Dogs that knock bars when jumping, for example, often have issues that involve the pelvic limbs.
- **Amount and type of exercise the patient experiences in a typical week.** The client

should be asked for specific details about how much strength, endurance, proprioception, flexibility, and skill training the patient undertakes during an average week. This gives the canine sports medicine and rehabilitation professional an idea of the knowledge of the client about exercise and the commitment of the client to the patient's success in athletics.

- **Diet and supplements.** It is important to be sure that the patient is being provided with nutrients and supplements that are appropriate for its physical tasks. This information also provides the canine sports medicine and rehabilitation professional with information regarding the level of knowledge and commitment of the client, since developing a strong base of knowledge regarding nutrition requires time and commitment on the part of the client.

- **Goals for the dog.** This information helps the sports medicine and rehabilitation professional to appropriately direct their clinical efforts toward the client's goals. For example, a conditioning program designed for a dog whose owner wants to do agility for fun and relaxation would be quite different from that of an aspiring world class competitor.

References

Brown, C. M. 1986. *Dog Locomotion and Gait Analysis*. Wheat Ridge, CO: Hoflin Publishing.

Cooley, D. M., Beranek, B. C., Schlittler, D. L., Glickman, N. W., Glickman, L. T., & Waters, D. J. 2002. Endogenous gonadal hormone exposure and bone sarcoma risk. *Cancer Epidemiol Biomarkers Prev*, 11, 1434–1440.

Cullen, K. L., Dickey, J. P., Bent, L. R., Thomason, J. J. & Moëns, N. M. M. 2013. Internet-based survey of the nature and perceived causes of injury to dogs participating in agility training and competition events. *J Am Vet Med Assoc*, 243, 1010–1018.

Duerr, F. M., Duncan, C. G., Savicky, R. S., Park, R. D., Egger, E. L., & Palmer, R. H. 2007. Risk factors for excessive tibial plateau angle in large-breed dogs with cranial cruciate ligament disease. *J Am Vet Med Assoc*, 231, 1688–1691.

Dugan, M. & Dugan, C. 2011. Seven secrets of dog show success. Part 4. Have a lot of money or know where to find it. DogChannel.com.

Dupertuis, C. W., & Sheldon, W. H. 1947. Anthropometric differences between somatotype groups. *Am J Phys Anthropol*, 2, 240.

Duval, J. M., Budsberg, S. C., Flo, G. L., & Sammarco, J. L. 1999. Breed, sex, and body weight as risk factors for rupture of the cranial cruciate ligament in young dogs. *J Am Vet Med Assoc*, 215, 811–814.

Elliott, R. P. 2009. *Dogsteps: A New Look*, 3rd edn. Irvine, CA: Fancy Publications.

Frantz, L. A., Mullin, V. E., Pionnier-capitan, M., Lebrasseur, O., Ollivier, M., Perri, A., et al. 2016. Genomic and archaeological evidence suggest a dual origin of domestic dogs. *Science*, 352, 1228–1231.

Galibert, F., Quignon, P., Hitte, C., & Andre, C. 2011. Toward understanding dog evolutionary and domestication history. *C R Biol*, 334, 190–196.

Hart, B. L., Hart, L. J., Thigpen, A. P. & Willits, N. H. 2014. Long-term health effects of neutering dogs: comparison of Labrador Retrievers with Golden Retrievers. *PLoS ONE*, 9(7), e102241.

Levy, I., Hall, C. Trentacosta, N. & Percival, M. 2009. A preliminary retrospective survey of injuries occurring in dogs participating in canine agility. *Vet Comp Orthop Traumatol*, 22, 321–324.

Miller, M. E., Christensen, G. C., & Evans, H. E. 1979. *Miller's Anatomy of the Dog*. Philadelphia: W.B. Saunders.

Ovodov, N. D., Crockford, S. J., Kuzmin, Y. V., Higham, T. F., Hodgins, G. W., & Van Der Plicht, J. 2011. A 33,000-year-old incipient dog from the Altai Mountains of Siberia: evidence of the earliest domestication disrupted by the Last Glacial Maximum. *PLoS ONE*, 6, e22821.

Priester, W. A. & Mckay, F. W. 1980. The occurrence of tumors in domestic animals. *Natl Cancer Inst Monogr*, 54, 1–210.

Ru, G., Terracini, B., & Glickman, L. T. 1998. Host related risk factors for canine osteosarcoma. *Vet J*, 156, 31–39.

Salmeri, K. R., Bloomberg, M. S., Scruggs, S. L., & Shille, V. 1991. Gonadectomy in immature dogs: effects on skeletal, physical, and behavioral development. *J Am Vet Med Assoc*, 198, 1193–1203.

Shannon, L. M., Boyko, R. H., Castelhano, M., Corey, E., Hayward, J. J., Mclean, C., et al. 2015. Genetic structure in village dogs reveals a Central Asian domestication origin. *Proc Natl Acad Sci U S A*. 112, 13639–13644.

Slauterbeck, J. R., Pankratz, K., Xu, K. T., Bozeman, S. C., & Hardy, D. M. 2004. Canine ovariohysterectomy and orchiectomy increases the prevalence of ACL injury. *Clin Orthop Relat Res*, 429, 301–305.

Spain, C. V., Scarlett, J. M., & Houpt, K. A. 2004. Long-term risks and benefits of early-age gonadectomy in dogs. *J Am Vet Med Assoc*, 224, 380–387.

Steiss, J. E. 2002. Muscle disorders and rehabilitation in canine athletes. *Vet Clin North Am Small Anim Pract*, 32, 267–285.

Thalmann, O., Shapiro, B., Cui, P., Schuenemann, V. J.,Sawyer S. K., Greenfield, D. L., et al. 2013. Complete mitochondrial genomes of ancient canids suggest a European origin of domestic dogs. *Science*, 342, 871–874.

Vanek, J. 2010. The sled dog harness. In: Duran, M. P. (ed.), *10th Biennial Meeting & Congress of the International Sled Dog Veterinary Medical Association*. Duluth, MN: ISDVMA, pp. 16–22.

VAN Hagen, M. A., Ducro, B. J., Van Den Broek, J., & Knol, B. W. 2005. Incidence, risk factors, and heritability estimates of hind limb lameness caused by hip dysplasia in a birth cohort of boxers. *Am J Vet Res*, 66, 307–312.

Vidoni, B., Sommerfeld-stur, I., & Eisenmenger, E. 2005. Diagnostic and genetic aspects of patellar luxation in small and miniature breed dogs in Austria. *Eur J Companion Anim Pract*, 16, 149–158.

Whitehair, J. G., Vasseur, P. B., & Willits, N. H. 1993. Epidemiology of cranial cruciate ligament rupture in dogs. *J Am Vet Med Assoc*, 203, 1016–1019.

Yong, E. 2016. A new origin story for dogs. The first domesticated animals may have been tamed twice. *Atlantic Monthly*, June.

2 Locomotion and Athletic Performance

Chris Zink, DVM, PhD, DACVP, DACVSMR, CCRT, CVSMT, CVA, and Brittany Jean Carr, DVM, CCRT

Summary

It is critical for the canine sports medicine and rehabilitation professional to understand canine gait and to recognize the differences in gait between different breeds of dogs to be able to recognize subtle lamenesses, which are quite common in canine athletes and working dogs. Structurally, dogs are quite different from horses. Their flexible spine (13 ribs as compared with the 17 or 18 of horses), relatively empty gastrointestinal tract, separate radius/ulna and tibia/fibula, and feet that can grip mean that canine locomotion is quite different from that of horses. Dogs use six basic gaits: walk, trot, transverse canter, rotary canter, transverse gallop and rotary gallop. The walk and trot use the same order of footfall as the horse. However, whereas horses almost exclusively use the transverse canter and gallop, dogs prefer the rotatory canter and gallop. There are several tools that can be used to accurately analyze and quantify gait abnormalities, including high-speed digital video cameras and kinematic, kinetic, and temporospatial analysis systems.

Introduction

Equine gait has been studied much more intensively than canine gait. As a result, there is a tendency for veterinarians and rehabilitation professionals to apply knowledge about equine gait to dogs. This is generally inadvisable because the musculoskeletal anatomy of horses is very different from that of dogs, and as a result, there are several major differences in the ways that the two species move. Dogs have a much more flexible spine than horses, partly because they have just 13 ribs as compared with the horse's 17 or 18, depending on breed. In addition, dogs have a separate radius and ulna as well as tibia and fibula, allowing them to rotate their limbs on their axes; they also have feet that grip. Horses also have six lumbar vertebrae in comparison to the

Canine Sports Medicine and Rehabilitation, Second Edition. Edited by Chris Zink and Janet B. Van Dyke.
© 2018 John Wiley & Sons, Inc. Published 2018 by John Wiley & Sons, Inc.

dog's seven. Another factor that further reduces the flexibility of the equine spine is the large amount of digesta in their voluminous gastrointestinal tract.

There are four main gaits that both dogs and horses use: the walk, trot, canter, and gallop (Elliott, 2009). Dogs and horses use the same movements and order of footfall when walking and trotting, but when cantering and galloping, the gaits that dogs use are substantially different from those of horses.

When evaluating a dog's gait, it is important to keep in mind the original purpose for which the dog was bred. For example, a racing Greyhound, with its arched lumbar spine, at the trot will look quite different from a Labrador Retriever, which has a level topline (Figure 2.1). The arched spine of the Greyhound allows the dog to reach far cranially with the pelvic limbs when the spine is flexed, giving this breed a much longer stride length at the gallop. However, it also reduces the Greyhound's step length at a trot because the more vertical slant of the pelvis prevents full rearward extension of the pelvic limb unless the spine is in full extension.

Different performance events require dogs to use their full range of gaits. Table 2.1 shows the gaits that dogs most commonly use in various types of canine athletic activities. It is critical for the rehabilitation professional to recognize how dogs use their bodies when performing each of the normal gaits so that they can recognize abnormalities, not just in the clinic but when viewing videos of dogs training or competing

Table 2.1   Gaits used by performance/working dogs

Event	1[a]	2	3
Agility	Canter/gallop	Trot	Walk
Obedience	Trot	Canter	Walk
Rally	Trot	Walk	Canter
Hunting	Gallop	Canter	Trot
Tracking	Walk	Trot	
Lure coursing	Gallop		
Police dogs	Walk	Trot	Canter/gallop
Detection dogs	Walk	Trot	

[a] Numbers 1 through 3 indicate the first through third most common gaits used in each performance event.

sent to them by clients. The value of viewing videos of clients' dogs moving cannot be overemphasized. Subtle changes in gait such as a slight shortening of stride, not visible to the naked eye, often can be captured with a simple smartphone set on video mode, and viewed in slow motion. In video footage it is possible to identify injuries long before the dog is lame.

Normal gaits

The walk

The walk is the slowest canine gait. The order of footfall is as follows: left rear foot (LR), left fore

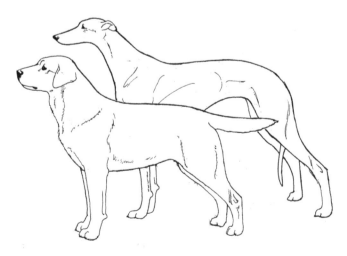

Figure 2.1   Arched spine of a Whippet compared to the level topline of a Labrador Retriever. These arrangements of the vertebral column and its musculature serve different purposes in the dog's movement. Source: Illustration by Marcia Schlehr.

foot (LF), right rear foot (RR), right fore foot (RF), repeat. In other words, a pelvic limb always makes the first move, followed by the thoracic limb on the same side. The dog places the rear foot down on the ground in a spot just ahead of the location where the ipsilateral front foot (which has now been lifted and moved forward) had been located. The footprints of a walking dog appear as diagrammed in Figure 2.2. When a dog is walking, there are alternately two feet then three feet on the ground. The walk is the only gait in which there are moments during which there are three feet on the ground, making this gait easy to recognize (Figure 2.3).

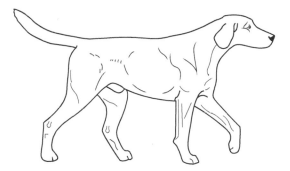

Figure 2.3   The walk is the only gait in which there are moments during which there are three feet on the ground. Source: Illustration by Marcia Schlehr.

The trot

In the trot, the dog moves diagonally opposite thoracic and pelvic limbs (e.g., RF and LR, then

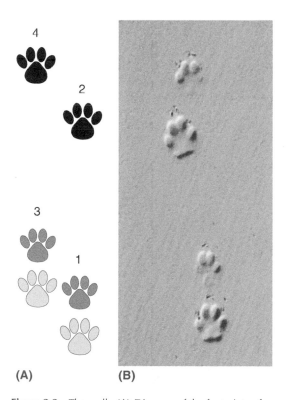

(A)   **(B)**

Figure 2.2   The walk. (A) Diagram of the footprints of a dog walking. The black prints represent the front feet and the gray prints represent the rear feet. The numbers represent the order of footfall. In this diagram, the light-gray prints represent the prints of the front feet from the previous stride. (B) Footprints in the sand left by a walking Dingo. Each rear foot is moved forward and placed in a spot just ahead of where the front foot (which has now lifted and moved forward) was previously.

LF and RR) forward, and they strike the ground at the same time. There is a moment of suspension after each pair of diagonal legs lifts off and before the other pair strikes the ground (Elliott, 2009). This is true for most breeds, although breeds with extremely angulated pelvic limbs, such as the German Shepherd Dog, may use a continuous support trot, in which one thoracic or pelvic limb remains on the ground during the period when other breeds would have a moment of suspension (Lyon, 1968; Brown, 1986).

When a dog is trotting, the foot of the pelvic limb that is moving forward should step into the spot where the ipsilateral front foot left the ground a moment before. This results in footprints as shown in Figure 2.4A. When viewing a trotting dog from the side, the front foot should be seen lifting just before the rear foot lands (Figure 2.4B).

The trot should be an efficient, ground-covering gait. Viewed from the side, a dog that is trotting efficiently will swing the thoracic limbs forward to touch the ground at a point under the tip of the dog's nose and kick the pelvic limbs back with full extension of the coxofemoral joints (Figure 2.5). When viewed from the front, the thoracic and pelvic limbs should be straight from the shoulder or pelvis to the ground, and should converge on a center point under the dog's body for the best biomechanical efficiency (Figure 2.6). This is called *single-tracking*. This prevents the dog's center of gravity from shifting from side to side, allowing the dog to use all its muscular energy to drive the body forward.

There are some breeds, however, that sacrifice efficiency at the trot to excel at other aspects of performance. For example, many herding breeds, and most notably Border Collies, have

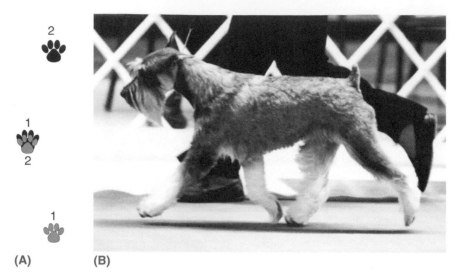

(A) **(B)**

Figure 2.4 **(A)** When a dog is trotting, the pelvic limb that is moving forward steps into the spot where the thoracic limb on the same side just left the ground a moment before. **(B)** When viewed from the side, the front foot can be seen lifting just before the rear foot lands. Source: Photo by Diane Larsen.

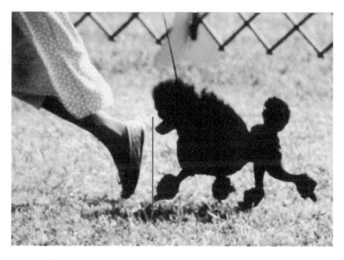

Figure 2.5 This dog is moving efficiently at the trot, swinging the thoracic limb well forward and kicking the pelvic limbs back.

pelvic limbs with adducted and internally rotated tarsi and abducted/externally rotated feet such that the tarsi are closer together than the feet, sometimes referred to as *cow hocks* (Figure 2.7). This may be an adaptation for herding; having this type of rear conformation is thought to provide improved stability for lying down and standing up (to reduce or increase pressure on the sheep, respectively) and to help the pelvic limbs push off when turning.

Another adaptation of the trot gait seen in Border Collies is a relatively reduced forward reach and rearward extension (drive) when the limbs are viewed from the side. It is thought that this apparent lack of reach and drive is an adaptation that allows the dog to turn more rapidly, much as a spinning figure skater turns more rapidly when their arms are closer to the body (Carr *et al.*, 2015).

The trot is the gait that is best used to detect lameness, because it is the only gait for which

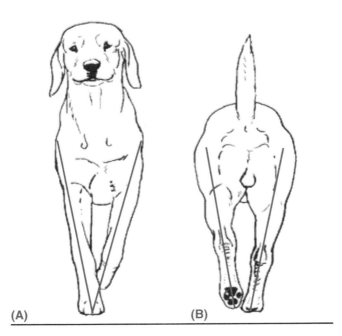

(A)   **(B)**

Figure 2.6 (**A, B**) When viewed from the front or the rear, the limbs should be straight and should converge on a center point under the dog's body for the best biomechanical efficiency. This prevents the dog's center of gravity from shifting from side to side, allowing the dog to use all of its muscular energy to drive the body forward. Source: Illustrations by Marcia Schlehr.

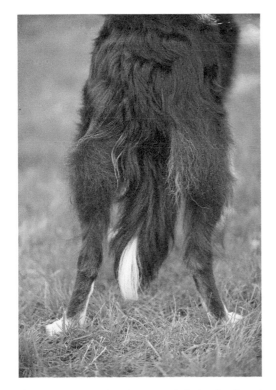

Figure 2.7 Some breeds, particularly herding breeds, have pelvic limbs with internally rotated tarsi, sometimes referred to as being *cow hocked*. Source: Photo by George Brown.

the thoracic limbs and pelvic limbs are never assisted in bearing weight by the contralateral limb. Thus, when a dog is experiencing pain or lack of stability in one limb, it is more clearly revealed by a head nod (most obvious in thoracic limb lameness) or asymmetrical motions of the pelvis (pelvic limb lameness). In addition, the trot is a gait that is symmetrical and is slow enough for the experienced human eye to observe stride length and foot placement.

The canter

The canter is a somewhat complex gait, made more so by the fact that dogs use two different styles of canter, the transverse and the rotary canter. Dogs preferentially use the rotary canter whereas horses should always use the transverse canter.

The order of footfall for the transverse canter is as follows: RR, LR and RF together (the thoracic limb actually strikes the ground a little after the pelvic limb), and LF (Figure 2.8A). When cantering or galloping, the second of either the thoracic or pelvic limbs to strike the ground is called the front or rear *lead leg*, respectively. It is referred to as the lead leg because the second leg strikes the ground in a location cranial to the first leg to strike the ground. In the case of the transverse canter, the dog uses the same lead leg for both the thoracic and pelvic limbs. In Figure 2.8.A, for example, the lead legs are the left pelvic limb and the left thoracic limb. If the dog were using the right legs as lead in a transverse canter, the order of footfall would be LR, RR and LF, then RF.

Interestingly, dogs as well as wild canids much more commonly use a rotary canter than a transverse canter. The order of footfall for the rotary canter is: RR, LR and LF, then RF (Figure 2.8B). Note that while, on the second step, the thoracic and pelvic limbs are considered to strike the ground together, in fact the thoracic limb strikes the ground just after the pelvic limb. In the rotary canter, the dog uses

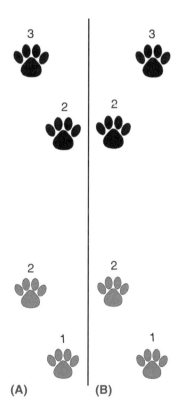

(A)   **(B)**

Figure 2.8   The canter. **(A)** Footprints of a dog using the transverse canter, in which the thoracic limb and the pelvic limb are both on the same lead (in this case the left). **(B)** Footprints of a dog using the more common rotary canter, in which the dog uses a different lead in the rear (in this case, the left) and the front.

opposite leads on the pelvic limb (in this example, the left lead) and the thoracic limb (in this example, the right lead). If the dog were using the right lead on the pelvic limb and the left lead on the thoracic limb, the order of footfalls would be LR, RR and RF, then LF.

The rotary canter gives the dog a rolling appearance, particularly when the dog is viewed from the rear, as the two ipsilateral legs frequently abduct as they swing forward together. This motion should not be mistaken for lameness. The rotary canter provides dogs with a distinct advantage in gaiting, particularly when turning. Regardless of whether a dog is using a transverse or rotary canter, when turning it uses the thoracic limb on the side to which the dog is turning as the lead leg. In other words, if a dog is turning to the right, it uses the right thoracic limb as lead. During the rotary canter, dogs can turn with greater efficiency and accuracy. Using the front lead leg that is on the side to which the dog is turning, the dog abducts that thoracic limb and pulls itself in the direction of the turn. Then, because there is a point at which both pelvic limbs are on the ground in the rotary canter, the dog effectively pushes off with both pelvic limbs in the direction of the turn (Figure 2.9).

The gallop

At the gallop, the dog uses the power of its highly muscular and flexible spine and abdomen to produce two moments of suspension, one after the thoracic limbs and one after the pelvic limbs leave the ground. Starting with the dog in the air after the thoracic limbs have left the ground, the dog flexes the entire spine, bringing the pelvic limbs forward under its body (Figure 2.10). The two pelvic limbs strike the ground, one foot slightly before the other. The dog then pushes off with the pelvic limbs in extension and extends the spine, reaching forward with the two thoracic limbs. There is a moment of suspension as the dog is driven through the air with its spine in full extension, then the thoracic limbs land on the ground, one slightly ahead of the other. The dog then pulls the thoracic limbs under

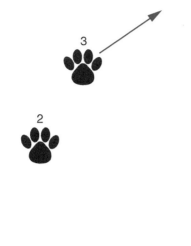

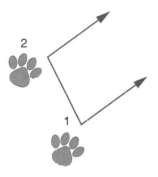

Figure 2.9   A dog that is using the rotary canter can easily abduct the right thoracic limb to pull itself in the direction to which it is turning, and also can push off in that direction when both pelvic limbs are on the ground.

the body and pushes off from the ground, experiencing a second period of suspension as it flexes the spine and brings the pelvic limbs forward to initiate the next stride. This is why the dog's gallop is often termed a *double suspension gallop*.

As in the canter, dogs most often use different lead legs on the thoracic and pelvic limbs when galloping. In contrast, horses use the ipsilateral thoracic and pelvic legs as lead. The pattern of footfall for the canine rotary gallop using the RF leg as lead would be RR and LR, then LF and RF (Figure 2.11).

The amble

When a dog is walking and begins to speed up gradually, the thoracic limb swings forward very soon after the pelvic limb swings forward, and it starts to appear as if ipsilateral limbs are forward together. As long as there are moments, however brief, when there are three feet on the ground, this gait is still considered a walk. This fast walk is often referred to as an amble. The amble is a normal, although not generally preferred gait. Dogs tend to use this gait when they are tired but want to move quickly, to use a different set of muscles from the trot, or when they are not fit enough or have not been trained to trot at a slower speed.

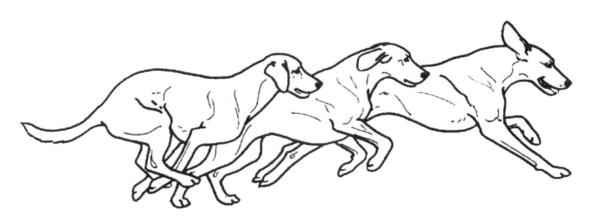

Figure 2.10   In the gallop, the dog uses the power of its highly muscular and flexible spine and abdomen, producing two moments of suspension, each followed alternately by the thoracic limbs or the pelvic limbs striking the ground. Source: Illustration by Marcia Schlehr.

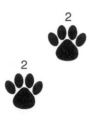

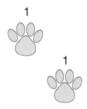

Figure 2.11 The pattern of footfall for the rotary gallop. In this example, the dog is using the right lead in the front and the left lead in the rear.

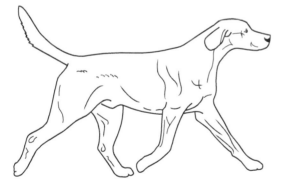

Figure 2.12 In the pace, both limbs on the same side of the body move forward together until there are only two feet on the ground, followed by a period of suspension. Source: Illustration by Marcia Schlehr.

The pace

If the ambling dog continues to increase its speed, it might begin to pace. In the pace, ipsilateral thoracic and pelvic limbs swing forward together and then strike the ground. This is followed by a period of suspension, and then the contralateral thoracic and pelvic limbs strike the ground together (Figure 2.12). The order of footfall is LR and LF, followed by a short period of suspension, then RR and RF. The pace is a very ungainly gait, with the dog's center of gravity shifting from side to side, requiring the dog to waste effort recentering the body, when it could use that muscular effort to drive forward. Most dogs are not able to change speed or turn very effectively when pacing, which is why it is considered an abnormal gait in dogs, particularly in performance/working dogs. Dogs that routinely pace have either been inadvertently trained to gait this way by consistently walking on leash at speeds that are between their ideal walk and trot speeds, or they have a physical problem that prevents them from feeling comfortable at a trot.

Interference at the trot

Another gait abnormality is referred to colloquially as *crabbing* or *side-winding*. Some dogs will crab when heeling because as they raise their head up and look at the handler, the rear naturally swings outward. This is generally correctable through training. However, a far more common reason for crabbing is related to an imbalance of angulation between the thoracic and pelvic limbs, and for that reason is not amenable to retraining. The most common form of imbalance of angulation consists of a dog with a very angulated rear and a straighter front. The less angulated thoracic limb has a shorter step length and, therefore, a faster gait cycle time than the more angulated pelvic limb. This makes it difficult for diagonally opposite thoracic and pelvic limbs to strike the ground at the same time as they should when a dog is trotting.

There are four common ways that dogs attempt to correct for this disparity. Some dogs will use what is called a *hackney gait*, in which, after swinging forward, the thoracic limbs are held high in the air, waiting until the more angulated pelvic limbs have finished their swing phase so that the thoracic and pelvic limbs can strike the ground together. This gait is commonly seen in the Miniature Pinscher

Case Study 2.1   Gait retraining

Signalment: 4 y.o. M/I Shetland Sheepdog that is training and competing in obedience and agility.

History: Twice in the last 18 months, the patient has had surgery to remove interdigital cysts, first between P4 and P5, then between P3 and P4 on the left thoracic limb. Pathology reports indicate that both cysts consist of granulomatous inflammation secondary to keratin and hairs that had been driven through the interdigital epidermis. Client notes that she is losing points in obedience competition because patient is lagging during heeling exercise, especially when client is doing an about turn. Client wonders whether this is related to pain or discomfort in the left forefoot after the two surgeries.

Examination: Patient is a large Sheltie (18" at the withers; breed standard indicates maximum height should be 16") and is moderately overweight, but otherwise, all body systems are normal. Surgical sites are completely healed and other than small scars, there is no evidence of the previous interdigital cysts. No evidence of lameness or pain/discomfort on examination. However, when moving at a trotting speed, patient paces. When client moves faster or pulls on patient's collar to off-balance him, he trots for two to three strides then drifts back into a pace.

Diagnosis: Gait abnormality—pacing.

Recommendation: A gait retraining and reconditioning program was developed. Patient trotted daily through ground poles elevated approximately 3" off the ground and placed parallel to each other approximately 18" apart. After 3 weeks of daily short training sessions, patient was weaned off ground poles over a period of another 3 weeks. In addition, client started placing the poles on hills, facing both up and down and sideways on the hill. Approximately a week after initiating the program, patient stopped pacing while heeling in obedience, and after approximately 4 weeks on the retraining program he stopped pacing whenever he was moving. Scores for the obedience heeling exercise improved by 50%.

Comments: Many obedience dogs are inadvertently trained to pace because their client starts off walking slowly during training and gradually speeds up. When pacing, a dog's center of gravity shifts from side to side, making the dog less able to adapt to the client's gait changes. This also can put abnormal stress on the feet and might have contributed to the interdigital cysts that developed in this dog.

and has been accepted as correct for this breed. A second way that dogs adapt is by *paddling* or *flipping* the front feet at the extreme end of forward extension. Again, this keeps the thoracic limbs in the air longer to allow for the pelvic limbs to finish the swing phase. Another accommodation is for the dogs to abduct the thoracic limbs on the swing phase of the trot, again keeping the thoracic limbs in the air for a longer period of time.

But by far the most common adaptation is for the dog to keep the thoracic limb on the ground longer during the stance phase of gait. Because the dog keeps the thoracic limb on the ground at the end of the stance phase, the ipsilateral pelvic limb swings forward and strikes the thoracic limb, which has remained on the ground. To avoid this, dogs will move the pelvic limbs to one side or the other of the ipsilateral thoracic limb—hence, crabbing or side-winding. When viewing the dog gaiting from the side, the pelvic limbs can be seen bypassing the thoracic limbs under the dog's abdomen (Figure 2.13). This gait causes the spinal musculature on one side of the dog's body to move differently from the musculature on the other side, creating an imbalance. Surprisingly, this gait abnormality is largely accepted in the conformation ring, possibly because many breed judges admire the image of a dog with abundant rear angulation and a straighter front with the head held high, which makes the dog appear to be alert.

A recent observation of dogs at the Westminster Dog Show, the premier conformation event in the United States, revealed that

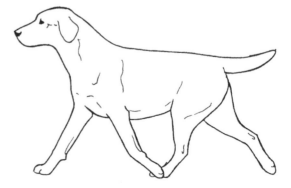

Figure 2.13   When viewed from the side, the distal thoracic and pelvic limbs of a dog that is crabbing can be seen bypassing each other. Source: Illustration by Marcia Schlehr.

more than half of the sporting and working dogs exhibited this abnormality (Chris Zink, personal communication, 2017). Having said that, it is not uncommon to see wolves in the wild crabbing, but only when they are trotting at maximal speed. Thus, this gait pattern should be considered abnormal only when seen consistently at slow or moderate speeds.

Occasionally, to avoid interference, a dog will either widen the thoracic limbs to allow the pelvic limbs to pass between them medially or will widen the pelvic limbs to allow each pelvic limb to pass on the lateral side of its ipsilateral thoracic limb. This is the most common reason why some dogs can be seen to be moving wide with the thoracic or pelvic limbs when trotting, rather than single-tracking.

Gait training/retraining

Many canine athletes are presented to the canine sports medicine/rehabilitation professional with very subtle alterations of gait—so subtle that they may not be defined as lameness. An intimate understanding of the complexities of canine gait can go a long way in helping identify and appropriately treat early musculoskeletal problems.

Dogs first begin to be conscious of gaiting and of putting their feet down in an ordered pattern at about 6 months of age, although with training they can improve their gaits and transitions between gaits at any age. Surprisingly, the gait with which dogs most often struggle is the one that seems the simplest to us—the trot. This is considered the most natural gait for most breeds and is the gait that wild canids such as wolves and foxes use for traveling long distances in an energy-efficient manner. Dogs that consistently amble or pace in preference to trotting should first be thoroughly examined to rule out injuries that may make it difficult for the dog to trot. This would include most injuries that cause pain when bearing weight on one or more limbs, since at a trot the dog's weight is never shared by the contralateral limb.

If physically sound, these patients should be trained to trot correctly so that they understand how to use this energy-conserving gait when appropriate. In addition, a form of the trot gait can be used as an effective whole body conditioning exercise. The trot is the most effective gait for conditioning because it forces the dog to bear all its weight on only one thoracic and the contralateral pelvic limb at a time, thus requiring the dog to use the muscles on both sides of the body equally. Dogs that have lost condition after surgery or a long period of lameness and rest benefit tremendously from being retrained to trot once they have completed rehabilitation.

Training or retraining a dog to trot is a simple matter requiring minimal equipment. It does, however, require regular, preferably daily, repetition over a period of several weeks to establish or re-establish the neuronal pathways for this pattern of movement (Zink, 2008). What we commonly refer to as muscle memory is, in fact, the strengthening of existing synapses and establishment of new synapses along the neuronal pathway, and is thus more accurately referred to as neurological memory (Zehr, 2006). It takes 4–6 weeks of daily, brief training sessions to teach a young dog to trot consistently, and 6–8 weeks of daily sessions to retrain a dog to trot if it has been habitually pacing. Interestingly, gait training has long been an established component of training for young horses, whereas young canine athletes are generally left to establish gait patterns on their own. With increasing confinement and leash laws for dogs, this frequently results in dogs that are unfamiliar with even basic gait patterns.

To train or retrain a dog to trot, place eight 5-foot long, 1-inch diameter PVC poles on the ground parallel to one another approximately as far apart as the dog's height measured from the ground to the top of the scapula. The ends of the poles can be rested on empty soda cans that have been dented and laid on their sides or on any other holder that will elevate them to a height of 2 to 4 inches above the ground, depending on the size of the dog. The cans keep the poles from rolling out of place and provide auditory feedback when the dog knocks a pole.

Have the client start with the dog on leash about 20 feet from one end of the poles and move at a moderate speed toward the poles with the arm that is holding the leash outstretched so that the handler runs beside the poles while the dog trots over them as shown in Figure 2.14. Have the handler continue about 20 feet past the poles so that the dog practices trotting over

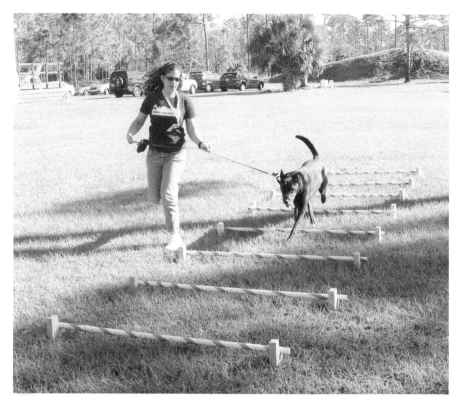

Figure 2.14   To train dogs to trot, poles can be laid parallel to each other about as far apart as the dog's height at the most dorsal point of the scapula. The dog is then trotted over them, starting 20 ft away from the poles and continuing 20 ft past.

ground without poles, after which they should stop, turn toward the dog, and stop again prior to making the next pass. This is important because the dog needs to learn to start moving immediately at a trot, so stopping at the end of each pass gives the dog experience with multiple starts in any given training session. The poles will force the dog to move in an efficient trot gait, picking its feet up and balancing its center of gravity. The client should be encouraged not to look at the dog so that the dog will then look forward at the poles.

During the early stages of training many dogs will amble or pace toward the poles. However, the poles will force the dog to trot. If the dog continues to amble or pace over the poles, this can be rectified by elevating the poles to carpus height or in some cases, a little higher. Once the dog is consistently approaching the poles at a trot, the client can give the dog a cue word as they start trotting. That word should be different from any previous cue word used for gaiting.

Have the client move the dog in both directions over the poles, working with the dog on both the right and left sides. One training session consists of 10–12 passes. The dog should practice on different surfaces and with a variety of distractions. After 15–20 training sessions, the dog can begin to be weaned off the poles by having the client move one pole from the middle to the end, leaving a double-sized gap that requires the dog to take two strides across the gap.

After another three to five training sessions, have the client move a second pole to the end, leaving another gap. Continue until there are double-length spaces between each pair of poles, at which time the poles can be randomly removed every three to five training sessions until all are removed. At this point, when cued, the dog should trot forward a few feet without the handler moving.

Once the dog understands the basic trot, the same eight-pole exercise can be used as a conditioning exercise for the thoracic limb, pelvic limb, and core musculature. Just have the client increase the distance between the poles by 0.5 to 1 inch (depending on the size of the dog) every one to two training sessions. Once the poles are at a distance that the dog finds difficult as indicated by taking two steps between poles, have the client reduce the inter-pole distance by 1 inch, then train for 7–10 days (10–12 passes/day). During this time, the dog develops the musculature to be able to continue increasing the distance. Have the client keep increasing the distance between poles and reducing by 1 inch when necessary until the dog cannot progress to a further distance. By this point, the dog's musculature will have been optimized, and its ability to trot will be completely second nature.

Gait analysis

Visual observation of gait

A systematic and disciplined approach should be used to clinically evaluate a patient's gait. To document this clinical evaluation in the medical record, findings are often semi-quantified using a numerical rating scale (Table 2.2) or visual analog scale.

Both the numerical rating scale and visual analog scale were developed to provide a systematic approach to visual observation of gait. However, it is important to realize that, while visual or subjective gait analysis is often helpful in identifying lameness, the gold standard for characterizing lameness is quantification of gait characteristics with a form of objective gait analysis, such as force plate analysis.

Evans and colleagues compared visual observation of gait with force plate analysis (Evans et al., 2005). This study evaluated 148 Labrador Retrievers—131 that were 6 months post-surgery for unilateral cranial cruciate ligament injury and 17 that were free of orthopedic disease. The observer identified only 11% of the 131 dogs that were 6 months post-surgery as being abnormal, whereas force plate analysis revealed that 75% of the 131 dogs failed to achieve ground reaction forces consistent with sound Labrador Retrievers.

While force plate analysis has been shown to be superior to visual observation, visual observation is still a practical tool in clinical practice, and its importance should not be discounted.

Videography for gait analysis

The camera is a readily accessible, underutilized tool for lameness assessment, and is particularly useful for identifying subtle injuries. Most standard smartphones have cameras that will take video at 120 frames per second, which is ideal for slow motion examination of a dog's footfalls and gait patterns. Videos should be taken in as high resolution as possible, and many phones are large enough to view the video with the client without having to upload to a computer.

The dog should be recorded from the side and while going toward and away from the camera; however, the best information often comes from the side view. Always video the dog on a flat, hard surface like concrete; outdoors is preferable because there is adequate space and lighting to maximize the camera's frames per second. The trot is the most useful gait to video. Dogs that are short striding on the thoracic limb can often be seen placing one front foot down prior to the landing of the contralateral rear foot (Figure 2.15). It is also useful to have the client send you high-resolution videos of the patient either training or competing at both recent trials and prior to recognition of the injury. Performance videos will often reveal a dog avoiding the use of the correct front lead leg when turning, or flinching on landing from a jump or when turning at speed.

Table 2.2 Numerical rating scale for visual assessment of gait

Lameness grade	Description
Grade 1	Sound at the walk, but weight shifting and mild lameness noted at trot
Grade 2	Mild weight-bearing lameness noted with the trained eye
Grade 3	Weight-bearing lameness, typically with distinct head nod
Grade 4	Significant weight-bearing lameness
Grade 5	Toe-touching lameness
Grade 6	Non-weight-bearing lameness

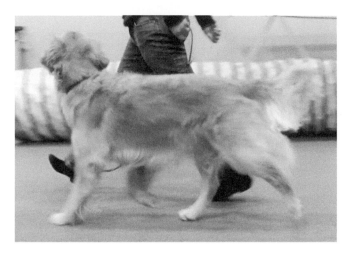

Figure 2.15   This image taken from a video shows a Golden Retriever's left front foot on the ground, but the right rear foot only just about to touch down. When seen repeatedly, this is evidence of short-striding, in this case of the left front foot.

Objective gait analysis in performance dogs

Performance dogs can be stoic and do not always show overt signs of pain or lameness. Early signs of lameness may be as subtle as a shortened stride or shorter stance time on the injured leg and often cannot be seen by visual observation alone, and thus need to be objectively quantified. Gait analysis is an important tool to establish a diagnosis, monitor the progress of treatment and determine when the dog has achieved full recovery.

Every performance or working dog should have a baseline objective gait analysis performed prior to training and performing. Having a baseline objective gait analysis provides data to refer to in the event of injury or change in performance, and is especially important given individual- or breed-related variation in gait patterns. Additionally, if a pre-existing orthopedic condition is suspected, objective gait analysis provides an easy opportunity to objectively screen for and measure any lameness or gait abnormalities, which can also then be monitored.

Objective gait analysis tools

Normal locomotion requires proper functioning of the musculoskeletal system coordinated by the nervous system. In the past, canine gait was usually evaluated subjectively. Such analysis was limited mainly to the walk and the trot because of their slower speeds, and analysis was still limited due to the inability of the human eye to follow rapid movements. While subjective gait analysis still has a very important role in clinical practice, validated objective gait analysis technologies have recently become available to help veterinarians quantitate gait characteristics in the clinical setting. This can greatly assist in the detection of a subtle lameness and in monitoring response to various treatments.

While there are multiple quantitative gait analysis methods that can be used to establish a diagnosis and to monitor treatment efficacy, it is important to establish normal parameters for accurate interpretation of gait analysis results. Quantitative analysis of canine locomotion most commonly involves the measurement of temporospatial characteristics, kinematics of limb segments, and/or kinetics of the foot connecting with the substrate. The advantages and disadvantages of each type of gait analysis system are summarized in Table 2.3.

Gait analysis should always be performed in a quiet space where the patient has minimal distractions because velocity, head turning, and changes in acceleration have all been shown to affect gait (Gillette & Angle, 2008; Maes *et al.*, 2008; Gordon-Evans, 2012). Additionally, it is

Table 2.3   Comparison of commonly used objective canine gait analysis systems

	Advantages	Disadvantages
Kinematic gait analysis	Collects positions, velocities, acceleration/ deceleration, and angles of various anatomic structures in space Can be performed in 2-D or 3-D	Skin movement affects marker placement Difficult to establish consistent positioning with breed variation Technically challenging to operate
Kinetic gait analysis	Measures forces in three dimensions Very well studied Most widely used quantitative gait application	Only collects a single reading per single pass Technically challenging to operate Size restrictions can apply
Temporospatial gait analysis	Provides multiple readings from a single pass Determines stride and step length Provides information on limb placement User-friendly software Portable No size restrictions	Can only measure total ground reaction force

recommended that gait analysis be performed with the patient wearing a collar with a loose leash attached as harnesses and other external apparatuses have been reported to affect gait (Carr & Zink, 2016). Finally, it is important to have the handler on the same side of the dog each time data are recorded as handler side has also been shown to affect gait characteristics (Keebaugh et al., 2015).

Kinetic systems

Kinetic systems measure forces in three dimensions: vertical, craniocaudal, and mediolateral. These systems generally are ground-based, with the traditional system based on force plates, which measure forces (Box 2.1) by incorporating strain gauges as sensing elements or quartz crystals to generate piezoelectric signals. The measured forces are often presented graph-

ically, with the peak forces as the maximum forces generated in the described phase of gait, represented by the force–time curve. The impulse is then represented as the area under the force–time curve.

Peak vertical force (PVF) is the single largest force during the stance phase and represents only a single data point on the force–time curve. Vertical impulse (VI) can be derived by calculating the area under the vertical force curve using time. PVF and VI are the two most commonly used indices to detect lameness. In general, a lame dog has a lower PVF and VI in the affected limb (Nunamaker & Blauner, 1985; Gillette & Angle, 2008; Gordon-Evans, 2012). While braking, propulsion, and mediolateral forces may be useful in evaluating mechanisms of locomotion, they are not used commonly for diagnostic purposes or to assess outcome (Gillette & Angle, 2008).

A typical report from a force plate is seen in Figure 2.16, which shows the forces produced by the thoracic limb (first peak) and the pelvic limb (second peak) in each of the three dimensions. Force plate measurements are the most widely used quantitative gait application in veterinary medicine to date (Voss et al., 2007). Thus, force plate analysis is currently viewed as the gold standard for quantification of gait characteristics by objective gait analysis.

Limitations of kinetic systems include the potential for habituation of dogs to the system,

---

Box 2.1   Types of ground reaction forces

- Peak vertical force
- Vertical impulse
- Rising and falling slope
- Braking force
- Braking impulse
- Propulsive force
- Propulsive impulse
- Mediolateral force

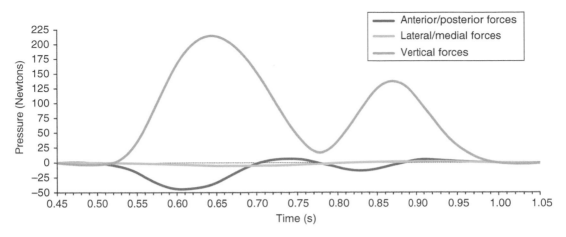

Figure 2.16   Typical force plate report, showing the forces produced by the thoracic limb (first peak) and the pelvic limb (second peak) in each of the three dimensions. Source: Adapted from Gillette & Angle, 2008.

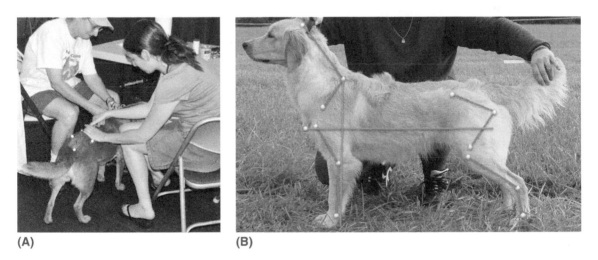

(A)   **(B)**

Figure 2.17   The typical kinematic analysis system uses colored, retroreflective, or light-emitting diode (LED) markers (**A**) that identify specific anatomic landmarks on the dog that are associated with the limb or joint under study. Distances between any pairs of markers and angles between groups of three markers (**B**) are calculated by computer.

resulting in gait changes (Rumph *et al.*, 1997), the need to standardize the velocity of the subject, and the extreme variability in the morphology of different breeds of dogs (Molsa *et al.*, 2010). As with other systems, the time required to acquire and analyze kinetic data means that these systems are generally not useful in a clinical context.

Kinematic analysis

Kinematics is the science of the motion of objects, and kinematic gait analysis quantifies the positions, velocities, acceleration/decelera-

tion, and angles of various anatomic structures in space. Kinematic analysis can be performed in two dimensions, which record data in the x and y axes normal to the camera lens, or three dimensions, which include data that are out-of-plane to the lens, thus providing rotational and circumduction data. Three-dimensional (3-D) data are proportionately more accurate and more complex to obtain and analyze. These systems can be used to characterize normal gait in dogs of various sizes and breeds, to analyze lameness of any cause, and to monitor response to surgical, medical, and rehabilitation therapy (Lee *et al.*, 2007; Off & Matis, 2010).

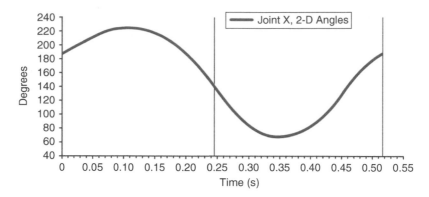

Figure 2.18   Two-dimensional (2-D) kinematic analysis of carpal range of motion during the trot. Source: Adapted from Gillette & Angle, 2008.

The typical kinematic analysis system uses colored, retroreflective, or light-emitting diode (LED) markers that identify specific anatomic landmarks on the dog that are associated with the limb or joint under study (Figure 2.17). The movements of these markers when the dog is gaited are followed by a series of cameras (minimum of three) that place the markers in space relative to a control 3-D standard. The locations of the markers over time are then used to create a 2-D or 3-D model of how the dog moves, with accurate calculations of bone and joint excursion.

Kinematic parameters include displacements, angular velocities, and range of motion. Displacement is the distance recorded when a marker changes position. Angular velocity is the speed at which this change occurs. Range of motion is calculated from the displacement at a specific joint.

An example of a 2-D kinematic measurement is shown in Figure 2.18, which shows carpal range of motion (ROM) during the trot (Gillette & Angle, 2008). In contrast, 3-D kinematic data generate three graphs for every anatomic structure. For example, the angles of excursion of the hip joint in a trotting dog are shown in the sagittal (flexion-extension), transverse (internal-external rotation), and frontal (abduction-adduction) planes, as in Figure 2.19 (Fu et al., 2010).

A major limitation of data from kinematic analysis systems is the tremendous breed variation in the structure of dogs, as well as variation between individual dogs of the same breed, such as in the amount of pelvic limb angulation (Bertram et al., 2000). This significantly limits comparisons between studies. In addition,

there is some uncertainty as to whether healthy dogs truly have right and left symmetry (Gillette & Zebas, 1999; Colborne et al., 2011). Further, there can be limitations with respect to the accurate placement of markers, and the potential for skin movement can add significant error to measurements. Several techniques have been proposed to mitigate or correct for skin movement in humans and horses (van Weeren et al., 1992; Sha et al., 2004; Guo et al., 2005). It remains to be seen how these might apply to dogs with their generally more mobile skin.

Several other kinematic systems are under development, including radiostereometric analysis, dynamic magnetic resonance imaging, dynamic computed tomography, accelerometer systems, and electromagnetic motion tracking (Gillette & Angle, 2008). The next decade should provide the canine sports medicine/rehabilitation professional with many advanced tools for gait analysis.

There are now systems that will analyze and integrate methodologies using 3-D kinematic (motion) analysis (i.e., which includes analysis of the third coordinate axis), kinetic (forces) analysis, and electromyography simultaneously in one system (Ritter et al., 2001; Gillette & Angle, 2008).

Temporospatial gait analysis

Pressure-sensing walkways have been validated to analyze gait characteristics in dogs and to aid in diagnosing orthopedic, muscular, and neurological disorders that affect gait. Studies have established protocols for the collection of data using these systems and have

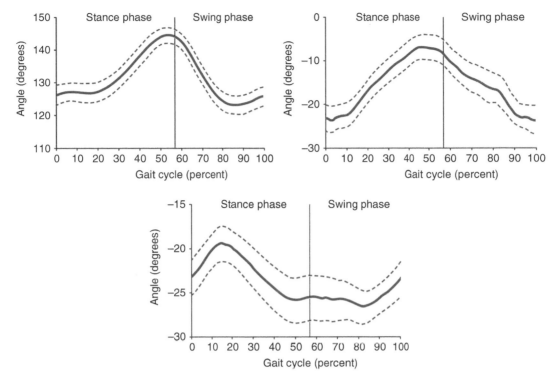

Figure 2.19   Kinematic report showing the angles of excursion of the hip joint in a trotting dog in the sagittal (flexion-extension; top left), transverse (internal-external rotation; top right), and frontal (abduction-adduction; bottom) planes. Source: Adapted from Fu *et al.*, 2010.

determined reference values and symmetry ratios for various breeds (Webster *et al.*, 2005; Lascelles *et al.*, 2006; Gordon-Evans *et al.*, 2009; Light *et al.*, 2010;).

Table 2.4   Temporospatial gait analysis parameters

Temporal (timing) gait parameters	Spatial (distance) gait parameters
Gait cycle time is the elapsed time between the first contacts of two consecutive footfalls of the same foot, measured in seconds (s)	*Stride length* is measured on the line of progression between the heel points of two consecutive footprints of the same foot (e.g., left front foot to left front foot)
Stance time is the time elapsed between the first contact and the last contact of one identified foot, expressed in seconds (s)	*Step length* is the distance between the heel point of one foot to the heel point of the contralateral foot (e.g., left front foot to the right front foot)
Stride time is the time elapsed between the first contacts of two consecutive footfalls of the same foot, measured in seconds (s)	

Pressure-sensing walkway measurement systems objectively analyze gait data quickly and provide several temporal (timing) and spatial (distance) gait parameters (Table 2.4). Temporal (timing) gait analysis is the assessment of average velocities of the various gaits as well as time durations for the two phases of gait for each leg: the stance phase and the swing phase. The stance phase is the weight-bearing portion of each gait cycle. It is initiated by central pad contact and ends when the toe of the same foot lifts off the mat. The swing phase is the non-weight-bearing portion of each gait cycle, during which the foot is in the air.

Spatial (distance) gait analysis is the assessment of the progression of gait. Two commonly assessed spatial parameters are stride length and step length. Stride length is measured on the line of progression between the central pad points of two consecutive footprints of the same foot (e.g., left front foot to left front foot). Step length is the distance between the central pad point of one foot to the central pad point of the contralateral foot (e.g., the left front foot to the right front foot).

Table 2.5 Temporospatial gait analysis advantages and disadvantages

Advantages	Disadvantages
Multiple readings can be obtained from a single pass	Ability to only measure total ground reaction forces
Determination of stride and step length	Inability to separate the three force vectors (dorso-ventral, craniocaudal and mediolateral) as with force plate analysis
Information on limb placement	
User-friendly software	
Portability	

Most pressure-sensing walkways do not measure total ground reaction forces but rather compute an indirect measure of these forces. One of the most important measurements collected is the total pressure placed on each foot. Dogs place more of their weight on their thoracic limbs compared to their pelvic limbs. For most breeds, this distribution is approximately 60% of the dog's weight on the thoracic limbs (30% on each thoracic limb) and 40% on the pelvic limbs (20% on each pelvic limb). However, recent studies have shown this can vary among breeds (Carr et al., 2015).

As with any other gait analysis system, there are advantages and disadvantages to using a pressure-sensing walkway (Table 2.5). All the above quantitative gait analysis systems have the potential to provide substantial information regarding most areas of locomotion research. However, for several reasons, only certain aspects of these technologies can be harnessed by the practicing veterinarian. Many of these systems are very expensive, in the hundreds of thousands of dollars. In addition, they frequently have a significant learning curve, not only for the acquisition of data, but even more so for their analysis. Some systems require significant numbers of repeat measures on a single dog, which is not practical in the clinical setting, and accurate analysis of the data is often not possible in real time.

Nonetheless, several 2-D computer-assisted videographic gait analysis systems are finding their way into specialty practices. These systems can be operated by trained technical staff

and provide a videographic presentation of the dog's gait that can be understood by the educated client. New developments will continue to increase our ability to quantify the kinematics and kinetics of canine gait.

Accelerometry in dogs

Recently, accelerometers have been validated for use in dogs (Hansen et al., 2007; Brown et al., 2010; Michel & Brown, 2011; Wrigglesworth et al., 2011; Yam et al., 2011; Preston et al., 2012; Clark et al., 2014; Morrison et al., 2014; Bruno et al., 2015; Vitger et al., 2016). In fact, recent studies have demonstrated their use in managing weight loss plans for overweight patients (Morrison et al., 2014; Vitger et al., 2016). One study demonstrated that accelerometers could be used to measure physical performance and potentially differentiate between on-lead activity, off-lead activity, and playing activity in healthy dogs versus dogs with osteoarthritis (Bruno et al., 2015). These inexpensive and small units are under development for use in clinic-based objective gait analysis systems.

Breed variation in gait

Studies have compared the gaits of various breeds and found differences in ground reaction forces (Bertram et al., 2000; Besancon et al., 2004;Colborne et al., 2005; Molsa et al., 2010; Voss et al., 2010; Agostinho et al., 2011; Kano et al., 2016; Volstad et al., 2016). These differences were attributed to variations in conformation and/or body weight. One recent study evaluated temporospatial gait characteristics of Border Collies and Labrador Retrievers (Carr et al., 2016). Labrador Retrievers were shown to place significantly more weight on the pelvic limbs at both the walk and the trot than Border Collies. Border Collies were also shown to have a significantly shorter gait cycle and stride length, even when accounting for differences in body size and weight.

That study proposed that the differences in quantitative gait characteristics identified could be related to differences in the original purposes for which these dogs were bred. Border Collies were originally bred for herding sheep, a job that requires rapid changes in movement and speed. In contrast, Labrador Retrievers were bred for hunting, a job that requires them to run straight to retrieve game and return directly to the hunter. However, regardless of possible functional reasons for quantitative differences in dog gaits, both breed- and structure-related differences in quantitative gait characteristics should be established and accounted for when assessing the gaits of different breeds.

References

Agostinho, F. S., Rahal, S. C., Miqueleto, N. S. M. L., Verdugo, M. R., Inamassu, L. R., & EL-warrak, A. O. 2011. Kinematic analysis of Labrador retrievers and Rottweilers trotting on a treadmill. *Vet Comp Orthop Traumatol*, 24, 185–191.

Bertram, J. E. A., Lee, D. V., Case, H. N., & Todhunter, R. J. 2000. Comparison of the trotting gaits of Labrador Retrievers and Greyhounds. *Am J Vet Res*, 61, 832–838.

Besancon, M. F., Conzemius, M. G., Evans, R. B., & Ritter, M. J. 2004. Distribution of vertical forces in the pads of Greyhounds and Labrador Retrievers during walking. *Am J Vet Res*, 65, 1497–1501.

Brown, C. M. 1986. *Dog Locomotion and Gait Analysis*. Wheat Ridge, CO: Hoflin Publishing.

Brown, D. C., Michel, K. E., Love, M., & Dow, C. 2010. Evaluation of the effect of signalment and body conformation on activity monitoring in companion dogs. *Am J Vet Res*, 71, 322–325.

Bruno, E. A., Guthrie, J. W., Ellwood, S. A., Mellanby, R. J., & Clements, D. N. 2015. Global positioning derived performance measures are responsive indicators of physical activity, disease, and the success of clinical treatments in domestic dogs. *PLoS ONE*, 10(2), e0117094.

Carr, B. J. & Zink, M. C. 2016. The effects of five commercially available harnesses on canine gait. *American College of Veterinary Surgeons 2016 Surgical Summit*, Seattle, Washington.

Carr, B. J., Canapp, S. O., & Zink, M. C. 2015. Quantitative comparison of the walk and trot of border collies and Labrador retrievers, breeds with different performance requirements. *PloS ONE*, 10(12), e0145396.

Carr, B. J., Canapp, S. O., Meilleur, S., Christopher, S. A., Collins, J., & Cox, C. 2016. The use of canine stifle orthotics for cranial cruciate ligament insufficiency. *Vet Ev*, 1(1).

Clark, K., Caraguel, C., Leahey, L., & Beraud, R. 2014. Evaluation of a novel accelerometer for kinetic gait analysis in dogs. *Canadian Vet J*, 78, 226–232.

Colborne, G. R., Innes, J. F., Comerford, E. J., Owen, M. R. & Fuller, C. J. 2005. Distribution of power across the hindlimbs in Labrador Retrievers and Greyhounds. *Am J Vet Res*, 66, 1563–1571.

Colborne, G. R., Good, L., Cozens, L. E., & Kirk, L. S. 2011. Symmetry of hind limb mechanics in orthopedically normal trotting Labrador Retrievers. *Am J Vet Res*, 72, 336–344.

Elliott, R. P. 2009. *Dogsteps: A New Look*, 3rd edn. Irvine, CA: Fancy Publishing.

Evans, R., Horseman, C., & Conzemius, M. 2005. Accuracy and optimization of force platform gait analysis in Labradors with cranial cruciate disease evaluated at a walking gait. *Vet Surg*, 34, 445–449.

Fu, Y.-C., Torres, B. T., & Budsberg, S. C. 2010. Evaluation of a three-dimensional kinematic model for canine gait analysis. *Am J Vet Res*, 71, 1118–1122.

Gillette, R. L. & Angle, T. C. 2008. Recent developments in canine locomotor analysis: a review. *Vet J*, 178, 165–176.

Gillette, R. L. & Zebas, C. J. 1999. A two-dimensional analysis of limb symmetry in the trot of Labrador Retrievers. *J Am Vet Med Assoc*, 35, 515–520.

Gordon-evans, W. J. 2012. Gait analysis. In: Tobias, K. M. & Johnston, S. A. (eds), *Veterinary Surgery: Small Animal*. St Louis: Elsevier, pp. 1190–1196.

Gordon-evans, W. J., Evans, R. B., & Conzemius, M. G. 2009. Accuracy of spatiotemporal variables in gait analysis of neurologic dogs. *J Neurotrauma*, 26, 1055–1060.

Guo, Z., Wang, G., Ding, H., & Ding, H. 2005. Algorithm for recognizing marker in human motion detection. *J Biomed Eng*, 22, 312–315.

Hansen, B. D., Lascelles, B. D., Keene, B.W., Adams, A. K., & Thomson, A. E. 2007. Evaluation of an accelerometer for at-home monitor of spontaneous activity in dogs. *Am J Vet Res*, 68(5), 468–475.

Kano, W. T., Rahal, S. C., Agostinho, F. S., Mesquita, L. R., & Santos, R. R. 2016. Kinetic and temporospatial gait parameters in a heterogenous group of dogs. *BMC Vet Res*, 12, 2.

Keebaugh, A. E., Redman-bentley, D., & Griffon, D. J. 2015. Influence of leash side and handlers on pressure mat analysis of gait characteristics in small-breed dogs. *J Vet Med*, 246, 1215–1221.

Lascelles, B. D., Roe, S. C., Smith, E., Reynolds, L., Markham, J., Marcellin-little, D., *et al.* 2006. Evaluation of a pressure walkway system for measurement of vertical limb forces in clinically normal dogs. *Am J Vet Res*, 67, 277–282.

Lee, J. Y., Kim, G., Kim, J.-H., & Choi, S. H. 2007. Kinematic gait analysis of the hind limb after tibial plateau levelling osteotomy and cranial tibial wedge osteotomy in ten dogs. *J Vet Med*, 54, 579–584.

Light, V. A., Steiss, J., Montgomery, R. D., Rumph, P.F., & Wright, J. C. 2010. Temporal-spatial gait analysis by use of a portable walkway system in healthy Labrador Retrievers at a walk. *Am J Vet Res*, 71, 997–1002.

Lyon, M. 1968. *The Dog in Action*. New York: Howell Book House, Inc.

Maes, L. D., Herbin, M., Hackert, R., Bels, V. L., & Abourachid, A. 2008. Steady locomotion in dogs: temporal and associated spatial coordination patterns and the effect of speed. *J Exp Biol*, 211, 138–149.

Michel, K. E. & Brown, D. C. 2011. Determination and application of cut points for accelerometer-based activity counts of activities with differing intensity in pet dogs. *Am J Vet Res*, 72(7), 866–870.

Molsa, S. H., Hielm-bjorkman, A. K., & Laitinen-vapaavuoir, O. M. 2010. Force platform analysis in clinically healthy Rottweilers: comparison with Labrador Retrievers. *Vet Surg*, 39, 701–707.

Morrison, R., Reilly, J. J., Penpraze, V., Pendlebury, E., & Yam, P. S. 2014. A 6-month observational study of changes in objectively measured physical activity during weight loss in dogs. *J Small Anim Pract*, 55, 566–570.

Nunamaker, D. M. & Blauner, P. D. 1985. Normal and abnormal gait. In: Newton, C. D. & Nunamaker, D. M. (eds), *Textbook of Small Animal Orthopaedics*. Philadelphia: JB Lippincott, pp. 1084–1085.

Off, W. & Matis, U. 2010. Excision arthroplasty of the hip joint in dogs and cats. Clinical, radiographic, and gait analysis findings from the Department of Surgery, Veterinary Faculty of the Ludwig-Maximilians-University of Munich, Germany, 1997. *Vet Comp Orthop Traumatol*, 23, 297–305.

Preston, T., Baltzer, W. & Trost, S. 2012. Accelerometer validity and placement for detection of changes in physical activity in dogs under controlled conditions on a treadmill. *Res Vet Sci*, 93(1), 412–416.

Ritter, D. A., Nassar, P. N., Fife, M., & Carrier, D. R. 2001. Epaxial muscle function in trotting dogs. *J Exp Biol*, 204, 3053–3064.

Rumph, P. F., Steiss, J., & Montgomery, R. D. 1997. Effects of selection and habituation on vertical ground reaction force in greyhounds. *Am J Vet Res*, 59, 375–378.

Sha, D. H., Mullineaux, D. R., & Clayton, H. M. 2004. Three-dimensional analysis of patterns of skin displacement over the equine radius. *Equine Vet J*, 36, 665–670.

van Weeren, P. R., Sloet Van Oldruitenborgh-oosterbaan, M. M., & Clayton, H. M. 1992. Correction models for skin displacement in equine kinematic gait analysis. *J Equine Sci*, 12, 178–192.

Vitger, A. D., Stallknecht, B. M., Nielsen, D. H., & Bjornvad, C. R. 2016. Integration of a physical training program in weight loss plan for overweight pet dogs. *J Am Vet Med Assoc*, 248, 174–182.

Volstad, N., Nemke, B., & Muir, P. 2016. Variance associated with the use of relative velocity for force platform gait analysis in a heterogenous population of clinically normal dogs. *Vet J*, 207, 80–84.

Voss, K., Imhol, J., Kaestner, S., & Montavon, P. M. 2007. Force plate gait analysis at the walk and trot in dogs with low-grade hindlimb lameness. *Vet Comp Orthop Traumatol*, 20, 299–304.

Voss, K., Galeandro, L., Wiestner, T., Haessig, M., & Montavon, P. M. 2010. Relationships of body weight, body size, subject velocity, and vertical ground reaction forces in trotting dogs. *Vet Surg*, 39, 863–869.

Webster, K. E., Wittwer, J. E., & Feller, J. A. 2005. Validity of the GAITRite walkway system for the measurement of averaged and individual step parameters of gait. *Gait Posture*, 22, 317–321.

Wrigglesworth, D. J., Mort, E. S., Upton, S. L. & Miller, A. T. 2011. Accuracy of the use of triaxial accelerometry for measuring daily activity as a predictor of daily maintenance energy requirement in healthy adult Labrador Retrievers. *Am J Vet Res*, 72(9), 1151–1155.

Yam, P. S., Penpraze, V., Young, D., Todd, M. S., Cloney, A. D., Houston-callaghan, K. A., & Reilly, J. J. 2011. Validity, practical utility and reliability of Actigraph accelerometry for the measurement of habitual physical activity in dogs. *J Small Anim Pract*, 52, 86–92.

Zehr, E. P. 2006. Training-induced adaptive plasticity in human somatosensory reflex pathways. *J Appl Physiol*, 101, 1783–1794.

Zink, M. C. 2008. *The Agility Advantage: Health and Fitness for the Canine Athlete*. South Hadley, MA: CleanRun Productions.

3 Musculoskeletal Structure and Physiology

Stuart Bliss, DVM, PhD, DACVS, CCRP

Summary

The musculoskeletal system consists of a diverse set of specialized tissues that define overall body shape, and provide for coordinated movement. Structural integrity, health, and appropriate functional conditioning of the musculoskeletal system are essential for athletic performance. The response of musculoskeletal tissues to injury and disease, disuse, or conditioning forms the basis upon which all athletic training and physical rehabilitation programs are based. Effective sports medicine and rehabilitation practice depends on an understanding of musculoskeletal tissue structure, physiological adaptations to exercise, and maladaptive responses to injury and disease. This chapter provides an overview of key concepts in musculoskeletal tissue structure and physiology as they pertain to athletic performance and recovery from injury. The molecular and histologic structure, development, and functional properties of bone, cartilage, synovium, tendon and ligament, and skeletal muscle are reviewed. Basic mechanisms underlying injury and loss of function of musculoskeletal tissues as well as healing responses are outlined. Emphasis is placed on structure–function relationships and physiological concepts that are relevant to the performance and rehabilitation of the canine athlete.

Basic organization of musculoskeletal connective tissues

With the exception of skeletal muscle, the tissues that make up the musculoskeletal system are generally classified as dense connective tissues. Connective tissues are composed of tissue-specific mesenchymal cells distributed throughout a specialized extracellular matrix (ECM).

Dense connective tissues consist predominantly of ECM and contain relatively few cells. The ECM contains an array of structural fibers made up of cross-linked fibrillar proteins, along with a hydrated gelatinous interfibrillar matrix containing a variety of nonfibrillar proteins, proteoglycans, glycoproteins, proteolipids, and polysaccharides. The composition and molecular organization of the ECM define the

Canine Sports Medicine and Rehabilitation, Second Edition. Edited by Chris Zink and Janet B. Van Dyke.
© 2018 John Wiley & Sons, Inc. Published 2018 by John Wiley & Sons, Inc.

mechanical properties and functionality of a given tissue. These properties vary greatly amongst tissues, reflecting the diverse functional roles to which different structures are adapted.

Cellular components of musculoskeletal tissues

Musculoskeletal tissues contain a variety of cell types. The tissue-specific cells within musculoskeletal structures are named in accordance with the tissues they inhabit (tenocytes within tendon, chondrocytes within cartilage, etc.). The majority of these are fully differentiated cells that are responsible for the synthesis and lifelong turnover of the ECM that surrounds them. All connective tissues also contain small numbers of progenitor cells that represent variable stages of lineage commitment from multipotent mesenchymal stem cells to tissue-specific blast forms (osteoblasts, tenoblasts, etc.). Progenitor cells play important roles in repair, regeneration, and adaptive remodeling of connective tissues.

With the exception of articular chondrocytes, musculoskeletal tissue cells are highly interconnected through adherens and gap junctions (Chi et al., 2005; Civitelli, 2008). These interconnections are established during development and allow close intercellular communication. The broad connectivity of the cellular network enhances the ability of tissues to mount regional responses to specific biological or mechanical stimuli (Ko & McCulloch, 2001; Wall & Banes, 2005). Connective tissue cells are also highly responsive to mechanical stimuli. Mechanotransduction is the process by which cells mount biological responses to mechanical stimuli (Ramage et al., 2009). The mechanical stresses imposed upon musculoskeletal tissues are borne primarily by the ECM. The resulting strains within the ECM may trigger cellular responses through a variety of mechanisms, including direct deformation of the plasma membrane and alteration of transmembrane ion conductance, deflection of the primary cilium, activation of cell-surface receptors by extracellular fluid shears, or ligand-independent activation of signaling receptors (Silver & Siperko, 2003; Bonewald, 2006). The response of a tissue to a mechanical

stimulus may be either physiological or pathological, depending on the state of the tissue and the nature of the stimulus. Physiological responses result in appropriate adaptive changes of the ECM that enhance a tissue's ability to meet the demands placed upon it. An example of adaptive remodeling is the hypertrophy and mitochondrial biogenesis that occurs within skeletal muscle in response to athletic conditioning.

Molecular components of extracellular matrix

Collagen

Collagen is the most abundant protein in the body, and is a ubiquitous component of all connective tissues. All collagens are triple helical proteins made up of three individual polypeptides called alpha chains. Homotypic collagens are composed of three identical alpha chains. Heterotypic collagens are composed of various combinations of alpha chains that differ in amino acid sequence. In mammals, there are 34 known alpha chain genes and at least 28 distinct collagen types. Use of alternative transcription start sites as well as alternative splicing of individual alpha chain transcripts results in a wide variety of collagen configurations with diverse structures and unique mechanical properties (Hulmes, 2002).

Collagens may be divided into several major groups: The fibrillar collagens are of primary importance in the musculoskeletal system as they are the major structural components of connective tissues such as tendon, ligament, cartilage, and bone. The major fibrillar collagens are types I, II, and III. Type I collagen forms linear and extensively crosslinked macromolecular structures that impart high tensile strength to tendons and ligaments. It is also the most abundant collagen type in bone. Type II collagen is the predominant collagen in hyaline cartilage. Within articular cartilage, type II collagen fibrils are crosslinked into extensive three-dimensional networks that provide resistance to deformation in a multitude of directions. Other collagen groups include the fibril-associated collagens with interrupted triple helices (FACIT collagens, types IX, XII,

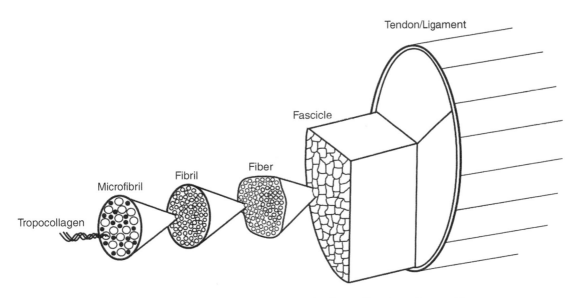

Figure 3.1   Schematic depiction of the hierarchical structuring of collagen fibers in tendons and ligaments.

XIV, XVI, XIX, XX, XXI, and XXII), filamentous collagens (type VI), short-chain collagens (types VIII and X), and basement membrane collagens (types IV, VII, XV, and XVIII). Nonfibrillar collagens do not assemble into discrete fibrils; however, many associate with fibrillar collagens and regulate fibril assembly, fibril diameter, and interfibrillar interactions (FACIT collagens) (Kadler *et al.*, 1996; Zhang *et al.*, 2005). Others contribute to the unique mechanical properties of specific tissues (filamentous and basement membrane collagens).

Biosynthesis of collagen involves transcription and translation of the alpha chain gene, and production of a pre-pro-collagen peptide. During translation, specific proline and lysine residues within this molecule are hydroxylated by ascorbic acid- and iron-dependent prolyl- and lysyl-hydroxylases. Hydroxylated pre-pro-alpha chains undergo intracellular self-assembly into triple helical procollagen. The globular amino- and carboxy-termini of the procollagen molecules are subsequently cleaved by various metalloproteinases resulting in the formation of tropocollagen. Tropocollagen molecules are secreted from the cell where they assemble into a variety of higher order structures according to specific tissue requirements. Extracellular tropocollagen molecules are further stabilized by intermolecular crosslinks as well as noncovalent association with other ECM components.

Within the ECM, fibrillar tropocollagen molecules further assemble in a staggered fashion into nascent fibrils. These fibrils are stabilized by intermolecular crosslinks catalyzed by lysyl-oxidase enzymes. Numerous nonfibrillar collagens, other proteins, proteoglycans, and proteolipids associate closely with the surfaces of collagen fibrils and regulate interfibrillar cohesion and interactions (Chapman, 1989). Groups of fibrils are further organized in hierarchical fashion into fibers, which are themselves further bundled into fascicles (Figure 3.1). Collagen fibers are the basic macroscopic structural units of many musculoskeletal structures such as tendons and ligaments.

Elastin

Elastin is an important component of many musculoskeletal tissues, including tendons, ligaments, myofascial structures, joint capsule, and articular cartilage. Elastin provides tissues with elasticity, which refers to the ability of a tissue to undergo reversible deformation. The content of elastin within musculoskeletal tissues varies greatly depending on the requirement for elasticity. Elastin is a minor component of bone, where it occurs predominantly with the walls of blood vessels; however, it is particularly abundant within the ECM of structures that undergo repeated cycles of elongation and elastic recoil such as joint capsules or the nuchal ligament.

Elastin is a high-molecular weight insoluble protein biopolymer made up of numerous tropoelastin subunits (Mithieux & Weiss, 2005). Tropoelastin is a 65 kDa hydrophobic protein. Biosynthesis of elastin involves transcription and translation of a single tropoelastin gene. Tropoelastin is secreted from the cell as a complex with specific elastin-binding proteins. Within the extracellular environment, tropoelastin undergoes temperature-dependent conformational changes that expose hydrophobic residues within the molecule that allow its incorporation into a developing elastin macromolecule through hydrophobic interactions (Indik et al., 1989; Vrhovski & Weiss, 1998). This process is facilitated by many ECM components, most notably the glycoproteins fibrillin and fibronectin. Following assembly, elastin polymers are stabilized by covalent intermolecular crosslinks, the formation of which is catalyzed by various copper-dependent lysyl oxidases. Groups of elastin polymers are further assembled in hierarchical fashion into higher order fibers that consist of a central core of crosslinked elastin surrounded by an organized coat of microfibrillar glycoproteins rich in fibrillin.

Elastic fibers are highly extensible and can withstand up to 200% increases in length from the resting state. Elastic fibers are also extremely durable, and are capable of virtually unlimited numbers of cycles of elongation and elastic recoil without loss of strength (Keeley et al., 2002). Production of elastin (elastogenesis) is prominent during growth, as well as during the repair and remodeling phases of tissue healing. However, once formed, elastic fibers are extraordinarily stable and may persist throughout adulthood without turnover.

Proteoglycans

Proteoglycans (PGs) are glycosylated proteins that are prominent components of the extracellular matrix of all connective tissues. The basic structure of a PG consists of a core protein to which a variable number of glycosaminoglycan (GAG) side chains are covalently attached (Figure 3.2). Core proteins vary greatly in length and amino acid sequence. The GAG side chains are long, linear polysaccharide polymers composed of repeating disaccharide units. The disaccharide units are composed of two six-carbon sugars, the first of which is either a hexose or a hexuronic acid, and the second

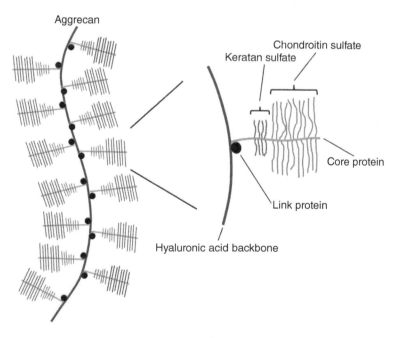

Figure 3.2 Aggrecan structure. Multiple proteoglycan monomers are bound by specific link proteins to a backbone of hyaluronic acid to form macromolecular aggregating proteoglycans.

Table 3.1 Chemical composition of major glycosaminoglycans

Glycosaminoglycan	Hexose/hexuronic acid	Hexosamine
Chondroitin sulfate	(2-sulfo-) glucuronic acid	(4/6-sulfo-) *N*-acetyl-glucosamine
Dermatan sulfate	Glucuronic acid, or (2-sulfo-) iduronic acid	(4/6-sulfo-) *N*-acetyl-glucosamine
Heparan sulfate	Glucuronic acid, or (2-sulfo-) iduronic acid	(6-sulfo-) *N*-acetyl-glucosamine, or (6-sulfo-) *N*-sulfo-glucosamine
Keratan sulfate	(6-sulfo-) galactose	(6-sulfo-) *N*-acetyl-glucosamine
Hyaluronic acid	Glucuronic acid	*N*-acetyl-glucosamine

of which is an amino sugar (hexosamine) (Table 3.1). The sugars within most GAGs are sulfated, which renders the polysaccharide chains highly negatively charged. Glycosaminoglycans are covalently linked to serine residues within a core protein. Hyaluronic acid (HA), a ubiquitous component of ECMs throughout the body, is unique within the family of GAGs since it is neither sulfated nor covalently linked to proteins.

Several classes of PGs are recognized, the most thoroughly characterized of which are the interstitial PGs. This class includes the aggregating PGs and the small leucine-rich PGs (SLRPs; Hardingham & Fosang, 1992). The aggregating proteoglycans include aggrecan, versican, brevican, and neurocan. These PG species are massive macromolecular complexes in which many individual proteoglycan molecules are assembled in a brush-like array along a backbone of hyaluronic acid (see Figure 3.2). Due to their extreme negative charge, aggregating PGs have a high affinity for water. Aggregating PGs are immobilized within a given tissue through association with collagen fibrils. Their high degree of hydration underlies the turgidity and resistance to compression of several musculoskeletal tissues such as hyaline articular cartilage, meniscal fibrocartilage, and the nucleus pulposus of the intervertebral disc.

The SLRPs are a structurally diverse group of PGs with variable degrees of GAG conjugation and that are expressed in tissue-specific patterns. SLRPs associate with fibrillar elements of the ECM such as collagen and elastin and have many functions, including modulation of the assembly and interaction of collagen and elastin fibers, modulation of ion transport through the ECM, and regulation of growth factor effects on connective tissue cells (Schaefer & Iozzo, 2008).

Proteoglycan synthesis involves transcription and translation of a core protein, GAG conjugation of the protein, and secretion of mature PG into the extracellular environment. In comparison to the fibrillar components of the ECM, PGs undergo rapid turnover. Existing PGs are degraded by a variety of proteases and polysaccharidases. In turn, PG biosynthesis is a highly regulated anabolic process that can be triggered by exposure of cells to a variety of biological mediators as well as some pharmacological agents. The ability to alter the types and concentrations of PGs within the ECM in response to specific stimuli allows resident cells to adjust many properties of the ECM in accordance with tissue demand. PG turnover thus represents an important mechanism of tissue adaptation, and targeted stimulation of PG production *in vivo* is an area of great clinical therapeutic interest.

Musculoskeletal ontogeny

Regeneration is the re-establishment of the original form and function of a tissue after injury or loss. Within the musculoskeletal system, bone and muscle are capable of regeneration, while the healing of tendon, ligament, and cartilage results in mechanically inferior tissues. Currently, there is great interest in clinical strategies, including rehabilitative programs, designed to promote or accelerate regenerative healing (Ambrosio *et al.*, 2010). Tissue regeneration often involves a close recapitulation of developmental morphogenesis; thus, an understanding of basic developmental processes is relevant to physical rehabilitation. A thorough review of musculoskeletal development is beyond the scope of this chapter; however, several key concepts are outlined as they relate to rehabilitation, especially of the canine athlete.

The mammalian musculoskeletal system derives predominantly from mesoderm. During development, mesoderm is established during gastrulation, as cells of the deep surface of the epiblast delaminate from the ectodermal portion of the primitive streak to populate the mesenchyme between the ectodermal and endodermal germ layers. During neurulation, these cells organize along the lateral aspects of the developing neural tube to form the paraxial mesoderm. Secretion of morphogens by cells of the neural tube and adjacent ectoderm triggers segmentation of the paraxial mesoderm into somites. The ventromedial aspect of the somite forms the sclerotome, from which vertebrae and ribs derive. The dorsolateral aspect of the somite forms the dermomyotome, which further organizes into superficial dermotomal and deep myotomal components. The cells of the myotome undergo myoblastic differentiation and give rise to the axial musculature. The lateral aspect of the paraxial mesoderm develops into the lateral plate mesoderm, which divides into superficial somatic and deep splanchnic layers (Figure 3.3). The limbs originate as focal thickenings of the somatic lateral plate mesoderm (limb buds). The early limb bud is populated by myoblastic cells that migrate into the lateral plate mesoderm from the somitic myotomes, and that ultimately give rise to the appendicular musculature. Outgrowths of cells of the neural tube enter the limb bud in conjunction with myoblasts to innervate developing limb structures. Outward growth and patterning of the limb is guided by gradients of signaling molecules produced by the surrounding ectoderm.

Myoblastic differentiation within the myotome is the earliest musculoskeletal fate specification to occur during development. Muscle development is triggered by the activation of a myogenic transcriptional program that culminates in the expression of a core set of myogenic factors including myogenic factor 5 (MYF5), muscle-specific regulatory factor-4 (MRF-4), myoblast determination protein (MYOD), and myogenin (Pownall *et al.*, 2002). The timing and sequence of expression of these myogenic factors varies with anatomic site during development. Contractile myofibers first appear in the limbs at approximately mid-gestation, prior to limb innervation. These

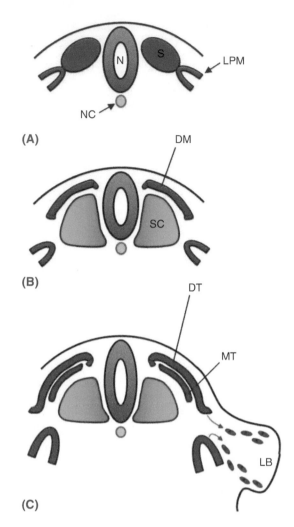

Figure 3.3   Schematic cross-sectional depiction of embryological origins of musculoskeletal structure. **(A)** Segmentation of paraxial mesoderm adjacent to the neural tube (N) and notochord (NC) leads to the formation of somites (S) and lateral plate mesoderm (LPM). **(B)** Each somite segregates into a ventromedial sclerotome (SC) and a dorsolateral dermomyotome (DM). **(C)** The dermomyotome separates into a dorsolateral dermatome (DT, red) and a ventromedial myotome (MT, blue). Appendicular musculoskeletal structures derive from mesodermal precursors that migrate into the limb bud (LB) from the ventrolateral dermomyotome and lateral plate mesoderm (arrows). Axial musculoskeletal structures derive from the sclerotome.

primary fibers persist as type I (slow-twitch, or oxidative) fibers in the adult. Secondary myofibers develop later concomitant with the establishment of limb innervation and become type II (fast-twitch, or glycolytic) fibers.

Muscle contractility is robust throughout the latter half of gestation, and the mechanical forces produced by developing muscle are essential to the appropriate development of all other musculoskeletal structures.

With the exception of the craniofacial skeleton, which is largely of neural crest origin, bones originate as condensations of mesenchymal cells that initially differentiate into chondrocytes to form a cartilaginous model of the developing skeleton. As the chondrocytes undergo interstitial growth, hypoxia develops within the central region of the avascular cartilaginous precursor. This triggers hypertrophy of chondrocytes, and stimulates production of angiogenic growth factors and vascular invasion of the cartilage model. Vascularization marks the onset of endochondral ossification as the cartilage model becomes populated with osteoprogenitors and as chondroid matrix is resorbed and replaced with osteoid. Endochondral ossification continues throughout postnatal growth, primarily within the physes of the long bones. This process of developmental endochondral ossification is recapitulated with remarkable fidelity during indirect fracture healing (see later).

The initial mesenchymal condensation that precedes appendicular bone formation is initially continuous along the length of the elongating limb bud. As chondrogenic differentiation occurs, this mesenchymal column undergoes a process of segmentation marked by the appearance of discrete interzones that mark the sites of future diarthrodial joints. Apoptosis of cells within the interzone leads to the formation of a fluid-filled joint space, a process termed cavitation (Khan et al., 2007). Wnt14 is a key morphogen expressed at these interzones (Archer et al., 2003). Separation of the articular surfaces and development of a fully mobile synovial joint requires continuous mobilization of the nascent joint by contraction of associated developing musculature, as well as distention of the joint cavity with hyaluronic acid. The hyaluronic acid within the interzone is initially secreted by cells of the articular surfaces and later by the developing synovium. Mechanical strain of joint tissues stimulates production of hyaluronic acid through upregulation of some isoforms of hyaluronic acid synthase, an effect that persists through adulthood (Itano & Kimata, 2002; Momberger et al., 2005).

Tendon and ligament primordia arise as condensations of mesenchymal cells that initially reside immediately subjacent to the basal lamina of the developing dermis (Benjamin & Ralphs, 1995). These cells initially organize into parallel longitudinal rows and subsequently become separated as they elaborate collagen-rich ECM. During differentiation, they develop long cytoplasmic processes by which cell-to-cell contact is maintained despite deposition of large quantities of intercellular ECM. The bony prominences that form attachment sites for tendons and ligaments are defined during formation of the cartilaginous anlage of a bone; however, full maturation of both the bony tuberosities at which tendons and ligaments insert, as well as their enthesial architecture, is dependent upon traction forces exerted on these sites by developing muscles. In the proximal portion of the limbs, connections with bone are established during the early stages of tendon differentiation. In contrast, distal tendons initially lack connection with bone but establish insertions later in development through fusion with enthesial outgrowths of a target bone.

During development, all musculoskeletal tissues are populated with small but significant numbers of undifferentiated progenitor cells, or mesenchymal stem cells (Figure 3.4). These cells include osteoblasts of bone, satellite cells of skeletal muscle, and stem cells of tendon, ligament, and cartilage. Mesenchymal stem cells are multipotent, capable of undergoing osteogenic, chondrogenic, adipogenic, or neurogenic differentiation in response to appropriate signals. They also are capable of self-renewal through asymmetric cell division. They are activated by injury or conditioning stimuli, and play important roles in the healing and functional adaptation of tissues (Wu et al., 2007; Fan et al., 2009; Tapp et al., 2009; Lim et al., 2010; Reich et al., 2012). Stem cell therapy involving harvest and orthotopic implantation of autologous mesenchymal stem cells is an area of active orthopedic research and has become an accepted treatment for progressive osteoarthrosis in the dog (Black et al., 2007, 2008; Guercio et al., 2012) (see Chapter 16).

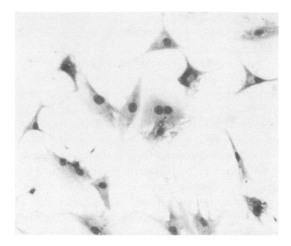

Figure 3.4 Canine bone marrow-derived mesenchymal stem cells in primary culture show characteristic mesenchymal morphology. These cells area capable of chondrogenic, osteogenic, adipogenic, or neurogenic differentiation in response to specific signals.

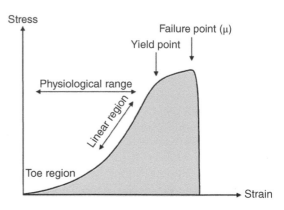

Figure 3.5 Idealized stress–strain curve highlighting key mechanical parameters of musculoskeletal tissues. The slope of the linear region describes the stiffness (modulus) of the material. The area under the curve (shaded region) represents the total energy introduced into the material to cause mechanical failure.

Structure–function relationships of musculoskeletal tissues

Basic concepts

The tissues of the musculoskeletal system are highly responsive to mechanical strains. From a biomechanical perspective, physiologic adaptation refers to the process by which musculoskeletal tissues adjust their biochemical composition, molecular architecture, and mechanical properties in accordance with the demands placed upon them. Both athletic training and rehabilitative therapy involve the application of controlled forces to the musculoskeletal system to facilitate physiologic adaptations that are specifically suited to a given athletic or therapeutic objective. Here we introduce several basic concepts related to the mechanical properties and functional adaptations of musculoskeletal tissues.

The body is subject to two basic categories of force. Intrinsic forces originate from within the body due to muscular contractions or the inherent elasticity of connective tissues such as ligaments or myofasciae. Extrinsic forces arise from outside the body and include ground reaction forces due to gravity as well as forces imposed on the body through contact with other objects.

When subjected to force, objects deform. This relationship can be represented graphically as a force-deformation curve, which describes the structural properties of a given object. When normalized to the cross-sectional area of an object, the applied force and resulting deformation are referred to as stress and strain, respectively. Stress–strain relationships thus describe the mechanical properties of a particular material. An idealized stress–strain curve pertaining to musculoskeletal tissues is illustrated in (Figure 3.5). The initial nonlinear portion of the curve is the toe region and represents an early phase of deformation that occurs as stress is first applied to the material. In connective tissues, the toe region typically reflects the straightening of crimped collagen fibrils, or the elongation of elastin fibers. The linear portion of the curve represents a zone of elastic deformation, where the material will return to its original state upon removal of the applied stress. The slope of this region of the curve is called the modulus, and describes the stiffness of the material. The yield point represents the transition from elastic to plastic deformation; beyond the yield point, structural alterations within the material prevent it from returning to its original state despite removal of the applied stress. The failure point represents complete loss of structural integrity and macroscopic breakdown of the material such as would occur with bone fracture or tendon rupture. The area under the curve represents the total amount of energy introduced into the material to cause failure. The maximum strength of the material is indicated by *mu*, the level of applied stress at the point of failure.

Musculoskeletal tissues are anisotropic and viscoelastic. Mechanical properties of aniso-tropic materials vary depending upon the direction of applied stress. For example, tendons are capable of resisting high tensile loads, but deform readily when subjected to compressive stress. Mechanical properties of viscoelastic materials vary depending upon the rate at which stress is applied. Viscoelasticity is a melding of the basic properties of viscosity and elasticity. Viscosity is a property of fluids that reflects the resistance of molecules to strain (flow) in response to a given force. Highly viscous fluids are resistant to flow, but will flow linearly and irreversibly over time in response to a constant force. Elasticity is a property of solids that deform instantly in response to an applied stress but that return to their original state following removal of the stress. Viscoelastic materials demonstrate elastic deformation in response to rapid loading but undergo perma-nent change of shape in response to sustained stress. The progressive strain that occurs in viscoelastic materials in response to a constant stress is called creep. Stress relaxation is a related property that refers to the gradual dis-sipation of internal stress that occurs in response to a constant strain.

The viscoelasticity of musculoskeletal tissues derives from their composite structure: within the ECM, collagen and elastin fibrils form the solid component and impart tensile resistance and elasticity, while the hydrated proteoglycan-rich extrafibrillar matrix behaves as a viscous fluid that allows gradual interfibrillar shear and permanent strain in response to sustained stress (Elliott *et al.*, 2003). Under normal condi-tions, the responses of musculoskeletal tissues to physiological stresses are primarily elastic. Strains experienced by the ECM are neverthe-less sensed by resident cell populations and trigger constitutive ECM remodeling activity by which the structural integrity of a given tis-sue is maintained (Kjaer, 2004). In tissues such as muscle, tendon, and ligament, sustained or high-intensity activity, such as occurs during athletic training or performance, may cause greater degrees of plastic deformation of the ECM. This type of strain represents a form of ECM microinjury (Kjaer, 2004; Mackey *et al.*, 2008). Mild inflammatory responses may occur in vascularized tissues in response to stress-induced plastic deformations of the ECM. Inflammatory mediators may in turn trigger anabolic cellular responses that result in adaptive changes in ECM composition and a net gain in tissue strength (Vierck *et al.*, 2000). This type of cellular response underlies the physiological adaptation of musculos-keletal tissues and is the basis for athletic conditioning.

Skeletal muscle

Organization and motor activity

Collectively, the skeletal musculature is the largest organ in the body. Skeletal muscle is a complex and highly organized tissue composed of repeating units called sarcomeres. Individual muscles are organized into beds containing numerous fascicles surrounded by perimysium, and each fascicle is composed of multinucleated myofibers enclosed by an endomysium (Figure 3.6). The epimysium is the collagen-rich sheath that surrounds a whole muscle; epimysium is continuous with the dense aponeurotic fascial sheets that enclose some muscle groups. The perimysium is the primary component of the ECM through which the force of contraction is transferred from a muscle to its associated tendon.

Single myofibers act in concert through the sliding filament model of actin and myosin within organized sarcomeres (Figure 3.7). Within the sarcomere, structural proteins anchor actin, troponins and tropomyosin to the Z-line that contains actinin. Multimeric myosin proteins are suspended as intercalating filamentous strands with globular head units that function as ratchets along adjacent actin filaments. Binding of acetylcholine to receptors on the surface of the myofiber sets off a cascade of intracellular signaling events resulting in calcium release from the sarcoplasmic reticulum. Intracellular free calcium interacts with troponin C, which is bound to the actin, troponin complex (I, C, and T), and tropomyosin

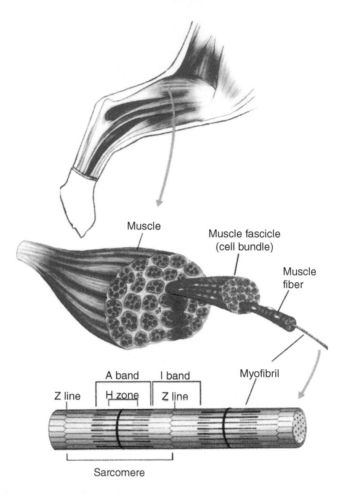

Figure 3.6   Hierarchical organization of skeletal muscle. Source: Used with permission from Hand *et al.*, 2010.

(Figure 3.8). This interaction drives a conformational change in the tropomyosin allowing exposure of a groove that allows myosin heads to interact with the actin filament. This interaction causes the adenosine triphosphate (ATP) bound to the myosin head interacting with the actin to undergo hydrolysis (Moczydlowski & Apkon, 2009). The ADP is then released from the myosin head allowing a conformational shift in the myosin head from an open to a closed position leading to a shortening of the myofiber. Muscle contraction is dependent upon ATP hydrolysis, and generation of ATP is a key rate-limiting step in muscle contractility. This is discussed in more detail in Chapter 4.

Skeletal muscle performance is dependent on fiber type. The traditional classification system is type I (oxidative) and type II (glycolytic). This classification is based on mitochondrial enzymatic machinery and ATPase staining in acidic and alkaline conditions. ATPase staining is commonly used to differentiate these fiber types in histologic sections and is based on myosin isoform ATPase activity as being either slow (oxidative—type I) or fast (glycolytic—type II) (Armstrong *et al.*, 1982). Postural muscles like the quadriceps femoris contain highly oxidative type I fibers that generate slow and sustained contraction. In contrast, muscles adapted to rapid and forceful contractions such as the gracilis contain higher proportions of type II fibers. Several forms of type II fibers have been described, which reflect amino acid sequence differences in sarcomeric myosin ATPase. The type IIC isoform is commonly expressed in canine muscle and represents a capacity for oxidative metabolism that is intermediate between type I and type IIB fibers.

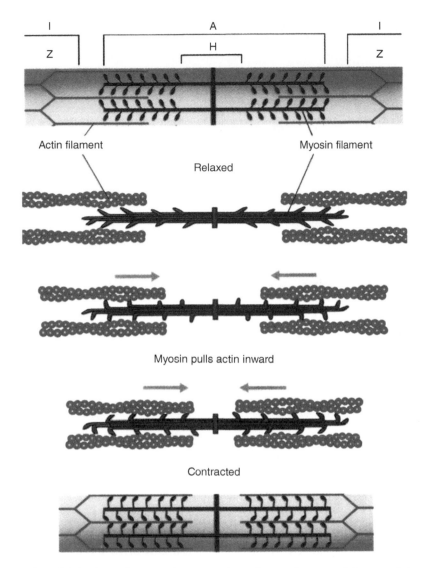

Figure 3.7   Contraction of skeletal muscle occurs due to ATP-dependent conformational changes of the globular heads of myosin proteins that cause myosin to slide along adjacent actin filaments. Source: Used with permission from Hand *et al.*, 2010.

However, this fiber type difference is of low functional significance as the metabolic capability of the differing type II fibers is not dramatically different. In general, canine skeletal muscle has high mitochondrial density and oxidative capacity and is adapted to endurance activities (Wakshlag *et al.*, 2004).

Overall muscling and fiber type differences have been observed between breeds of dogs; these are exemplified by the observed differences between Greyhounds and other breeds. The Greyhound has approximately 15%

more muscle mass, and higher overall muscle-to-bone ratios than other breeds (Gunn, 1978b). Greyhounds also have unique fiber type distributions, with approximately 75–100% type II fibers in the semitendinosus while other breeds typically have fewer than 50% type II fibers (Gunn, 1978a). These differences explain why Greyhounds are sprinters unlike the majority of other breeds. Little work has been performed across breeds to examine the energetics of muscle and how training affects performance.

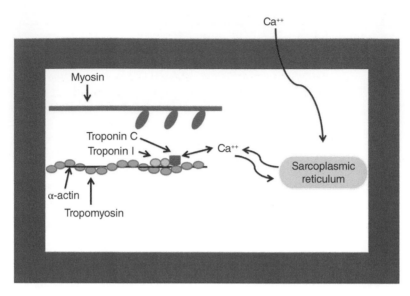

Figure 3.8   Calcium released from the sarcoplasmic reticulum binds to troponin C, triggering myosin–actin interaction through conformational changes in tropomyosin. Source: Used with permission from Hand *et al.*, 2010.

Hypertrophy and sarcopenia

Muscle mass is governed by a complex combination of mediators including insulin, insulin-like growth factors, androgens, myostatin, cytokine/myokines, and plasma amino acids (Solomon & Bouloux, 2006; Spangenburg, 2009). From a veterinary perspective, muscle hypertrophy has been a desired phenotype in agriculture and performance arenas. Selective breeding has perpetuated a genetic mutation in the myostatin gene that is associated with constitutive muscle hypertrophy. Myostatin is a negative regulator of myofiber differentiation, satellite cell maturation and muscle biosynthetic activity, and its inactivation leads to hypertrophy (Bradley *et al.*, 2008). Heterozygotes for the myostatin loss-of-function mutation have shown improved racing performance, which has led to perpetuation of this trait within the Whippet population (Mosher *et al.*, 2007).

Androgens and other anabolic mediators such as growth hormone play a role in the control of muscle mass; however, the effects of these compounds on musculoskeletal homeostasis are highly species-specific. Normal physiological concentrations of canine gonadal steroids may augment the stimulatory effects of exercise on skeletal myofiber synthesis; however, their impact on the development and maintenance of overall muscle mass is less pronounced than in other species (West & Phillips, 2010). Although banned within organized canine athletics, exogenous anabolic steroids and growth hormone can induce supraphysiological muscle hypertrophy. In combination with appropriate conditioning, this may confer some performance advantage to canine athletes involved in resistance events such as weight pulling or sprinting. However, augmentation of muscle mass is unlikely to be beneficial in canine endurance activities.

Sarcopenia refers to the progressive decrease in muscle mass and strength that occurs with aging. Sarcopenia reflects loss of myofibers due to apoptosis, as well as decreases in myofiber size. Overall muscle circumference is often maintained during early sarcopenia, as lost myofibers are replaced with adipose and fibrous tissue (Freeman, 2012). Declining performance may be the only early clinical indicator of this condition. Muscle loss becomes measurable as sarcopenia progresses and is common in the geriatric population. Until recently, this phenomenon had not been documented in dogs, but recent biochemical assessment of aging canine muscle has confirmed that the upregulation of autophagy is occurring in elderly dogs leading to myofiber loss (Pagano *et al.*, 2015). Concentric, but not eccentric, exercise can retard sarcopenia. Concentric activity includes weight training and isometrics. Aquatic therapy, limb weighting, and balance board exercises emphasize concentric activity and might be useful components of rehabilitation and fitness programs for elderly sarcopenic animals.

Cytokines and skeletal muscle

Skeletal muscle is highly responsive to a wide variety of cytokines, chemokines and growth factors, and the prevailing milieu of biological mediators controls many aspects of muscle growth, repair, and adaptation. Infiltrating leukocytes, particularly macrophages, are an important source of many cytokines that influence muscle homeostasis. Myofibers produce a variety of cytokines, termed myokines, that exert local autocrine and paracrine effects (Pedersen *et al.*, 2007). The effects of cytokines upon skeletal muscle homeostasis are mediated by complex and highly integrated intracellular signaling, transcriptional, and translational processes within the myofiber. These dynamic signaling systems are further influenced by a wide range of mechanical stimuli, pharmacological agents, and diet (Sakamoto & Goodyear, 2002; Tisdale, 2007).

Exercise leads to enhanced skeletal muscle myofibril deposition and hypertrophy (Miyazaki & Esser, 2009; Gundersen, 2011). This involves mechanoreceptor stimulation, but also relies on increased insulin-like growth factor 1 (IGF-1) expression, decreased myostatin synthesis, and enhanced satellite cell differentiation. Exercise increases insulin-independent glucose transport and insulin sensitivity, which in turn leads to myofibril protein synthesis (Spangenburg, 2009). Exercise also stimulates the production of myokines. The myokine interleukin 15 (IL-15) has received considerable attention due to its ability to abrogate myofibril proteolysis, maintaining the myofiber in a hypertrophic state (Argiles *et al.*, 2009). IL-15 also enhances skeletal muscle energetics through stimulation of lipolysis in both muscle and adipose tissue. The anabolic effects of IL-15 on muscle and adipose tissue metabolism suggest the activity of this cytokine may open an interesting pharmacological avenue for improving lean body mass (LBM), especially in age-related sarcopenia.

Interleukin 6 (IL-6) appears to play an interesting role in exercise as it is directly made by skeletal muscle during exercise. There appear to be strong correlations between plasma and muscle IL-6 concentrations and glycogen depletion during prolonged exercise (Nieman *et al.*, 2015). This increase in IL-6 is currently thought to be a systemic signal that allows for hepatic upregulation of glucose synthesis as part of a complex milieu of events that lead to cross-talk between skeletal muscle and hepatic tissues to ensure homeostasis during exercise (Knudsen *et al.*, 2016).

Cytokines play a key role in the repair and regeneration of muscle after injury. Following acute traumatic injury such as strain or laceration, skeletal muscle has a strong capacity for regeneration; however, this is dependent upon the nature and duration of the post-traumatic inflammatory response as well as the mechanical strains present at the site. The inflammatory response that occurs following muscle injury is biphasic (Tidball & Villalta, 2010). The initial phase is an innate immune response characterized by infiltration of damaged muscle by neutrophils and proinflammatory M1 macrophages that elaborate Th1 cytokines such as tumor necrosis factor α (TNFα) and interferon γ (IFNγ). Production of oxidants by leukocytes during this phase leads to additional secondary muscle injury. During the early inflammatory phase, local satellite cells become activated and begin to proliferate. Approximately 24 hours post-injury, M1 macrophages begin gradually to be replaced by a second population of counter-inflammatory M2 macrophages, which downregulate the acute inflammatory process through production of cytokines such as IL-4, IL-10, and IL-13. Many mitogenic and differentiating signals are produced during this later phase including hepatocyte growth factor, insulin-like growth factor-1 (IGF-1), fibroblast growth factors and vascular endothelial growth factor. These signals can stimulate the expression of myogenic transcription factors within proliferating satellite cells, marking the onset of myoblastic differentiation (Ten Broek *et al.*, 2010). Myostatin is also upregulated during this phase, which slows proliferation of satellite cells and promotes differentiation of regenerating myoblasts. Low-grade mechanical strains are stimulatory for early myogenic differentiation and muscle regeneration. However, loss of the endomyseal and perimyseal ECM leaves healing muscle fragile and susceptible to reinjury. Aggressive early stretching of injured muscles, or rapid return to high-intensity activity after muscle injury commonly leads to re-injury and re-initiation of an acute inflammatory response. Recurrent or sustained monocytic infiltration of injured or diseased muscle ultimately triggers fibroblast activation, collagen deposition, and excessive fibrosis, leading to permanent loss of muscle function.

Examination of exercising sled dogs before an endurance race, 5 days into racing, and at the finish showed there were no elevations in the any of the cytokines (IL-6, TNFα, IL-8, or IL-15) other than monocyte chemoattractant protein 1 (MCP-1), which was elevated at the mid-point and finish of the race. The lack of cytokine response was thought to be due to the often transient nature of the inflammation of exercise as an early event as this response had never been examined in ultra-endurance exercise such as endurance sled dog racing (Yazwinski *et al.*, 2013). More recent examination of this response in exercising sled dogs 2 days into an endurance event suggested mild elevations in IL-6 and IL-10, thought to be part of the M1 and M2 responses to exercise, but these were far lower than the IL-6 response seen after prolonged daily exercise in people, suggesting that this metabolic response may be dampened in these unique canine athletes (Von Pfeil *et al.*, 2015)

Bone

Structural and functional organization of bone

Bone is a complex and highly dynamic tissue that serves many functions throughout the body. The bony skeleton provides a mechanical frame that supports locomotion by organizing and directing the forces of muscular contraction. In the adult, hematopoiesis takes place primarily within a highly specialized bone marrow niche, and is regulated by resident bone cells. Bone is also a storehouse for calcium and other minerals as well as fat, and plays important roles in mineral homeostasis and energetics.

Cortical bone has a dense structure, and is made up of overlapping Haversian units or osteons. The basic Haversian unit has a cylindrical organization with a central vascular channel (central, or Volkmann's canal) surrounded by several layers of concentrically organized bone matrix (circumferential lamellae) populated by osteocytes (Figure 3.9). Trabecular, or cancellous bone is present only within the medullary cavity and consists of an interconnected system of thin bony shelves and struts called trabeculae. Trabecular bone has an extensive surface area and is organized into a vast number of microcompartments that contain fat and islands of hematopoietic cells (Figure 3.10). The external and medullary surfaces of a bone are covered by thin periosteal and endosteal membranes, respectively. These membranes are highly vascular, richly innervated and populated by osteoblasts and smaller numbers of osteoprogenitor cells. The ECM of the periosteal and endosteal membranes contains primarily type I collagen, large amounts of elastin, and a variety of proteoglycans. Bone can also be classified according to the organization of the type I collagen fibrils within the matrix. Woven bone is an intermediate form of bone with random orientation of collagen fibrils that occurs during the initial phase of endochondral ossification or fracture healing. Lamellar bone is a mature form of bone with greater density in which the collagen fibrils are deposited in a highly ordered, multidirectional, layered pattern. Mature cortical bone is a form of lamellar bone.

The chemical composition and molecular organization of bone is highly conserved. Living bone contains approximately 70% mineral, up to 20% organic matrix, and 5–10% water. Bone mineral is primarily calcium hydroxyapatite—$Ca_{10}(PO_4)_6(OH)_2$. Other minerals such as magnesium, carbonate, and phosphate are present in small amounts. The organic matrix is made up of 90% type I collagen. The remainder is composed of other collagen types (types III and V), a variety of proteoglycans, several bone-specific proteins such as bone sialoprotein and osteocalcin, and a variety of growth factors elaborated during osteogenesis

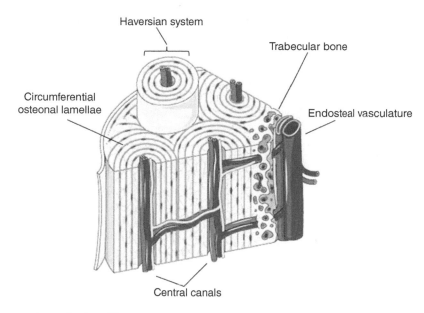

Figure 3.9   Structural organization of bone.

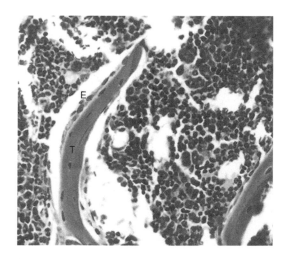

Figure 3.10 Cancellous bone is composed of thin bony shelves, or trabeculae (T), covered with an endosteal membrane (E).

that are immobilized through their association with other components of the bone matrix (Kim *et al.*, 2011).

The major cells in bone include osteoblasts, osteocytes, and osteoclasts. Osteoblasts are osteogenic cells that reside within periosteal and endosteal membranes. They are a heterogeneous population of cells representing various stages of differentiation including mesenchymal stem cells, osteogenic progenitors,

preosteoblasts, and osteoblasts. Mesenchymal stem cells and osteogenic progenitor cells are capable of self-replication, which is important for maintenance of a pool of progenitors that can participate in osteosynthesis during growth, physiological remodeling, and healing of bone. Osteoblasts are responsible for biosynthesis, deposition, and mineralization of bone matrix, as well as synthesis and secretion of growth factors and biological mediators that are deposited within the matrix during bone formation. Osteocytes are terminally differentiated bone cells that form as osteoblasts become surrounded by bone matrix during osteosynthesis. In mature bone, osteocytes reside within lacunae within the concentric lamellae of a Haversian unit. They communicate with neighboring osteocytes and osteoblasts by direct contact via long cytoplasmic projections that extend through canaliculi within the bone matrix. Osteoclasts are multinucleated cells derived from hematopoietic precursors; they resorb bone matrix.

The tightly packed crystalline organization of bone mineral imparts high stiffness and strength. Bone is nevertheless a highly anisotropic material that is able to withstand large compressive loads but is comparatively weak when subjected to tensile stress. Compressive loads are borne by the mineral component of the ECM while tensile stresses are resisted by the organic component of the bone matrix, primarily the collagen fibrils (Currey, 2008). The walls of cellular lacunae and canaliculi as well as the interfaces between individual lamellae of osteons are important sites of stress concentration within cortical bone. Most fractures are thought to develop as tensile stresses within the bone matrix lead to delamination of osteonal lamellae, and subsequent propagation and expansion of cortical microcracks.

Bone remodeling

Bone is a dynamic tissue that undergoes continual turnover throughout life. This remodeling process involves a highly regulated balance between resorption of existing bone and deposition of new bone (Sims & Gooi, 2008). Adaptive remodeling is the process by which the morphology and mechanical properties of a bone are adjusted in response to regional mechanical strains. Adaptive remodeling of bone is often referred to as Wolff's law.

Bone remodeling involves the coordinated activities of osteocytes, osteoclasts, and osteoblasts (Figure 3.11). This triad of cells is termed the *basic multicellular unit* (BMU). Osteocytes are the primary mechanosensors within bone. Mechanical strains within the bone matrix cause pressure changes and fluid flows within the canaliculi of Haversian systems; these are transduced by osteocytes into biological signals. Osteocytes form a highly interconnected cellular network and communicate both with adjacent osteocytes and with nearby endosteal or periosteal osteoblasts through gap junctions as well as through release of soluble mediators. Physiological strains are trophic for osteocytes and elicit release of the osteocyte-specific protein sclerostin (Robling *et al.*, 2008). Sclerostin is an inhibitory mediator that downregulates the activity of osteoblasts. The remodeling process is triggered by the loss of osteocytes. This may occur through direct trauma. Osteocytes may also be lost by apoptosis, which is triggered by supraphysiological strains, or by conditions of very low strain such as occur with disuse and

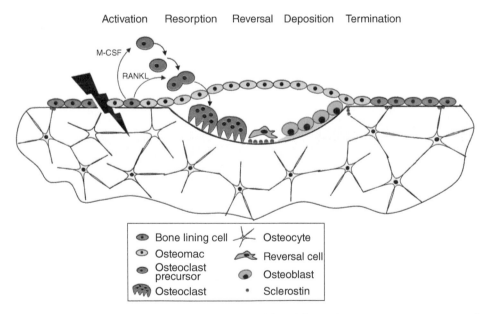

Figure 3.11 Bone remodeling proceeds in five phases (depicted from left to right). During activation, matrix damage causes loss of osteocytes and interruption of sclerostin signaling. Expression of RANKL (receptor activator of NFκB ligand) and M-CSF (monocyte colony-stimulating factor) by bone lining cells leads to recruitment and differentiation of osteoclast precursors. During resorption, mature osteoclasts demineralize and hydrolyze bone matrix within a compartment lined by specialized mononuclear cells called osteomacs. Reversal involves enzymatic modification of the surface of the resorption pit by reversal cells. During deposition, osteoblasts fill the bone defect with new osteoid. The remodeling cycle is terminated when new osteocytes resume negative regulatory sclerostin signaling to adjacent lining cells and osteoblasts.

immobilization. Loss of osteocytes facilitates activation, proliferation, and differentiation of osteoblasts. Activation of osteoblasts involves expression of mediators such as monocyte colony-stimulating factor (M-CSF) and the receptor activator of NFκB ligand (RANKL), which cause recruitment and differentiation of osteoclastic precursors (Sims & Gooi, 2008). Osteoclasts home to a target region and their activity leads to the formation of a resorption pit, or Howship's lacuna. During resorption, numerous growth factors are released from the matrix, and further stimulate biosynthetic activity of osteoblasts. Osteoclasts ultimately undergo apoptosis, and the lacuna is then filled in with new bone by osteoblasts. As osteoblasts become encased in new osteoid, they differentiate into osteocytes and re-establish their inhibitory effects upon nearby osteoblasts, thereby ending the remodeling cycle.

Most remodeling occurs on the surfaces of trabecular bone. However, a similar process of remodeling also occurs within cortical bone. Here, osteoclasts are recruited to areas of osteocyte loss through the vasculature of the Haversian systems. Several osteoclasts advance as a unit through the cortical matrix forming a cutting cone, and creating a longitudinal tunnel of resorption (Figure 3.12). In the wake of the osteoclasts, ostoblasts line the tunnel and deposit concentric layers of osteoid forming a new Haversian system. Cutting cones play a major role in the remodeling of fracture callus into mature cortical bone, as well as in direct healing of rigidly stabilized fractures.

Bone healing

Fracture healing is a regenerative process in which the original morphology and mechanical properties of a fractured bone can be fully re-established. Two basic forms of bone healing are recognized. Primary, or direct healing occurs when a fracture is anatomically reduced and rigidly stabilized. Primary healing may also occur in some stable hairline fractures. Direct interfragmentary contact and rigid stabilization of fragments subverts the normal stimulus for intermediary callus formation and the remodeling response dominates the healing process. Cutting cones traverse the fracture site and re-establish bony continuity by direct deposition of mature lamellar bone. Gap healing is a variation of primary bone healing in which very small but stable interfragmentary gaps are initially filled with woven bone before being remodeled to lamellar bone by the activity of cutting cones. Lack of interfragmentary motion is a prerequisite for both forms of primary healing.

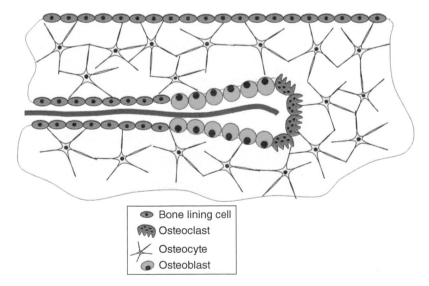

Bone lining cell
Osteoclast
Osteocyte
Osteoblast

Figure 3.12   Cutting cones consist of small clusters of osteoclasts that create longitudinal resorption tunnels within cortical bone. New Haversian systems are formed in the wake of a cutting cone through the deposition of concentric layers of bone matrix by osteoblasts.

Bone healing as it occurs in the absence of surgical intervention is referred to as secondary, or indirect healing, and occurs in several overlapping phases. The initial injury causes soft tissue damage and acute hemorrhage and results in the formation of a fracture hematoma that fills the fracture site and that may encompass displaced fragments. Within several hours, an acute inflammatory response develops and the area is infiltrated by neutrophils and macrophages. Following the clearance of necrotic tissue debris, the reparative phase begins, marked by capillary outgrowth from surrounding soft tissues and vascularization of the fracture hematoma. Vascularization converts the fracture hematoma to granulation tissue and forms the extraosseous blood supply of healing bone. This is a critical step in the initiation of secondary healing, and preservation of this developing blood supply is a major goal in the clinical management of fractures. Proliferation and influx of progenitor cells from the soft tissue envelope surrounding the fracture occurs. Periosteum and muscle are major sources of mesenchymal stem cells that undergo chondroblastic and osteoblastic differentiation in response to the growth factor milieu within the granulation bed at the fracture site. Mechanical strains within the granulation tissue of the fracture site elicit the deposition of chondroid matrix and woven bone in a disorganized fashion resulting in the formation of soft callus. This occurs over several weeks. Mineralization of this early matrix produces hard callus, which is the earliest radiographically detectable phase of secondary healing (Figure 3.13). Bridging of the fracture gap with mineralized hard callus re-establishes bony continuity and marks the transition from the reparative phase to the remodeling phase.

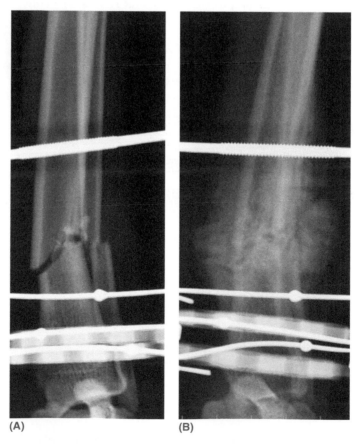

(A)   (B)

Figure 3.13   Radiographic appearance of a distal radial fracture in a dog (**A**), and mineralized callus of secondary bone healing bridging the fracture site 7 weeks after repair (**B**).

Case Study 3.1 Delayed union

Signalment: 7 y.o. M/C Terrier mix. Presented for evaluation of non-healing fracture of right radius.

History: Original fracture occurred 4 years prior, repaired successfully with plate and screw fixation. Three years later, draining tract appeared on distal aspect of right antebrachium. Culture yielded methicillin-resistant *Staphylococcus pseudintermedius*. Plate removed. Six months later, radius refractured at original site. Type II external fixator applied. After 12 weeks of fixation, fracture site not healed (Figure 3.14A). Referred for second opinion.

Examination: Patient bearing minimal weight on right forelimb. Disuse atrophy of right forelimb

musculature. Copious drainage from proximal pin tracts.

Treatment: Fixator removed. Fracture ends debrided to reopen medullary cavity. Autogenous cancellous bone graft placed at fracture site. Ring fixator applied (Figure 3.14B). Postoperatively, intensive rehabilitation designed to promote limb use. Eight weeks postoperatively, radiographs demonstrated bridging osteosynthesis at fracture site (Figure 3.14C). Circular external fixation technique allows axial interfragmentary micromotion, which is highly stimulatory for mechanosensitive osteoblasts. Successful healing in this case was attributed to the combined effects of bone graft, fixation method, and a rehabilitation program emphasizing rapid return to function.

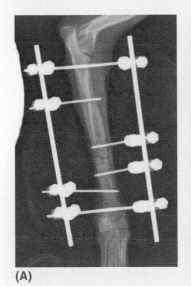
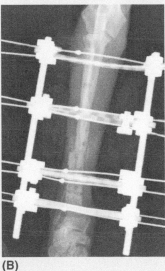
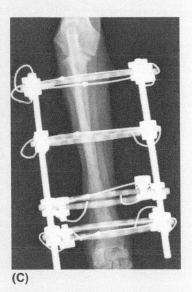

(A) (B) (C)

Figure 3.14 Delayed union. **(A)** After 12 weeks of fixation, the fracture site has not healed. **(B)** An autogenous cancellous bone graft was placed at the fracture site and a ring fixator applied. **(C)** Eight weeks postoperatively, radiographs demonstrated bridging osteosynthesis at the fracture site.

During remodeling, the woven bone of the callus is gradually resorbed and replaced with denser and more organized lamellar bone, and the medullary compartment is also reformed.

Cartilage

Cartilage is an avascular connective tissue composed of chondrocytes suspended in a specialized ECM containing type II collagen, elastin, variable amounts of type I collagen, and a diverse array of proteoglycans. The three basic forms of cartilage—hyaline, fibrocartilage, and elastic cartilage—differ in composition and organization of the ECM and are adapted to specific roles and mechanical environments within the body. Hyaline cartilage forms the contact surface of synovial joints (Figure 3.15A). Fibrocartilage is a tougher form

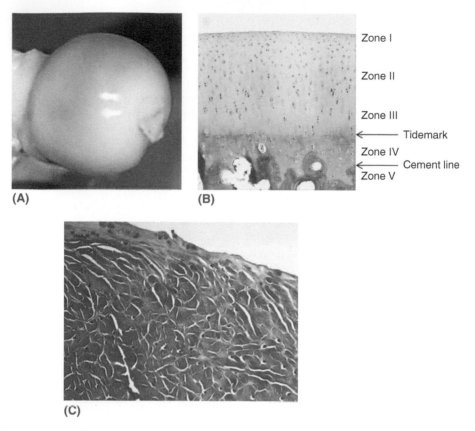

(A)   **(B)**

Zone I

Zone II

Zone III

Tidemark

Zone IV

Cement line

Zone V

(C)

Figure 3.15   Gross (**A**) and histological (**B**) appearance of normal articular cartilage with zonal labeling, and histological appearance of meniscal fibrocartilage (**C**).

of cartilage with a dense ECM that is adapted to resist compressive stress. Fibrocartilage is found in menisci, the annulus fibrosis of intervertebral discs, and occurs as a specialization within some regions of tendon that experience high compressive loads (Figure 3.15B,C). Elastic cartilage is a flexible and elastin-rich cartilage found in the larynx, epiglottis, and pinna. Elastic cartilage is not a significant component of the musculoskeletal system.

Articular cartilage is a smooth and translucent tissue with high water content (approximately 70%) and a delicate collagen fibrillar network. It consists of approximately 50% collagen and 35% proteoglycan on a dry weight basis. The remaining 10% includes nonstructural proteins and glycoproteins, along with various minerals and lipids. Chondrocytes account for approximately 10% of the volume of articular cartilage.

The collagen in articular cartilage is predominantly type II, which forms a complex three-dimensional network within the ECM and accounts for the tensile strength of articular cartilage. The massive aggregating PG aggrecan is the most abundant PG in articular cartilage on a dry weight basis. The aggrecan core protein has a molecular mass of approximately 240 kDa. Monomers are rich in chondroitin sulfate and keratan sulfate side chains and are made up of approximately 90% carbohydrate. Many aggrecan monomers may be linked to a single backbone molecule of hyaluronic acid, generating molecular complexes that may reach 2×10^5 kDa in mass. Articular cartilage also contains several species of SLRPs, including decorin, biglycan, and fibromodulin (Roughley, 2006). SLRPs make up a small proportion of the proteoglycan mass of articular cartilage; however, due to their small size, they can be abundant on a molar basis. The functions of articular cartilage SLRPs are not completely understood. SLRPs bind many components of the ECM, including collagen and fibronectin, and play roles in collagen and elastin fibrillogenesis as well as serving to sequester growth factors within the ECM.

Chondrocytes make up a small proportion of articular cartilage yet they are responsible for the biosynthesis, maintenance, and turnover of the entire ECM compartment throughout life. Collagen within canine articular cartilage is extremely stable and most lasts for the life of the individual. In contrast, the rate of turnover of cartilage PG is more rapid (approximately 300 days; Maroudas, 1980). Under normal conditions, chondrocytes maintain a highly regulated balance of matrix biosynthesis and degradation that is precisely adjusted to meet functional requirements of the tissue. ECM turnover is influenced by the prevailing mechanical environment, along with a plethora of cytokines and growth factors produced by leukocytes, synovial lining cells, and chondrocytes. Mechanical load and cytokines elicit the production of catabolic enzymes that can degrade ECM components. This degradative process is normally counterbalanced by production of enzyme inhibitors and anabolic growth factors. Imbalance between anabolic and catabolic functions of the chondrocyte can result in detrimental changes in ECM composition and loss of mechanical integrity of the ECM. This basic imbalance underlies most processes of joint degeneration. Loss of moderate amounts of PG from cartilage ECM can be restored by de novo biosynthesis; however, extensive loss of PG or breakdown of the collagen network is irreversible and invariably leads to progressive joint degeneration.

Articular cartilage is a heterogeneous tissue the organization of which differs between joints, as well as between different contact regions within a given joint. Articular cartilage is subdivided into five discrete zones (Figure 3.15B). Zones I through III are the more superficial and unmineralized zones. Zone III is separated from the calcified cartilage of zone IV by the tidemark. The deep limit of the articular cartilage is the cement line that forms at the conclusion of endochondral ossification of the articular portion of the epiphysis.

Zone I (tangential) chondrocytes have flattened morphology, and are oriented parallel to the articular surface. Zone II (transitional) chondrocytes assume a more globoid shape. Zone III (radiate) cells become oriented with their axes perpendicular to the articular surface. The chondrocytes within articular cartilage are arranged in close coordination with the orientation of the collagen fibrils within the matrix. Fibril organization varies with different regions of the tissue, in accordance with the local mechanical stresses that are generated by joint loading. In zone I, stresses develop parallel to the plane of the articular surface, and collagen fibrils here are largely parallel or tangential to the articular surface. Zones II and III experience complex patterns of shear, tension, and compression, and collagen fibrils in these zones are arranged in a three-dimensional cross-linked isotropic web adapted to resist multidirectional tension. Compressive stresses prevail in the deeper zones. Collagen fibrils in zones IV and V are larger in diameter and, as in bone, mineralization enhances the ability of the tissue to withstand compressive stress. Collagen concentration is highest at the articular surface, where tensile stresses are greatest, and decreases within the deeper layers of the cartilage. In contrast, PG concentration in articular cartilage is greatest within the deep zones, and decreases toward the articular surface.

Articular cartilage undergoes significant deformation during normal activity, but these strains are elastic and fully reversible. As a composite tissue, articular cartilage has overall low modulus of elasticity (stiffness); its deformability enhances both the congruity and the contact area of opposing articular surfaces during joint loading. This results in dynamic improvements in joint stability and reduced stress per unit area of the articular surface. In addition, cartilage surface deformation drives fluid away from compressed regions into adjacent regions of matrix, as well as into the surrounding synovial fluid (Figure 3.16). This bulk exchange of fluid between the cartilage matrix and the synovial fluid is a major route by which nutrients are delivered to the chondrocyte and underscores the importance of early joint mobilization and controlled cartilage loading during rehabilitation from

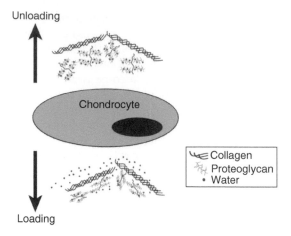

Figure 3.16   Loading of articular cartilage causes displacement of water from highly anionic aggregating proteoglycans. Upon release of load, the hygroscopic proteoglycans draw water into the matrix. Load-induced bulk flow of water through the matrix is a major mechanism by which nutrients are delivered to chondrocytes.

joint trauma or surgery. Compressive loads applied to articular cartilage are distributed among the different components of the matrix. The osmotic properties of the highly hydrated aggregating PGs establish a relatively incompressible fluid compartment that resists volumetric compression. Collagen fibrils resist tensile stresses, and tether the PGs within the matrix. In healthy cartilage, the hydraulic swelling pressure of the aggregating PGs is finely balanced by the tensile resistance of the collagen network. Swelling pressure varies with the density and distribution of the charged GAG side chains of the PGs. The magnitude of the resisting tensile counterforce depends in turn on the stiffness and strength of the collagen network. Imbalance between the osmotic and tensile components of the cartilage matrix leads to compromises in the mechanical integrity of the cartilage and results in cartilage degeneration, osteoarthritis, and decreased joint function (Lai *et al.*, 1991).

Fibrocartilage is made up of chondrocytes suspended in an ECM that is denser than that of articular cartilage. The ECM of fibrocartilage is rich in type I collagen and contains smaller quantities of PGs. Like articular cartilage,

fibrocartilage contains appreciable quantities of elastin. Fibrocartilage is a tough and flexible tissue with a rubbery consistency. The collagen fibrils in fibrocartilage have a variable orientation that is specifically suited to an individual tissue. For example, the circumferential orientation of fibrils in the peripheral regions of menisci is adapted to accommodate the hoop stresses that concentrate in these tissues in response to compressive loads (Masouros *et al.*, 2008). Likewise, fibrocartilage develops within the pulley regions of certain tendons where compressive stresses become concentrated within the ECM (Benjamin *et al.*, 2008). Disorganized fibrocartilage develops readily as a sequel to the degeneration or healing of many musculoskeletal tissues, including bone, tendon, and ligament. It also forms following vascularization of naturally occurring or iatrogenic articular cartilage defects that communicate with the trabecular bone subjacent to the subchondral bone plate.

Synovium

The synoviae form the capsular enclosures of diarthrodial joints, as well as tendon sheaths and the walls of bursae (Figure 3.17). All synovial membranes share a common histologic structure and consist of a thin lining of intimal synovial cells supported by a vascular fibroelastic subintima. The synovial lining is a discontinuous layer of two types of synovial

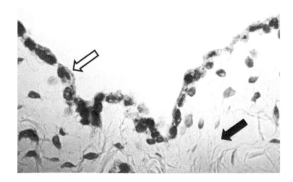

Figure 3.17   Histological appearance of normal synovial membrane. The synovial cells (white arrow) overlie a richly vascularized and innervated fibroelastic subintima (black arrow).

cells. Type B synoviocytes are fibroblastic cells with a slightly flattened morphology and are primarily responsible for production of hyaluronic acid, proteoglycans, surfactants, and matrix metalloproteinases. Type A synoviocytes are intimal macrophages that form within the bone marrow and traffic to the joint. They are responsible for immune surveillance within the joint, and phagocytosis of intra-articular debris. Both cell types communicate continuously with chondrocytes through the elaboration into the synovial fluid of cytokines, growth factors, and other mediators that reach the chondrocytes by diffusion through the matrix. The synovial lining lacks a basal lamina. The synovium is therefore an inefficient barrier, and the trafficking of cells and mediators between the subintimal vasculature and the synovial fluid, or between periarticular tissues and the joint space, is relatively unconstrained. Hence, periarticular tissues are often affected by primary joint pathology, and likewise, periarticular lesions can cause significant bystander-type joint injury.

The subintima is a richly vascularized and innervated tissue that forms the fibrous component of joint capsules. Normal subintima is a highly flexible tissue that helps guide and constrain joint motion and that may merge with adjacent ligaments. It often forms extensive villi and areolar folds that project the synovium deep into the joint space in close proximity with the surface of the articular cartilage. The margins of diarthrodial joints are delineated by the enthesial attachments of fibrous capsules to adjacent bone.

Synovial joint degeneration

Osteoarthritis (OA) is the most prevalent musculoskeletal disease in dogs, and is a significant cause of decreased performance in canine athletes. OA is often considered to be primarily a disease of articular cartilage. However, current thinking recognizes the diarthrodial joint as an organ, and describes progressive joint degeneration as a form of organ failure (Loeser *et al.*, 2012). Thus, while mechanical failure of articular cartilage is a defining element of OA, the trajectory of cartilage loss is affected by concurrent maladaptive changes involving both synovium and subchondral bone.

Cartilage damage may occur in normal joints as a result of either traumatic injury or chronic overuse. Cartilage injury may also occur when physiological loads are placed upon a joint that suffers from inherent anatomic incongruity, such that the applied force is concentrated upon a small contact area. The latter scenario occurs in dogs with developmental joint disease such as elbow incongruity or hip dysplasia. Cartilage overloading can lead to death of chondrocytes and rupture of the collagen network of the matrix. This can result in loss of proteoglycans by diffusion into the synovial fluid and matrix collapse. Once the mechanical properties of the matrix are compromised, cartilage becomes less capable of withstanding load, and even physiological stresses can cause further structural matrix damage. At the histological level, this is manifest as irregularity and fissuring of the articular surface, cartilage thinning, mineralization of the intermediate zones, and ultimately complete cartilage loss and exposure of the subchondral bone (eburnation) (Figure 3.18).

Chondrocytes are sensitive to the mechanical properties of the matrix, and changes in matrix structure are detected by chondrocytes as altered patterns of force. Chondrocytes initially respond to matrix disruption by upregulating anabolic activities and increasing biosynthesis of collagen and proteoglycans. This represents a reparative response; however, the regenerative capabilities of cartilage are limited, and

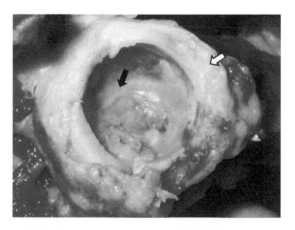

Figure 3.18   Gross appearance of end-stage synovial joint degeneration showing severe capsular fibrosis (white arrow) and subchondral bone eburnation and sclerosis (black arrow).

abnormal loading ultimately shifts the chondrocyte toward a catabolic phenotype (Goldring, 2006). This involves elaboration of a cadre of proinflammatory mediators and matrix metalloproteinases. Proinflammatory mediators can feed back in an autocrine or paracrine manner to further augment catabolic activity of chondrocytes. They may also be released into the synovial fluid where they can activate the synovium. Enzymatic digestion of collagen and proteoglycan components of the matrix by metalloproteinases leads to further mechanical compromise, and can lead to a progressive cascade of matrix collapse (Kurz *et al.*, 2005).

The ability of articular cartilage to withstand physiological loading is dependent upon the compliance of the subchondral bone (Goldring, 2006). Primary diseases or remodeling processes of bone that affect the stiffness of subchondral bone can lead to stress concentration within overlying cartilage and can render the matrix susceptible to injury even under physiological conditions. Conversely, as cartilage matrix is lost, altered patterns of loading are experienced by the subchondral bone itself, which can lead to secondary maladaptive remodeling and loss of underlying trabeculae. This interplay between cartilage and subchondral bone can establish an independent self-perpetuating cascade of joint degeneration.

The synovium is highly responsive to changes in the cartilage and may affect cartilage degeneration at several levels (Sellam & Berenbaum, 2010). Inflammatory diseases of the joint involve rapid activation of the synovium and typically lead to joint effusion and intra-articular recruitment of leukocytes. Matrix metalloproteinases released by leukocytes and synovial cells may initiate a cascade of cartilage degradation by direct attack upon matrix components. Release of proinflammatory cytokines by the synovium may also enhance the catabolic activities of chondrocytes. Degradation of cartilage matrix causes the release into the synovial fluid of small proteolytic fragments of many matrix components, including collagen, fibronectin, proteoglycan core and link proteins, and many others. These fragments can function as potent biological mediators. Matrix fragments (or matrikines) bind to synovial cell surface receptors and can alter patterns of synovial

fluid production, elicit the production of proinflammatory mediators and growth factors, and increase production of matrix metalloproteinases by the synovium.

The complex interplay that develops between cartilage, synovium, and subchondral bone leads to synovial hyperplasia and villous hypertrophy, sustained decreases in the quality of synovial fluid, sclerosis of subchondral bone, and persistent capsular inflammation and fibrosis. Alterations in the thickness and compliance of the joint capsule lead to joint stiffness and loss of range of motion (common clinical manifestations of progressive OA) and also may contribute to OA progression by further altering patterns of cartilage loading.

Tendons, ligaments, and entheses

Tendons are bands of collagen-rich tissue that link muscle to bone and that transfer forces of muscle contraction to the skeleton. Several forms of tendon are recognized. Positional tendons (e.g., the tendon of origin of the biceps brachialis) are dense cord-like structures with discrete sites of osseous attachment and are primarily involved in muscular control of joint position. Positional tendons are frequently contained within a fluid-filled sheath that provides for low-friction sliding motion. Wrap-around tendons (e.g., digital extensor tendons) are positional tendons that undergo a sharp change of direction as they cross a joint. They often pass through specialized bony grooves that function as pulleys during joint motion. The portion of a wrap-around tendon that traverses a joint is usually stabilized by a fibrous retinaculum, and the tendon itself may contain fibrocartilage that provides resistance to the compressive stresses that concentrate at the site of the pulley. Energy-storing tendons (tarsal extensors and carpal flexors) are adapted to weight-bearing and maintenance of posture, and contain higher concentrations of elastin than other tendon types. Aponeuroses are flattened sheet-like structures that often link muscles to other fascial structures (e.g., insertional aponeuroses of the abdominal wall muscles).

Ligaments are connective tissue bands with osseous origins and insertions and that typically cross a joint. Some ligaments (e.g., the transverse acetabular ligament) originate and insert on the same bone. Ligaments function primarily to stabilize joints and direct and constrain joint motion. Two basic forms of ligaments are recognized. Capsular ligaments (e.g., collateral ligaments of most joints) are collagen-rich thickenings of a joint capsule. Intra-articular ligaments (e.g., the round ligament of the femoral head) cross joints within synovial compartments. Intra-articular ligaments are surrounded with a thin epiligament that merges with the periosteum at both origin and insertion.

Tendons and ligaments have similar histological structure and biochemical composition (Figure 3.19). Both contain small numbers of fibroblastic cells that are aligned with the direction of the collagen fibrils. The ECM is rich in type I collagen and contains a variety of PGs and variable quantities of elastin. The diameter of collagen fibrils within tendons and ligaments is usually bimodally distributed (Frank *et al.*, 1999). Larger diameter fibrils provide higher tensile strength, while small diameter fibrils increase the overall fibrillar surface area. A bimodal distribution of fibril diameters leads to increased density of fibril packing within a given tendon cross-sectional area and allows the mechanical properties of a tendon to be fine tuned through variations in interfibrillar

crosslinking as well as the composition of the interfibrillar matrix.

Tendons and ligaments are highly anisotropic and viscoelastic. They have high strength and stiffness when loaded in tension but buckle readily when loaded in compression. The stress–strain relationships in tendons and ligaments have been well characterized (Figure 3.20). The initial elongation at the toe region of the curve results from the straightening of fibrillar crimps. The linear elastic region describes reversible elongation that occurs due to direct fibrillar elongation or interfibrillar shear; rapid loading causes fibrillar elongation, while slow or sustained loading results in interfibrillar shear and either stress relaxation or creep. The yield point represents rupture of interfibrillar bonds and permanent distortion of collagen alpha-helices. Macroscopic failure of a tendon or ligament involves complete mechanical disruption of the interfibrillar matrix and radical interfibrillar shear with pullout of individual fibers (Benjamin *et al.*, 2008).

Entheses are specialized structures at the attachment sites of tendons or ligaments upon bone (Benjamin *et al.*, 2006; Shaw & Benjamin, 2007). Two basic forms of entheses are recognized. Fibrous entheses occur where muscles attach directly to diaphyseal bone. Fibrous entheses are made up of collagen fibers

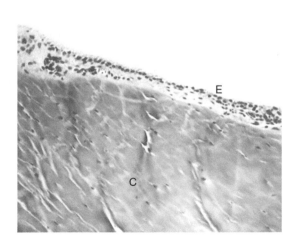

Figure 3.19 Histological appearance of canine cranial cruciate ligament. Organized fascicles of collagen fibers (C) are covered by a thin synovial epiligament (E). Tendons have a similar structure and histological appearance.

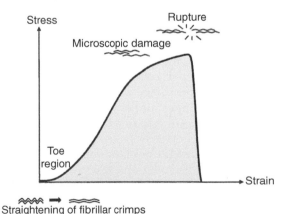

Figure 3.20 Stress–strain relationships of tendons and ligaments. Initial elongation at the toe region reflects straightening of the crimped collagen fibrils. Irreversible deformation at the yield point occurs due to interfibrillar shear. Failure involves loss of interfibrillar adhesion and pullout of collagen fibers.

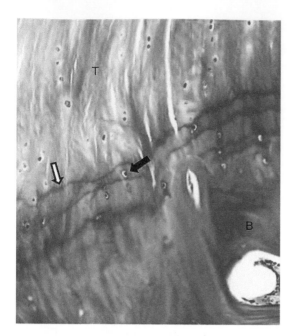

Figure 3.21 Histological appearance of a fibrocartilaginous enthesis. Collagen fibers within the body of the tendon (T) transition through a zone of fibrocartilage before intercalating into the collagen structure of the bone matrix (B). Multiple tidemarks (white arrow) and chondrocytes isolated with lacunae (black arrow) are present within the fibrocartilage zone.

(Sharpey's fibers) that blend with the periosteum and are anchored directly into cortical bone. Fibrocartilaginous entheses contain a zone of fibrocartilage at the tendon or ligament attachment site that serves as a transition zone between the parallel collagen fibers of the tendon/ligament and the bone matrix (Figure 3.21). As in the deeper zones of articular cartilage, enthesial fibrocartilage contains deep mineralized and more proximal nonmineralized regions that are separated by a tidemark. The interface between the bone matrix and the deep mineralized zone of the enthesial fibrocartilage has an irregular and wavy configuration that presents an extensive surface area along which collagen fibrils cross to merge with the bone matrix.

Entheses form a transition between two structures (tendon/ligament and bone) that differ greatly in mechanical properties and that are adapted to resist different forms of loading (tensile loads for tendon/ligament, and compressive loads for bone) (Thomopoulos *et al.*, 2003).

Entheses are also subjected to multidirectional stresses since conditions of load are often present throughout the full range of motion of an associated joint. The structure of fibrocartilaginous entheses in particular has evolved to dissipate the complex stresses that would otherwise concentrate at the osteotendinous or osteoligamentous interface. The complex patterns of loading and high-intensity stresses that occur at many entheses during locomotion underlie the susceptibility of these structures to both acute injury and chronic pathology (Shaw & Benjamin, 2007; Slobodin *et al.*, 2007).

Case Study 3.2   Calcanean tendon repair

Signalment: 4 y.o. F/S Chesapeake Bay Retriever. Presented for evaluation of right pelvic limb lameness.

History: Patient showed intermittent performance deficits while hunting for 3 months; lameness worsened acutely during recent training.

Examination: II-III/IV right pelvic limb lame with plantigrade stance, 170-degree standing angle at stifle. Right calcanean tendon thick and mildly painful on palpation just proximal to insertion. Ultrasonographic examination: fiber disorganization consistent with tendon rupture and enthesiopathy.

Treatment: Surgical reattachment of tendon to calcaneus. For 12 weeks postoperatively, tarsus was maintained in extension with dynamic supportive bracing. Patient received regular hydrotherapy. Site treated daily with low-level laser. Low-intensity pulsed ultrasound treatment once every 3 days. Local injections of platelet-rich plasma performed at 1, 2, and 4 weeks postoperatively. Six months postop., patient's function improved; however, lameness developed consistently after moderate exercise. Standing angles of stifle and tarsus:162 and 129 degrees, respectively. The gastrocnemius insertion remained palpably thick.

Discussion: This case highlights the extraordinary difficulty associated with management of enthesial disruptions. Fibrocartilaginous entheses are highly specialized structures that dissipate multidirectional stresses at osteotendinous junctions. Surgical reattachment of tendons produces a mechanically inferior fibrous enthesis that is incapable of resisting large and complex osteotendinous loads.

References

Ambrosio, F., Wolf, S. L., Delitto, A., Fitzgerald, G. K., Badylak, S. F., Boninger, M. L., & Russell, A. J. 2010. The emerging relationship between regenerative medicine and physical therapeutics. *Phys Ther*, 90, 1807–1814.

Archer, C. W., Dowthwaite, G. P., & Francis-west, P. 2003. Development of synovial joints. *Birth Defects Res C Embryo Today*, 69, 144–155.

Argiles, J. M., Lopez-soriano, F. J., & Busquets, S. 2009. Therapeutic potential of interleukin-15: a myokine involved in muscle wasting and adiposity. *Drug Discov Today*, 14, 208–213.

Armstrong, R. B., Saubert, C. W. T., Seeherman, H. J., & Taylor, C. R. 1982. Distribution of fiber types in locomotory muscles of dogs. *Am J Anat*, 163, 87–98.

Benjamin, M. & Ralphs, J. R. 1995. Functional and developmental anatomy of tendons and ligaments. In: Gordon, S. L., Blair, S. J., & Fine, L. J. (eds), *Repetitive Motion Disorders of the Upper Extremity*. Rosemont, IL: American Academy of Orthopaedic Surgeons, pp. 185–203.

Benjamin, M., Toumi, H., Ralphs, J. R., Bydder, G., Best, T. M., & Milz, S. 2006. Where tendons and ligaments meet bone: attachment sites ('entheses') in relation to exercise and/or mechanical load. *J Anat*, 208, 471–490.

Benjamin, M., Kaiser, E., & Milz, S. 2008. Structure-function relationships in tendons: a review. *J Anat*, 212, 211–228.

Black, L. L., Gaynor, J., Gahring, D., Adams, C., Aron, D., Harman, S., et al. 2007. Effect of adipose-derived mesenchymal stem and regenerative cells on lameness in dogs with chronic osteoarthritis of the coxofemoral joints: a randomized, double-blinded, multicenter, controlled trial. *Vet Ther*, 8, 272–284.

Black, L. L., Gaynor, J., Adams, C., Dhupa, S., Sams, A. E., Taylor, R., et al. 2008. Effect of intraarticular injection of autologous adipose-derived mesenchymal stem and regenerative cells on clinical signs of chronic osteoarthritis of the elbow joint in dogs. *Vet Ther*, 9, 192–200.

Bonewald, L. F. 2006. Mechanosensation and transduction in osteocytes. *Bonekey Osteovision*, 3, 7–15.

Bradley, L., Yaworsky, P. J., & Walsh, F. S. 2008. Myostatin as a therapeutic target for musculoskeletal disease. *Cell Mol Life Sci*, 65, 2119–2124.

Chapman, J. A. 1989. The regulation of size and form in the assembly of collagen fibrils in vivo. *Biopolymers*, 28, 1367–1382.

Chi, S. S., Rattner, J. B., Sciore, P., Boorman, R., & Lo, I. K. 2005. Gap junctions of the medial collateral ligament: structure, distribution, associations and function. *J Anat*, 207, 145–154.

Civitelli, R. 2008. Cell-cell communication in the osteoblast/osteocyte lineage. *Arch Biochem Biophys*, 473, 188–192.

Currey, J. 2008. Collagen and the mechanical properties of bone and calcified cartilage. In: Fratzl, P. (ed.), *Collagen: Structure and Mechanics*. New York, NY: Springer Science – Business Media, pp. 397–420.

Elliott, D. M., Robinson, P. S., Gimbel, J. A., Sarver, J. J., Abboud, J. A., Iozzo, R. V., & Soslowsky, L. J. 2003. Effect of altered matrix proteins on quasilinear viscoelastic properties in transgenic mouse tail tendons. *Ann Biomed Eng*, 31, 599–605.

Fan, J., Varshney, R. R., Ren, L., Cai, D., & Wang, D. A. 2009. Synovium-derived mesenchymal stem cells: a new cell source for musculoskeletal regeneration. *Tissue Eng Part B Rev*, 15, 75–86.

Frank, C. B., Hart, D. A., & Shrive, N. G. 1999. Molecular biology and biomechanics of normal and healing ligaments—a review. *Osteoarthritis Cartilage*, 7, 130–140.

Freeman, L. M. 2012. Cachexia and sarcopenia: emerging syndromes of importance in dogs and cats. *J Vet Intern Med*, 26, 3–17.

Goldring, M. B. 2006. Update on the biology of the chondrocyte and new approaches to treating cartilage diseases. *Best Pract Res Clin Rheumatol*, 20, 1003–1025.

Guercio, A., Di Marco, P., Casella, S., Cannella, V., Russotto, L., Purpari, G., et al. 2012. Production of canine mesenchymal stem cells from adipose tissue and their application in dogs with chronic osteoarthritis of the humeroradial joints. *Cell Biol Int*, 36, 189–194.

Gundersen, K. 2011. Excitation-transcription coupling in skeletal muscle: the molecular pathways of exercise. *Biol Rev Camb Philos Soc*, 86, 564–600.

Gunn, H. M. 1978a. Differences in the histochemical properties of skeletal muscles of different breeds of horses and dogs. *J Anat*, 127, 615–634.

Gunn, H. M. 1978b. The proportions of muscle, bone and fat in two different types of dog. *Res Vet Sci*, 24, 277–282.

Hand, M. S., Thatcher, C. D., Remillard, R. L., Roudebush, P., & Novotny, B. J. (eds). 2010. *Small Animal Clinical Nutrition*, 5th edn. Topeka, KS: Mark Morris Institute.

Hardingham, T. E. & Fosang, A. J. 1992. Proteoglycans: many forms and many functions. *FASEB J*, 6, 861–870.

Hulmes, D. J. 2002. Building collagen molecules, fibrils, and suprafibrillar structures. *J Struct Biol*, 137, 2–10.

Indik, Z., Yeh, H., Ornstein-goldstein, N., Kucich, U., Abrams, W., Rosenbloom, J. C., & Rosenbloom, J. 1989. Structure of the elastin gene and alternative splicing of elastin mRNA: implications for human disease. *Am J Med Genet*, 34, 81–90.

Itano, N. & Kimata, K. 2002. Mammalian hyaluronan synthases. *IUBMB Life*, 54, 195–199.

Kadler, K. E., Holmes, D. F., Trotter, J. A., & Chapman, J. A. 1996. Collagen fibril formation. *Biochem J*, 316(1), 1–11.

Keeley, F. W., Bellingham, C. M., & Woodhouse, K. A. 2002. Elastin as a self-organizing biomaterial: use of recombinantly expressed human elastin polypeptides as a model for investigations of structure and self-assembly of elastin. *Philos Trans R Soc Lond B Biol Sci*, 357, 185–189.

Khan, I. M., Redman, S. N., Williams, R., Dowthwaite, G. P., Oldfield, S. F., & Archer, C. W. 2007. The development of synovial joints. *Curr Top Dev Biol*, 79, 1–36.

Kim, S. H., Turnbull, J., & Guimond, S. 2011. Extracellular matrix and cell signalling: the dynamic cooperation of integrin, proteoglycan and growth factor receptor. *J Endocrinol*, 209, 139–151.

Kjaer, M. 2004. Role of extracellular matrix in adaptation of tendon and skeletal muscle to mechanical loading. *Physiol Rev*, 84, 649–698.

Knudsen, J.G., Joensen, E., Bertholdt, L., Jessen, H., Van Hauten, L., Hidalgo, J., & Pilegaard, H. 2016. Skeletal muscle IL-6 and regulation of liver metabolism during high-fat diet and exercise training. *Physiol Rep*, 4(9). pii: e12788.

Ko, K. S. & Mcculloch, C. A. 2001. Intercellular mechanotransduction: cellular circuits that coordinate tissue responses to mechanical loading. *Biochem Biophys Res Commun*, 285, 1077–1083.

Kurz, B., Lemke, A. K., Fay, J., Pufe, T., Grodzinsky, A. J., & Schunke, M. 2005. Pathomechanisms of cartilage destruction by mechanical injury. *Ann Anat*, 187, 473–485.

Lai, W. M., Hou, J. S., & Mow, V. C. 1991. A triphasic theory for the swelling and deformation behaviors of articular cartilage. *J Biomech Eng*, 113, 245–258.

Lim, J. H., Boozer, L., Mariani, C. L., Piedrahita, J. A., & Olby, N. J. 2010. Generation and characterization of neurospheres from canine adipose tissue-derived stromal cells. *Cell Reprogram*, 12, 417–425.

Loeser, R. F., Goldring, S. R., Scanzello, C. R., & Goldring, M. B. 2012. Osteoarthritis: a disease of the joint as an organ. *Arthritis Rheum*, 64, 1697–1707.

Mackey, A. L., Heinemeier, K. M., Koskinen, S. O., & Kjaer, M. 2008. Dynamic adaptation of tendon and muscle connective tissue to mechanical loading. *Connect Tissue Res*, 49, 165–168.

Maroudas, A. 1980. *Metabolism of Cartilaginous Tissues: A Quantitative Approach*. Tunbridge Wells: Pitman.

Masouros, S. D., Mcdermott, I. D., Amis, A. A., & Bull, A. M. 2008. Biomechanics of the meniscus-meniscal ligament construct of the knee. *Knee Surg Sports Traumatol Arthrosc*, 16, 1121–1132.

Mithieux, S. M. & Weiss, A. S. 2005. Elastin. *Adv Protein Chem*, 70, 437–461.

Miyazaki, M. & Esser, K. A. 2009. Cellular mechanisms regulating protein synthesis and skeletal muscle hypertrophy in animals. *J Appl Physiol*, 106, 1367–1373.

Moczydlowski, E. & Apkon, M. 2009. Cellular physiology of skeletal, cardiac, and smooth muscle. In: Boron, W. F. & Boulpaep, E. L. (eds), *Medical Physiology: A Cellular and Molecular Approach*, 2nd edn. Philadelphia, PA: Saunders-Elsevier.

Momberger, T. S., Levick, J. R., & Mason, R. M. 2005. Hyaluronan secretion by synoviocytes is mechanosensitive. *Matrix Biol*, 24, 510–519.

Mosher, D. S., Quignon, P., Bustamante, C. D., Sutter, N. B., Mellersh, C. S., Parker, H. G., & Ostrander, E. A. 2007. A mutation in the myostatin gene increases muscle mass and enhances racing performance in heterozygote dogs. *PLoS Genet*, 3, e79.

Nieman, D.C., Zwetzloot, K.A., Meaney, M.P., Lomiwes, D.D., Hurst, S.M., & Hurst, R.D. 2015. Post-exercise skeletal muscle glycogen related to plasma cytokines and muscle IL-6 protein content, but not muscle cytokine mRNA expression. *Front Nutr*, 2, 27.

Pedersen, B. K., Akerstrom, T. C., Nielsen, A. R., & Fischer, C. P. 2007. Role of myokines in exercise and metabolism. *J Appl Physiol*, 103, 1093–1098.

Pagano, T. B., Wojcik, S., Costagliola, A., De Biase, D., Iovino, S., Iovane, V., et al. 2015. Age related skeletal muscle atrophy and upregulation of autophagy in dogs. *Vet J*, 206, 54–60.

Pownall, M. E., Gustafsson, M. K., & Emerson, C. P., Jr. 2002. Myogenic regulatory factors and the specification of muscle progenitors in vertebrate embryos. *Annu Rev Cell Dev Biol*, 18, 747–783.

Ramage, L., Nuki, G., & Salter, D. M. 2009. Signalling cascades in mechanotransduction: cell-matrix interactions and mechanical loading. *Scand J Med Sci Sports*, 19, 457–469.

Reich, C. M., Raabe, O., Wenisch, S., Bridger, P. S., Kramer, M., & Arnhold, S. 2012. Isolation, culture and chondrogenic differentiation of canine adipose tissue- and bone marrow-derived mesenchymal stem cells—a comparative study. *Vet Res Commun*, 36, 139–148.

Robling, A. G., Niziolek, P. J., Baldridge, L. A., Condon, K. W., Allen, M. R., Alam, I., et al. 2008. Mechanical stimulation of bone in vivo reduces osteocyte expression of Sost/sclerostin. *J Biol Chem*, 283, 5866–5875.

Roughley, P. J. 2006. The structure and function of cartilage proteoglycans. *Eur Cell Mater*, 12, 92–101.

Sakamoto, K. & Goodyear, L. J. 2002. Invited review: intracellular signaling in contracting skeletal muscle. *J Appl Physiol*, 93, 369–383.

Schaefer, L. & Iozzo, R. V. 2008. Biological functions of the small leucine-rich proteoglycans: from genetics to signal transduction. *J Biol Chem*, 283, 21305–21309.

Sellam, J. & Berenbaum, F. 2010. The role of synovitis in pathophysiology and clinical symptoms of osteoarthritis. *Nat Rev Rheumatol*, 6, 625–635.

Shaw, H. M. & Benjamin, M. 2007. Structure-function relationships of entheses in relation to mechanical load and exercise. *Scand J Med Sci Sports*, 17, 303–315.

Silver, F. H. & Siperko, L. M. 2003. Mechanosensing and mechanochemical transduction: how is mechanical energy sensed and converted into chemical energy in an extracellular matrix? *Crit Rev Biomed Eng*, 31, 255–331.

Sims, N. A. & Gooi, J. H. 2008. Bone remodeling: Multiple cellular interactions required for coupling of bone formation and resorption. *Semin Cell Dev Biol*, 19, 444–451.

Slobodin, G., Rozenbaum, M., Boulman, N. & Rosner, I. 2007. Varied presentations of enthesopathy. *Semin Arthritis Rheum*, 37, 119–126.

Solomon, A. M. & Bouloux, P. M. 2006. Modifying muscle mass—the endocrine perspective. *J Endocrinol*, 191, 349–360.

Spangenburg, E. E. 2009. Changes in muscle mass with mechanical load: possible cellular mechanisms. *Appl Physiol Nutr Metab*, 34, 328–35.

Tapp, H., Hanley, E. N., Jr, Patt, J. C., & Gruber, H. E. 2009. Adipose-derived stem cells: characterization and current application in orthopaedic tissue repair. *Exp Biol Med (Maywood)*, 234, 1–9.

Ten Broek, R. W., Grefte, S., & Von Den Hoff, J. W. 2010. Regulatory factors and cell populations involved in skeletal muscle regeneration. *J Cell Physiol*, 224, 7–16.

Thomopoulos, S., Williams, G. R., Gimbel, J. A., Favata, M., & Soslowsky, L. J. 2003. Variation of biomechanical, structural, and compositional properties along the tendon to bone insertion site. *J Orthop Res*, 21, 413–419.

Tidball, J. G. & Villalta, S. A. 2010. Regulatory interactions between muscle and the immune system during muscle regeneration. *Am J Physiol Regul Integr Comp Physiol*, 298, R1173–1187.

Tisdale, M. J. 2007. Is there a common mechanism linking muscle wasting in various disease types? *Curr Opin Support Palliat Care*, 1, 287–292.

Toll, P.W., Gillette, R.L., & Hand, M.S. 2010. Feeding working and sporting dogs. In: Hand, M.S., Thatcher, C.D., Remillard, R.L., Roudebush, P., & Novotny, B.J. (eds), *Small Animal Clinical Nutrition*, 5th edn. Topeka, KS: Mark Morris Institute.

Vierck, J., O'reilly, B., Hossner, K., Antonio, J., Byrne, K., Bucci, L., & Dodson, M. 2000. Satellite cell regulation following myotrauma caused by resistance exercise. *Cell Biol Int*, 24, 263–272.

Von Pfeil, D. J., Cummings, B. P., Loftus, J. P., Levine, C. B., Mann, S., Downey, R. L., Griffitts, C., &Wakshlag, J. J. 2015. Evaluation of plasma inflammatory cytokine concentrations in racing sled dogs. *Can Vet J*, 56, 1252–1256.

Vrhovski, B. & Weiss, A. S. 1998. Biochemistry of tropoelastin. *Eur J Biochem*, 258, 1–18.

Wakshlag, J. J., Cooper, B. J., Wakshlag, R. R., Kallfelz, F. A., Barr, S. C., Nydam, D. V., & Dimauro, S. 2004. Biochemical evaluation of mitochondrial respiratory chain enzymes in canine skeletal muscle. *Am J Vet Res*, 65, 480–484.

Wall, M. E. & Banes, A. J. 2005. Early responses to mechanical load in tendon: role for calcium signaling, gap junctions and intercellular communication. *J Musculoskelet Neuronal Interact*, 5, 70–84.

West, D. W. & Phillips, S. M. 2010. Anabolic processes in human skeletal muscle: restoring the identities of growth hormone and testosterone. *Phys Sportsmed*, 38, 97–104.

Wu, Y., Wang, J., Scott, P. G., & Tredget, E. E. 2007. Bone marrow-derived stem cells in wound healing: a review. *Wound Repair Regen*, 15 (Suppl. 1), S18 26.

Yazwinski, M., Milizio, J. G., & Wakshlag, J. J. 2013. Assessment of serum myokines and markers of inflammation associated with exercise in endurance racing sled dogs. *J Vet Intern Med*, 27, 371–376.

Zhang, G., Young, B. B., Ezura, Y., Favata, M., Soslowsky, L. J., Chakravarti, S., & Birk, D. E. 2005. Development of tendon structure and function: regulation of collagen fibrillogenesis. *J Musculoskelet Neuronal Interact*, 5, 5–21.

4 The Role of Nutrition in Canine Performance and Rehabilitation

Joseph J. Wakshlag, DVM, PhD, DACVN, DACVSMR

Summary

Nutrition plays an integral role in sports performance and rehabilitation. Performance dogs pursue a multitude of different activities that likely require dietary modifications for optimal performance that revolve around substrate utilization. Sprinting dogs require more carbohydrate while endurance athletes require fat as the major fuel for exercise. These principles are best employed in a well-trained, fit athlete in optimal body condition, which varies slightly depending on the athletic endeavor. However, many athletes, regardless of the task, are kept lean to ensure that they are not carrying excess weight. Due to popular feeding practices that often do not use commercial dog food as a portion of the ration there are risks of vitamin and mineral imbalances of which clients with performance dogs need to be aware. Rehabilitation often employs dietary principles that revolve around nutritional adequacy for wound healing and maintenance of lean body mass. The concepts of lean body mass and protein consumption are fundamental to obesity management, which can be a component of rehabilitation and gerontology as well. Additionally, the use of long-chain omega-3 fatty acids and other nutraceuticals for their anti-inflammatory properties and ability to dampen the chronic inflammation and improve mobility in canine osteoarthritis, a common sequela to many orthopedic procedures, is discussed.

Introduction

In canine performance, many variables such as conformation, genetics, and behavioral drive are determinants for success, yet controllable variables such as training and nutrition are important as well. Canine sporting venues and events have grown in the past 20 years, with limited physiological data on the numerous activities in which dogs partake. There are considerable nutritional physiology data from studying two athletic extremes: endurance dogs (sled dogs) and sprinting dogs (Greyhounds). Nutritional studies for more

Canine Sports Medicine and Rehabilitation, Second Edition. Edited by Chris Zink and Janet B. Van Dyke.
© 2018 John Wiley & Sons, Inc. Published 2018 by John Wiley & Sons, Inc.

popular activities, such as agility and field trial activities, have been largely ignored, leading to attempts to translate endurance and sprinting knowledge into sound nutritional principles for all athletic dogs. These principles are addressed here, focusing on three areas: energetics, nutrition for performance, and nutrition during rehabilitation.

Energetics and the myofiber

Conversion of substrate to energy

The generation of ATP is a universal process in all cells that occurs through the enzymatic machinery of the mitochondrial electron transport chain (ETC). In short, the ETC uses free hydrogen to create an electrochemical gradient between the inner and outer mitochondrial membrane. This generates a covalent bond between ADP and inorganic phosphate to make ATP, which is the storage form of energy.

ATP generation and hydrolysis becomes a central theme to appropriate muscle contraction. ATP is ultimately formed from the generation of hydrogenated nicotinamide adenine dinucleotide (NADH) and dihydrogenated flavin adenine dinucleotide ($FADH_2$) in the

citric acid cycle within mitochondria. The citric acid cycle is a complex of many enzymes that convert the byproducts of glucose, protein, and fat degradation as pyruvate (glucose and some amino acids) and acetate (fatty acids and some amino acids) into covalently bound coenzyme A (CoA) moieties to make acetyl CoA—the major entry point substrate for the citric acid cycle (Figure 4.1). No matter where substrates enter the citric acid cycle they are eventually turned into carbon dioxide with oxygen as the reactant in the process for generating ATP (Shulman & Petersen, 2009).

Glycolysis and beta-oxidation of fatty acids

ATP generation occurs through beta-oxidation of fat and glucose oxidation through glycolysis, both of which lead to acetyl CoA production. Beta-oxidation of fat is a critical process to normal daily energy metabolism because fat is considered the preferred fuel during rest. Glycolysis is a complex process that begins with fructose conversion to glucose or glucose's immediate entry into the glycolytic pathway. This breakdown of glucose results in one 6-carbon molecule, generating two 3-carbon precursors,

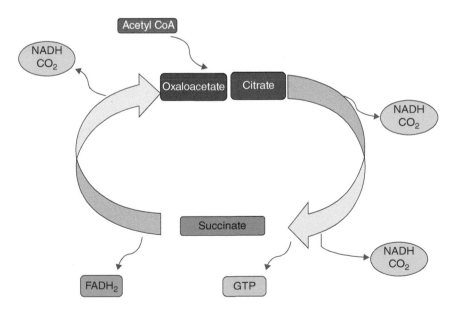

Figure 4.1 The citric acid cycle showing acetyl CoA entry and the formation of NADH and $FADH_2$ with the liberation of CO_2 and GTP. NADH and $FADH_2$ then enter the electron transport chain.

which eventually generate 2NADH and 4ATP and two pyruvate molecules (Figure 4.2). ATP is produced rapidly via glycolysis and does not require oxygen—the rate-limiting step in the citric acid cycle—making glycolysis a preferred system to generate ATP quickly and anaerobically. The excess pyruvate is converted to lactate under anaerobic metabolism. Glycogen stores for ATP generation, unlike fat in most cases, are limited.

Glycolysis occurs in the cytoplasm of all cells. During rest, glycolysis is inhibited causing a flux of glucose toward eventual glycogen formation (Figure 4.3). In times of need, increased glycogen phosphorylase activity induces glycogenolysis and generation of glucose 6-phosphate for glycolysis and entry into the citric acid cycle. Beta-oxidation of fat occurs in the mitochondria, and transport of free fatty acid into the inner mitochondria is required. Carnitine is bound to the carboxyl terminus of the free fatty acid in exchange for CoA (Figure 4.4). Once the carnitine is bound, the fatty acid is transported across the outer

mitochondrial membrane by carnitine acyl transferase I to the inner compartment, and then carnitine palmitoyl transferase II will transport the fatty acid–carnitine moiety into the mitochondrion. The fatty acid will become conjugated to acetyl CoA again, and then carnitine will undergo reverse transportation back to the cytoplasm. Interestingly during prolonged exercise, we often observe a decline in serum free fatty acids while acylated carnitine derivatives rise, suggesting that transport into mitochondria can be part of the rate-limiting process of beta-oxidation of fat (Shulman & Petersen, 2009).

Energetics of substrates

The unit of energy generated by metabolism of protein, carbohydrate, and fat is the calorie or joule. The kilocalorie (kcal) is the unit referred to in lay terminology when talking about calories, and is equivalent to 4.16 kilojoules (kJ). One gram of protein placed in a bomb

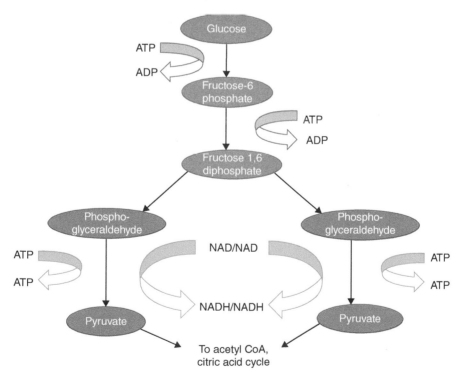

Figure 4.2 Basic anaerobic glycolysis showing glucose being split into two pyruvate molecules, which eventually become acetyl CoA for entry into the citric acid cycle. Note that 2ATP are utilized, but 4ATP are made in the reaction to provide quick anaerobic energy.

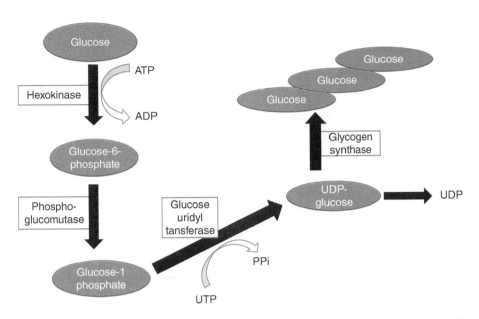

Figure 4.3   Glycogenolysis occurs when excessive glucose is taken into cells as reserve glucose stores, and is eventually broken down for glucose when needed. UDP, uridine diphosphate; UTP, uridine triphosphate.

calorimeter generates approximately 5.24 kcal. Fat generates 9.16 kcal/g, and carbohydrate 4.26 kcal/g. This is the gross energy (GE) of the substrate, and does not take into account the energy lost in feces due to incomplete digestion. This loss is reflected in the digestible energy (DE). Metabolizable energy (ME) as reported on pet food labels takes into account energy lost in urine, deamination of amino acids, and gases. ME is assumed to be significantly less than the GE or DE. Protein and carbohydrate are generally given a value of 4 kcal/g, and fat 9 kcal/g as calculated by the Atwater equation when evaluating human foods (Box 4.1). This equation is modified to adjust for slightly less digestible ingredients in a manufactured pet food, making protein and carbohydrate approximately 3.5 kcal/g, and fat 8.5 kcal/g (National Research Council, 2006a, 2006b).

Body condition, energy utilization at rest and during exercise

The National Research Council (NRC) has set forth energy and nutrient requirements for dogs. Two equations are used to represent resting energy requirement (Box 4.2). The linear equation closely mimics the results obtained from the exponential equation until the subject's weight reaches 25 kg, when the linear equation diverges, overestimating the energy requirements needed at rest. A multiplication factor of 1.0–2.0, based on activity, is applied to the linear equation's initial calculation of $(30 \times \text{kg body-weight}) + 70$, which is considered the resting energy requirement (RER). The exponential equation is (kg body-weight)$^{0.75}$ multiplied by 70, which is considered the resting energy requirement. For activity, this multiplication factor is increased up to approximately 140 to calculate maintenance energy requirements (MER) for active pet dogs. These equations are starting points for patients undergoing rehabilitation. When integrating exercise into a therapeutic plan, 20–30 minutes of rehabilitation activity 3–4 times a week would likely add in a negligible energy increase and should be recognized when making a diet plan for a rehabilitation patient.

Increasing physical activity and the effects of training have been extensively studied in dogs during treadmill exercise. The maximum oxygen consumption during exercise $(V_{O_2 \, max})$ reflects the energy that can be generated via oxygen utilization in the mitochondrial ETC. An average 20-kg Foxhound or Alaskan sled

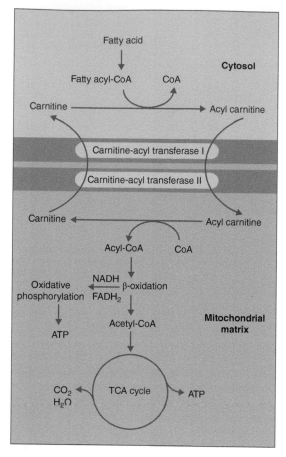

Figure 4.4   Fatty acid entry into the mitochondria is dependent on carnitine-mediated transport through both the outer and inner mitochondrial membranes via carnitine palmitoyl transferase 1 and carnitine acylcarnitine translocase. After fatty acid transport carnitine is recycled through the actions of carnitine palmitoyltransferase II. Fat within the mitochondria will then undergo beta-oxidation and entry of acetyl CoA into the citric acid cycle. Source: Picture reproduced from Hand *et al.*, 2010.

dog working at maximal oxygen consumption would need approximately 700–900 kcal per hour of work based on the experimental conditions set forth in simulated treadmill exercise (Ordway *et al.*, 1984; Musch *et al.*, 1985; Reynolds *et al.*, 1999). This oxygen consumption is directly related to skeletal muscle mitochondrial density and volume. In the field, there are many other factors to take into consideration such as external temperature, thermal regulation,

---

Box 4.1   Atwater's and modified Atwater's equations

The following formulas demonstrate the use of Atwater's formula and modified Atwater's formula, respectively, to calculate kcal in a pet food that consists of 24% protein, 12% fat, and 50% carbohydrates on a dry matter basis in 100 g. Note the modest differences between the two equations. The modified Atwater's equation is used to calculate most commercial pet foods and can potentially undercalculate the number of kilocalories in highly digestible foods.

Atwater's formula

Protein $= 4\,\text{kcal/g} \times 24 = 96\,\text{kcal}$
Fat $= 9\,\text{kcal/g} \times 12 = 108\,\text{kcal}$
Carbohydrate $= 4\,\text{kcal/g} \times 50 = 200\,\text{kcal}$
Total kcal $= 404\,\text{kcal}$

Modified Atwater's formula

Protein $= 3.5\,\text{kcal/g} \times 24 = 84\,\text{kcal}$
Fat $= 8.5\,\text{kcal/g} \times 12 = 102\,\text{kcal}$
Carbohydrate $= 3.5\,\text{kcal/g} \times 50 = 175\,\text{kcal}$
Total kcal $= 361\,\text{kcal}$

Box 4.2   Calculations for resting and active energy requirements

Linear equation for a 30-kg dog

Resting energy requirement $= 30 \times \text{BW}\,(\text{kg}) + 70 = 970\,\text{kcal}$
Active maintenance energy requirement $= 2\{(30 \times \text{BW}) + 70\} = 1940\,\text{kcal}$

Exponential equation for a 30-kg dog

Resting energy requirement $= 70 \times \text{BW}\,(\text{kg})^{0.75} = 897\,\text{kcal}$
Active maintenance requirement $= 140 \times \text{BW}\,(\text{kg})^{0.75} = 1794\,\text{kcal}$

variability in terrain and incline versus decline. Treadmill exercise reveals that there is a loss of efficiency in energy utilization with increased incline due to the need for vertical rise increasing overall kcal expenditure. Larger dogs need to exert more energy to break the fall that occurs on decline (Taylor *et al.*, 1972; Ordway *et al.*, 1984; Schmidt-Nielsen, 1984). Uneven footing or poor footing (snow and sand), as well as load bearing result in increased energy expenditure (Taylor, 1957).

Field studies examining energy expenditure of working Greyhounds have shown that the average 32–35-kg Greyhound expends approximately 2050 to 2160 kcal per day. These studies take into account the typical training regimen for a racing Greyhound, which includes being penned or caged with daily sprint training in enclosed paddocks for approximately 30 minutes and two races a week (Hill *et al.*, 1999, 2000). These findings translate to approximately 150–160 kcal/kg$^{0.75}$. This relatively high MER may be a reflection of the increased muscle mass in Greyhounds. One would expect that average agility dogs would have similar kilocalorie requirements for their proposed activities. However, recent evidence suggests that the average competitive agility dog consumes approximately 106 kcal/kg$^{0.75}$ to maintain a body condition of 4/5 out of 9 (J. Wakshlag, unpublished findings).

Interestingly studies by Hill and colleagues suggested that feed restriction during racing from the normal of approximately 155 kcal/kg$^{0.75}$ body-weight (BW) down to a restricted regimen of only 137 kcal/kg$^{0.75}$ resulted in decreased racing times making mild feed restriction advantageous (Hill *et al.*, 1999). There are numerous reports of caloric intake in racing sled dogs. Decombaz and colleagues (1995) suggested an intake of only 2100 kcal/day during an average of 79 km a day (228 kcal/kg$^{0.75}$), while Orr (1966) suggested an intake of approximately 4400 kcal when pulling a heavy load over ice for 32 km per day (270 kcal/kg$^{0.75}$). These discrepancies appear significant and may be related to climate, housing, and activity in and outside of the kennel. Additionally, these estimates did not factor in changes in lean and fat mass during these activities.

Two studies used double-labeled water with deuterium and ^{18}O (heavy oxygen) to assess total oxygen loss via urine versus that generated and lost through respiration as CO_2. This technique allows calculation of relative CO_2 loss, which is a rough estimate of total kilocalories consumed since the only route for CO_2 generation is the ETC. Dogs running an average of 79 km a day over 8 days expended approximately 438 kcal/kg$^{0.75}$ BW. However, the conditions and temperature during the field experiment were not reported (Decombaz *et al.*, 1995). A second study by Hinchliff and colleagues in extreme racing conditions with dogs running at a speed of approximately 7 km/h approximately 14 h per day over 5 days (total 490 km) at temperatures between –10 and –35°C suggested the kcal expenditure in 18 dogs averaged 1052 ± 192 kcal/kg$^{0.75}$ BW per day (Hinchcliff *et al.*, 1997b). This study and a more recent study examining food diaries of mushers suggests that metabolically these dogs would need approximately 9000–13,000 kcal per day to maintain body-weight (Loftus *et al.*, 2014). This intake is nearly impossible, and therefore many dogs in these conditions use body reserves to meet the caloric demands.

Most clients with performance dogs are acutely aware of their animals' body condition scores (BCS) and competitive body-weights. The traditional body condition scoring methods use a 5- or 9-point system. The 9-point system has been validated through comparison with dual X-ray absorptiometry analysis (Laflamme, 1997) and is preferred by the author (Purina, 2012). Typically, clients with performance dogs keep their dogs at a 4–5/9 BCS where ribs are easily palpable, there is an obvious abdomen tuck, and when viewed and felt from the top the spinous processes can be felt, while a waist can be visualized. In athletic dogs, particularly Greyhounds, field trial, hunting and sprint sled dogs, it may be more desirable to have a BCS between 3 and 4. In this paradigm, ribs can be visualized in shorter haired dogs, the spinous processes and wings of the ilia are prominent, but ample paralumbar musculature extends between the wings of the ilia so that the sacral spinous processes can be localized, but do not protrude. Dogs in sprinting and intermediate activity (10–30 minutes) need to be lean to achieve ideal performance (Figure 4.5), and restricted meal feeding is common. In endurance activities where speed is not as important

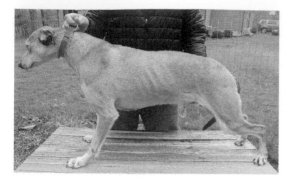

Figure 4.5 Appropriate body condition score (BCS) for a working sled dog—current BCS 4 of 9. Note that the musculature is defined and ribs are visible, which may not be the case in heavier coated dogs.

Table 4.1　Essential and non-essential amino acids

Dietary essential amino acids	Dietary non-essential amino acids
Isoleucine	Alanine
Leucine	Tyrosine
Lysine	Aspartic acid
Methionine	Asparagine
Phenylalanine	Glutamine
Tryptophan	Glutamic acid
Valine	Glycine
Histidine	Serine
Threonine	Cysteine
Arginine	Proline

and there is a greater chance for body condition loss during extended activity, a body condition score of 4–5 may be ideal before competition due to the potential for weight loss during competitive racing (Hinchcliff *et al.*, 1998).

Nutrition for performance

Dietary protein—beyond energy

In addition to essential amino acids supplied in the diet (Table 4.1), dogs can synthesize non-essential amino acids through amidation, deamination, and carboxylation reactions that convert carbon precursors and essential amino acids into nonessential amino acids. Nitrogen retention studies rely on nitrogen balance as the measure of adequacy; however, most canine nitrogen retention studies have never examined the consequences for lean mass. The NRC states that only 20 g/1000 kcal of protein is minimally required for maintenance, equating to approximately 10–12% crude protein in a typical dry commercial product.

Dietary protein helps maintain muscle integrity and appropriate total protein, albumin and red blood cell status. The hematocrit and serum albumin tend to decrease with training and racing, and such decreases appear to be a result of overtraining syndrome (Kronfeld *et al.*, 1989; Wakshlag *et al.*, 2010). This syndrome can be correlated to the acute phase response whereby the liver changes its protein production profile to proteins such as haptoglobin and C-reactive

protein, possibly at the expense of albumin (Wakshlag *et al.*, 2010; Kenyon *et al.*, 2011). The mechanism for these changes is poorly understood, but is thought to be due to acute inflammation of exercise and potential cytokine alterations resulting in accompanying decreases in red blood cell counts (Kronfeld *et al*, 1989; Wakshlag *et al.*, 2010; Kenyon *et al.*, 2011). Adequate protein intake may be helpful in ameliorating this condition.

Studies examining protein consumption and its role in maintaining red blood cell counts and hematocrit in training sled dogs have postulated that approximately 30% of the metabolizable energy (70–80 g protein/1000 kcal) should come from highly digestible animal-based protein (Kronfeld *et al.*, 1989). Four groups of sprint racing sled dogs exercising approximately 60 km in field work per week, plus treadmill training each week, on four diets comprising 18% ME protein (48 g/1000 kcal), 24% ME protein (60 g/1000 kcal), 30% ME protein (75 g/1000 kcal), and 36% ME protein (90 g/1000 kcal) from an initial diet of approximately 26% ME protein were examined. After 12 weeks of feeding each diet, routine complete blood counts, serum chemistries, $Vo_{2\,max}$ and physical assessment were performed. Six of eight dogs in the lowest protein diet (18% ME) sustained musculoskeletal injuries and showed a 25% drop in $Vo_{2\,max}$. Dogs in the highest protein group displayed a 10% increase in plasma volume, and there was a linear correlation between hematocrit, hemoglobin, and total blood volume and protein intake (Reynolds *et al.*, 1999). Querengaesser and colleagues examined diets of approximately 72 and 85 g/1000 kcal and showed that there was no difference in the hematocrit decline over a 6-month period of training, but the higher protein group had elevated post-exercise hematocrit, further suggesting that protein may affect parameters associated with performance (Querengaesser et al., 1994). An interesting study of mongrel dogs exercised 4 hours per day at 12 km/h compared soy protein versus fish meal-based protein at approximately 35% of the ME. After 3 weeks, this study showed decreased hematocrit, and increased red blood cell fragility in the dogs fed soybean meal (Yamada et al., 1987). These data suggested that endurance dogs should receive minimally 70 g/1000 kcal (approximately 26% of ME) of highly digestible animal-source protein with no upper limit yet defined.

In sprinting dogs, the picture may be slightly different as Hill and colleagues performed studies suggesting that racing Greyhounds perform better on lower protein diets of 63 g/1000 kcal versus 106 g/1000 kcal (Hill et al., 2001b). These diets substituted carbohydrates for the protein in an isocaloric exchange of nutrients; therefore the enhanced performance may have been due to the increased carbohydrate in the diet, not the lack of protein. Though it appears that approximately 60 g/1000 kcal may be adequate for racing Greyhounds, further decreases in protein have not been evaluated and are very contrary to current feeding practices. Most Greyhounds are provided 0.25–0.5 kg of meat mixed with dry commercial dog food, approaching 106 g/1000 kcal to meet their energy requirements (Kohnke, 1998; Hill, 1998). The differences noted in sprinting dogs and endurance dogs may be related to overall muscle turnover rates, as exercise leads to increased protein turnover, and increased muscle inflammation observed with increased duration of exercise (Wasserman et al., 1988, 1989, 1991; Wakshlag et al., 2002a). Without firm recommendations or studies in sprinting dogs, a reasonable recommendation is that most sprinting and intermediate activity dogs receive minimally 60 g/1000 kcal consumed (22–24% ME).

Dietary fat and carbohydrate—energy and demands

The respiratory quotient (RQ) is the ratio of oxygen consumed to CO_2 generated. If the RQ is close to 0.7, primarily fat is being consumed for CO_2 production, while if the RQ is closer to 1 primarily glucose is being consumed (Figure 4.6). Early in exercise (the first 20–30 minutes) protein oxidation is minimal, therefore substrate utilization and changes in oxygen

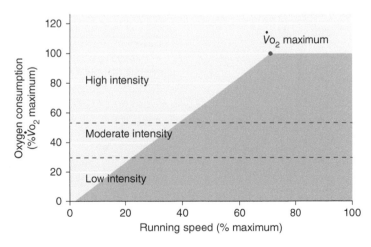

Figure 4.6 Depiction of running speed versus the maximal oxygen consumption. Note that the $Vo_{2\,max}$ is reached well before maximal speed is reached reflecting the generation of energy by anaerobic glycolysis, which can only be sustained for short periods of time. $Vo_{2\,max}$ is often reached at between 65 and 75% of maximal running capacity. Source: Picture reproduced from Hand et al., 2010.

consumption can be examined when feeding differing carbohydrate and fat diets (Toll & Gillette, 2010). A significant amount of work has been performed examining gradation of exercise and duration as they relate to $Vo_{2\,max}$ and RQ values (Wagner *et al.*, 1977; Grandjean, 1998). These studies have laid the groundwork for our understanding of oxygen consumption, showing that when dogs reach up to 40% of their $Vo_{2\,max}$, they primarily use fat for energy, while between 40 and 70% they use a mixture of glucose and fatty acids. Once an animal reaches 70% or higher oxygen consumption, they use primarily glucose for energy (Toll *et al.*, 1992; Reynolds *et al.*, 1995) (see Figure 4.6).

Animals working at maximal speed during the first few seconds of exercise rely upon immediate energy from the phosphocreatine system that generates ATP through shuttling inorganic phosphate to ADP. Glycogenolysis soon ensues, generating energy for typical sprinting or intermediate exercise. Generation of pyruvate and eventually lactic acid predominates if glycolysis is maintained, leading to pH alteration and intracellular dysfunction. Pyruvate incorporation into the citric acid cycle (carbohydrate oxidation) becomes a major source of energy for long-term exercise (20 minutes to 2 hours) as long as glycogen is present for glycogenolysis. Eventually protein oxidation will take place if glycogen is depleted in endurance exercise. As glycogen is depleted a dog will not be able to sustain oxygen consumption above 50–60% of $Vo_{2\,max}$. Fatty acid oxidation begins to rise by 30 minutes into an exercise bout and will be sustained at an oxygen consumption rate of between 30 and 50% of the maximum as the primary fuel. This provides acetyl CoA production for the citric acid cycle at a steady rate, allowing some dogs to exercise at this low to moderate oxygen consumption rate for multiple hours (Reinhart, 1998; Toll & Gillette, 2010) (Figure 4.7).

This understanding provides the basis for fat use as a major form of energy in canid diets, which is contrary to recommendations in human endurance exercise, which focuses on carbohydrate loading (Hargreaves *et al.*, 1984). One study showed that time to exhaustion during low-intensity exercise did not correlate with glycogen depletion in dogs (Downey *et al.*, 1980). The generation of energy from fat is up to 70% of the ME during long-duration exercise, suggesting a propensity for fat utilization, which may be due to the dog's high aerobic activity in skeletal muscle and increased mitochondrial density as compared to humans (Wakshlag *et al.*, 2004). Beagles running at low to moderate intensity increased their time to exhaustion by approximately 25% when provided diets with 55–81 g/1000 kcal of fat versus 33 g/1000 kcal (Downey *et al.*, 1980). Kronfeld, Hammel and colleagues showed that dogs performed equally well on diets containing absolutely no carbohydrate

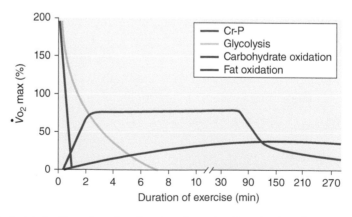

Figure 4.7   The graph depicts the $Vo_{2\,max}$ based on duration of exercise. Note that initially $Vo_{2\,max}$ is above 100%, reflecting anaerobic energy generated by creatine phosphate (Cr-P) reserves and glycolysis; this eventually plateaus in 2–4 minutes with carbohydrate oxidation. As glycogen stores are depleted beta-oxidation of fat occurs and sustains the exercise bout somewhere around 60–90 minutes, making fat the primary fuel for exercise in the endurance athlete. Source: Picture reproduced from Hand *et al.*, 2010.

compared to two diets with increasing carbohydrate content (Hammel et al., 1977; Kronfeld et al., 1977). Further studies in trained and untrained sled dogs showed that when comparing a high-carbohydrate (162 g/1000 kcal; 59% ME) low-fat (18 g/1000 kcal; 14% ME) diet to a high-fat (70 g/1000 kcal; 58% ME) low-carbohydrate (43 g/1000 kcal) diet, there was no difference in muscle glycogen storage (Reynolds et al., 1995). Interestingly, the dogs on the high-fat diet showed diminished glycogen consumption with exercise. Huskies racing approximately 100 km per day over 5 days showed immediate glycogen depletion, with an increase in skeletal muscle glycogen and gradual depletion (Reynolds et al., 1995) of skeletal muscle triglyceride, further suggesting that the longer these endurance dogs run, the more they adapt to fat utilization sparing muscle glycogen (McKenzie et al., 2008). More recently, trained and untrained endurance sled dogs were examined using carbon dioxide capture techniques to examine relative carbohydrate and fat oxidation during long-term treadmill exercise and, surprisingly, the trained and untrained dogs appeared to be using carbohydrate equally if not primarily as an energy source (Miller et al., 2015). These newer data suggest that although fat is an important fuel, in today's elite canine athlete carbohydrate is also an important fuel that should not be ignored. The more important question is where is the carbohydrate coming from. Recent data point toward amino acids since protein makes up over 30% of the metabolizable energy in many cases, and modest blood urea nitrogen (BUN) rises are observed in endurance sled dogs (Ermon et al., 2014; Loftus et al., 2014; Miller et al., 2015).

Fat consumption can supply approximately 60–70% of the ME in low-intensity exercise, and in times of extreme demand, fat may supply up to 85% of the ME, particularly in endurance sled dogs. Based on experience it is advisable to introduce fats to the diet over a period of 2–3 weeks for gastrointestinal adaptation. Metabolic adaptation to high-fat diets will take approximately 8–12 weeks to allow for mitochondrial adaptation (Reynolds et al., 1994; Reinhart, 1998). This helps to prevent steatorrhea, which is a common occurrence when feeding high-fat diets. Excess fat in the diet may also require an increase in divalent cation nutrients (calcium,

iron, zinc, copper, and manganese) due to soap formation with free fatty acids chelating these cations, particularly calcium, making them less available for absorption.

The amount of fat in the Greyhound diet is highly debated as studies by Toll and colleagues have shown that Greyhounds on a high-carbohydrate diet (46% ME vs 6% ME) ran 0.4 km/h faster (Toll et al., 1992). The high-carbohydrate diets contained only 31% ME fat, while the high-fat diet consisted of 75% ME as fat. Hill and colleagues showed slightly different results suggesting that Greyhounds fed 25% ME protein, 32% ME fat, and 43% ME carbohydrate performed better than those on a higher carbohydrate diet (21% ME protein, 25% ME fat, and 54 % ME carbohydrate; Hill et al., 1999). These results taken together with previous reports suggesting higher carbohydrate diets enhance performance imply that approximately 30% ME fat and 24% ME protein with the remaining ME from carbohydrate seems adequate for racing Greyhounds. Surprisingly, this type of dietary breakdown results in a product that would be approximately 24–28% dry matter protein, 12–14 % dry matter fat, and 45–50% carbohydrate, which is similar to many commercial adult pet foods on the market.

Very little information regarding optimal dietary fats for canine athletes is available, but there has been some speculation that chain length and saturation can affect a variety of issues, from inflammation to oxidative potential during exercise (Bauer, 2006). Medium-chain triglycerides when digested liberate 8- to 12-carbon fatty acids, which undergo some direct absorption into the bloodstream and are transported via albumin to cells for metabolism (Table 4.2). This has led to speculation that medium-chain triglycerides in the form of coconut and palm oils can be used more rapidly at the initiation of exercise leading to further glycogen sparing (Hawley, 2002; Jeukendrup & Aldred, 2004). This does not appear to be the case in other species, and one pilot study in athletic dogs showed limited utility; thus it cannot currently be recommended as a strategy in fat adaptation (Reynolds et al., 1998). Consideration of polyunsaturated fatty acids will be reserved for the discussion of nutrition for rehabilitation where their influence on inflammation may be more pertinent. Since many performance

Table 4.2   Differences between medium- and long-chain triglycerides

	Medium-chain triglycerides	Long-chain triglycerides
Chain length	10–14 carbons long	16–22 carbons long
Kilocalories per gram	Approx. 8 kcal	Approx. 9 kcal
Primary GI absorption	Direct enterocyte to portal blood	Synthesis into chylomicrons
Transport in blood	Carried via albumin	Chylomicrons and lipoproteins
Cell absorption	Diffusion	Lipase-dependent absorption

animals, including Foxhounds, hunting dogs, and service dogs, rely on detection capabilities, the potential use of polyunsaturated fatty acids in olfaction is of interest. A small study using only four dogs in a Latin square design showed that olfactory performance was affected by altering fat content in the diet by adding either corn oil rich in polyunsaturated fatty acids or medium-chain triglycerides from coconut/palm oils. This study suggested that corn oil and its high linoleic acid might enhance olfactory capability in pointers. More importantly, scent detection may decrease with the use of medium-chain triglycerides (Altom et al., 2003). More recently a study looking at dietary fat and protein:fat ratios in the diet suggested that detection of target in trained detection Labradors was slightly better on a high corn oil diet where 54% of the ME was fat and only 18% of the ME was protein (Angle et al., 2014). Whether this was due to substrate utilization or the high polyunsaturated nature of the fat affecting olfaction cannot be determined, but physiologically the dogs on the corn oil-based high-fat diet had better thermal recovery from exercise (Ober et al., 2016). Another study examining hunting dogs suggested that a diet with slightly higher protein and higher fat improved bird find rates (Davenport et al., 2001). Whether this was due to the altered substrates, differences in ingredients, or long-chain polyunsaturated fat enrichment could not be determined based on the experimental design.

Carbohydrates—timing and strategy

The use of carbohydrates as a major dietary substrate makes sense in sprinting animals like Greyhounds, with approximately 40–50% of the ME in the diet as highly digestible carbohydrates. Endurance sled dogs may need less than 15% of the ME as carbohydrates, as there are no definitive carbohydrate requirements (Reinhart, 1998; Hill et al., 2001b), although this is now up for debate with findings of robust glucose utilization in endurance sled dogs (Miller et al., 2015).

Carbohydrate loading is a principle used in human athletics, which can translate into the canine arena. It may be beneficial for sprinting and intermediate athletes, particularly over multiple-day events, where muscle glycogen is depleted daily and needs to be replenished (Reynolds et al., 1997; Wakshlag et al., 2002b; McKenzie et al., 2008). Studies performed in sled dogs have definitively shown that post-exercise supplementation with a maltodextrin supplement at 1.5 g/kg BW within 30 minutes of exercise increases skeletal muscle glycogen within 4 to 24 hours. In both studies, it was evident that this dosing returned muscle glycogen to baseline concentrations before exercise the following day, while without supplementation skeletal muscle glycogen content was only 50% of baseline concentrations (Reynolds et al., 1997; Wakshlag et al., 2002b). Based on this information, post-exercise carbohydrate repletion is recommended in dogs running anywhere between 5 minutes and 3 hours per day, particularly when expected to perform similarly the following day. The effectiveness of this strategy in endurance events is unknown and is not routinely recommended.

In the human athletic arena, protein with carbohydrate is often provided post exercise. The protein is thought to help curb skeletal muscle proteolysis after intermediate exercise (Betts & Williams, 2010). This approach has not been examined in the canine performance arena. In human athletics, the use of whey-based protein in young athletes post exercise appears to help in retention of lean mass and

Case Study 4.1   Hitting the wall

History: A highly competitive sled dog team racing in open sprint races ranging from 16 to 30 miles over 2- or 3-day heats was very successful. As the season progressed this team competed in two longer races near the end of the season and placed disappointing fifth and seventh places when expected to be within the top three, based on previous performances. Track times for various points along the trail showed an average of approximately 19 miles per hour for the 20-mile heats on days one and two. The team was in third place by day two with day one time being better than day two for the two 20-mile heats (one hour average time for top finishers). This team performed very well on day three, running a 30-mile heat while maintaining a speed of 18 miles per hour for the first 22 miles. Their speed for the last eight miles of the race dropped to 13 miles per hour, dropping this team into a seventh place overall finish.

Examination of feeding practices: High-quality commercial kibble and fresh meat with an ME of approximately 32% protein/62% fat and 8% carbohydrate. They did not use post-exercise carbohydrate repletion supplements. This poor performance was assumed to be due to skeletal muscle glycogen depletion during days 1 and 2, so that by day 3 the dogs could work at only 50–60% of their $Vo_{2\,max}$ late in the race due to lack of carbohydrate oxidation capabilities. The following year this team altered the diet to contain 30% protein, 50% fat, and 20% carbohydrate ME and used post-exercise carbohydrate supplementation on days 1 and 2 of racing, and again became competitive in longer distance sprint racing in Alaska.

possibly improves glycogen repletion in some situations (Betts & Williams, 2010), but firm recommendation in canine performance cannot be given at the time of writing.

Dietary fiber

Dietary fiber, regardless of its form, leads to fecal bulk. This increase in fecal bulk can lead to inappropriate defecation during competition and extra weight carried by the competitor, which may be detrimental. Fiber comes in two forms; insoluble (nonfermentable) and soluble (fermentable). Insoluble fiber results in fecal bulk and acts as a binding agent that can improve fecal quality when diarrhea is a problem. Soluble fiber has the capacity to alter the large intestinal microflora and potentially increase the absorptive surface of the small and large intestine through villous hypertrophy. This has been used strategically in canid athletes with stress-related diarrhea. Soluble fiber tends to be a matrix on which certain bacterial genera, including bifidobacteria, lactobacilli, and streptococci, thrive (Wakshlag *et al.*, 2011; Gagné *et al.*, 2013). These bacterial genera ferment soluble fiber sources and liberate volatile fatty acids (acetate, butyrate, propionate) that promote colonocyte regeneration and may improve recovery from diarrhea (Whelan & Schneider, 2011). Many of the enteric formulas of commercial dog food use small amounts of gums, soy fiber, fructo-oligosaccharides, other oligosaccharides and mixed insoluble and soluble fiber sources, to improve fecal quality and intestinal absorptive capabilities. The amount of soluble fiber added is generally less than 2% of dry matter in the diet since overfermentation can result in deteriorating fecal quality (Beloshapka *et al.*, 2011). Mixed soluble and insoluble sources commonly added to commercial dog foods to improve fecal quality are chicory root, beet pulp, and psyllium. In many instances the addition of psyllium husk powder to feed is used in exercising canines to improve exercise-related stress diarrhea. Psyllium husk fiber is unique since it is a mucilage with water-binding properties and, much like other mixed fiber sources, provides a modest fermentation value. It is often recommended to start with approximately 4 g of psyllium (1 rounded teaspoon of fine powder) per day, titrating upward, not exceeding 16 g per day in a typical 20–30-kg canine athlete (Leib, 2000).

Electrolytes, minerals, and the canine athlete

Minerals can be classified into major minerals and trace minerals (Table 4.3). The major minerals are of most importance since deficiencies in dogs fed nontraditional diets (meat base without bone) have been observed. If meats are being used it is often advised to have the bones ground into the meat supply to improve the calcium and phosphorus balance. Calcium

Table 4.3   Essential major and trace minerals

Major minerals	Trace minerals
Potassium	Iron
Calcium	Zinc
Phosphorus	Copper
Sodium	Manganese
Chloride	Iodine
Magnesium	Selenium

should be between 0.6 and 1.2% dry matter, with similar amounts of phosphorus to maintain calcium homeostasis for structural integrity of bone and appropriate cellular signaling and buffering capacities (National Research Council, 2006c). Magnesium is also a concern when bone is not a constituent in a nontraditional diet when commercial feed is not being used. Deficiency can manifest in exercising dogs as hyperextension of the carpus. Deficiencies of other major minerals including sodium, potassium, and chloride have never been observed in adult working dogs. However, nonclinical hyponatremia has been observed in endurance Huskies during races and simulated endurance races (Hinchcliff *et al.*, 1993, 1997a, 1997c; McKenzie *et al.*, 2007). It is believed that due to the high calorie meat consumption and high water turnover rate during these strenuous exercises, sodium conservation is heightened by increases in the renin/aldosterone/angiotensin system as well as modest sodium loss causing a mild hyponatremia and hypokalemia (Hinchcliff *et al.*, 1997a, 1997c). It must be noted that this chronic hyponatremia was observed in the Yukon quest in 1992 and simulated endurance events with a specific kennel (Burr *et al.*, 1993; Hinchcliff *et al.*, 1997a, 1997c). Studies examining this phenomenon in three teams participating in the 2012 Yukon Quest suggest that each team responded differently. One team was provided with sodium chloride in the diet and showed no signs of subclinical hyponatremia or hypokalemia (Ermon *et al.*, 2014). More recently, Frank and colleagues examined correlations of electrolytes to muscle creatine kinase (CK) 2 days into a race and found that the declines in potassium and sodium were both correlated to a CK rise, suggesting that hypokalemia is associated with muscle cell permeability (Frank *et al.*, 2015). These findings do not warrant use of electrolyte mixtures to sustain dogs who are eating commercial rations as these studies are in dogs being fed large amounts of meat, which is low in sodium and potassium compared to their normal training rations. Currently studies using electrolyte mixtures have shown no beneficial effects and/or potential gastrointestinal upset (diarrhea) after a day of activity (Young *et al.*, 1960; Mazin *et al.*, 2001). Most importantly, if sufficient commercial dog food formulated according to the Association of American Feed Controls Officials (AAFCO) regulations is provided, supplementation with any of these major minerals is not necessary; however, it should be noted that calcium availability will be hindered when providing fat at over 60% of the ME in a feed. Competitions where aggressive fat supplementation is used are usually a few days to a week in duration and should not affect long-term calcium homeostasis.

Trace mineral intake (see Table 4.3) will increase proportionally with intake of commercial dog food and will also increase to a lesser degree when using meat to supplement commercial diets. To date there has not been an observed clinical deficiency in copper, zinc, iron, manganese, iodine, or selenium in athletic canines being fed traditional commercial or commercial dog food/meat mix diets. This is likely due to the amounts of trace minerals incorporated into most pet foods being greater than the minimum amount legislated by AAFCO, and the increased intake of food in athletic dogs. Currently, it is unknown whether supplemental trace minerals are needed, or if the amounts deemed sufficient for pet dogs will meet the demands of performance canids.

Vitamins/antioxidants and the canine athlete

Vitamins are classified as either fat- or water-soluble (Table 4.4). Water-soluble vitamins are involved in metabolism as intermediates and coenzymes within the citric acid cycle or as carriers and coenzymes for carbon transfer. Sufficiency in these vitamins is absolutely required for metabolism. Many commercial dog foods and meats tend to be fairly rich in these vitamins. Most commercial pet food will contain two to ten times the minimum requirement

Table 4.4   Essential water-soluble and fat-soluble vitamins

Water-soluble vitamins	Fat-soluble vitamins
Thiamin (B1)	Vitamin A
Riboflavin (B2)	Vitamin D
Niacin (B3)	Vitamin E
Pantothenic acid (B5)	Vitamin K
Pyridoxine (B6)	
Folic acid	
Cobalamin (B12)	
Choline	

since the water-soluble vitamins have large margins of safety. Vitamin C is the most abundant water-soluble antioxidant found in the mammalian body, and dogs sustain their requirements through hepatic synthesis; however, dogs may not synthesize as much as other species (Chatterjee *et al.*, 1975). Lack of high hepatic synthesis taken with the fact that serum ascorbic acid concentrations decreased more than 50% after an undefined race distance of 1.5 hours duration has led experts to speculate that supplementation may be useful (Kronfeld *et al.*, 1989). Similar decreases have been observed in unsupplemented exercising Greyhounds (1.8–2.8 mg/L; Marshall *et al.*, 2002; Scott *et al.*, 2002). Supplementation of 1 g of ascorbic acid per day returns serum concentrations closer to what is considered a normal baseline concentration (5–6 mg/L), but similar supplementation in Greyhounds for 4 weeks resulted in slower racing times by 0.3 km/h. Therefore vitamin C supplementation, having shown no definitive benefit for athletic canines, is not routinely recommended at the time of writing, particularly for racing Greyhounds.

Fat-soluble vitamins (A, D, E, and K) have smaller margins of safety and are more concerning. Sufficient vitamin K is synthesized by indigenous bacteria in the gastrointestinal tract of normal dogs. Vitamin A may be of more concern if organ meats are used as a portion of the diet, and they should not exceed 15% of any meat mix used to feed. This is due to the high concentration of vitamin A found in liver. Excess vitamin A consumption may manifest as poor coat quality, perturbed bone mineralization and hepatic damage. Dogs, as a species, are very tolerant to high dietary vitamin A (Morris

et al., 2010). Vitamin D is also found in organ meats, particularly liver, making a small amount of organ meat desirable if using meat as part of the diet. Many commercial dog foods have at least twice the cholecalciferol needed in the diet, so with the increased energy consumption required by athletic dogs, the amount of cholecalciferol consumed is usually adequate.

Vitamin E is sufficient in commercial pet food, and most manufacturers add significantly more than the requirements, making vitamin E deficiency unlikely. Deficiency has been observed in hunting dogs fed an all meat diet and was associated with retinal degeneration (Davidson *et al.*, 1998). Vitamin E has been examined extensively in endurance sled dogs, and low serum vitamin E was associated with an increased risk of being dropped from the Iditarod (race event). Additionally, serum vitamin E dropped after a single day of endurance activity in two separate studies (Kronfeld *et al.*, 1989; Piercy *et al.*, 2001a, 2001b). Increased serum creatine kinase was never directly correlated to low vitamin E concentrations in dogs exhibiting exertional rhabdomyolysis (Piercy *et al.*, 2001a). Similarly, decreased serum vitamin E concentrations have been observed in Greyhounds racing 500 m (Scott *et al.*, 2001). These finding suggested that supplementation might be beneficial. A consensus statement made by the Iditarod trail committee in 1996 stated that endurance sled dogs should be supplemented with 400 IU of vitamin E daily during training and racing in an effort to reduce exertional rhabdomyolysis. However, there appears to be no decrease in the incidence of exertional rhabdomyolysis (Iditarod Veterinary Trail committee, personal communication). More compelling evidence for not supplementing vitamin E was provided when Scott and colleagues and Hill and colleagues showed that although supplementing with 100 to 1000 IU raised serum tocopherol concentrations, dogs receiving 1000 IU had slowed racing times (Hill *et al.*, 2001a; Scott *et al.*, 2001). Tocopherol supplementation is not recommended in canine athletes as long as they are being fed sufficient complete and balanced dog food, while supplementation should be considered for dogs being fed nontraditional diets (primarily meats)—vitamin E (200–400 IU for a typical athletic 20- to 40-kg dog)—to prevent deficiency.

Some hypothesize that use of antioxidant cocktails has the ability to quench free radicals more effectively than single agents, and there have been two separate studies examining this concept. The first study used a mixture of 475 IU of alpha-tocopherol, 706 mg of vitamin C, and 5.1 mg of beta-carotene per kilogram of food for 3 weeks. The other study used 400 IU of alpha-tocopherol, 3 mg of beta-carotene, and 20 mg of lutein per kilogram of food for 4 weeks (Baskin et al., 2000; Piercy et al., 2000). Both studies found no association with decreased muscle damage as evaluated by CK and limited antioxidant potential during recovery, while serum concentrations increased for all of the supplemented antioxidants. Other single agent studies examining astaxanthin (a carotenoid) and blueberries (flavonoids) have shown increased antioxidant potential in serum with no association with improved performance (Dunlap et al., 2006; Reynolds et al., 2010). Based on the limited information and lack of benefits for performance, supplementation is not recommended at the time of writing.

Feeding strategies in canine athletes

Feeding patterns can affect performance. Frequency and time of feeding become important not only to decrease fecal bulk, but also to maximize metabolites that are typically used for the activity. Sprinting dogs running for less than 10 minutes during a single bout of exercise will benefit from modest feed restriction 24 hours prior to exercise (decreasing total meal by 20%) during single-day events to decrease fecal bulk. Although some advocate small carbohydrate meals before exercise to provide glucose as fuel for impending exercise, there are few data to support this strategy in dogs (Hawley et al., 1997). Sprinting and intermediate athletes, particularly agility and field trial dogs that perform multiple bouts of exercise in a day, may benefit from carbohydrates in small amounts immediately after a bout of exercise when expected to undertake another bout within 2–3 hours. If repetitive bouts are close together this may not be advised to avoid vomiting or regurgitation (Hill, 1998). During multiple days of competition, post-exercise glycogen repletion is advised within 30 minutes of the last bout of exercise for the day to replenish muscle glycogen.

Intermediate athletes exercising typically once a day for 20 to 120 minutes typically rely on both glycogen and fat for energy generation; therefore it is recommended that they be fed diets moderate in fat (50% of ME) and carbohydrate (20% ME), and high in protein (30% ME). This diet allows adequate muscle glycogen repletion during training and helps increase mitochondrial volume. Fat will be used as a primary fuel at rest and within 20 minutes of exercise allowing for glycogen sparing when these athletes are asked to run above 60% of $Vo_{2\ max}$. These athletes will benefit from post-exercise carbohydrate supplementation to restore muscle glycogen concentrations particularly during multiple-day events (Reynolds et al., 1997; Wakshlag et al., 2002b). In an effort to promote fat use and lipolysis, feeding a single meal each day may be advantageous with that meal about 2 hours post exercise. Modest feed restriction (20% of meal) the day before racing will prevent defecation during exercise, promote lipolysis, and decrease fecal bulk (Hill et al., 1999; Toll & Gillette, 2010). Care should be taken not to feed larger meals immediately after exercise particularly in larger, deep-chested breeds prone to gastric dilatation and volvulus.

Endurance athletes (i.e., Foxhounds and sled dogs) tend to be fed one or two large meals each day during training, which will typically need to be approximately 300–500 kcal/kg$^{0.75}$ during heavy training (Ordway et al., 1984; Musch et al., 1985; Decombaz et al., 1995; Hinchcliff et al., 1997b). These meals should be approximately 30% ME protein, 60–70% ME fat, and negligible carbohydrate (<10% ME). The ration will likely comprise over 50% commercial dog food, with the rest as high-fat meat. This is necessary to achieve the caloric density and digestibility needed for competitive racing and hunting. As training intensifies there are back-to-back runs of 60 miles or greater on different terrains, thus increasing caloric demands. These are often met by using high-fat meats in small chunks during rest periods on the trail. Little is known about the nutrient composition, but these tactics appear successful during competitive endurance sled dog training and racing. During racing, dogs are fed significantly larger meals during 4–8-hour or longer rest stops. Since carbohydrate is not a primary fuel for exercise in these athletes, post-exercise carbohydrate supplementation for glycogen repletion is not recommended. Foxhounds that course through fields every day and pointing dogs asked to hunt for multiple hours may benefit from post-exercise carbohydrates since they will rest for significant times (>8 hours) between exercise bouts. However, the more recent findings by Miller and colleagues suggests we may be rethinking these strategies in the future and that intermediate and endurance feeding may not be all that different (Miller et al., 2014).

Feeding primarily meat is not routinely recommended for dogs due to the incomplete nature of this feed, yet it is commonly practiced and is likely not detrimental for short periods of time (1–2 weeks). Typically meat is provided raw but most veterinary professionals recommend cooking the meat. Cooking does not appear to decrease digestibility significantly (Kerr et al., 2012). The major biological difference between raw and cooked meat is pathogen contamination in the former; this can cause detrimental health effects in both owners and dogs when feeding raw meat (Chengappa et al., 1993; Morley et al., 2006 Kukanich, 2011). Studies examining therapy dogs in Ontario have revealed that zoonotic pathogen exposure risk is approximately seven-fold higher for salmonella and 14 times higher for enterogenic antibiotic-resistant E. coli species (Lefebvre et al., 2008). This risk has prevented raw-fed dogs from becoming therapy dogs in Canada. In addition to the zoonotic risk, the effects of high salmonella burden have led to the demise of Greyhound puppies and increased the risk of diarrhea in adult Greyhounds when using poor quality raw meats (Chengappa et al., 1993). There have also been salmonella outbreaks associated with commercial foods (Schotte et al., 2007; Behravesh et al., 2010), but the relative risk and level of contamination is far greater in raw meats; therefore cooking is advised (Freeman & Michel, 2001; Weese et al., 2005).

Nutrition and rehabilitation

There are three major areas of concern to the canine rehabilitation patient including obesity management, maintaining lean body mass (particularly geriatric rehabilitation patients with sarcopenia), and decreasing chronic inflammation associated with orthopedic disease.

Obesity and rehabilitation

Obesity is the leading disease of dogs in western society, with nearly 40% of dogs being overweight to obese. The exact reasons are multifaceted, including overfeeding, lack of exercise, and a misconception of appropriate body condition by most dog owners (Laflamme, 2006). Obesity as a disease or as a complicating factor to orthopedic injury requires attention. In many situations, the orthopedic injury may lead to a sedentary lifestyle increasing the predisposition toward obesity, but recent evidence suggests that owner activity patterns are directly correlated with dog activity, and changing those exercise patterns in owners can be difficult (Wakshlag et al., 2012). It has been well documented that weight loss of as little as 11% of body-weight can have a positive impact on clinical signs associated with osteoarthritis (Impellizeri et al., 2000). There are many company-related resources, publications, and nutrition texts for weight management plans (Wakshlag et al., 2012).

The ideal diet for achieving appropriate weight loss is one that helps to maintain lean mass at the expense of fat mass and creates some level of satiety to prevent excessive begging or food-seeking behaviors. Two major strategies are used including increased fiber intake and high-protein diets that promote lean body mass retention. Fiber has been used and can be an efficacious way to decrease the caloric density of food, while maintaining gastric fill. Unfortunately, it induces only short-term satiety (Butterwick & Markwell, 1997; Weber et al., 2007). More importantly, the use of high-fiber diets (>12% dry matter) allows owners to feed more volume. This can also be achieved by switching from dry food to wet food since most low-calorie, high-fiber dry foods have a higher caloric density per cup than the average low-calorie high-fiber therapeutic wet food. High-protein diets (>30% dry matter) may be beneficial in maintaining lean body mass when fed during weight reduction. Additionally, dogs fed higher protein appear to maintain lean mass while losing weight. Similarly, a structured rehabilitation exercise protocol shows maintenance of lean body mass during weight loss as well. Neither strategy has been shown to increase weight loss, but dogs that are more active can eat more calories during the weight loss protocol, possibly improving compliance better. This appears to be an effective strategy for improving health during weight loss (Diez *et al.*, 2002; Weber *et al.*, 2007; Wakshlag *et al.*, 2010; Vitgar *et al.*, 2016).

Diet and rehabilitation in the geriatric dog

It has been fairly well documented that aging dogs undergo a slow deterioration of skeletal muscle mass, known as sarcopenia (Freeman, 2012). This coupled with neurogenic atrophy in many geriatric dogs leads to a thin body condition warranting rehabilitation to help preserve lean body mass and increase mobility. Many senior dog foods restrict fat and protein as pre-emptive measures to decrease obesity. For most geriatric rehabilitation patients with lean body mass deterioration these low-protein and low-kilocalorie diets are inappropriate. Due to the decrease in digestive capabilities in most lean aging dogs the need for higher calorie and protein foods during the rehabilitative process is warranted. Studies in young versus old dogs suggest that the need for protein to maintain hepatic and skeletal muscle protein turnover may nearly double from 2.5 g to approximately 4 g of protein per kg body-weight (Wannemacher & McCoy, 1966). Unfortunately, evidence-based medicine regarding the effects of rehabilitation and diet in geriatric canine patients is lacking. Based on present information, the geriatric rehabilitation canine patient should receive approximately 5 g/kg body-weight in high-quality protein. This translates into a moderate fat food (12–16% dry matter) containing approximately 28–30% dry matter protein, making normal adult canine food or even performance rations the preferred choice when feeding the sarcopenic geriatric rehabilitation patient.

Feeding to mitigate inflammation and joint disease

Orthopedic surgical patients or patients with chronic joint pain due to early or chronic osteoarthritis are commonly prescribed rehabilitation to improve muscle tone and mobility. These patients should use foods with additional long-chain omega-3 fatty acids. The most common sources of fat in commercial dog foods come in the form of saturated, monounsaturated, and polyunsaturated fatty acids (Figure 4.8). The polyunsaturated fatty acids come from plant, animal, or marine sources. Plant sources supply either linoleic acid, an omega-6 fatty acid; or alpha-linolenic acid, an omega-3 fatty acid. The canine body has a limited ability to elongate these 18-carbon fatty acids into 20-carbon fatty acids including arachidonic acid (AA) and eicosapentaenoic acid

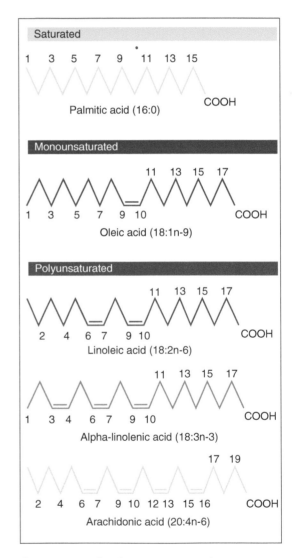

Figure 4.8 Fat classifications as saturated, monounsaturated, and polyunsaturated, which are divided into omega-3 and omega-6 fatty acids based on where the first double bond is found from the omega carbon, labeled as 1 in this diagram. Source: Picture reproduced from Hand *et al.*, 2010.

(EPA) in particular (Figure 4.9). AA is a precursor to the normal production of eicosanoids—prostaglandin E_2 (PGE_2) and leukotriene B_4 (LTB_4)—through the cyclooxygenase and lipoxygenase enzymes, which are involved in the inflammatory response as well as maintenance of mucosal integrity. Therefore, if EPA or its slightly longer omega-3 counterpart docosahexaenoic acid (DHA) is substituted for AA in the diet there is less production of the pro-inflammatory eicosanoids such as PGE_2 and LTB_4 (see Figure 4.9). This results in less cartilage degradation due to lower metalloprotease and local cytokine production, allowing for better

glycosaminoglycan and collagen production (Budsberg & Bartges, 2006). This supplementation of long-chain omega-3 fatty acids results in improved clinical outcomes in osteoarthritis (Fritsch et al.; 2010; Roush et al., 2010). The form of omega-3 fatty acid used is important since the shorter chain omega-3 fatty acid, often supplemented as alpha-linolenic acid (flaxseed oil), may not exert the same anti-inflammatory effects as the longer chain omega-3 fatty acids (EPA, DHA) found in marine oils (Bauer, 2006). The dose of fish oil in these cases may be more than what is traditionally used in over-the-counter commercial dog foods. Evidence suggests that

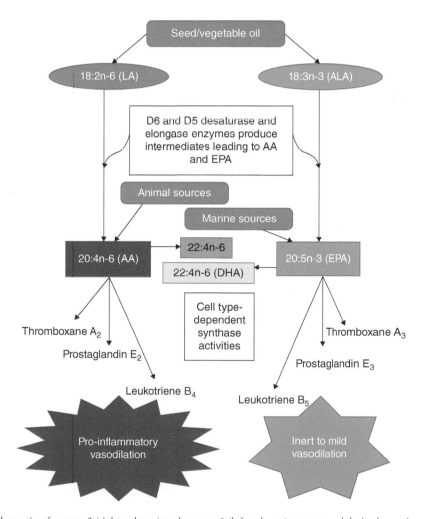

Figure 4.9 Schematic of omega-3 (right column) and omega-6 (left column) sources and their elongation and conversion into bioactive molecules during the inflammatory response. Note that the omega-3 fatty acids become odd-series eicosanoids (i.e., PGE_3), which are inert and that can inhibit the pro-inflammatory actions of the omega-6 fatty acid-generated eicosanoids designated by even numbers (i.e., PGE_2). LA, linoleic acid; ALA, alpha-linolenic acid; AA, arachidonic acid; EPA, eicosapentaenoic acid; DHA, docosahexaenoic acid.

a total dose of approximately 1 g of EPA/DHA per 10 kg body-weight is effective (Fritsch *et al.*, 2010, Roush *et al.*, 2010). Many clients will prefer to supplement with fish oil. The strength and number of capsules needed differ tremendously, so regular-strength liquid white fish or salmon oil that provides approximately 250 mg of EPA and DHA per gram is advised. One teaspoon contains approximately 1 g of EPA/DHA mixture. Dogs eating a typical over-the-counter adult commercial dog food should receive about one teaspoon of fish oil per 10 kg body-weight to achieve the dose needed for joint inflammation. Each teaspoon of fish oil contains approximately 45 kcal, and the food provided should be adjusted appropriately to avoid weight gain when multiple teaspoons are being used. Additionally, this dilutes the nutrient content of the food provided, therefore a higher protein food (>28% dry matter) is recommended.

Freeze dried *Perna cannaliculus*, also known as New Zealand green lipped mussel (GLM), contains glucosamine, chondroitin sulfate, and long-chain omega-3 fatty acids. Two clinical studies performed using a food enriched with GLM found improvement of joint crepitus and joint pain resulting in clinically improved joint scores when evaluated by veterinary surgeons (Bui & Bierer, 2001; Pollard *et al.*, 2006). GLM can be found in a variety of supplements. However, it is commonly thought that freeze-dried GLM is superior as this process preserves the fatty acid component. A clinically effective dose of GLM has not been elucidated, but based on data of GLM incorporated into a commercial pet food, and a non-commissioned study, 50–100 mg/kg body-weight may be an appropriate dose (Pollard *et al.*, 2006; Hielm-Borkman *et al.*, 2009).

Glucosamine and chondroitin sulfate (a larger conglomerate of glucosamine molecules) have been extensively studied in human clinical trials for osteoarthritis. The outcomes have been varied and the largest clinical trial in osteoarthritis did not reveal any benefits for joint pain or range of motion, except for chondroitin sulfate in the most severe cases of osteoarthritis (Towheed *et al.*, 2005; Hochberg & Clegg, 2008; Sawitzke *et al.*, 2010). This suggests that once osteoarthritis is present supplementation has no bearing on pain associated with the disease. Due to some evidence that glucosamine diminishes cartilage degeneration over time, it may still be prudent to initiate glucosamine and/or chondroitin sulfate treatment early in the disease process and continue it indefinitely as it has been proven safe (Sarzi-Puttini *et al.*, 2005; Aragon *et al.*, 2007). The only clinical studies examining its use in osteoarthritis show potential for benefits when assessed by clients and veterinarians, yet there were no differences in gait or subjective assessment in one study with placebo control (Moreau *et al.*, 2003; McCarthy *et al.*, 2007). In the age of evidence-based medicine there is no clinical evidence for its use. However, many orthopedists and rehabilitation therapists are proponents of its use. A range of other nutraceuticals including elk velvet, resin, curcumin, undenatured collagen type II, *Bosswelia serrata*, and hyperimmunized cow protein isolates, which have some clinical evidence supporting their use, have been reviewed elsewhere (Aragon *et al.*, 2007).

Case Study 4.2   Rehabilitation optimization

Signalment: 12 y.o. M/N 26-kg Siberian Husky in good body condition (5/9) with a right cranial cruciate rupture for over 19 months. Left cranial cruciate ligament ruptured and clients agreed to bilateral TTA surgery. Right stifle had chronic progressing severe osteoarthritis.

Evaluation for rehabilitation: Diet history noted that patient has been eating 3.5 cups of a senior dog food with 18% protein, 12% fat and has 375 kcal per cup. Ingredient list shows a chicken meal base with rice, barley, canola oil, and animal fat. Diet evaluation reveals that patient is getting only 3.0 g of protein per kg body-weight, and has no glucosamine or omega-3 fatty acids. Client resisted using therapeutic food due to cost so rehabilitation therapist looked to commercial over-the-counter products and supplementation. Therapist found a food that has 32% protein, 16% fat, and 405 kcal per cup. Feeding the patient approximately 3 cups per day, provides 4 g of protein per kg body-weight. Additional supplementation for inflammatory joint disease was instituted as fish oil at 2.5 teaspoons per day and 1000 mg of glucosamine/chondroitin sulfate mix daily during initiation of this patient's rehabilitation plan.

Webliography

Purina (2012) Understanding your Dog's Body Condition. Purina.com. http://www.library.tufts.edu/vet/images/bcs_dog.pdf

References

Altom, E. K., Davenport, G. M., Myers, L. J. & Cummins, K. A. 2003. Effect of dietary fat source and exercise on odorant-detecting ability of canine athletes. *Res Vet Sci*, 75, 149–155.

Angle, T. C., Wakshlag, J. J., Gillette, R. L., Steury, T., Haney, P., Barrett, J., & Fisher, T. 2014. The effects of exercise and diet on olfactory capability in detection dogs. *J Nutr Sci*, 3, e44.

Aragon, C. L., Hofmeister, E. H., & Budsberg, S. C. 2007. Systematic review of clinical trials of treatments for osteoarthritis in dogs. *J Am Vet Med Assoc*, 230, 514–21.

Baskin, C. R., Hinchcliff, K. W., Disilvestro, R. A., Reinhart, G. A., Hayek, M. G., Chew, B. P., *et al.* 2000. Effects of dietary antioxidant supplementation on oxidative damage and resistance to oxidative damage during prolonged exercise in sled dogs. *Am J Vet Res*, 61, 886–891.

Bauer, J. E. 2006. Facilitative and functional fats in diets of cats and dogs. *J Am Vet Med Assoc*, 229, 680–684.

Behravesh, C. B., Ferraro, A., Deasy, M., 3rd, Dato, V., Moll, M., Sandt, C., *et al.* 2010. Human Salmonella infections linked to contaminated dry dog and cat food, 2006-2008. *Pediatrics*, 126, 477–483.

Beloshapka, A. N., Wolff, A. K., & Swanson, K. S. 2012. Effects of feeding polydextrose on faecal characteristics, microbiota and fermentative end products in healthy adult dogs. *Br J Nutr*, 108(4), 638–644.

Betts, J. A. & Williams, C. 2010. Short-term recovery from prolonged exercise: exploring the potential for protein ingestion to accentuate the benefits of carbohydrate supplements. *Sports Med*, 40, 941–959.

Bierer, T. L. & Bui, L. M. 2004. High-protein low-carbohydrate diets enhance weight loss in dogs. *J Nutr*, 134, 2087S–2089S.

Budsberg, S. C. & Bartges, J. W. 2006. Nutrition and osteoarthritis in dogs: does it help? *Vet Clin North Am Small Anim Pract*, 36, 1307–1323, vii.

Bui, L. M. & Bierer, R. L. 2001. Influence of green lipped mussels (*Perna canaliculus*) in alleviating signs of arthritis in dogs. *Vet Ther*, 2, 101–111.

Burr, J. F., Reinhart, G. A., Swenson, R. A., Swaim, S. E., Vaughn, D. M., & Bradley, D. M. 1993 Serum biochemical values in sled dogs before and after competing in long-distance races. *J Am Vet Med Assoc*, 211, 175–179.

Butterwick, R. F. & Markwell, P. J. 1997. Effect of amount and type of dietary fiber on food intake in energy-restricted dogs. *Am J Vet Res*, 58, 272–276.

Chatterjee, I. B., Majumder, A. K., Nandi, B. K., & Subramanian, N. 1975. Synthesis and some major functions of vitamin C in animals. *Ann N Y Acad Sci*, 258, 24–47.

Chengappa, M. M., Staats, J., Oberst, R. D., Gabbert, N. H., & McVey, S. 1993. Prevalence of Salmonella in raw meat used in diets of racing greyhounds. *J Vet Diagn Invest*, 5, 372–377.

Davenport, G. M., Kelley, R. L., Altom, E. K., & Lepine, A. J. 2001. Effect of diet on hunting performance of English pointers. *Vet Ther*, 2, 10–23.

Davidson, M. G., Geoly, F. J., Gilger, B. C., McLellan, G. J., & Whitley, W. 1998. Retinal degeneration associated with vitamin E deficiency in hunting dogs. *J Am Vet Med Assoc*, 213, 645–651.

Decombaz, J., Jambon, M., Pigueet, C., Thelin, A., & Bellevre, O. 1995. Energy intake and expenditure of sled dogs during the Alpirod race 1995. In: Grandjean, D. & Vanek, J. (eds), *Second Annual International Sled Dog Veterinary Medical Association Symposium*, September 18–19, 1995, Reims, France, pp. 113–118.

Diez, M., Nguyen, P., Jeusette, I., Devois, C., Istasse, L., & Biourge, V. 2002. Weight loss in obese dogs: evaluation of a high-protein, low-carbohydrate diet. *J Nutr*, 132, 1685S–1687S.

Downey, R. L., Kronfeld, D. S., & Banta, C. A. 1980. Diet of Beagles affects stamina. *J Am Anim Hosp Assoc*, 16, 273–277.

Dunlap, K. L., Reynolds, A. J., & Duffy, L. K. 2006. Total antioxidant power in sled dogs supplemented with blueberries and the comparison of blood parameters associated with exercise. *Comp Biochem Physiol A Mol Integr Physiol*, 143, 429–434.

Ermon, V., Yazwinski, M., Milizio, J. G., & Wakshlag, J. J. 2014. Serum chemistry and electrolyte alterations in sled dogs before and after a 1600 km race: dietary sodium and hyponatraemia. *J Nutr Sci*, 25(3), e26.

Frank, L., Mann, S., Johnson, J., Levine, C., Downey, R., Griffits, C., & Wakshlag, J. 2015. Plasma chemistry before and after two consecutive days of racing in sled dogs: associations between muscle damage and electrolyte status. *Comp Exer Phys*, 11, 151–158.

Freeman, L. M. 2012. Cachexia and sarcopenia: emerging syndromes of importance in dogs and cats. *J Vet Intern Med*, 26, 3–17.

Freeman, L. M. & Michel, K. E. 2001. Evaluation of raw food diets for dogs. *J Am Vet Med Assoc*, 218, 705–709.

Fritsch, D., Allen, T. A., Dodd, C. E., Jewell, D. E., Sixby, K. A., Leventhal, P. S., & Hahn, K. A. 2010.

Dose-titration effects of fish oil in osteoarthritic dogs. *J Vet Intern Med*, 24, 1020–1026.

Gagné, J. W., Wakshlag, J. J., Simpson, K. W., Dowd, S. E., Latchman, S., Brown, D., *et al.* 2013. Effects of a synbiotic on fecal quality, short-chain fatty acid concentrations, and the microbiome of healthy racing sled dogs. *BMC Vet Res*, 9, 246.

Granjean, D. 1998. Nutrition for sled dogs. In: Bloomberg, M. S., Dee, J. F., & Taylor, R. A. (eds), *Canine Sports Medicine and Surgery*. Philadelphia, PA: Saunders, pp. 336–347.

Hammel, E. P., Kronfeld, D. S., Ganjam, V. K. & Dunlap, H. L., Jr. 1977. Metabolic responses to exhaustive exercise in racing sled dogs fed diets containing medium, low, or zero carbohydrate. *Am J Clin Nutr*, 30, 409–418.

Hand, M. S., Thatcher, C. D., Remillard, R. L., Roudebush, P., & Novotny, B. J. (eds). 2010. *Small Animal Clinical Nutrition*, 5th edn. Marceline, MO: Mark Morris Institute, pp. 323–357.

Hargreaves, M., Costill, D. L., Coggan, A., Fink, W. J., & Nishibata, I. 1984. Effect of carbohydrate feedings on muscle glycogen utilization and exercise performance. *Med Sci Sports Exerc*, 16, 219–222.

Hawley, J. A. 2002. Effect of increased fat availability on metabolism and exercise capacity. *Med Sci Sports Exerc*, 34, 1485–1491.

Hawley, J. A., Schabort, E. J., Noakes, T. D., & Dennis, S. C. 1997. Carbohydrate-loading and exercise performance. An update. *Sports Med*, 24, 73–81.

Hielm-borkman, A., Tulamo, R. M., Salonen, H., & Raekallio, M. 2009. Evaluating complementary therapies for canine osteoarthritis Part I: Green-lipped mussel (*Perna canaliculus*). *Evid-Based Compl Alt*, 6(3), 365–373.

Hill, R., Lewis, D., Scott, K., Randell, S., Sundstrom, D., Speakman, J., & Butterwick, R. 1999. Mild food restriction increases the speed of racing Greyhounds. *J Vet Int Med*, 13, 281.

Hill, R. C. 1998. The nutritional requirements of exercising dogs. *J Nutr*, 128, 2686S–2690S.

Hill, R. C., Bloomberg, M. S., Legrand-defretin, V., Burger, I. H., Hillock, S. M., Sundstrom, D. A., & Jones, G. L. 2000. Maintenance energy requirements and the effect of diet on performance of racing Greyhounds. *Am J Vet Res*, 61, 1566–1573.

Hill, R. C., Armstrong, D., Browne, R. W., Lewis, D. D., Scott, K. C., Sundstrom, D., & Harper, J. 2001a. Chronic administration of high doses of vitamin E appear to slow racing greyhounds. *FASEB J*, 15, A990.

Hill, R. C., Lewis, D. D., Scott, K. C., Omori, M., Jackson, M., Sundstrom, D. A., *et al.* 2001b. Effect of increased dietary protein and decreased dietary carbohydrate on performance and body composition in racing Greyhounds. *Am J Vet Res*, 62, 440–447.

Hinchcliff, K. W., Olson, J., Crusberg, C., Kenyon, J., Long, R., Royle, W., *et al.* 1993. Serum biochemical changes in dogs competing in a long-distance sled race. *J Am Vet Med Assoc*, 202, 401–405.

Hinchcliff, K. W., Reinhart, G. A., Burr, J. R., Schreier, C. J., & Swenson, R. A. 1997a. Effect of racing on serum sodium and potassium concentrations and acid-base status of Alaskan sled dogs. *J Am Vet Med Assoc*, 210, 1615–1618.

Hinchcliff, K. W., Reinhart, G. A., Burr, J. R., Schreier, C. J., & Swenson, R. A. 1997b. Metabolizable energy intake and sustained energy expenditure of Alaskan sled dogs during heavy exertion in the cold. *Am J Vet Res*, 58, 1457–1462.

Hinchcliff, K. W., Reinhart, G. A., Burr, J. R., & Swenson, R. A. 1997c. Exercise-associated hyponatremia in Alaskan sled dogs: urinary and hormonal responses. *J Appl Physiol*, 83, 824–829.

Hinchcliff, K. W., Shaw, L. C., Vukich, N. S., & Schmidt, K. E. 1998. Effect of distance traveled and speed of racing on body weight and serum enzyme activity of sled dogs competing in a long-distance race. *J Am Vet Med Assoc*, 213, 639–644.

Hochberg, M. C. & Clegg, D. O. 2008. Potential effects of chondroitin sulfate on joint swelling: a GAIT report. *Osteoarthritis Cartilage*, 16(Suppl. 3), S22–S24.

Impellizeri, J. A., Tetrick, M. A., & Muir, P. 2000. Effect of weight reduction on clinical signs of lameness in dogs with hip osteoarthritis. *J Am Vet Med Assoc*, 216, 1089–1091.

Jeukendrup, A. E. & Aldred, S. 2004. Fat supplementation, health, and endurance performance. *Nutrition*, 20, 678–688.

Kenyon, C. L., Basaraba, R. J., & Bohn, A. A. 2011. Influence of endurance exercise on serum concentrations of iron and acute phase proteins in racing sled dogs. *J Am Vet Med Assoc*, 239, 1201–1210.

Kerr, K. R., Vester Boler, B. M., Morris, C. L., Liu, K. J. & Swanson, K. S. 2012. Apparent total tract energy and macronutrient digestibility and fecal fermentative end-product concentrations of domestic cats fed extruded, raw beef-based, and cooked beef-based diets. *J Anim Sci*, 90, 515–522.

Kohnke, J. R. 1998. Nutrition in the racing Greyhound. In: Bloomberg, M. S., Dee, J. F., & Taylor, R. A. (eds), *Canine Sports Medicine and Surgery*. Philadelphia, PA: Saunders, pp. 328–336.

Kronfeld, D. S., Hammel, E. P., Ramberg, C. F., Jr, & Dunlap, H. L., Jr. 1977. Hematological and metabolic responses to training in racing sled dogs fed diets containing medium, low, or zero carbohydrate. *Am J Clin Nutr*, 30, 419–430.

Kronfeld, D. S., Adkins, T. O., & Downey, R. L. 1989. Nutrition, anaerobic and aerobic exercise and stress. In: Burger, I. H. & Rivers, J. P. W. (eds), *Nutrition of the Dog and Cat: Waltham Symposium*.

New York, NY: Cambridge University Press, pp. 133–145.

Kukanich, K. S. 2011. Update on Salmonella spp. contamination of pet food, treats, and nutritional products and safe feeding recommendations. *J Am Vet Med Assoc*, 238, 1430–1434.

Laflamme, D. P. 1997. Development and validation of a body condition score system for dogs. In: *Canine Practice*. Santa Barbara, CA: Veterinary Practice Publishing Co., 22, pp. 10–15.

Laflamme, D. P. 2006. Understanding and managing obesity in dogs and cats. *Vet Clin North Am Small Anim Pract*, 36, 1283–1295.

Lefebvre, S. L., Reid-smith, R., Boerlin, P., & Weese, J. S. 2008. Evaluation of the risks of shedding salmonellae and other potential pathogens by therapy dogs fed raw diets in Ontario and Alberta. *Zoonoses Public Hlth*, 55, 470–480.

Leib, M. S. 2000. Treatment of chronic idiopathic large-bowel diarrhea in dogs with a highly digestible diet and soluble fiber: a retrospective review of 37 cases. *J Vet Intern Med*, 14, 27–32.

Loftus J. P., Yazqinski, M., Milizio, J. G., & Wakshlag, J. J. 2014. Energy requirements for racing endurance sled dogs. *J Nutr Sci*, 3, e34.

Marshall, R. J., Scott, K. C., Hill, R. C., Lewis, D. D., Sundstrom, D., Jones, G. L., & Harper, J. 2002. Supplemental vitamin C appears to slow racing greyhounds. *J Nutr*, 132, 1616S–1621S.

Mazin, R. M., Fordyce, H. H., & Otto, C. M. 2001. Electrolyte replacement in urban search and rescue dogs: a field study. *Vet Ther*, 2, 140–147.

McCarthy, G., O'donovan, J., Jones, B., McAllister, H., Seed, M., & Mooney, C. 2007. Randomised double-blind, positive-controlled trial to assess the efficacy of glucosamine/chondroitin sulfate for the treatment of dogs with osteoarthritis. *Vet J*, 174, 54–61.

McKenzie, E. C., Hinchcliff, K. W., Valberg, S. J., Williamson, K. K., Payton, M. E., & Davis, M. S. 2008. Assessment of alterations in triglyceride and glycogen concentrations in muscle tissue of Alaskan sled dogs during repetitive prolonged exercise. *Am J Vet Res*, 69, 1097–1103.

McKenzie, E. C., Jose-cunilleras, E., Hinchcliff, K. W., Holbrook, T. C., Royer, C., Payton, M. E., *et al.* 2007. Serum chemistry alterations in Alaskan sled dogs during five successive days of prolonged endurance exercise. *J Am Vet Med Assoc*, 230, 1486–1492.

Miller, B. F., Drake, J. C., Peelor, F. F., Biela, L. M., Geor, R., Hinchcliff, K., *et al.* 2015. Participation in a 1,000-mile race increases the oxidation of carbohydrate in Alaskan sled dogs. *J Appl Physiol*, 118, 1502–1509.

Moreau, M., Dupuis, J., Bonneau, N. H., & Desnoyers, M. 2003. Clinical evaluation of a nutraceutical,

carprofen and meloxicam for the treatment of dogs with osteoarthritis. *Vet Rec*, 15; 152(11), 323–9.

Morley, P. S., Strohmeyer, R. A., Tankson, J. D., Hyatt, D. R., Dargatz, D. A. & Fedorka-cray, P. J. 2006. Evaluation of the association between feeding raw meat and Salmonella enterica infections at a Greyhound breeding facility. *J Am Vet Med Assoc*, 228, 1524–1532.

Morris, P., Salt, C., Raila, J., Breten, T., Kohn, B., Schweigert, F., & Zentek, J. 2010. The effects of feeding vitamin A to puppies up to 52 weeks of age. In: *The Waltham International Science Symposium: Pet Nutrition–Art or Science?* Cambridge, UK, p. 52.

Musch, T. I., Haidet, G. C., Ordway, G. A., Longhurst, J. C. & Mitchell, J. H. 1985. Dynamic exercise training in foxhounds. I. Oxygen consumption and hemodynamic responses. *J Appl Physiol*, 59, 183–189.

National Research Council. 2006a. Comparative digestive physiology of dogs and cats. In: *Nutrient Requirements of Dogs and Cats*. Washington, DC: National Academy Press, pp. 5–21.

National Research Council. 2006b. Energy. In: *Nutrient Requirements of Dogs and Cats*. Washington, DC: The National Academies Press, pp. 29–48.

National Research Council. 2006c. Minerals. In: *Nutrient Requirements of Dogs and Cats*. Washington, DC: National Academy Press, pp. 145–192.

Ober, J., Gillete, R. L., Angle, T. C., Haney, P., Fletcher, D. J., & Wakshlag, J. J. 2016. The effects of varying concentrations of dietary protein and fat on blood gas, hematologic serum chemistry, and body temperature before and after exercise in Labrador Retrievers. *Front Vet Sci*, 3, 59.

Ordway, G. A., Floyd, D. L., Longhurst, J. C., & Mitchell, J. H. 1984. Oxygen consumption and hemodynamic responses during graded treadmill exercise in the dog. *J Appl Physiol*, 57, 601–607.

Orr, N. W. 1966. The feeding of sledge dogs on Antarctic expeditions. *Br J Nutr*, 20, 1–12.

Piercy, R. J., Hinchcliff, K. W., Disilvestro, R. A., Reinhart, G. A., Baskin, C. R., Hayek, M. G., *et al.* 2000. Effect of dietary supplements containing antioxidants on attenuation of muscle damage in exercising sled dogs. *Am J Vet Res*, 61, 1438–1445.

Piercy, R. J., Hinchcliff, K. W., Morley, P. S., Disilvestro, R. A., Reinhart, G. A., Nelson, S. L., Jr, Schmidt, K. E., & Craig, A. M. 2001a. Vitamin E and exertional rhabdomyolysis during endurance sled dog racing. *Neuromuscul Disord*, 11, 278–286.

Piercy, R. J., Hinchcliff, K. W., Morley, P. S., Disilvestro, R. A., Reinhart, G. A., Nelson, S. L., *et al.* 2001b. Association between vitamin E and enhanced athletic performance in sled dogs. *Med Sci Sports Exerc*, 33, 826–833.

Pollard, B., Guilford, W. G., Ankenbauer-perkins, K. L., & Hedderley, D. 2006. Clinical efficacy and tolerance of an extract of green-lipped mussel (*Perna canaliculus*) in dogs presumptively diagnosed with degenerative joint disease. *N Z Vet J*, 54, 114–118.

Querengaesser, A., Iben, C., & Leibetseder, J. 1994. Blood changes during training and racing in sled dogs. *J Nutr*, 124, 2760S–2764S.

Reinhart, G. A. 1998. Nutrition for sporting dogs. In: Bloomberg, M. S., Dee, J. F., & Taylor, R. A. (eds), *Canine Sports Medicine and Surgery*. Philadelphia, PA: Saunders, pp. 348–356.

Reynolds, A. J., Fuhrer, L., Dunlap, H. L., Finke, M. D., & Kallfelz, F. A. 1994. Lipid metabolite responses to diet and training in sled dogs. *J Nutr*, 124, 2754S–2759S.

Reynolds, A. J., Fuhrer, L., Dunlap, H. L., Finke, M., & Kallfelz, F. A. 1995. Effect of diet and training on muscle glycogen storage and utilization in sled dogs. *J Appl Physiol*, 79, 1601–1607.

Reynolds, A. J., Carey, D. P., Reinhart, G. A., Swenson, R. A., & Kallfelz, F. A. 1997. Effect of post exercise carbohydrate supplementation on muscle glycogen repletion in trained sled dogs. *Am J Vet Res*, 58, 1252–1256.

Reynolds, A. J., Hayek, M. G., Lepine, A. J., & Sunvold, G. D. 1998. The role of fat in the formulation of performance rations: Focus on fat sources. In: Carey, D. P. & Reinhart, G. A. (eds), *Recent Advances in Canine and Feline Nutrition: 1998 Iams Nutrition Symposium Proceedings*. Wilmington, OH: Orange Frazer Press, Vol II, pp. 277–281.

Reynolds, A. J., Reinhart, G. A., Carey, D. P., Simmerman, D. A., Frank, D. A., & Kallfelz, F. A. 1999. Effect of protein intake during training on biochemical and performance variables in sled dogs. *Am J Vet Res*, 60, 789–795.

Reynolds, A. J., Jackson, J., Waldron, M. E., Leavitt, Y. E., Bailey, K. K., Milbury, P. E., & Blumberg, J. 2010. Comparison of astaxanthin, alpha tocopherol and placebo treatments on post exercise indices of oxidative stress in dogs. *Nestle Purina Nutrition Forum–Advances in Nutrition*, 74.

Roush, J. K., Cross, A. R., Renberg, W. C., Dodd, C. E., Sixby, K. A., Fritsch, D. A., *et al.* 2010. Evaluation of the effects of dietary supplementation with fish oil omega-3 fatty acids on weight bearing in dogs with osteoarthritis. *J Am Vet Med Assoc*, 236, 67–73.

Sarzi-puttini, P., Cimmino, M. A., Scarpa, R., Caporali, R., Parazzini, F., Zaninelli, A., *et al.* 2005. Osteoarthritis: an overview of the disease and its treatment strategies. *Semin Arthritis Rheum*, 35, 1–10.

Sawitzke, A. D., Shi, H., Finco, M. F., Dunlop, D. D., Harris, C. L., Singer, N. G., *et al.* 2010. Clinical efficacy and safety of glucosamine, chondroitin sulphate, their combination, celecoxib or placebo

taken to treat osteoarthritis of the knee: 2-year results from GAIT. *Ann Rheum Dis*, 69, 1459–1464.

Schmidt-nielsen, K. 1984. *Scaling, Why is Animal Size So Important?* Cambridge, UK: Cambridge University Press.

Schotte, U., Borchers, D., Wulff, C., & Geue, L. 2007. Salmonella Montevideo outbreak in military kennel dogs caused by contaminated commercial feed, which was only recognized through monitoring. *Vet Microbiol*, 119, 316–323.

Scott, K. C., Hill, R. C., Lewis, D. D., Boning, A. J., Jr, & Sundstrom, D. A. 2001. Effect of alpha-tocopheryl acetate supplementation on vitamin E concentrations in Greyhounds before and after a race. *Am J Vet Res*, 62, 1118–1120.

Scott, K. C., Hill, R. C., Lewis, D. D., Gronwall, R., Sundstrom, D. A., Jones, G. L., & Harper, J. 2002. Serum ascorbic acid concentrations in previously unsupplemented greyhounds after administration of a single dose of ascorbic acid intravenously or per os. *J Anim Physiol Anim Nutr*, 86, 222–228.

Shulman, G. I. & Petersen, K. F. 2009. Metabolism. In: Boron, W. F. & Boulpaep, E. L. (eds), *Cellular Medical Physiology: A Cellular and Molecular Approach*, 2nd edn. Philadelphia, PA: Saunders-Elsevier, pp. 1170–1174.

Taylor, C. R., Caldwell, S. L., & Rowntree, V. J. 1972. Running up and down hills: some consequences of size. *Science*, 178, 1096–1097.

Taylor, R. J. 1957. The work output of sledge dogs. *J Physiol*, 137, 210–217.

Toll, P. W. & Gillette, R. L. 2010. The canine athlete. In: Hand, M. S., Thatcher, C. D., Remillard, R. L., Roudebush, P., & Novotny, B. J. (eds), *Small Animal Clinical Nutrition*, 5th edn. Marceline, MO: Mark Morris Institute, pp. 323–357.

Toll, P. W., Pieschl, R. L., & Hand, M. S. 1992. The effect of dietary fat and carbohydrate on sprint performance in racing greyhound dogs. In: *Proceedings of the 8th International Racing Greyhound Symposium, North American Veterinary Conference*. Gainesville, FL: North American Veterinary Conference, pp. 1–3.

Towheed, T. E., Maxwell, L., Anastassiades, T. P., Shea, B., Houpt, J., Robinson, V., *et al.* 2005. Glucosamine therapy for treating osteoarthritis. *Cochrane Database Syst Rev*, CD002946.

Vitgar, A. D., Stallknecht, B. M., Nielsen, D. H., & Bjornvad, C. R. 2016. Integration of a physical activity in a weight loss plan for overweight pet dogs. *J Am Vet Med Assoc*, 248, 174–182.

Wagner, J. A., Horvath, S. M., & Dahms, T. E. 1977. Cardiovascular, respiratory, and metabolic adjustments to exercise in dogs. *J Appl Physiol*, 42, 403–407.

Wakshlag, J. J., Kallfelz, F. A., Barr, S. C., Ordway, G., Haley, N. J., Flaherty, C. E., *et al.* 2002a. Effects of exercise on canine skeletal muscle proteolysis: an investigation of the ubiquitin-proteasome pathway and other metabolic markers. *Vet Ther*, 3, 215–225.

Wakshlag, J. J., Snedden, K. A., Otis, A. M., Kennedy, C. A., Kennett, T. P., Scarlett, J. M., *et al.* 2002b. Effects of post-exercise supplements on glycogen repletion in skeletal muscle. *Vet Ther*, 3, 226–234.

Wakshlag, J. J., Cooper, B. J., Wakshlag, R. R., Kallfelz, F. A., Barr, S. C., Nydam, D. V., & Dimauro, S. 2004. Biochemical evaluation of mitochondrial respiratory chain enzymes in canine skeletal muscle. *Am J Vet Res*, 65, 480–484.

Wakshlag, J. J., Stokol, T., Geske, S. M., Greger, C. E., Angle, C. T., & Gillette, R. L. 2010. Evaluation of exercise-induced changes in concentrations of C-reactive protein and serum biochemical values in sled dogs completing a long-distance endurance race. *Am J Vet Res*, 71, 1207–1213.

Wakshlag, J., Struble, A., Simpson, K., & Dowd, S. 2011. Negative fecal characteristics are associated with pH and fecal flora alterations during dietary change in dogs. *Int J App Res Vet Med*, 9, 278–283.

Wakshlag, J. J., Struble, A. M., Warren, B. S., Maley, M., Panasevich, M. R., Cummings, K. J., *et al.* 2012. Evaluation of dietary energy intake and physical activity in dogs undergoing a controlled weight-loss program. *J Am Vet Med Assoc*, 240, 413–419.

Wannemacher, R. W., Jr & McCoy, J. R. 1966. Determination of optimal dietary protein requirements of young and old dogs. *J Nutr*, 88, 66–74.

Wasserman, D. H., Williams, P. E., Lacy, D. B., Green, D. R., & Cherrington, A. D. 1988. Importance of intrahepatic mechanisms to gluconeogenesis from alanine during exercise and recovery. *Am J Physiol*, 254, E518–525.

Wasserman, D. H., Spalding, J. A., Lacy, D. B., Colburn, C. A., Goldstein, R. E. & Cherrington, A. D. 1989. Glucagon is a primary controller of hepatic glycogenolysis and gluconeogenesis during muscular work. *Am J Physiol*, 257, E108–117.

Wasserman, D. H., Geer, R. J., Williams, P. E., Becker, T., Lacy, D. B. & Abumrad, N. N. 1991. Interaction of gut and liver in nitrogen metabolism during exercise. *Metabolism*, 40, 307–314.

Weber, M., Bissot, T., Servet, E., Sergheraert, R., Biourge, V., & German, A. J. 2007. A high-protein, high-fiber diet designed for weight loss improves satiety in dogs. *J Vet Intern Med*, 21, 1203–1208.

Weese, J. S., Rousseau, J., & Arroyo, L. 2005. Bacteriological evaluation of commercial canine and feline raw diets. *Can Vet J*, 46, 513–516.

Whelan, K. & Schneider, S. M. 2011. Mechanisms, prevention, and management of diarrhea in enteral nutrition. *Curr Opin Gastroenterol*, 27, 152–159.

Yamada, T., Tohori, M., Ashida, T., Kajiwara, N., & Yoshimura, H. 1987. Comparison of effects of vegetable protein diet and animal protein diet on the initiation of anemia during vigorous physical training (sports anemia) in dogs and rats. *J Nutr Sci Vitaminol*, 33, 129–149.

Young, D. R., Schafer, N. S., & Price, R. 1960. Effect of nutrient supplements during work on performance capacity in dogs. *J Appl Physiol*, 15, 1022–1026.

5 Introduction to Canine Rehabilitation

Amy Kramer, PT, DPT, CCRT, Amie Lamoreaux Hesbach, PT, DPT, MS, CCRP, CCRT, and Shari Sprague, MPT, CCRT, FP-ME, CCKTP

Summary

As the practice of canine rehabilitation and sports medicine continues to evolve, roles of practitioners are more specialized as approaches become more advanced. Clinical reasoning, care pathways, and specific applied interventions are adopted from the inter-professional practice of human sports medicine, requiring knowledge and understanding of the art and science of physical rehabilitation and related medical sciences. Contributing to a multifaceted team, the rehabilitation professional must be able to synthesize information related to the integrity and efficiency of the neuromusculoskeletal system, in coordination with other body systems, to affect the functional abilities of the patient. This is accomplished through the examination and evaluation of the patient with the purpose of identifying medical comorbidities, specific impairments, functional limitations, and disabilities. Understanding the interplay between the objective information collected during the rehabilitation examination and evaluation, patient-specific factors, and knowledge of basic sciences, physics, and biomechanics will guide the therapist in establishing a treatment plan that will ultimately contribute to the patient's return to an optimal level of function following injury, illness, or onset of a medical disorder or disease.

The purpose of this introductory chapter is to:
- Define the practice of canine rehabilitation.
- Describe various contributions of the different members of the interprofessional canine rehabilitation team.
- Discuss the history and evolution of the practice of canine rehabilitation in the United States and internationally.
- Describe the practice of physical therapy as it pertains to the management of the canine rehabilitation patient.
- Discuss specific physiological considerations for the canine rehabilitation therapist when planning rehabilitation interventions.
- Describe patient management and treatment planning methods by which the canine rehabilitation therapist coordinates the implementation of treatment strategies and interventions.

Canine Sports Medicine and Rehabilitation, Second Edition. Edited by Chris Zink and Janet B. Van Dyke.
© 2018 John Wiley & Sons, Inc. Published 2018 by John Wiley & Sons, Inc.

Defining the practice of canine rehabilitation

One of the challenges in establishing a new specialty is defining the specific characteristics of the practice as well as identifying the requisite level of knowledge, professional skills, clinical reasoning, and professional behaviors necessary for practitioners to safely and effectively provide specialized care. Canine rehabilitation has evolved from the practice of both veterinary medicine and human rehabilitation medicine, specifically, physical therapy. Professional and regulatory organizations are now faced with the task of defining this new collaborative specialty, in which both veterinarians and physical therapists practice, while examining the contributions from both fields as well.

Traditionally, the field of rehabilitation medicine has been driven by an interprofessional team that manages the individual needs of the patient and includes physical medicine and rehabilitation physicians, physical therapists, occupational therapists, speech language pathologists, nurses, physician extenders and other medical professionals.

Physical medicine and rehabilitation (PM&R), also referred to as physiatry, is a medical specialty with a focus on the management of physical and/or cognitive impairments that affect disability throughout the life span (American Board of Physical Medicine and Rehabilitation, 2016). Physiatrists are trained in the rehabilitation of disorders of the neurological, musculoskeletal, and other organ systems and in the long-term management of patients with disabling conditions. This specialty involves the secondary and tertiary prevention of disease and injury through the medical management of pain, comorbidities, and contextual factors specific to the individual patient. This is accomplished through diagnostic and therapeutic injection and electro-diagnostic procedures, as well as medication management. Physiatrists provide leadership to the interprofessional team concerned with the restoration of physical, psychological, social, occupational, and vocational function in patients whose abilities have been limited by disease, trauma, congenital disorders, or pain. The interdisciplinary team collaborates with the physiatrist to enable the patient to maximize functional abilities (American Board of Physical Medicine and Rehabilitation, 2016).

Physical therapy or physiotherapy, as defined by the World Confederation for Physical Therapy (WCPT), is a rehabilitation specialty with a focus on the restoration, maintenance, and promotion of optimal physical function throughout the life span. Physical therapy is provided by physical therapists to individuals who have or may develop impairments, activity limitations, and participation restrictions related to conditions of the musculoskeletal, neuromuscular, cardiovascular, pulmonary, and/or integumentary systems; or the negative effects attributable to unique individual and environmental factors as they relate to performance. Physical therapy might be used in circumstances in which movement and function are reduced by aging, injury, pain, diseases, disorders, conditions, or environmental factors. Physical therapists, also known as physiotherapists, provide a functional assessment to identify pain or loss of function caused by a physical injury, disorder, or disability and develop treatment plans to reduce pain, improve movement quality, address individual patient needs, and restore normal muscular control, for improvements in motor performance and function (McGowan, 2007; American Physical Therapy Association, 2015).

Sports medicine, in human medicine, is a subspecialty of both medicine and physical therapy. A primary care sports medicine specialist is a physician with training in the treatment and prevention of illness and injury who has completed 1 to 2 years of additional fellowship training in sports medicine. The sports medicine specialist helps patients to maximize function and minimize disability and time away from sports, work, or school. The sports medicine physician is also board-certified in Emergency Medicine, Family Medicine, Internal Medicine, Pediatrics, or Physical Medicine and Rehabilitation and is a leader of the sports medicine team, which might also include other specialty physicians and surgeons, athletic trainers, physical therapists, coaches, strength and conditioning professionals, nutritionists, sport psychologists, neuropsychologists, and the athlete (American Medical Society for Sports Medicine, 2016).

In physical therapy, a sports medicine specialist is a physical therapist who is qualified through completion of an internship, externship, research and publication, and specialty examination in Sports Physical Therapy through the American Board of Physical Therapy Specialties (ABPTS) and is provided the designation of Board-Certified Sports Clinical Specialist (SCS).

The *practice of veterinary medicine*, as defined by the American Veterinary Medical Association (AVMA) Model Practice Act, originally in 2012, is "to diagnose, prognose, treat, correct, change, alleviate, or prevent animal disease, illness, pain, deformity, defect, injury, or other physical, dental, or mental conditions by any method or mode, including the:

● Performance of any medical or surgical procedure, or
● Prescription, dispensing, administration, or application of any drug, medicine, biologic, apparatus, anesthetic, or other therapeutic or diagnostic substance, or
● Use of complementary, alternative, and integrative therapies, or
● Use of any procedure for reproductive management, including but not limited to the diagnosis or treatment of pregnancy, fertility, sterility, or infertility, or
● Determination of the health, fitness, or soundness of an animal, or
● Rendering of advice or recommendation by any means including telephonic and other electronic communications with regard to any of the above.
● To represent, directly or indirectly, publicly and privately, an ability and willingness to do an act described.
● Use of any title, words, abbreviation, or letters in a manner or under circumstances that induce the belief that the person using them is qualified to do any act described" (American Veterinary Medical Association, 2017).

Canine rehabilitation is the application of the science of rehabilitation medicine as it is adapted to canine patients. Canine sports medicine is a subspecialty of both veterinary medicine and canine rehabilitation, with an emphasis on the primary care management of the canine athlete by a veterinarian, as well as the management of nutrition, conditioning, rehabilitation, and injury prevention by the interdisciplinary and interprofessional canine rehabilitation team. This team may consist of doctors of veterinary medicine, physical therapists, and veterinary technicians. These veterinarians might be board certified by the American College of Veterinary Sports Medicine and Rehabilitation (ACVSMR) as well as other specialty colleges.

There are adjunctive specialists, including integrative veterinary medical professionals, who use acupuncture, chiropractic, and massage in the treatment of the canine rehabilitation patient. In 2001, the AVMA House of Delegates defined "complementary and alternative veterinary medicine (CAVM)" as treatments including "aromatherapy, Bach flower remedy therapy, energy therapy, low energy photon therapy, magnetic field therapy, orthomolecular therapy, veterinary acupuncture, acutherapy, acupressure, veterinary homeopathy, veterinary manual or manipulative therapy (similar to osteopathy, chiropractic or physical medicine and therapy), veterinary nutraceutical therapy, and veterinary phytotherapy." The House of Delegates was specific in its declaration that CAVM be "held to the same standards as traditional veterinary medicine, including validation of safety and efficacy by the scientific method."

The interdisciplinary rehabilitation team

Acknowledging that a variety of professionals contribute to the canine rehabilitation team, a challenge is the coordination of these practitioners, each of whom fills an important role in the management of the canine patient. Optimal outcomes are achieved when the team is coordinated and collaborative, thus exploiting each team member's knowledge, skill, experience, and expertise while leaving ego at the door for an appropriately balanced and patient-focused approach to management, whether the patient is an athlete, working dog, or pet.

The veterinarian serves as the primary care practitioner or case manager (*managing veterinarian* or *veterinarian of record*), providing necessary medical management of the canine patient and leading the rehabilitation team by coordinating referrals within the team and providing veterinary medical clearance for various rehabilitative and CAVM services. The veterinarian might provide a specific knowledge and skill set, directly contributing to the rehabilitation of the patient as well, whether qualified as a boarded specialist (in surgery, neurology, internal medicine, nutrition, or sports medicine and rehabilitation) or certified or trained in acupuncture, chiropractic, myofascial trigger point therapy, rehabilitation, or regenerative medicine.

In the United States, a doctor of veterinary medicine or veterinarian (DVM, VMD) completes 4 years of doctoral-level professional education following completion of prerequisites in a bachelor's degree program. Veterinarians who choose to further qualify in one of 21 specialties complete an internship and a 3-year residency, publish research, and take a specialty examination (McGowan, 2007).

A veterinary technician may or may not have an associate's or bachelor's degree and might be certified, registered, or licensed (in 47 of 50 states, at the time of this publication) to practice directly under the supervision of a veterinarian. Veterinary technicians can attend canine rehabilitation certification programs in the United States and are valued members of the rehabilitation team (McGowan, 2007; National Association of Veterinary Technicians in America, 2017).

The physical therapist might be involved directly in the evaluation and treatment of the canine rehabilitation patient by referral or after receiving veterinary medical clearance, indirectly as a consultant to the rehabilitation team, or as a team leader, orchestrating the various members of the rehabilitation team. Physical therapists do not work in canine rehabilitation autonomously, as they might when practicing with human patients. However, it is important that they continue to practice within, and be regulated by, their own profession and regulatory and licensure boards (McGowan, 2007). Having received additional training and education in canine anatomy, physiology, biomechanics, pathology, orthopedics, and neurology, the physical therapist might be certified in canine rehabilitation or may complete an advanced master's degree in animal physiotherapy in one

of several programs available worldwide. The physical therapist might provide skill, knowledge, or expertise to the rehabilitation management of the canine patient, for example, in manual therapy (mobilization, manipulation, and other specialized techniques), myofascial trigger point therapy, kinesiotaping, or neurofacilitation (neurodevelopmental training or proprioceptive neuromuscular facilitation).

Physical therapists are neuromusculoskeletal rehabilitation specialists who have a defined role in the current medical model under the World Health Organization (WHO). In the United States, physical therapists (PTs) complete a 3–4-year doctoral-level professional education program (DPT) at an accredited college or university following completion of prerequisites in the basic sciences and a bachelor's degree program. They are required to pass a national board examination for licensure. As in medicine, postgraduate professional development can continue with specialized residency training and, beyond that, fellowship training, which allows for board certification as a specialist in one of eight specialties designated by the American Board of Physical Therapy Specialties (ABPTS). Physical therapists are also active researchers, contributing to the science of rehabilitation related to the primary, secondary, and tertiary prevention of injuries, diseases, and disorders of all body systems (American Physical Therapy Association, 2015).

In practice, physical therapists direct their evaluation and treatment through the disablement model rather than the medical model of disease (World Health Organization, 1997). This focuses physical therapy interventions on the overall ability, disability, or function of the individual by directly addressing the impairments that relate to the specific needs of the patient. The therapist does not directly treat the pathology or medical diagnosis, but rather the impairments caused by them. An example of this is the use of treatment interventions that address pain, altered joint biomechanics, altered muscle length-tension and motor control, and altered joint range of motion in a patient with the medical diagnosis of a scapular body fracture, rather than directly treating the scapular body fracture itself. Through this approach, physical therapists can reduce the risk of exacerbation (or recurrence) of an injury and/or subsequent injury of a different structure (joint, muscle, tendon, etc.) in the future (American Physical Therapy Association, 2010).

Physical therapy has been identified as contributing to reduced costs associated with neuromusculoskeletal injury as well as reducing hospital readmission rates in neurologically compromised human patients. Early movement has proven to be paramount for many medical conditions, and physical therapists are the health-care providers who understand how to accomplish this safely, even in the most medically complex patients (Ries, 2015).

Physical therapist assistants (PTAs) complete an associate's or bachelor's degree from an accredited college prior to taking a board examination for licensure and, in all states, work under the direct or indirect supervision of a physical therapist. PTAs do not evaluate, determine, or alter a rehabilitation plan of care. Physical therapist assistants may attend some canine rehabilitation certification programs in the United States and are valued members of the rehabilitation team.

Adjunctive practitioners involved in the rehabilitation team might include acupuncturists, chiropractors, or massage therapists who have received additional training and/or certification in animal practice. Veterinary assistants and trainers may also assist the canine rehabilitation team in some facilities but are not qualified to attend canine rehabilitation certification programs. When appropriate, an occupational therapist, orthotist, or prosthetist may be consulted to assist with brace, splint, orthosis, or prosthetic fabrication for a canine rehabilitation patient.

As the practice of canine rehabilitation has evolved, this novel collaborative practice has been acknowledged by each profession's parent organization through discussion as well as official position statements. In 1993, the House of Delegates of the American Physical Therapy Association (APTA) released a collaborative practice statement. This statement has since been revised, and suggests that "Physical therapists may establish collaborative, collegial relationships with veterinarians for the purposes of providing physical therapy services or consultation. However, the APTA opposes the use of the terms 'physical therapy' or 'physiotherapy'

in veterinary practice unless services are performed by a physical therapist or physical therapist assistant under the direction and supervision of a physical therapist." Each state's practice act, which supersedes any other legislation, ultimately dictates the appropriate language to be used by practitioners in this field (American Physical Therapy Association, 2009.

The Board of Directors of the American Association of Rehabilitation Veterinarians (AARV) released the Model Standards for Veterinary Physical Rehabilitation Practice in February 2011, a statement of "guiding principles for the ideal practice of veterinary physical rehabilitative medicine" including definitions, scope and standards of practice, communication, referral, and continuing education (American Association of Rehabilitation Veterinarians, 2009–2017).

Clear communication and continued collaboration between these professional organizations and on the part of the professionals themselves will be necessary to ensure that the field of canine rehabilitation continues to evolve and grow in future years. Recognition of each discipline's value and contribution to the overarching goal of providing the best care will result in the best possible outcome for every canine rehabilitation patient and client.

The evolution of canine rehabilitation and sports medicine

Historically part of the skill set of trainers at horse and dog racetracks, rehabilitation and sports medicine has become not only more commonplace, but also integral and complementary to the practice of veterinary medicine. The earliest known publication regarding canine rehabilitation, *Physical Therapy for Animals: Selected Techniques*, a text by Ann Downer, a physical therapist at Ohio State University, introduced traditional rehabilitation techniques to the world of veterinary medicine in 1978. *Care and Training of the Racing Greyhound*, published in 1994 by veterinarians Linda L. Blythe and James R. Gannon, was the first text directly addressing topics pertinent to canine sports medicine (McGonagle *et al.*, 2014). There are now no fewer than a dozen textbooks regarding animal rehabilitation, sports medicine, and

Case Study 5.1   Rehabilitation of T3-L3 nonsurgical paraparesis through collaborative efforts of a veterinary neurologist, veterinary acupuncturist, and physical therapist

Signalment: 15 y.o. F/S Golden Retriever.

Presenting complaint: Patient referred by primary care veterinarian to veterinary neurologist with chief complaint of weakness in pelvic limbs following a fall from a step between house and yard. Ambulatory with thoracolumbar kyphosis. Clients elected against diagnostic imaging. Presumptive diagnosis through physical examination: T3-L3 lesion. Prednisone (15 mg b.i.d.) prescribed. Clients instructed in use of Help 'Em Up Harness™ by rehabilitation-certified veterinary technician. Patient referred to veterinary acupuncturist, where evaluated 3 weeks later. Patient had progressed to nonambulatory, paraplegic status. Veterinary acupuncturist performed acupuncture, prescribed tramadol (50 mg b.i.d.) for neck pain, initiated low-level laser therapy (class IIIb) and amoxicillin, 500 mg b.i.d., for bilateral greater trochanteric pressure injuries (grade 3), and suggested clients obtain a wheelchair. Four weeks following initiation of acupuncture treatment, patient referred to a physical therapist certified in canine rehabilitation.

Current treatment: Medications (prednisone, tramadol, amoxicillin), dry needle and electro-acupuncture, and low-level laser therapy to pressure injuries.

Rehabilitation evaluation: Patient unable to rise from lateral recumbency to standing without complete body-weight support/assistance. Able to lift head independently. When supported in standing via harness, standing frame, quad cart or wheelchair, patient actively steps with thoracic limbs, though with internal rotation and frequent adduction (scissoring). No tail wag with sensory stimulation, laser therapy, or during mobility activities. Withdrawal weak and delayed (>2 s) in pelvic limbs, though slightly more responsive medially than laterally and in left vs right. PROM within functional limits (WFL) with some tightness noted at bilateral teres major, bilateral iliopsoas, and bilateral pelvic limb interosseus muscles. Girth not objectively measured, however, atrophy observed at scapular, triceps, epaxial, cranial, quadriceps, and hamstring muscles. Greater trochanteric pressure injury sites grade 3 (defined by the National Pressure Ulcer Advisory Panel as full-thickness skin loss involving damage to, or necrosis of, subcutaneous tissue that may extend down to, but not through, underlying fascia, 2–3 cm in diameter, pink to red without eschar and without drainage noted). Patient nonpainful with palpation, PROM, and during functional mobility activities.

Home environment: The patient lives in a two-story home with tile and hardwood floors with area rugs/runners. Four wooden stairs to enter the home. No other pets and no children. Client telecommutes from home.

History: Patient previously very active (hiking with the client regularly).

Table 5.1   Summary for Case Study 5.1 using disablement model

Diagnosis	T3-L3 nonsurgical paraparesis
Disability	Unable to participate in activities (hiking) with clients
Functional limitation	Unable to rise from lying and walk from indoors to outdoors without body-weight assistance
Impairment	Nonambulatory, requires assistance for all functional mobility/transfers, reduced sensory awareness, reduced strength, pain
Goals	● Clients will be compliant and competent with home exercises/activities in 2 weeks ● Patient will tolerate standing (in the cart, over a physioroll/peanut, or over the standing frame) for up to 10 minutes in 4 weeks ● Patient will step with thoracic limbs while in the quad cart for at least 50 feet with minimal assistance in 4 weeks ● Patient will assist with transitions from lateral to sternal and sternal to sitting in 4 weeks
Rehabilitation plan, strategy, and tactics	● Home-based physical therapy sessions, weekly ● Acupuncture sessions, weekly ● Strategy: strengthening, sensory stimulation, neuromuscular facilitation/stimulation, pain management, promoting increased independence with function ● Tactics: therapeutic exercise, neuromuscular facilitation, manual therapy, laser therapy, neuromuscular electrical stimulation (NMES), and functional mobility facilitation

related topics, as well as clinical and academic research articles regularly published in journals including *Veterinary Surgery*, the *Journal of the American Veterinary Medical Association* (*JAVMA*), *Veterinary Clinics of North America*, the *American Journal of Veterinary Research* (*AJVR*), and *Orthopaedic Physical Therapy Practice* (*OPTP*), amongst others.

The practice of canine rehabilitation and sports medicine continues to evolve, the result of scientific, medical, and technological advancements, increased visibility and accessibility, and increased demand.

The exponential progress in research and technology in recent years has led to growth in medicine, veterinary medicine, and rehabilitation and sports science. Advancements in genetic and pharmaceutical research have resulted in the use of medications that are more specific to the patient, and, as a result, more effective. Diagnostic imaging is more technologically advanced, allowing for more specific diagnostics and for treatment to be more targeted and efficient. The use of minimally invasive surgical techniques has allowed for quicker procedure (and anesthesia) time resulting in quicker recovery time with fewer intraoperative and postoperative complications. Further, the use of and research into regenerative medicine treatments, including stem cell and platelet-rich plasma (PRP) injections, are expanding (McGowan, 2007; McGonagle *et al.*, 2014).

The predictable growth in canine rehabilitation is reflective of the parallel growth in rehabilitation in human medicine, with use of services pre- and post-operatively, as a conservative, nonoperative option, and to assist with management of medical conditions not traditionally addressed by rehabilitation medicine (i.e., oncological rehabilitation, vestibular rehabilitation) becoming more commonplace (McGonagle *et al.*, 2014).

There is increased accessibility to specialties in veterinary medicine, not only at academic teaching hospitals, but also at private specialty and referral practices (McGowan, 2007; McGonagle *et al.*, 2014). Some veterinary specialists, especially surgeons and neurologists, have an expectation that rehabilitation be an integral component of postoperative care, whether on site or in a nearby facility. There are free-standing, independent rehabilitation facilities in many areas, making rehabilitation more accessible to the client.

Veterinarians, veterinary technicians, and physical therapists trained in canine rehabilitation are becoming more numerous, as programs provide education not only in professional continuing education, but also for physical therapy and veterinary medicine professionals during the professional education curriculum. Early in the evolution of the field of canine rehabilitation and sports medicine, the Animal Rehabilitation Special Interest Group (AR-SIG) of the Orthopaedic Section of the American Physical Therapy Association (APTA) continuing education programs in canine and equine physical therapy evolved into the Northeast Seminars/University of Tennessee Canine Rehabilitation Practitioner (CCRP) Certification Program. This Program has graduated practitioners from varied medical and veterinary backgrounds since 2003. The Canine Rehabilitation Institute has provided a postgraduate education program collaborating the efforts of physical therapy and veterinary medicine clinicians, certifying over 1000 therapists and veterinary professionals since 2003. Both programs have offered their education programs internationally as well as in the United States. Alternately, there are at least seven postgraduate certification, degree, or diploma programs for physical therapists in animal physiotherapy, based in Canada, Europe, Africa, and Australia. Although the pathways by which practitioners enter the field are varied, each can provide specialized treatment through unique knowledge and skill, resulting in a valued service to the collaborative canine rehabilitation and sports medicine team (McGonagle *et al.*, 2014).

The field of canine rehabilitation and sports medicine has seen increased demand as there are more pets who live longer and who are more active, and, thus, more likely to be injured and potentially benefit from canine rehabilitation services. The average life span of the dog has been extended, similar to that of the human population. Along with this extended life span, there is increased awareness of treatment options available in veterinary medicine (McGonagle *et al.*, 2014). According to the American Pet Products Association National Pet Owners Survey (2015–2016), 54.4 million US households owned at least one dog, with coordinated increases in expenditures on pets, including medical services (American Pet Products Association, 2016).

Professional organizations and conferences

As the number of clinicians, both physical therapy and veterinary medical professionals, specializing in the field of canine rehabilitation and sports medicine grows, the need for organizations representing clinical, legislative, and educational interests grows as well. There has also been a more urgent call to establish legislation and regulation in this new specialty, especially when using personnel, treatment strategies, and modalities that are not considered conventional in veterinary medicine, to ensure safe and ethical practice. These professional organizations work primarily as lobbying, political, and legislatively active organizations, but also provide annual scientific conferences and continuing education to members. Many have newsletters with clinically or legislatively relevant information, scientific journals, and online social media forums for collaboration and professional discussion.

Animal Rehabilitation Special Interest Group (AR-SIG)

The Animal Rehabilitation Special Interest Group (AR-SIG), a special interest group (SIG) of the Orthopaedic Section of the American Physical Therapy Association (APTA), was established in 1993. The purpose of the ARSIG is to provide a forum for physical therapists and physical therapist assistants to discuss, promote, and advance the practice of animal rehabilitation. The ARSIG presents annually at the APTA Combined Sections Meeting and provides continuing education to members (Animal Rehabilitation Special Interest Group, 2016).

The goals of the ARSIG are to:

- Promote the role of physical therapists in the field of animal rehabilitation.
- Share information and resources with members of the physical therapy community and veterinary medical professions.

- Establish collegial relationships with veterinary medical professionals to promote the highest standards of quality and care in animal rehabilitation.
- Develop and provide educational programming and other learning opportunities to benefit members of the SIG.
- Foster research to support evidence-based practice on topics related to animal rehabilitation.
- Develop and promote contemporary practice guidelines for animal rehabilitation.
- Provide resources and support for SIG members involved in the political process of codifying legislative language directed at enhancing, advancing, and protecting physical therapist practice in animal rehabilitation.
- Participate as active members in the International Association of Physical Therapists in Animal Practice of the World Confederation of Physical Therapy.

American Association of Rehabilitation Veterinarians (AARV)

The American Association of Rehabilitation Veterinarians (AARV) was established in 2007. The mission of the AARV is to "advance the art and science of veterinary rehabilitation through education, advocacy and a commitment to research." The organization's objectives are to:

- Spread awareness of the practice and benefits of rehabilitation to primary care veterinarians, veterinary specialists, veterinary students and the public.
- Advocate for the inclusion of rehabilitation as part of comprehensive veterinary care,
- Promote model standards for best veterinary rehabilitation practices.
- Provide high-quality continuing education in veterinary rehabilitation.
- Advocate for legislation consistent with the AARV's goals and best practice guidelines.
- Strive to improve the practice of veterinary rehabilitation by promoting and supporting clinical research.
- Create partnerships with other organizations, companies and educational institutions to advance the field (American Association of Rehabilitation Veterinarians, 2009–2017).

The AARV affiliate organization, the American Association of Rehabilitation Veterinary Technicians (AARVT), was established in April 2011, and the Academy of Physical Rehabilitation Veterinary Technicians (APRVT) is a specialty organization for technicians approved in 2017.

American College of Veterinary Sports Medicine and Rehabilitation (ACVSMR)

The American College of Veterinary Sports Medicine and Rehabilitation (ACVSMR) was approved as a new College under the American Board of Veterinary Specialties (ABVS) by the American Veterinary Medical Association (AVMA) in April 2010. The first diplomates were installed in 2012 and included veterinarians from North America and Europe, although application is open worldwide. Specialties include certificates in either canine or equine rehabilitation and sports medicine. There are two routes to qualification, either a nontraditional or a traditional residency. The purpose of the ACVSMR is to "meet the unique needs of athletic and working animals and all animals in need of rehabilitation." The growth of the ACVSMR has led to parallel growth of rehabilitation and sports medicine education and clinical programs in teaching hospitals and specialty and referral practices as 3–6-year ACVSMR residencies are established in these facilities (American College of Veterinary Sports Medicine and Rehabilitation, 2010–2017).

International Association of Veterinary Rehabilitation and Physical Therapy (IAVRPT)

In August 1999, the first International Symposium for Physical Therapy and Rehabilitation in Veterinary Medicine was held at Oregon State University, with 300 participants from 21 countries. The International Association of Veterinary Rehabilitation and Physical Therapy (IAVRPT) was officially established in July 2008, in coordination with the International Symposium, "to provide a forum for the presentation of clinical and research information and discussion of topics related to animal rehabilitation, to further scientific investigation, and to promote the continued development of this specialty area to provide improved quality of care based on sound evidence" (McGonagle

et al., 2014). These symposia continue to occur every two years with different countries hosting each subsequent meeting (International Association of Veterinary Rehabilitation and Physical Therapy, 2017).

Internationally, there are organizations for physical therapists practicing in animal rehabilitation in 11 countries: Australia, Belgium, Canada, Finland, Germany, The Netherlands, New Zealand, South Africa, Sweden, the United Kingdom, and the United States (McGowan, 2007; McGonagle et al., 2014). In April 2011, the International Association of Physical Therapists in Animal Practice (IAPTAP) was established as a subgroup of the World Congress for Physical Therapy (WCPT) to "foster collaboration among physical therapists worldwide and to share information relating to research, education, and practice" (McGonagle et al., 2014; World Confederation for Physical Therapy, 2017).

Canine rehabilitation and sports medicine professionals have presented at conferences worldwide, including the International Racing Greyhound Symposium (now the International Canine Sports Medicine Symposium at the Veterinary Meeting and Expo, VMX), APTA Annual Conference and Combined Sections Meeting (CSM), American College of Veterinary Surgeons (ACVS) Symposium, Symposium on Therapeutic Advances in Animal Rehabilitation (STAAR), and Veterinary Orthopedic Society conference (McGonagle et al., 2014).

Physical therapy principles of patient management

Disablement model

Management of the canine rehabilitation and sports medicine patient is through means of the Disablement Model, as established by the World Health Organization, focusing on the factors affecting an individual's ability to perform daily tasks that are usual, customary, essential, and desirable to that being. This results in a more functional emphasis than pathological or medical diagnostic focus of evaluation and treatment. Efforts are geared toward optimizing the patient's response to rehabilitation interventions with eventual resolution of the patient's functional limitation.

The following terms pertinent to implementation of the disablement model in practice are operationally defined as described by the World Health Organization's International Classification of Impairments, Disabilities, and Handicaps (ICIDH) (World Health Organization, 1997; Levine *et al.*, 2004):

Active pathology: The interruption of or interference with normal processes and the simultaneous efforts of the organism to restore itself to a normal state by mobilizing the body's defense and coping mechanisms (Jette, 1994).
Impairment: Any loss or abnormality of anatomic, physiological, mental, or psychological structure or function (Jette, 1994).
Functional limitation: The restriction of the ability to perform a physical action, task, or activity in an efficient, typically expected, or competent manner at the level of the whole organism or person (Jette, 1994).
Disability: An inability to perform or a limitation in the performance of routine actions, tasks, behaviors, and activities in the manner or range considered normal for that individual, resulting from an impairment (Jette, 1994).

In rehabilitation, the impairment is addressed through treatment interventions with the intent to improve functional abilities (and resolve functional limitations). Not all impairments are functionally limiting or lead directly to disability in all patients. For example, two Labrador Retrievers of similar age, size, and conformation might have fragmented medial coronoid processes resulting in restrictions in elbow range of motion. One dog is a house pet who rarely encounters stairs and the other works in search and rescue and must scramble over varied terrain and frequently climb piles of rubble, stairs, and other obstacles. The loss in elbow range of motion is a rather minor limitation to the house pet, but is a functional limitation and, potentially, a disability for the search and rescue dog. Rehabilitation (as well as potential surgical and medical) interventions would vary in these cases, although both share the same active pathology. Thus, it is essential for the rehabilitation therapist to perform a thorough examination and evaluation to identify the impairments that will be addressed through appropriate rehabilitation interventions (or referral).

The rehabilitation evaluation

The rehabilitation or neuromusculoskeletal evaluation can serve to:

- Identify the pathoanatomic source of the patient's pain and/or functional impairments, and rule out any non-neuromusculoskeletal system disease or disorder causing the patient's symptoms (i.e., red flags).
- Assess the integrity and performance (i.e., strength, length, flexibility) of the involved tissues and structures as well as surrounding tissues and structures involved in movement.
- Determine the patient's functional abilities, functional limitations, impairments, and physical performance requirements essential for full participation in their normal physical or athletic activities.

The rehabilitation therapist can determine an appropriate plan of care, including selection of interventions, only following completion of a thorough and thoughtful evaluation, critically appraising or assessing the patient with regards to impairments, functional limitations, and disability. Each step in the evaluation is valuable to the end result and eventual outcome of the rehabilitation plan of care.

The first step in the evaluation is gathering a detailed *subjective report and history*, potentially from a variety of sources, including the veterinarian providing referral or veterinary medical clearance, any veterinary specialists involved in the care of the patient, and the client. This interview and information-gathering will provide an initial problem list that will guide the rehabilitation examination and, together, will create a roadmap and strategy for implementation of rehabilitation interventions.

Some significant elements of the subjective report and history include:

- Past medical history, including surgical procedures and outcome.
- History of present illness (i.e., injury, disorder, chief complaint, concern), including medications and other concurrent treatments.
- Diet and supplements.

- Prior level of functioning, for long-term goal or outcome projections, for safe and appropriate progression of rehabilitation activities, and for treatment planning.
- Home and work environment, including barriers and/or the potential need for modifications during the rehabilitation episode of care. (Additionally, knowledge about the home environment can assist the therapist in setting goals and selecting home exercise program activities, e.g., using stairs for a pelvic limb weight-bearing exercise.)
- Client goals.
- Work or athletic training history, possible causative factors (including overtraining and client resistance to recovery periods during training), work or athletic requirements, and potential for return to work or play.

The second step is the *objective examination*, including outcome measurements, but also importantly, an in-depth analysis of movement. The objective examination might include measurement of or description of:

- Measurement of passive range of motion (PROM) with end-feel and observation of functional range of motion, which is used during functional activities.
- Soft tissue flexibility, especially of multi-joint muscles (e.g., the hamstrings).
- Lameness/gait, including the use of lameness scores or scales, or, if available, kinematic documentation of gait characteristics (i.e., step length, stride length, velocity, ground reaction forces, functional range of motion).
- Neurological status, including level of arousal, spinal reflexes, reactions, sensation, pain sensation, sensory integration, coordination, balance, and cranial nerve function.
- Functional mobility, including analysis of movement strategies and assessment for the potential use of assistive devices.
- Motor control and strength.
- Results of palpatory assessment for pain, effusion, or edema, muscle tone, or muscle spasm.
- Cardiovascular or cardiorespiratory status, aerobic capacity/endurance, including baseline vital signs.

- Skin, nail, and fur or hair coat quality and integrity and, if applicable, incisional healing status.
- Joint motion, integrity, and stability via accessory motion testing and other special tests.

Although the rehabilitation therapist is most concerned with impairments and disability related to the patient's injury, the examination can also be used to provide a working hypothesis and to gain an understanding of the pathoanatomic cause of the patient's impairments and disability. If possible, knowledge of the differential diagnosis can guide the therapist with regards to the proper management of the patient's injury. For example, a patient who presents with pelvic limb lameness who is identified as having a cranial cruciate ligament rupture with medial meniscal involvement would warrant a referral to a boarded surgeon, while one who is identified as having a stable stifle, but a painful muscle strain could be managed conservatively through rehabilitation. Moreover, knowledge of a definitive diagnosis will offer more options with regards to use of potential rehabilitation interventions. Many physical electromagnetic and thermodynamic modalities are contraindicated if malignancy is suspected.

In the case of a sports or traumatic injury, based on the history, the impairments revealed in the rehabilitation examination, and the therapist's knowledge and understanding of the requirements of the functional or sports activity, the therapist can *reconstruct the crime* and guide recovery through rehabilitation to include interventions that might help to prevent further injury or recurrence of the injury in the future. Disability due to a canine sports-related injury will be specific to each individual patient due to individual factors including body structure and conformation, movement strategies or habits used during functional or sports activities (e.g., two-on-two-off contacts with the A-frame in agility), and factors related to the specific environment in which the injury occurred (i.e., flooring surfaces, angle of inclination of a jump or turn).

In-depth observation and analysis of movement, especially postures, transitions or transfers, and gait, can reveal evidence of movement dysfunction secondary to the injury, causative of the injury, or that might potentiate the risk of re-injury or subsequent injury. Movement dysfunction can be defined as incompetent movement that requires compensation to complete a functional task or that results in an inability to complete the task. Understanding the causes of (or impairments leading to) a movement dysfunction is paramount in selection of an intervention (e.g., manual therapy, therapeutic exercise with neuromuscular facilitation techniques) that will correct the movement dysfunction.

An example of a movement dysfunction is a dog who performs a stand to sit or sit to stand transitional movement with the right pelvic limb externally rotated and abducted. Further examination reveals that he has reduced tarsal flexion passive range of motion (PROM), reduced stifle flexion PROM, pain on flexion of the right pelvic limb (hip, stifle, and tarsus), stifle effusion, right pelvic innominate caudal rotation, reduced weight bearing of the right pelvic limb in standing, and muscle atrophy (reduced girth or muscle mass) at the right thigh. This movement dysfunction could have implications in higher level functioning tasks, such as stair climbing or jumping. The beginning of a jump requires the dog to function in a preparatory, *spring loaded* hip, stifle, and tarsal flexed position, releasing this potential energy in an explosive launch out of this position into one that is extended. In essence, these are the same joint positions required to sit correctly. Movement dysfunction in a stand-to-sit or sit-to-stand transitional movement will have implications in the performance of a jump that requires a higher level of control to manage significantly higher ground reaction forces. Moreover, the muscle tension created immediately prior to initiation of the jumping motion creates compressive forces on the joints, especially the stifle, as the muscle groups cross this intermediate joint. If the dog cannot sit without compensation, he will be unable to jump without compensation, putting the stabilizing ligaments and musculotendinous tissues at risk for injury with higher and asymmetric loads.

Case Study 5.2   Rehabilitation Grade 2 medial patellar luxation through collaborative efforts of a board-certified veterinary surgeon, massage therapist, and physical therapist

Signalment: 3 y.o. F/S miniature Poodle who competes in agility.

Presenting complaint: Patient intermittently three-legged (non-weight bearing left pelvic limb) lame for past 2 years, walking it off after a couple steps. Recently, lameness has progressed in frequency and interferes with agility training and competition. Patient has had massage therapy, by a massage therapist certified in canine massage techniques, every other month for the past 1½ years to treat tight muscles from her agility performances and the *muscle spasm* believed to cause the lameness. Patient presented to surgeon who diagnosed a Grade 2 medial patellar luxation and performed tibial tuberosity transposition due to the recent increased frequency of symptoms and client's desire to return to agility as quickly as possible. Prescribed Clavamox®, tramadol, and Rimadyl® upon discharge from the surgical hospital and referred to physical therapist certified in canine rehabilitation at suture removal (10 days post-op).

Current treatments: Medications as prescribed by the surgeon.

Rehabilitation evaluation

Gait/stance: Decreased weight bearing on the left pelvic limb with grade 5/6 lameness at walk, grade 6/6 at trot. Shortened stride on left pelvic limb with decreased hip extension at terminal stance phase of gait. Standing toe-touch weight bearing. Client reports patient holds limb non-weight bearing when going up two steps into house.

Appearance/posture: Incision healing well with no drainage, heat, or redness. Patient holds left pelvic limb in slight hip and stifle flexion and tarsal extension. Postures with kyphotic lumbar spine with pelvis rotated.

Palpation: Mild effusion at the peripatellar region with tenderness over incision. Moderate muscle tension/tone at left hamstrings, rectus femoris, iliopsoas, quadriceps, and lumbar epaxial region. Left anterior iliac rotation relative to right.

Transfers: To sit and sternal from standing with weight shifted slightly off the left pelvic limb. Does not use left pelvic limb to push off when transferring to or from sit or sternal.

(Continued)

Special tests: Grade I R medial patellar luxation. Negative tibial thrust and cranial drawer tests. Muscle atrophy of left gluteals, hamstrings, and quadriceps with thigh circumference reduced by 1 cm on left. With rear feet placed on scales, weight-bears 2 pounds on left and 6 pounds on right.

Home environment: Patient lives in single-story home with tile, hardwood flooring, area rugs, and runners. Two steps to enter home, and yard is fenced

with a pool. Two other dogs. Clients have a high bed with two steps for ease of access by dogs. Patient has not been allowed onto bed per surgeon's orders.

History: Patient was previously very active, competing in agility trials approximately twice monthly with two agility classes weekly and informal practice 2–3 times per week. Regularly walked 20–30 minutes 4–5 times per week, and swam in pool on occasion.

Table 5.2   Summary for Case Study 5.2 using disablement model

Diagnosis	Post-operative left grade 2 medial patellar luxation
Disability	Unable to participate in activities (agility, walks) with clients or play with other dogs
Functional limitation	Unable to rise from sit or down using pelvic limbs symmetrically; unable to climb stairs properly; unable to use the left pelvic limb properly with ambulation or in standing
Impairment	Pain, decreased strength, decreased weight bearing and improper use of the left pelvic limb with gait and movements, compensatory techniques with movements
Goals	(1) Clients will be compliant and demonstrate competency with home exercises/activities and all precautions and contraindications in 2 weeks (2) Patient will demonstrate symmetrical use of pelvic limbs to transfer from stand to sit/down and down/sit to stand in 4 weeks (3) Patient will have 0.5 cm increased left thigh muscle girth in 6 weeks (4) Patient will stand with 2 pounds more weight bearing on the left pelvic limb in 6 weeks for improved standing symmetry (5) Patient will ambulate without lameness on left pelvic limb in 8 weeks (6) Patient will ambulate up and down steps using the left pelvic limb properly in 8 weeks
Rehabilitation plan, strategy, and tactics	• Physical rehabilitation sessions weekly for 6 weeks and then every other week for 8 weeks, then begin a return to agility training once cleared by surgeon • Massage therapy to assist with tightness due to compensatory issues • Strategy: Strengthening, weight shifting, neuromuscular facilitation/stimulation, pain management, promote improved posture, body awareness/proprioception, and use of limb, and decrease compensatory techniques • Tactics: Therapeutic exercise with focus on progressive strengthening and weight-bearing program, neuromuscular facilitation techniques, manual therapy (massage, stretching, and joint mobilizations to stifle for pain and to pelvis to correct dysfunction), laser therapy, neuromuscular electrical stimulation (NMES), postural/core/functional task retraining

Range of motion (ROM) and goniometry

Objective measurement of active, passive, and resisted motions allows for identification of impairments that may relate to the patient's functional limitations and disability. These measurements may provide a valuable baseline as well as being an efficient method of re-evaluation, demonstrating progression in rehabilitation. Deficits or asymmetry in range of motion (ROM) measurements in combination with other examination information (e.g., pain on palpation, reduced joint accessory motion) might assist in identification and localization of impairment.

Active ROM is motion performed independently by the power of the individual's muscles without assistance. Active ROM can be limited due to weakness, pain, swelling, joint mobility limitations, or soft tissue extensibility limitations. *Passive ROM* is motion performed on the individual by an external force. The subject's muscles are relaxed, and no contraction is generated. This passive production of osteokinematic motion may be limited due to an intra-articular lesion, pain, swelling, contracted joint capsule, or soft tissue extensibility limitations. True passive ROM is difficult to perform in the conscious canine patient. *Resisted ROM* is motion performed independently through all or part of the range by the power of the individual's muscles against an opposing force.

The goniometer is used for the precise measurement of angles created by joints to gain objective measurement of joint ROM. Measurements are recorded in degrees and use specific bony landmarks for each joint (Table 5.3 and Figures 5.1–5.7). There are three parts of the goniometer: the stable or proximal arm, the fulcrum or axis, and the moving or distal arm.

Table 5.3   Landmarks for goniometry

Joint	Proximal arm	Axis	Distal arm	End feel
Shoulder flexion/extension (Figure 5.1)	Spine of the scapula	Acromion	Lateral humeral epicondyle	Soft or firm/firm
Shoulder abduction (Figure 5.2)	Spine of the scapula	Greater tubercle	Bisecting the lateral humerus	Firm
Elbow flexion/extension (Figure 5.3)	Greater tubercle	Lateral epicondyle	Lateral styloid process	Soft or firm/hard
Carpal flexion/extension (Figure 5.4)	Radial head	Lateral styloid	Fifth metacarpal	Firm/firm
Hip flexion/extension (Figure 5.5)	Bisecting the iliac wing	Greater trochanter	Lateral femoral condyle	Soft or firm/firm
Stifle flexion/extension (Figure 5.6)	Greater trochanter	Lateral femoral condyle	Lateral malleolus	Soft or firm/firm
Tarsal flexion/extension (Figure 5.7)	Fibular head	Lateral malleolus	Fifth metatarsal	Firm/firm

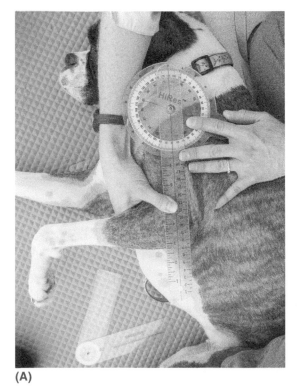

(A)

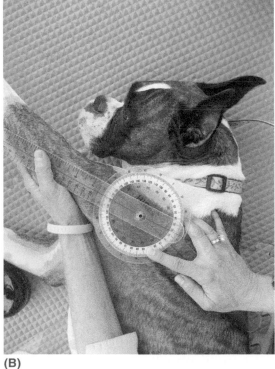

(B)

Figure 5.1   (A) Measuring shoulder flexion. (B). Measuring shoulder extension.

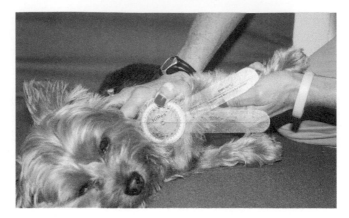

Figure 5.2   Measuring shoulder abduction.

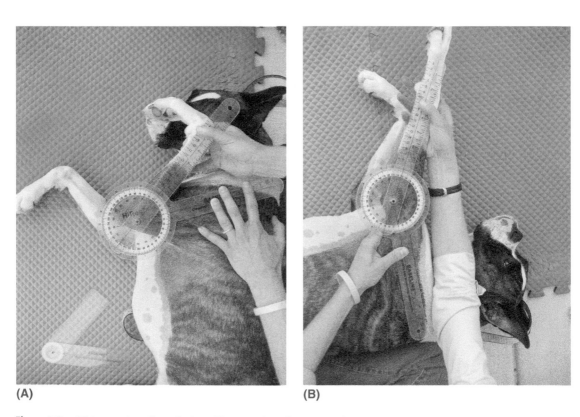

(A)   (B)

Figure 5.3   (A) Measuring elbow flexion. (B) Measuring elbow extension.

The axis is placed over the center of the joint, which changes depending upon the position of the joint, whether flexed or extended. The proximal arm is placed over the proximal segment, aligned with a proximal landmark, and the distal arm is placed over the distal segment, aligned with a distal landmark. Mean goniometric measurements for each joint can be found in Table 5.4. These measurements are based on sedated Labrador Retrievers. Other studies have noted that there is some variability from breed to breed (Benson *et al.*, 2004). In general, intrarater reliability, which is better than interrater reliability, even when using the same technique, has a 1–5-degree margin of error (Jaegger *et al.*, 2002).

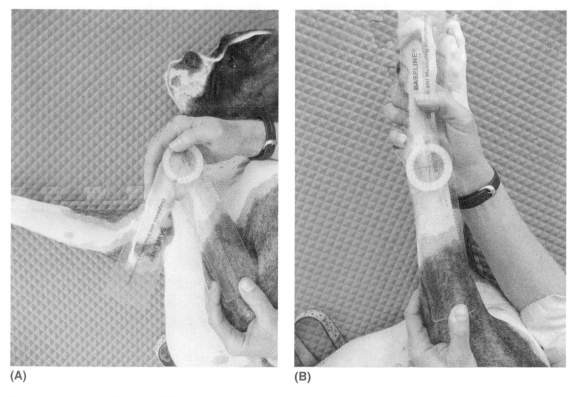

(A)   (B)

Figure 5.4   (A) Measuring carpal flexion. (B) Measuring carpal extension.

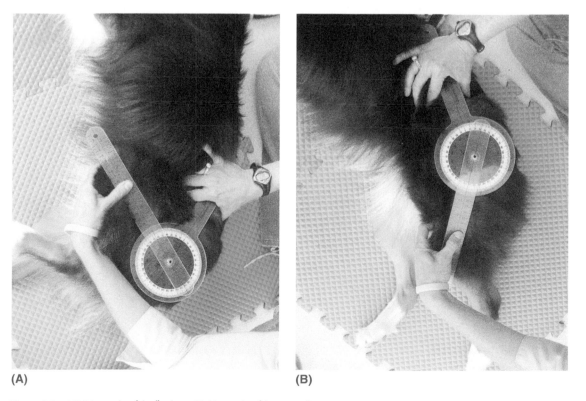

(A)   (B)

Figure 5.5   (A) Measuring hip flexion. (B) Measuring hip extension.

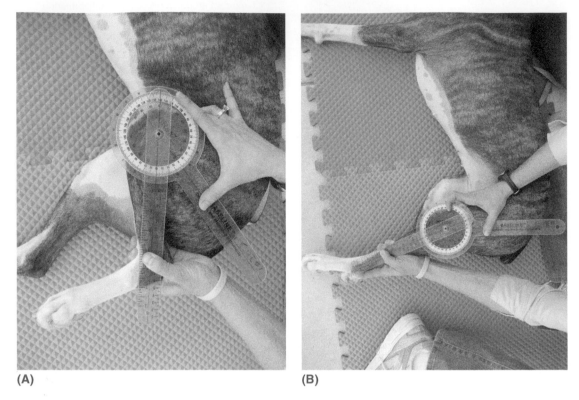

Figure 5.6 (**A**). Measuring stifle flexion. (**B**) Measuring stifle extension.

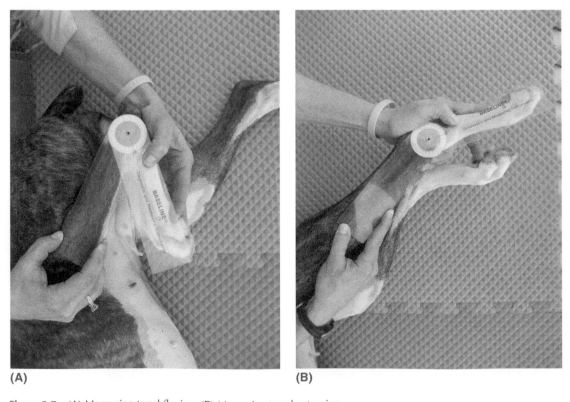

Figure 5.7 (**A**) Measuring tarsal flexion. (**B**) Measuring tarsal extension.

Table 5.4 Mean goniometric passive range of motion (PROM) measurements

Joint	Motion	Measurement
Shoulder	Flexion	57
	Extension	165
Elbow	Flexion	36
	Extension	165
Carpus	Flexion	32
	Extension	196
	Varus	7
	Valgus	12
Hip	Flexion	50
	Extension	162
Stifle	Flexion	42
	Extension	162
Tarsus	Flexion	39
	Extension	164

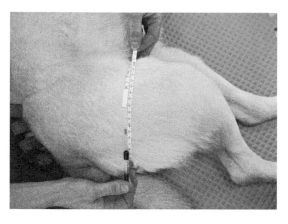

Figure 5.8 Girthometry of the pelvic limb muscles: Option 1.

Girth measurement

Girth measurements are circumferential measurements taken with a tape measure at standard anatomic sites around the body and used to document muscle size, body composition, and swelling, and to monitor changes in these objective measurements. The amount of tension on the tape, correct use of landmarks, altered joint or body position, and use of different testers or raters can affect reliability. There are different methods for taking girth measurements depending on the purpose of the measurement. If measuring swelling, the tape measure is usually placed around the affected area. If measuring for body composition or muscle size, consistent landmarks are important to increase reliability. One method is to pull the tape measure as high into the groin or axilla as possible and hold it in place using the fifth digit (Figure 5.8). However, this method may not be completely reliable as the tape can slip and therefore not be in the exact same place as a previous measurement.

The author (A.K.) prefers to use a method incorporating the same landmarks each time for improved accuracy. For example, when measuring thigh muscle size, the tape measure is placed at the greater trochanter with the tape wrapped tightly around the thigh as proximally as possible, and the tape ending at the greater trochanter (Figure 5.9). This technique can be reproduced, using the acromion,

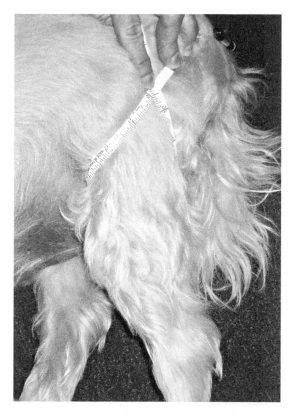

Figure 5.9 Girthometry of the pelvic limb muscles: Option 2.

for forelimb measurement. The measurement is rechecked for accuracy, compared to the opposite leg, and the patient's position (recumbent vs weight-bearing) is documented.

Physiological considerations

Regardless of professional background, the canine rehabilitation and sports medicine therapist must have the ability to consolidate the history, physical examination, and evaluation, and synthesize a rehabilitation plan based on a number of factors, including:

- Patient-specific considerations, including prior medical history, comorbidities, and red flags.
- The diagnosis or disorder being treated, as well as the expected response of the body's tissues to injury, especially with regards to healing and pain.
- The treatment strategies and tactics, and their effect on the various systems of the body, including neuromuscular, musculoskeletal, integumentary, cardiovascular, and cardiopulmonary and considering indications, precautions, and contraindications.
- The physics of potential rehabilitation interventions.

Patient-specific considerations

Characteristics of the patient need to be considered when setting the rehabilitation plan, especially with regards to physiological responses to interventions. Interventions in which forces are applied by the body or to the body will have varied effects on the body depending upon the patient breed and conformation, weight, body condition, and general level of conditioning. Patient age, prior level of functioning, nutritional status, duration of immobilization or activity restriction (and therefore, phase of healing of tissues), and prior medical history and comorbidities will alter the patient's tolerance of an activity or therapeutic procedure. The patient's stress and anxiety level and/or familiarity with the therapeutic procedure or environment in which it is applied, will also be a predictor of his success and tolerance of a therapeutic activity. For example, attempts to walk a dog in an underwater treadmill might be challenged when the patient reportedly "hates the water" or in a rehabilitation facility that is housed within the emergency hospital in which he was previously treated, leading to a fear response or heightened level of anxiety.

Comorbidities, or medical conditions that exist simultaneously but independently with another or a related medical condition, may cause unforeseen complications and affect the outcome of the rehabilitation interventions applied. Of significant concern are disorders that affect healing (i.e., diabetes mellitus, kidney disease, and use of corticosteroids), the efficiency of the cardiovascular/cardiorespiratory systems, and/or the ability of another limb to accept weight during functional activities or gait (i.e., hip dysplasia, elbow dysplasia, prior peripheral nerve injury due to being hit by a car).

Red flags are indicators of possible serious problems, such as inflammatory or neurological conditions, structural musculoskeletal damage or disorders, circulatory problems, infection, tumors, or systemic disease. If suspected, these require further investigation with immediate referral to the managing veterinarian (veterinarian of record or primary care practitioner or case manager), with potential for referral to a specialist. There are certain signs that, when observed in a patient's examination or history, might alert the rehabilitation therapist to the potential for a serious or potentially emergent condition. For this reason, the rehabilitation therapist must maintain open communication with the referring/managing veterinarian, and potentially, with a nearby veterinary emergency facility (Physiopedia, 2017b). Physical therapists are trained to recognize the presence of disease or impairment that may present as an injury to the neuromusculoskeletal system; however, they are not expected to diagnose the specific pathological process. They are trained to recognize when a referral to another healthcare provider is required.

Tissue healing response to injury

The canine rehabilitation therapist must not only consider the diagnosis (disorder, disease, injury, or surgical procedure) that has brought the patient and client to consult the rehabilitation team, but also the tissues involved. Skin, fascia, nerves, blood vessels, muscle, tendon, ligament, bone, and cartilage heal at different rates and with varied outcomes with regards to strength of the repair. The animal's age, nutritional status, comorbidities, and activity level can greatly affect the healing time during the recovery and rehabilitation phase. Of additional consideration is pain management and the use of regenerative medicine and other concurrent medical treatments that might accelerate or slow the healing timeframe.

There is a somewhat predictable progression of the body's tissues through the healing process. The time frame for each phase is variable depending upon the factors discussed above. The *inflammatory phase* occurs from day 0 until approximately day 6 and includes a complex series of physiological events. Initially, the chemically mediated vascular responses of vasodilation and vascular permeability occur, allowing for white blood cell migration and platelet aggregation to the site of tissue damage. This allows for phagocytic processes to clean cellular debris and fight against foreign pathogens, and causes fibrin clot formation to reduce bleeding and repair endothelial cell wall damage. Pain responses are associated with tissue damage from the production of pain-mediating substances such as prostaglandins and bradykinins. Vasoconstriction follows with a resulting reduction in blood flow. The goal of this phase of healing is to reduce blood loss, protect against foreign pathogens, clean debris from damaged tissue cells, and begin stabilization of the injury site. The *reparative* or *proliferative phase* begins day 3 to day 5 and lasts until about day 14, with fibroplasia and granulation tissue formation, epithelialization, angiogenesis, and contraction of the wound bed. This phase provides a weak scaffold upon which the scar tissue forms. The *maturation* or *remodeling phase* occurs anywhere from weeks to months following the injury and is dependent upon the type of tissue that is involved in the injury. In the natural healing process, without surgical or regenerative medicine intervention, complete recovery of the strength of the original tissue rarely occurs because the repaired tissue, or scar, is less organized than the noninjured tissue. Of note is that the presence of inflammation, although initially protective, chronically (or without the ability to progress healing to the proliferative phase) will extend healing times, possibly delay or cause nonunion or nonhealing of tissues, and result in weak, disorganized scar tissue formation (National Pressure Ulcer Advisory Panel, 2016; Physiopedia, 2017a).

Bony injuries heal in a similar fashion; however, osteoclasts and osteoblasts form a soft callus in the reparative or proliferative phase at about 2 weeks from the onset of the injury. This phase continues for 6 to 12 weeks during which time the soft callus is replaced by a hard callus. The maturation or remodeling phase can last for months during which the hard callus is remodeled and strengthened as it is gradually replaced by lamellar bone (Marsell & Einhorn, 2011; Physiopedia, 2017a).

Pain response to injury

Although pain is a subjective sensation defined as "an unpleasant sensory and emotional experience associated with actual or potential tissue damage," pain management is a consideration in the rehabilitation treatment of the canine patient with regards to the presence of tissue damage and/or inflammation. The rehabilitation therapist might use rehabilitation modalities and manual therapies, in combination with traditional pharmacological and medical management, to assist in the management of pain and inflammation. Furthermore, the rehabilitation therapist might direct interventions, such as therapeutic exercise, toward progressively increasing functional capacity and return of the patient to full activity as efficiently and safely as possible, so as to redirect the patient's perception of pain (Prentice, 2013).

Of concern in this return to activity are the alterations in central and peripheral neuromuscular processes, which are influenced by the presence of joint effusion, inflammation, and pain. As a result of these alterations, normal muscular contractions and motor control can be inhibited. Left unattended, these neuromuscular changes can lead to biomechanical alterations and subsequent aberrant forces on the injured and surrounding tissues. To complicate matters, these alterations in neuromuscular control are present after pain has resolved and tissue healing takes place. Long term, these biomechanical faults can lead to further injury and contribute to degenerative processes along the kinetic chain. The rehabilitation therapist should be aware of the potential for these changes and be prepared to apply interventions that can assist in the restoration of normalized neuromuscular functioning through manual therapy, manual mechanical correction or facilitation of joint position, and neuromuscular re-education/retraining (Soderberg, 1986; Hodges & Tucker, 2011; Tsao *et al.*, 2011). See Chapter 19 for more on the management of pain in dogs.

Rehabilitation intervention effects, indications, precautions, and contraindications

Related to the discussion on comorbidities and physiological response of the body to treatment, the rehabilitation therapist must consider the effects, indications, precautions, and contraindications of the various modalities and interventions included in the treatment plan. Although some might be indicated in the case of a specific diagnosis, due to other considerations (i.e., comorbidities, red flags), the therapist might use caution and/or choose to not use an intervention with a patient, thus making the rehabilitation plan individualized and patient-specific. The rehabilitation therapist should consider the application of physical rehabilitation interventions as potentially harmful as medications, requiring knowledge, skill, and experience in prescribing, dosage, and combining therapeutic procedures.

The reader should refer to chapters specific to the interventions (manual therapies, therapeutic exercise, physical modalities, etc.) for guidelines, discussion of the basic science of the intervention, more specific physiological effects, indications, precautions, and contraindications.

Physics of rehabilitation interventions

Biomechanics is the study of forces and their effects on human and animal bodies both during movement (dynamics) and at rest (statics) (O'Sullivan & Schmitz, 1994; TenBroek, 2005). The rehabilitation therapist must understand the biomechanical effects of forces applied to the patient's body when using specific rehabilitation interventions. These forces might result in acceleration, deceleration, or tissue deformation, with changes in length, shape, or orientation of the tissue, stressing the tissue, and resulting in strengthening or weakening (and/or repair) of the tissue. Such interventions include manual therapy techniques (Chapter 6) and therapeutic exercises, both on land (Chapters 8 and 10) and in the aquatic

environment (Chapter 9), and orthotics and prosthetics (Chapter 11). The physics involved in specific physical electromagnetic and thermodynamic modalities, including therapeutic ultrasound, electrical stimulation, laser therapy, heat, and ice, is discussed in detail in Chapter 7. Specialized knowledge and skill are necessary for safe application of these techniques.

Treatment planning in canine rehabilitation and sports medicine

Following completion of the canine rehabilitation or sports medicine evaluation, the therapist should consolidate impairments and functional limitations in an assessment statement and suggest a rehabilitation prognosis based on physiological considerations. Functional goals will help to determine the canine rehabilitation plan of care, including general treatment strategies and more specific treatment tactics or interventions.

Goal setting

The overall focus of rehabilitation is to meet functional goals that are realistic for the patient and meaningful to the client. Long-term goals include the restoration, maintenance, and promotion of maximal and optimal function and quality of life as related to movement. Determining realistic and appropriate treatment goals drives the clinician in planning, monitoring, prioritizing, progressing, and measuring the effectiveness of the current treatment strategy. It is a difficult process, requiring skill in the interpretation of objective data collected during the rehabilitation evaluation and subsequent re-evaluation, professional judgment, scientific knowledge, and skill in facilitating patient (and client) participation in the process.

The functional limitations and impairments apparent in the evaluation of the canine patient guide the therapist in setting appropriate goals, with additional consideration for the client's goals, physiological considerations (including comorbidities, contraindications, and precautions) and the patient's prior level of function. Rehabilitation goals are SMART:

- **S**pecific
- **M**easurable and meaningful
- **A**cceptable and action-oriented
- **R**easonable and relevant
- **T**imely.

As an example: within 4 weeks, the patient will demonstrate improved tarsal, stifle, and hip joint mobility and quadriceps and gluteal muscle strength to be able to transfer from sit to stand on a nonskid surface independently 90% of the time when called by the client.

Establishing the rehabilitation plan of care

The rehabilitation plan of care (POC) is initially set at the time of the evaluation; however, it is a fluid plan and can be altered or revised on subsequent visits (following re-evaluation by the physical therapist or veterinarian) based on careful observation and monitoring of the patient's response to treatment and the client's needs. The plan of care should include treatment strategies and interventions as well as the proposed treatment frequency and duration.

The rehabilitation treatment strategy is the general plan of action whereby impairments or functional limitations are improved, resolved, reversed, or ameliorated. For example, if impairments include reduced hip and stifle extension joint mobility, reduced tarsal flexion joint mobility, reduced gluteal strength, and reduced quadriceps strength, and functional limitations include the inability to rise from sitting to standing without assistance, then the treatment strategy will focus on improving joint mobility, increasing strength, and improving sit-to-stand abilities.

Plans for eventual treatment progression might be introduced, and specific activity or mobility precautions and contraindications might be outlined in the initial plan of care. The therapist should ensure that the plan of care is appropriate for the patient and client and focused on the established impairments and functional limitations, considerate of the previ-

ously stated rehabilitation goals. The plan of care should include suggestions with regards to potential referrals, to adjunctive professionals including CAVM providers, orthotists, or prosthetists, as well as recommendations on assistive devices, equipment, or home modifications that might be appropriate during or following the rehabilitation episode of care.

Client involvement and compliance

The therapist should make every effort to involve the client throughout the rehabilitation process. Through this involvement, the client is empowered and invested in the patient's recovery, increasing the likelihood that the rehabilitation process will be more successful. Clients should be encouraged to assist in setting functional goals and the plan of care, to give positive feedback to the patient during rehabilitation treatments, and to be compliant with the home exercise program and prescribed activity and movement restrictions. The therapist can take advantage of the time during visits to educate the client with regards to the etiology of the patient's disorder and potential outcome, encouraging better understanding by the client and, again, increasing the likelihood of compliance. To avoid confusion and conflict, in the case of multiple clients and involved, active family members, one person should act as the primary client and/or spokesperson. This person is able to be most consistent and compliant with regards to ensuring attendance at follow-up visits, performance of the home exercise program, and compliance with activity and movement restrictions, if warranted. This person will also be the primary communicator for the family, thus eliminating the potential confusion of multiple iterations of instructions and reports.

Rehabilitation interventions and tactics

When collaborating with a rehabilitation team with wide-ranging experience and skill, the plan of care might include more specific instruction with regards to manipulation or progression of variables of specific interventions.

The specific interventions used in rehabilitation treatment may include manual therapy techniques (Chapter 6), therapeutic exercises, both on land (Chapters 8 and 10) and in the aquatic environment (Chapter 9), physical electromagnetic and thermodynamic modalities (Chapter 7), and orthotics and prosthetics (Chapter 11). Additional consideration for incorporation of specialized techniques and treatments such as myofascial trigger point therapy, regenerative medicine interventions, and medical pain management is appropriate when considering the rehabilitation therapist's scope of practice or when referring to a specialist with this specific skill set.

Webliography

American Association of Rehabilitation Veterinarians. 2009–2017. Model standards. Available at: http://rehabvets.org/model-standards.lasso (accessed October 24, 2017).

American Board of Physical Medicine and Rehabilitation. 2016. Our Mission: Serving our diplomates, protecting the public. Available at: https://www.abpmr.org/About (accessed October 24, 2017).

American College of Veterinary Sports Medicine and Rehabilitation. 2010–2017. Our Mission. Available at: http://vsmr.org (accessed October 24, 2017).

American Medical Society for Sports Medicine. 2016. What is a sports medicine specialist? Available at: https://www.amssm.org/Content/pdf%20files/WhatisSMSpec-Patient-broch.pdf (accessed October 24, 2017).

American Pet Products Association. 2016. Pet industry market size and ownership statistics. Available at: http://www.americanpetproducts.org/press_industrytrends.asp (accessed October 24, 2017).

American Physical Therapy Association. 2009. Practice of physical therapists in animal rehabilitation. BOD P03-05-17-44. Available at: https://www.apta.org/uploadedFiles/APTAorg/About_Us/Policies/BOD/Practice/PracticeofPTinAnimalRehab.pdf (accessed October 24, 2017).

American Physical Therapy Association. 2010. Who are physical therapists and what do they do? Guide to physical therapist practice. Available at: www.mhprofessional.com/downloads/products/0071486410/dutton_ch01_0071486410.pdf (accessed October 24, 2017).

American Physical Therapy Association. 2015. The physical therapist scope of practice. Available at: http://www.apta.org/ScopeOfPractice/ (accessed October 24, 2017).

Animal Rehabilitation Special Interest Group. 2016. Animal rehabilitation special interest group. Available at: http://www.orthopt.org/content/special-interest-groups/animal-rehabilitation (accessed October 24, 2017).

American Veterinary Medical Association. 2017. Model veterinary practice act—July 2017. Available at: https://www.avma.org/KB/Policies/Pages/Model-Veterinary-Practice-Act.aspx#definitions (accessed October 24, 2017).

International Association of Veterinary Rehabilitation and Physical Therapy. 2017. Home page. Available at: http://www.iavrpt.org (accessed October 24, 2017).

LEVINE, D. L., MILLIS, D., & MARCELLIN-LITTLE, D. J. 2004. Proposed functional stifle scale. In: Kortekaas, P. M. (ed.), *Osteopathic Approach to Lumbo-Pelvic Dysfunctions in Canines*. Available at: www.orthopt.org/downloads/8767.pdf (accessed October 24, 2017).

National Association of Veterinary Technicians in America. Credentialing. Available at: https://navta.site-ym.com/?page=credentialing&hhSearchTerms=%22veterinary+and+technician+and+definition%22g (accessed November 9, 2017).

National Pressure Ulcer Advisory Panel. 2016. National Pressure Ulcer Advisory Panel (NPUAP) announces a change in terminology from pressure ulcer to pressure injury and updates the stages of pressure injury. Available at: https://www.npuap.org/national-pressure-ulcer-advisory-panel-npuap-announces-a-change-in-terminology-from-pressure-ulcer-to-pressure-injury-and-updates-the-stages-of-pressure-injury/ (accessed October 24, 2017).

Physiopedia. 2017a. Soft tissue healing. Available at: http://www.physio-pedia.com/Soft_Tissue_Healing (accessed October 24, 2017).

Physiopedia. 2017b. The flag system. Available at: http://www.physio-pedia.com/The_Flag_System (accessed October 24, 2017).

Ries, E. There's no place like home: reducing hospital readmission rates. PT in Motion. Available at: http://www.apta.org/PTinMotion/2015/11/Feature/HospitalReadmission/ (accessed November 10, 2017).

TenBroek, T. 2005. Introduction KIN335 Biomechanics Spring 2005. Available at: www.asu.edu/courses/kin335tt/Lectures/Introduction/Introduction.pdf (accessed October 24, 2017).

World Confederation for Physical Therapy. 2017. Home page. Available at: http://www.wcpt.org (accessed October 24, 2017).

World Health Organization. 2017. Home page. Available at: http://www.who.int/en/ (accessed October 24, 2017).

References

Benson, C., Lakey, S., Smith, M. & Hummel-Berry, K. 2004. A comparison of canine range of motion measurements between two breeds of disparate body types. Proceedings of the APTA. *J Orthop Sports Phys Ther*, 34(1), A39.

Blythe, L. L. & Gannon, J. R. 1994. *Care and Training of the Racing Greyhound: A Guide for Trainers*. American Greyhound Council.

Downer, A. H. 1978. *Physical Therapy for Animals: Selected Techniques*. Thomas Publishers.

Hodges, P. W. & Tucker, K. 2011. Moving differently in pain: a new theory to explain the adaptation to pain. *Pain*, 152(3S), S90–98.

Jaegger, G. L., Marcellin-Little, D. J. & Levine, D. 2002. Reliability of goniometry in Labrador Retrievers. *Am J Vet Res*, 63(7), 979–986.

Jette, A. M. 1994. Physical disablement concepts for physical therapy research and practice. *Phys Ther*, 74, 380–386.

Marsell, R. & Einhorn, T. A. 2011. The biology of fracture healing. *Injury*, 42(6), 551–555.

McGonagle, L., Blythe, L. & Levine, D. 2014. Introduction to physical rehabilitation, history of canine physical rehabilitation. In: Millis, D. & Levine, D. (eds), *Canine Rehabilitation and Physical Therapy*, 2nd edn. St Louis: Saunders, pp. 1–7.

McGowan, C. 2007. Introduction. In: McGowan, C., Goff, L., & Stubbs, N. (eds), *Animal Physiotherapy: Assessment, Treatment, and Rehabilitation of Animals*. Ames, IA: Blackwell Publishing, pp. 1–2.

O'Sullivan, S. B. & Schmitz, T. J. 1994. *Physical Rehabilitation: Assessment and Treatment*, 3rd edn. Philadelphia: F.A. Davis, chapters 1, 5, 10, & 11.

Prentice, W. 2013. Tissue response to injury. In: Prentice W. (ed.), *Principles of Athletic Training: A Competency-Based Approach*, 15th edn. New York: McGraw-Hill, pp. 265–284.

Soderberg, G. L. 1986. *Kinesiology: Application to Pathological Motion*, 7th edn. Baltimore, MD: Williams & Wilkins.

Tsao, H., Danneels, L. A. & Hodges, P. W. 2011. Smudging the motor brain in young adults with recurrent low back pain. *Spine*, 36(21), 1721–1727.

World Health Organization. 1997. *International Classification of Diseases*, 9th edn. New York: WHO.

6

Manual Therapy

Judy C. Coates, MEd, MSPT, CCRT

Summary

Specialized manual skills are used extensively in both evaluating and treating the canine patient. Manual techniques are used in an assessment to identify soft tissue abnormalities, muscle length tightness, limitations in passive range of motion (PROM), and restrictions in arthrokinematic motion. When assessing soft tissues, we must be able to distinguish between normal and pathological tissue characteristics. Flexibility is assessed with particular sensitivity to multijoint muscles. PROM provides information regarding quality and quantity of joint ROM with the use of end-feels and goniometry. Joint play is used to assess arthrokinematic or accessory joint motion. Identification and interpretation of abnormal findings will direct the therapist in determining the most appropriate and most efficient treatment techniques. Manual treatment involves a variety of soft tissue techniques, specific stretching techniques, PROM with overpressure and joint mobilization, including glides and traction. Soft tissue treatment techniques are designed to address a specific tissue type and pathology. For example, techniques used to increase circulation are different than techniques used to reduce adhesions or eliminate trigger points. Decreased flexibility is treated with direct and nondirect stretching techniques designed to optimize patient tolerance and effectiveness. Treatment of limited PROM depends on information gathered from end-feel assessment. Motion limited by an elastic end-feel will require different treatment techniques than motion that is limited by a boggy end-feel. Finally, joint mobilization consists of glides and traction. Different grades and techniques of mobilization are used to treat pain versus hypomobility.

Manual skills are critical to successful evaluation and treatment of the canine rehabilitation patient. Manual techniques are used in assessment and treatment of soft tissue abnormalities, osteokin- ematic and arthrokinematic dysfunction, and pain. In this chapter manual skills are divided into four categories: soft tissue mobilization, passive range of motion (PROM), stretching, and joint mobilization.

Canine Sports Medicine and Rehabilitation, Second Edition. Edited by Chris Zink and Janet B. Van Dyke.
© 2018 John Wiley & Sons, Inc. Published 2018 by John Wiley & Sons, Inc.

Soft tissue mobilization

Soft tissue mobilization (STM) or massage is the systematic application of manual pressure and movement of soft tissues, including skin, tendons, ligaments, fascia, and muscle. Soft tissue treatment techniques have been used for medical conditions since the 1800s; however, these techniques are a source of some controversy, as their value has not been well documented (Hertling & Kessler, 1990; Crawford *et al.*, 2016).

Some authors suggest that STM has positive effects on the circulatory, muscular, lymphatic, and endocrine systems (Fritz & Grosenbach, 2009; Salvo, 2012). More specifically, STM is presumed to create circulatory effects that drive fluid from the interstitial space to the vessels with movement toward the lymph nodes and heart (Millis *et al.*, 2004). Mobilization of connective tissue is used to increase the extensibility of the tissue and to prevent or reduce adhesion formation. Soft tissue techniques have been shown to increase ROM (Sefton *et al.*, 2011), promote healing (Zusman, 2011) and reduce pain (van den Dolder *et al.*, 2010; Sefton *et al.*, 2011). Sefton and colleagues (2011) demonstrated that soft tissue mobilization decreased the motor unit activity of the muscle, increased tissue extensibility, and increased range of motion. Abbott and colleagues (2015) demonstrated that STM combined with therapeutic exercise is more effective than exercise alone in the treatment of osteoarthritis, particularly if the treatments are spread out over an 11-month period of time. However, Bervoets and colleagues (2015) found no additional benefit when adding STM to a therapeutic exercise treatment. As a stand-alone treatment, however, STM was effective in increasing function and decreasing pain.

STM has been compared to therapeutic ultrasound (US) in its effect on range of motion (ROM) and pain with upper extremity neurodynamics (nerve tension testing) in humans. This study demonstrated greater improvements in mobility with STM than with US (Costello *et al.*, 2016). STM is frequently used to enhance post-exercise recovery. However, a recent meta-analytical review suggests that the effects are unclear and provide unimpressive, temporary effects (Poppendieck *et al.*, 2016).

Soft tissue assessment

To determine the appropriateness of STM as a treatment, an evaluation of the soft tissues must be performed. A thorough soft tissue assessment will identify the presence of soft tissue pathology, swelling, and pain. With this information, the most effective soft tissue treatment technique(s) can be chosen.

Soft tissues are evaluated by palpation of specific tissues and structures. A variety of techniques are used to assess soft tissue depending on tissue type. For example, fascial restrictions are evaluated using techniques quite different from those used for muscle or tendon. It is important to be cognizant of the properties of each type of tissue, understanding that normal muscle feels different than normal tendon, ligament, or fascia. The contralateral side is used for comparison. Documentation includes a description of the tissue that can be characterized by texture, shape, tone, and density. Abnormal soft tissue can be described as thick, soft/firm, boggy, tight, tender, in spasm, warm/cold/clammy, or as having crepitus.

Assessing swelling

The terms edema and swelling are often used interchangeably. In the strict sense, however, swelling does not include pitting. Swelling is the abnormal build-up of fluid in tissues (intracellular, extracellular, intracapsular, and extracapsular). When pressure is applied to a swollen area and an indentation remains once the pressure is removed, it is referred to as pitting edema. Table 6.1 lists several characteristics of swelling.

Resolution of swelling is a common treatment goal, as swelling will retard the recovery process. Swelling can result in pain, loss of ROM, and reflex inhibition of the surrounding muscles, leading to atrophy and weakness. Swelling

Table 6.1   Characteristics of swelling

Type of swelling	Characteristic
Fluid swelling	Soft and mobile
Edematous synovial swelling	Boggy
Pitting edema	Thick and slow moving

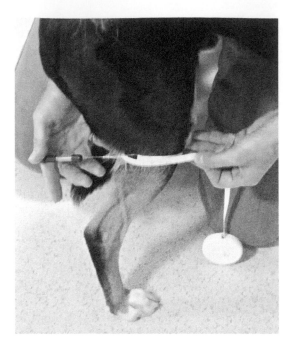

Figure 6.1   Measurement of stifle joint swelling using a Gulick girthometer.

can be measured with a Gulick girthometer and documented in centimeters (Figure 6.1) or it can be palpated and documented as minimal, moderate, or severe.

Soft tissue treatment

Varying physiological states are treated using different STM techniques. For example, effusion is most effectively treated with longitudinal strokes of moderate pressure; whereas a muscle spasm will respond better to ischemic compression. Once the goal of your soft tissue treatment is established, the most appropriate technique(s) can be applied.

Treatment goals

The following are common treatment goals:

- Increase circulation.
- Decrease swelling.
- Increase tissue extensibility.
- Reduce adhesions.
- Increase scar mobility.
- Eliminate trigger points or tender points.
- Promote tendon and ligament healing.

- Increase ROM.
- Decrease pain.
- Decrease muscle spasm.
- Facilitate or inhibit neuromuscular activity.

Techniques

The choice of technique for a particular condition will depend upon the goal of treatment, the size and shape of the muscle, tendon, ligament, or fascia, and the pathological state of the tissue.

Effleurage consists of long slow strokes, generally light to moderate pressure, usually parallel to the direction of the muscle fibers (Figure 6.2).

Petrissage involves short, brisk strokes, moderate to deep pressure, parallel, perpendicular, or diagonally across the direction of the muscle fibers. It may include kneading, wringing, or skin rolling (Figure 6.3).

Tapotement is rhythmic, brisk percussion often administered with the tips of the fingers; primarily used as a stimulating stroke to facilitate a weak muscle (Figure 6.4).

Cross-friction massage (also known as *deep friction massage*) was made popular by one of the foremost specialists in the diagnosis and treatment of musculoskeletal injury and pain syndromes, British physician James Cyriax. He proposed that the goals of cross-friction massage were to enhance tissue mobility, prevent scar tissue build-up, and increase circulation (Chamberlain, 1982). Cross-friction massage is performed by applying moderate digital pressure perpendicularly across the desired tissue (Figure 6.5). Pressure is maintained in such a way that the finger does not slide across the skin, but rather takes the skin with it. In so doing, the force is transmitted directly to deeper tissues. Cross-friction massage is commonly used on tendons, ligaments, and well-healed scars in order to promote realignment of noncontractile fibers. It has been shown to be effective in enhancing pain reduction and ROM when used as an adjunct therapy to therapeutic exercise (Sonkusale et al., 2016).

Ischemic compression is performed by applying sustained moderate to deep pressure to an area of localized hyperactivity. It is a therapeutic technique in which blood flow to a local area is intentionally blocked. It is believed that a resurgence of local blood flow will occur upon release. Once discomfort is reduced, increased pressure is applied. Ischemic compression is thought to

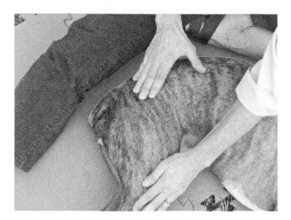

Figure 6.2   Effleurage to the gluteal muscles. Effleurage consists of long slow strokes, generally light to moderate pressure, usually parallel to the direction of the muscle fibers.

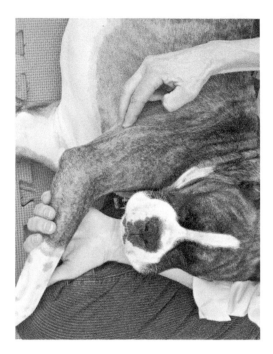

Figure 6.4   Tapotement to the triceps muscle. Tapotement is rhythmic, brisk percussion often administered with the tips of the fingers, primarily used as a stimulating stroke to facilitate a weak muscle.

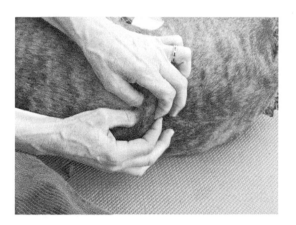

Figure 6.3   Petrissage (skin rolling) of the paravertebral muscles. Petrissage involves short, brisk strokes, moderate to deep pressure, parallel, perpendicular, or diagonally across the direction of the muscle fibers. It may include kneading, wringing, or skin rolling.

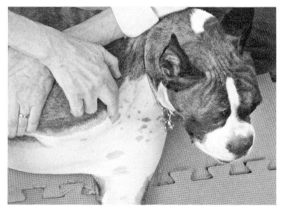

Figure 6.5   Cross-friction massage of the supraspinatus tendon. Cross-friction massage involves applying moderate pressure perpendicularly across the desired tissue. Pressure is maintained in such a way that the finger does not slide across the skin, but rather takes the skin with it.

restore circulation, inhibit the muscle, reduce muscular tension, and promote healing.

Trigger point release/trigger point pressure release techniques were popularized by Dr Janet Travell in the early 1940s in conjunction with her extensive work on myofascial pain. Myofascial pain or myofascial pain syndrome (MPS) is a musculoskeletal pain condition characterized by deep, achy pain (local or referred) and the presence of trigger points (TrPs; Saavedra *et al.*, 2014). Travell defines a TrP as a hyperirritable point within a taut band of skeletal muscle (Travell & Simons, 1983). A TrP can be active or latent. If active, it is tender to palpation and has a predictable pattern of referred pain that often occurs "within the same dermatome, myotome or sclerotome" as the muscle in which it is embedded (Travell & Simons, 1983).

If a TrP is latent, it is nontender to palpation and may persist. The presence of a TrP can result in muscle tightness and/or weakness leading to motor dysfunction (McPartland, 2004). Gordon and colleagues (2016) demonstrated decreased pain, increased flexibility, and improved mobility with the use of TrP release in patients with chronic shoulder pain.

Travell and Simons originally recommended a TrP treatment technique similar to ischemic compression. However, after further research in the late 1990s they modified their technique, recommending the use of gentle digital pressure. This change in approach was based on what Travell referred to as the "ATP energy crisis model." This model characterized a TrP as an area of tissue hypoxia for which ischemic compression was contraindicated (Simons *et al.*, 1999). Their modified technique was named "trigger point pressure release" (TTPR) and was based on the "barrier-release concept." This technique uses gentle digital pressure on the TrP, allowing the practitioner's finger to *follow* the releasing tissue (McPartland, 2004). As the TrP tissue is released, the digital pressure moves deeper into the TrP until it is resolved. Deactivation of TrPs can also be achieved with other techniques such as dry needling, positional release therapy, spray and stretch, and injection (McPartland, 2004). It should be noted that further scrutiny of trigger point theory and practice is ongoing and is necessary for a better understanding of the science behind this phenomenon.

Positional release therapy (PRT), also referred to as *strain-counterstrain* (SCS), is a technique used to treat tissue dysfunction (pain, tightness, spasm). The technique was developed in the 1950s by Dr Lawrence Jones, an osteopathic physician, who created a map of commonly occurring tender points throughout the body (Simons *et al.*, 1999). He believed that tender points were associated with nerve root innervations (Speicher, 2016). Jones proposed that PRT/SCS inhibited the muscle spindle activation, which decreases the amount of afferent impulses to the brain and, thus, efferent impulses to the same muscle. By interrupting this pathway, the patient's muscle is allowed to relax and assume a normal resting tone (Kuchera, 2008). Tender points were described as discrete areas of tissue tenderness that can occur anywhere in the body (Speicher, 2016). This is in contrast to a TrP, which is a hyperirritable band of tissue. A tender point is used diagnostically to indicate the location of the dysfunction (D'Ambrogio & Roth, 1997). PRT/SCS is a gentle, passive technique that is generally well tolerated in acute, subacute, and chronic somatic dysfunction in people of all ages (Speicher & Draper, 2006). The technique consists of precise positioning of the body part or joint such that the tissue is maximally relaxed or shortened. While gently palpating the tender point, positional micro-movements or "fine-tuning" are performed until decreased tenderness of the point is subjectively reported and a reduction of firmness of the point is objectively noted (D'Ambrogio & Roth, 1997). The position is held for 60–90 s (3 minutes for the neurological patient) after which the patient is slowly and passively returned to the anatomically neutral position without firing of the muscle spindle.

Additional manual techniques that are outside the scope of this text but merit acknowledgement are as follows.

Myofascial release (MFR) addresses myofascial connective tissue restriction with the intention of eliminating pain and restoring motion. Elongation of restricted fascial tissue is achieved by applying a slow, low load (gentle pressure) to the target viscoelastic medium (fascia). The load is applied in three planes of motion using either direct (into the direction of restriction) or indirect (away from the direction of restriction) techniques. This technique requires advanced training from a therapist specializing in MFR.

Acupressure is based on the ancient healing art of acupuncture. Using the same pressure points and meridians, acupressure employs finger pressure rather than needles to specific points on the body.

Manual lymphatic drainage therapy (MLD) focuses on specific lymph nodes and the natural flow of the lymphatic system. Given that the lymphatic system does not have its own pumping mechanism, MLD is intended to promote free-flowing lymphatic drainage. The technique uses specific rhythmic hand strokes taught by an MLD therapist.

Treatment design

With knowledge of the above treatment techniques, one can determine which technique(s) will most effectively address the patient's issues (Table 6.2). It is important that the underlying cause or the root of the soft tissue abnormality

Table 6.2   Treatment guidelines by goal

Goals	Techniques
Increase circulation	Effleurage, petrissage, tapotement
Decrease swelling	Effleurage; lymphatic drainage
Increase soft tissue extensibility	Effleurage, petrissage, cross-friction massage, positional release, trigger point release, MFR
Reduce adhesions	Cross-friction massage
Increase scar mobility	Cross-friction massage, MFR
Eliminate trigger or tender points	Trigger point release, positional release, ischemic compression
Promote tendon and ligament healing	Cross-friction massage
Increase ROM	All of the above
Decrease pain	Effleurage, petrissage, cross-fiber massage, trigger point release, MFR, ischemic compression
Decrease muscle spasm	Ischemic compression, effleurage, petrissage, tapotement

MFR, myofascial release; ROM, range of movement.

be identified and addressed for long-standing resolution of the problem.

For example, upper trapezius or scalene muscle pain is a common complaint in human medicine. On evaluation, tenderness, trigger points, and decreased flexibility are noted. Is this an isolated muscle strain or is something else causing the muscles to react? In humans, a forward head posture commonly results in upper trapezius and scalene overuse and pain. If this is the case, local treatment of the muscles will not resolve the issue. The root of the problem must be addressed. The effective treatment must involve changing the gravitational effect on these muscles. This can be accomplished with postural correction and exercise. A canine example is the patient with a suspected iliopsoas strain. Is this an isolated muscle strain or is the root of the problem elsewhere? Due to its attachments on the spine, the iliopsoas muscle can become activated with thoracolumbar

dysfunction. If that is the case, local treatment of the iliopsoas muscle will provide temporary relief at best. The spinal dysfunction must be addressed in order for full resolution of the iliopsoas pain.

There are a few contraindications to soft tissue mobilization. Patients with mast cell tumors, phlebitis, or infectious/parasitic dermatitis in the affected area should not be treated with this technique. With these precautions in mind, the therapist can determine the best techniques to apply to the patient, based upon the indicated treatment goals.

Range of motion (ROM)

Normal range of motion (ROM) is required for normal function. When ROM is compromised, the body naturally compensates by increasing movement at another segment. Thus, hypomobility at one segment may result in hypermobility at an adjacent segment. Hypermobility can lead to abnormal localized stress, causing pain and, eventually, laxity. Although there are numerous effective options for treating hypomobility, hypermobility can be difficult to stabilize, often requiring splinting or surgery. Therefore, it is important to thoroughly assess ROM and treat accordingly to establish normal mechanics of the joint and soft tissues. Normal ROM varies considerably among breeds and is affected by age and other factors. Norms for average ROM for all joints have not been well established for the canine population; therefore, comparison with the contralateral side is required.

Passive ROM (PROM)

PROM is used as an assessment tool as well as a treatment technique. PROM is passive, osteokinematic movement of bony segments around a joint axis performed by the therapist. The patient is noncontributory. Normally PROM is slightly greater than active range of motion (AROM) because each joint has a small amount of involuntary, end-range joint play motion that the therapist can create with overpressure (Norkin & White, 1985). Joint PROM is the ability of the joint to move through its normal ROM without restriction of muscles that

Case Study 6.1   Manual therapy for postoperative FHO

Signalment: 9 y.o. M/N Brittany Spaniel.

Presenting complaint: 1 month post-op L FHO with decreased ROM, decreased weight bearing, and weakness.

Evaluation: Physical exam WNL except:
Gait: (walk) PWB L pelvic limb, decreased L stride length and stance time, compensatory spinal side bend.
Palpation: decreased STM, trigger point and tenderness at L iliopsoas.
PROM: hip extension L 125, R 150.
Flexibility: L iliopsoas moderately tight; R NL.
Atrophy: moderate+ at L gluteals, moderate at L hamstrings, and quadriceps.
Strength: 3-leg strength test: fair (3/5); diagonal limb strength test: poor (<3/5).

Assessment: 1 month post-op L FHO with expected limitation in ROM, flexibility and strength.

Problem list:

- Limited L hip extension.
- Tight L iliopsoas.
- R pelvic limb weakness.
- Inadequate weight bearing.
- Altered gait.

Goals:

- Symmetrical walking gait in 6 weeks.
- Symmetrical sit-to-stand transfers in 6 weeks.
- Ability to walk on stairs without difficulty in 8 weeks.
- Return to 1-hour hikes in 10 weeks.

Treatment:
Modalities: laser to L iliopsoas.
Manual therapy: gentle passive stretch of L iliopsoas with simultaneous STM of muscle belly, trigger point release L iliopsoas, joint compressions in standing, passive gait simulation in standing.
PROM: gentle hip extension with STM of sartorius, rectus femoris, iliopsoas.
Therapeutic exercise:
- Weight bearing: weight-shifting exercises, slow walking with head elevated, counterclockwise circle walking, low cavaletti walking.
- Strengthen: 3-leg stands, backward walking, front feet on wobble disc.
- Home Exercise Plan (HEP): joint compressions and PROM per above; slow walking on flat and inclines, backward walking, side stepping, thoracic limbs on wobble board or disc.

cross two or more joints. Therefore, an assessment of passive joint ROM is distinguished from an assessment of muscle flexibility or joint arthrokinematics. If PROM is restricted, it is important to identify the limiting structure in order to direct the treatment appropriately. This is accomplished by noting end-feel.

End-feel

The restriction to further motion as perceived by the therapist is called end-feel. It is the sensation in the therapist's hands when overpressure is applied at the end-range of osteokinematic motion. End-feel is assessed by passively moving the joint through its available ROM, slowly applying moderate *overpressure* at the end-range, and noting the feel of the resistance. PROM can be limited by pain or swelling as well as musculotendinous tissue, bone, joint capsule, muscle spasm, fascial tissue, soft tissue approximation, or intra-articular derangement. Each structure has a characteristic feel that can be detected by the examiner (Norkin & White, 1985).

Table 6.3   Characteristics of different types of end-feel

End-feel/block	Sensation
Soft tissue approximation	Soft, yielding
Muscle/tendon	Firm, slight give, elastic
Capsule	Very firm
Muscle spasm	Abrupt stop, hard
Edema	Soft and boggy
Bone	Hard, unyielding
Empty	Pain before resistance
Springy	Rebound

Practice is necessary in order to develop the ability to sense the different characteristics of the limiting structure (Table 6.3). A pathological end-feel is the presence of restriction prematurely in the ROM.

By identifying the limiting structure, the treatment can be designed to affect the particular characteristics of that structure. For example, if joint ROM is restricted by joint capsule, the treatment of choice will be joint mobilization. However, if ROM is restricted by muscle spasm, the treatment of choice may be a soft tissue technique such as ischemic compression. Table 6.3 shows a list of end-feels with their associated sensations.

Assessment of PROM

In addition to end-feel, assessment of PROM provides the examiner with information about the quantity of joint osteokinematic motion. Quantity of motion is measured with a goniometer and documented in degrees. Goniometry provides a baseline measurement from which the effectiveness of the treatment can be determined. If the contralateral side is without pathology, its ROM can be used as normal.

A goniometer consists of a fulcrum, a proximal arm (stable arm), and a distal arm (moving arm). When measuring the quantity of joint ROM, the fulcrum is lined up with the approximate joint axis, the proximal arm is lined up with a specific proximal bony landmark, and the distal arm is lined up with a specific distal bony landmark. Each joint has specific bony landmarks to insure reproducibility. See Chapter 5 for the landmarks for each joint.

Technique

When assessing PROM, the proximal bony segment is stabilized and the distal bony segment is mobilized. In order for the measurement to be accurate, the patient's muscles must be relaxed. The limb is positioned such that joint motion is not restricted by multijoint muscle tightness. For example, shoulder flexion ROM must be performed with the elbow in flexion. If the elbow were extended, ROM would be limited by the biceps muscle becoming taut. Proper sequencing for PROM includes moving the joint through the available PROM, applying overpressure, noting the end-feel, and measuring ROM with a goniometer (Figure 6.6). Once end-feel is determined, the goniometer is placed on the limb and the angle is measured. The therapist must be careful not to block motion with the stabilizing or mobilizing hand. If a restriction is noted, the contralateral side is measured.

Treatment of limited PROM

As a treatment, PROM is used as a general technique to maintain or increase ROM. The

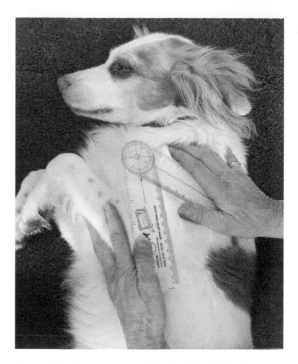

Figure 6.6 Measurement of the shoulder in flexion. The joint is moved through the available passive range of motion (PROM) noting the end-feel. The goniometer is then placed on the limb and the angle is measured.

assessment and treatment techniques are identical except that during treatment the end range of the movement is held for 10–20 seconds and repeated 3–5 times. With proper client instruction, this treatment can be added to the home program.

Flexibility

Flexibility refers to muscle length and should not be confused with joint PROM. It is assessed separately and is an important component of a thorough musculoskeletal exam. Clinically, two-joint or multijoint muscles are most commonly tight and/or injured.

Assessment of muscle flexibility

Muscle flexibility is assessed by placing the limb in the position that is opposite of the action(s) of the muscle being tested. For example, the actions of the biceps brachii muscle are to extend the shoulder and flex

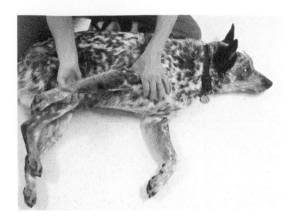

Figure 6.7   Biceps brachii muscle stretch. Moving the shoulder into flexion and the elbow into extension tests biceps flexibility.

the elbow. Therefore, moving the shoulder into flexion and the elbow into extension tests biceps flexibility (Figure 6.7). Documentation of abnormal flexibility can be noted as minimally, moderately, or severely restricted or can be measured with a goniometer.

Treatment of decreased flexibility

Increasing muscle extensibility is accomplished by stretching the tight muscle. Stretching can be performed passively, in combination with soft tissue mobilization or actively with specific exercises. Similar to the muscle flexibility assessment position, a passive stretch is performed with the limbs placed in a position that is opposite to the actions of the muscle. Typically, the origin of the muscle is stabilized and the insertion is moved away from the origin.

The stretch should be moderate (palpable muscle tension) and within the patient's comfort range. The stretch must be effective but not painful. If pain is produced, the patient will splint (involuntary rigid contraction of the muscles in response to pain), resulting in a shortening of the muscle fibers. Human research has shown that carryover is more effective with a 30-second passive, static stretch than a 15-second stretch. Gains with an additional 30 seconds (60 seconds total) were shown to be minimal (Bandy & Irion, 1994). For added effectiveness, the stretch can be combined with

soft tissue mobilization of the muscle being stretched. A muscle can also be stretched dynamically. This is performed by instructing the patient to actively move into a position that stretches the muscle. Dynamic stretching may not be as effective as static stretching in increasing flexibility (O'Sullivan *et al.*, 2009) but may be more effective in increasing athletic performance (McMillian *et al.*, 2006).

Joint mobilization

Attention to the intrinsic movement of joints reaches back to the days of Hippocrates (460–370 BC). Joint manipulation, referred to as bone setting, spread in Europe between the seventeenth and early twentieth centuries; however, no formal training was established until Andrew Still founded the first school of osteopathy in 1874. Physical therapists began studying joint mobilization and manipulation in manual therapy programs established by leaders in the field, Freddy Kaltenborn, Geoffrey Maitland, and Stanly Paris in the early 1960s. Research has demonstrated both biomechanical and neurophysiological effects of joint mobilization; however, the mechanism of change is still under scrutiny (Brantingham *et al.*, 2009; Zusman, 2010).

Joint play (or joint mobility) is passive, involuntary arthrokinematic motion that occurs between two joint surfaces during movement. It is required for normal osteokinematic motion. Joint play consists of two passive movements: traction/separation and translatoric gliding, both of which are required to prevent compression and/or subluxation of a joint (Kaltenborn *et al.*, 1999). Loss of joint play may be the result of capsular tightness that blocks the normal arthrokinematic gliding within the joint. Capsular tightness can be identified by assessing the end-feel during PROM and by assessing joint play.

The goals of joint mobilization are to increase arthrokinematic range of motion, improve joint alignment and tracking, decrease pain, and reduce muscle spasm by stimulating articular sensory receptors (Maitland, 1977). Joint mobilization has been shown to have mechanical effects on the joint capsule (i.e., stretch the capsule) that correspond with improved ROM

(Landrum *et al.*, 2008). Some research suggests that a primary effect of joint mobilization is enhancement of the sensorimotor system (Maitland, 1977; Kaltenborn *et al.*, 1999).

The following discussion of joint mobilization principles and techniques is based on the teachings of Freddy Kaltenborn, a Norwegian physical therapist who specialized in orthopedic manipulative therapy (OMT). He was certified in the United States as an instructor of orthopaedic medicine by James Cyriax, the British physician and professor of osteopathy. Additionally, Kaltenborn was an instructor of chiropractic in Germany. He was the first clinician to integrate the theory and practice of orthopedic medicine with the practice of osteopathy, and he authored several books related to manual techniques of the peripheral joints and spine.

Assessing joint play

Joint play is evaluated with an assessment glide. Kaltenborn defines a glide as the movement that occurs when the same point on one surface of the joint comes into contact with new points of its opposing surface (Kaltenborn *et al.*, 1999). The purpose of the assessment glide is to evaluate the quantity (amount of translation) and quality of joint accessory motion. It is an advanced skill requiring a thorough understanding of joint anatomy and mechanics. Tightening or injury of the capsule and/or its associated ligaments can limit joint play (Figure 6.8).

Technique—assessment glide

The assessment glide is a single translatoric glide in which one bony surface is stabilized and the other is mobilized. It is performed close to the joint line so that a pure translatory motion occurs without compression. The glide is performed in the loose-packed or resting position. This is the position in which the joint capsule and associated ligaments are most relaxed and the most amount of joint play is possible (Kaltenborn *et al.*, 1999). If this position is unattainable due to pain or pathology, the position of greatest comfort is used.

The angle of the glide is determined by the position of the joint surfaces and is referred to as the treatment plane. The treatment plane "passes through the joint and lies at a right angle to a line running from the axis of rotation (in the convex bony partner) to the middle of the contacting articular surface" (Kaltenborn *et al.*, 1999) (Figure 6.9). The treatment plane lies across the concave articular surface and moves with the concave joint partner (Kaltenborn *et al.*, 1999).

The glide is performed by applying slow, steady pressure along the treatment plane (Figure 6.10). Movement is continued until a

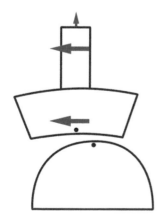

Figure 6.8 Motion involved in a joint glide. Source: Adapted from Kaltenborn *et al.*, 1999.

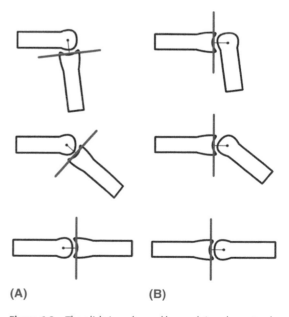

(A)   **(B)**

Figure 6.9 The glide is performed by applying slow, steady pressure along the treatment plane. The treatment plane lies across the concave articular surface. surface whether the concave surface is on the mobile **(A)** or stationary **(B)** segment. Source: Adapted from Kaltenborn *et al.*, 1999.

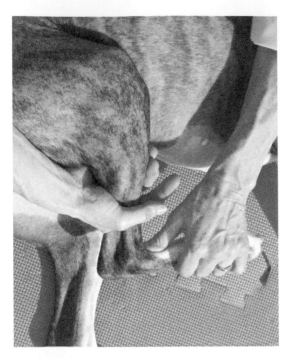

Figure 6.10   Assessment glide—caudal glide of the talus with stabilization of the distal tibia and fibula.

barrier (or restriction) is appreciated and no further translation is possible. The quantity of motion is graded on a scale of 0–6 (see below). Assessment glides can be performed in multiple directions (caudal, cranial, dorsal, ventral, medial, and lateral). The glide must be pain free as splinting in reaction to pain will skew the results. The quantity of motion is compared with the contralateral side.

Assessment glides are graded on a 0–6 scale (Kaltenborn *et al.*, 1999):

0 No movement (ankylosis)
1 Severely restricted
2 Moderately restricted
3 Normal
4 Moderately hypermobile
5 Severely hypermobile
6 Complete instability.

Joint mobilization (treatment)

Joint mobilization is a passive therapeutic technique intended to increase arthrokinematic motion and to relieve pain. When ROM is limited by capsular tightening, joint mobilization is the treatment of choice.

Because joint surfaces are rounded, physiological movement occurs around several axes simultaneously. Although a predominant movement plane is noted (sagittal, frontal, or transverse), osteokinematic motion is not pure and occurs in more than one movement plane. The mechanics of the convex and concave joint surfaces moving on one another involves rotational and translatory movements that coincide with rolling and gliding of the bony segments. The more congruent the surfaces are, the greater the amount of glide. Conversely, the more incongruent they are, the more rolling is required in order to avoid joint compression or subluxation. The direction of rolling and gliding depends on which surface is moving, the convex or concave.

Understanding the convex-concave rule is important for proper use of joint mobilization techniques. This rule states that when a concave surface moves on a stabilized convex surface, the arthrokinematic glide will occur in the *same* direction as the osteokinematic movement of the bony segment (Figure 6.11). For example, during osteokinematic stifle extension, the shaft of the tibia moves cranially. Arthrokinematically the concave proximal tibia (concave menisci) will

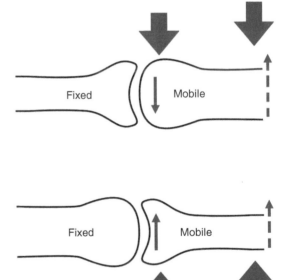

Figure 6.11   The convex-concave rule states that when a concave surface moves on a stabilized convex surface, the arthrokinematic glide will occur in the *same* direction as the osteokinematic movement of the bony segment. Source: Adapted from Kaltenborn *et al.*, 1999.

move in the *same* cranial direction on the stabilized convex distal femur. Conversely, if a convex surface moves on a stable concave surface, the arthrokinematic glide will occur in the *opposite* direction of the osteokinematic movement of the bony segment. For example, during osteokinematic shoulder extension, the shaft of the humerus moves cranially while arthrokinematically, the convex surface of the humerus moves in the *opposite* direction (caudally) on the stabilized concave glenoid fossa.

In summary, the therapist moves a bone with a *convex* joint surface *opposite* to the direction of the restricted bone movement, and a *concave* joint surface in the *same* direction as the direction of the restricted bone movement (Kaltenborn *et al.*, 1999).

Treatment variables include: (1) position of joint, (2) type of mobilization, (3) direction of mobilization, and (4) grade of mobilization. As with the assessment glide, treatment is initiated with the joint in the loose-pack or resting position. There are two types of mobilizations—a glide or oscillation and a sustained traction. A glide is performed parallel to the treatment plane and uses graded oscillations, while traction is performed perpendicular to the treatment plane and involves a graded sustained pull (Figure 6.12). The direction of the glide will depend on the specific restriction of the joint. The grade of mobilization will depend on the goal of your treatment (pain vs mobility).

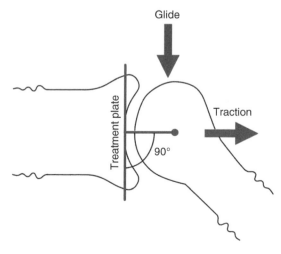

Figure 6.12 Glides are performed parallel to the treatment plane. Traction is performed at a right angle to the treatment plane. Source: Adapted from Kaltenborn *et al.*, 1999.

Treatment glide

A treatment glide is essentially a graded assessment glide that is performed in the treatment plane (parallel to the joint line). Grade I and II glides are used to treat pain. Grade III–IV glides are used to increase or maintain motion. All grades are used to stimulate mechanoreceptors and stimulate proprioceptive fibers. Grading is outlined in Table 6.4.

Geoffrey Maitland proposed that different grades of mobilization produce selective activation of different mechanoreceptors in the joint (Maitland, 1977).

Grade I activates type I mechanoreceptors with a low threshold that respond to very small increments of tension. This grade will activate cutaneous mechanoreceptors. Oscillatory motion will selectively activate the dynamic, rapidly adapting receptors (i.e., Meissner's and Pacinian corpuscles).

Grade II activates some type I mechanoreceptors. By virtue of the large amplitude of movement it will affect type II mechanoreceptors to a greater extent.

Grade III is similar to grade II but selectively activates more of the muscle and joint mechanoreceptors as it goes into resistance, and fewer of the cutaneous ones as the slack of the subcutaneous tissues is taken up.

Grade IV has a more sustained movement at the end of range and thus activates the static, slow-adapting type I mechanoreceptors whose resting discharge rises in proportion to the degree of change in joint capsule tension.

Table 6.4   Grading of treatment glides

Grade	Characteristics
I	Small-amplitude fast oscillations performed at the beginning of the available range
II	Large-amplitude slow oscillations performed throughout the first half of the available range
III	Large-amplitude slow oscillations performed throughout the second half of the available range
IV	Small-amplitude fast oscillations performed at the end of the available range

Traction

Traction is a sustained force that separates joint surfaces. It is performed at a right angle to the treatment plane. It is considered a more general technique than glides since it has a global effect on the capsule rather than affecting a particular aspect of the capsule. Grade I and II tractions are used for treating pain; grade III is used to stretch the surrounding tissues. Kaltenborn recommends intermittent traction with 10-second holds and a rest between each repetition. Other authors propose maintaining the traction for 20–30 seconds (Kaltenborn *et al.*, 1999). Grading of traction is shown in Table 6.5.

The *technique* for performing glides or traction involves starting with the joint in a position of maximal comfort in order to minimize muscle tension. This is the resting position. The therapist places the stabilizing hand on the nonmoving part (usually the proximal segment) as close to the joint space as possible. The mobilizing hand is on the joint partner to be moved, generally as close to the joint space as possible, though in some traction techniques a longer lever arm will be used, necessitating moving the mobilizing hand more distal on the limb.

Treatment *direction* depends upon the technique to be performed. Traction techniques are performed perpendicular to the treatment plane (grades I–III), while gliding techniques are performed parallel to the treatment plane (grades I–IV). The specific direction of the glide (dorsal, ventral, cranial, caudal, medial, lateral) will depend on the particular restriction determined by the assessment glide (arthrokinematic motion) and corresponding PROM/AROM (osteokinematic motion) limitations. Understanding the convex-concave rule allows the therapist to determine the best direction of the treatment glide. Treatment grade is based on the goal of the treatment (to decrease pain or to increase mobility) (Table 6.6).

Treatment example

Kaltenborn's techniques are based on an understanding of normal joint arthrokinematics. For example, glenohumeral extension is associated with a caudal glide of the humeral head, whereas glenohumeral abduction is associated with a medial glide of the humeral head. The arthrokinematic motion is opposite to the osteokinematic motion because the convex surface of the humeral head is moving on the concave surface of the scapula. Therefore, limited shoulder osteokinematic ROM into extension is associated with a restricted caudal assessment glide of the humerus due to a tight caudal capsule. Therefore, the appropriate treatment for restricted shoulder extension that is limited by capsular tightness is a grade III or IV caudal glide of the humerus (Table 6.7; Figure 6.13) and that for caudal mobilization of the tibiofemoral joint is provided in Table 6.8 (Figure 6.14).

Applying the convex-concave rule at the tibiofemoral joint:

- A caudal glide will promote stifle flexion.
- A cranial glide will promote stifle extension.
- Distraction promotes general joint mobility.

When using joint mobilization to increase ROM, consider how to maximize the treatment. This may include preparing the tissues. If the goal is to increase the extensibility of the capsule, warming the joint tissues may be an effective

Table 6.6 Determination of treatment grades

Problem	Treatment	Grade
Pain	Traction	Grades I, II
	Glide	Grades I, II
Hypermobility	Traction	Grade III
	Glide	Grades III, IV

Table 6.5 Grading of traction

Grade	Characteristics
I	No appreciable joint separation; eliminates compression forces
II	Slack is taken up, ligaments and capsule are taut
III	Slack has been taken up and more traction force is applied; surrounding tissues are stretched

Table 6.7 Technique for caudal mobilization of shoulder

Goal	To increase shoulder extension, decrease pain
Patient	Lateral recumbency; shoulder in resting position
Therapist	Stabilizing hand: thumb on caudal aspect of the acromion Mobilizing hand: index finger on the cranial aspect of the proximal humerus

precursor to joint mobilization. Exercise is the most effective means of warming the tissues; however, modalities may be used if the patient cannot tolerate exercise. Once joint mobilization is performed and improved PROM is noted, it is important that the patient actively uses the newly achieved ROM when possible. This can be accomplished with an exercise prescription that uses the new ROM. For example, in the case above where the treatment goal was to increase stifle flexion, the patient may perform sit-to-stand exercises or walk over high cavaletti poles in order to use the newly acquired ROM.

Figure 6.13 Caudal glide of the proximal humerus with scapular stabilization at the caudal aspect of the acromion.

Table 6.8 Technique for caudal mobilization of femorotibial joint

Goal	To increase stifle flexion, decrease pain
Patient	Lateral recumbency; stifle in resting position
Therapist	Stabilizing hand: web space at caudal distal femur Mobilizing hand: web space on tibial tuberosity

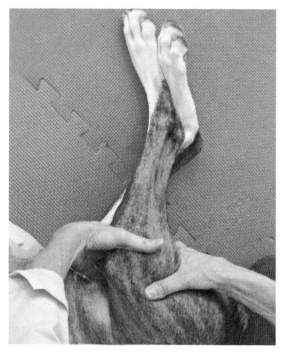

Figure 6.14 Caudal glide of the tibia with femoral stabilization.

Case Study 6.2   Manual therapy for postoperative TPLO

Signalment: 4 y.o. F/S Labrador.

Presenting complaint: 8 weeks post-op R TPLO with decreased ROM and weakness; radiographs reveal good bone healing.

Evaluation reveals: Physical exam WNL except:
Function: standing PWB R pelvic limb (approximately 40%).
Sitting R hip abducted/externally rotated; decreased stifle and tarsal flexion.
Gait: walk—PWB (approximately 65%) 100% of time; minimally+ shortened stride length and stance time.
Palpation: mild swelling at ventromedial and ventrolateral stifle joint.

PROM:

Stifle extension	L 165	R 150
Stifle flexion	L 40	R 50
Tarsal flexion	L 40	R 55

Flexibility: moderately tight R hamstrings, iliopsoas, sartorius.
Joint play: caudal tarsal glide—grade 2 hypomobility.
Atrophy: moderate at R gluteals and quadriceps, moderate at R hamstrings.

Strength:
- 3-leg standing test: good (3+/5)
- Diagonal leg standing test: fair (3/5)

(Continued)

Assessment: 2 months post-op R TPLO; behind schedule regarding ROM and weight bearing; nonpainful.

Problem list:

- Swelling
- Decreased weight bearing
- Asymmetrical sitting position
- Limited R stifle extension and flexion
- Limited R tarsal flexion
- Tight R hamstrings, quadriceps, sartorius
- R pelvic limb weakness – moderate
- Asymmetrical gait

Goals:

In 4 weeks:

- Normal sitting posture
- Normal ROM
- Normal flexibility
- FWB

In 8 weeks:

- Symmetrical walking gait
- Gradual return to off-leash activities
- Client independent in HEP

Modalities: Laser at ventromedial and ventrolateral stifle joint in loose-packed position.

Manual therapy:

Joint compressions: grade I–II at stifle in standing position.

Joint mobilization: grade III stifle joint traction followed by PROM into stifle flexion and extension.

Joint mobilization: grade IV, caudal tarsal glide followed PROM into tarsal flexion.

Passive stretch: hamstrings, quadriceps, sartorius with simultaneous soft tissue mobilization of the belly of affected muscle.

Therapeutic exercise:

Weight-bearing exercises such as clockwise circles, cavalettis.

R pelvic limb strengthening such as slow uphill walking; horizontal hill walking, backward walking, side stepping, exercise band resisted walking.

HEP

Instruct client in HEP to be performed 2×/day: joint compressions and PROM per above, petrissage of tight muscles per above; clockwise circles 5 reps; gradual progression of slow walking on flat surfaces with progression to inclines, backward walking and side stepping (3–6 feet × 5 reps).

Conclusion

Our hands are our most important rehabilitation tools. Using manual techniques to resolve soft tissue and joint issues will expedite the rehabilitation process and allow the therapist to progress to the next stage of the rehabilitation program.

References

Abbott, J. H., Chapple, C., Fitzgerald, G. K., Fritz, J. M., Childs, J. D., Harcombe, H., & Stout, K. 2015. The incremental effects of manual therapy or booster sessions in additions to exercise therapy for knee osteoarthritis: A randomized clinical trial. *Phys Ther*, 45, 975–983.

Bandy, W.D. & Irion, J.M. 1994. The effect of time on static stretch on the flexibility of the hamstring muscles. *Phys Ther*, 74(9), 845–850; discussion 850–852.

Bervoets, D. C., Luijsterburg, P. A., Alessie, J. J., Buijs, M. J., & Verhagen, A. P. 2015. Massage therapy has short-term benefits for people with common musculoskeletal disorders compared to no treatment: a systematic review. *Phys Ther*, 61, 106–116.

Brantingham, J. W., Globe, G., Pollard, H., Hicks, M., Korporaal, C., & Hoskins, W. 2009. Manipulative therapy for lower extremity conditions: expansion of literature review. *J Manipulative Physiol Ther*, 32, 53–71.

Chamberlain, G. J. 1982. Cyriax's friction massage: A review. *J Orthop Sport Phys*, 4(1), 16–22.

Costello, M., Puentedura, E., Cleland, J., & Ciccone, C. D. 2016. The immediate efects of soft tissue mobilization versus therapeutic ultrasound for patients with neck and arm pain with evidence of neural mechanosensitivity: a randomized clinical trial. *J Man Manip Ther*, 24, 128–140.

Crawford, C., Biyd, C., Paat, C. F., Price, A., Xenakis, L., Yang, E., Zhang, W., & the Evidence for Massage Therapy Working Group. 2016. The impact of massage therapy on function in pain popuulations – A systematic review and meta-analysis of randomized controlled trials: Part 1, Patients exeriencing pain in the general population. *Pain Med*, 17, 1353–1375.

D'Ambrogio, K. J. & Roth, G. B. 1997. *Positional Release Therapy*. St Louis, MO: Mosby.

Fritz, S. & Grosenbach, M. J. 2009. *Mosby's Essential Sciences for Therapeutic Massage*. St Louis, MO: Mosby.

Gordon, C-M., Andrasik, F., Schleip, R., Birbaumer, N., & Massimiliano, R. 2016. Myofascial triggerpoint release (mtr)for treating chronic shoulder pain: A novel approach. *J Bodywork Movement Ther*, 20, 614–622.

Hertling, D. & Kessler, R. M. 1990. *Management of Common Musculoskeletal Disorders: Physical Therapy Principles and Methods*, 2nd edn. Philadelphia, PA: Lippincott.

Kaltenborn, F. M., Evjenth, O., & Baldauf Kaltenborn, T. 1999. *Manual Mobilization of the Joints: The Kaltenborn Method of Joint Examination and Treatment: Vol. 1, The Extremities*, 5th edn. Minneapolis, MN: Orthopedic Physical Therapy Products.

Kuchera, M. L. 2008. Clinical application of counterstrain. *J Am Osteopath Assoc*, 108, 267–268.

Landrum, E. L., Kelln, C. B., Parente, W. R., Ingersoll, C. D., & Hertel, J. 2008. Immediate effects of anterior-to-posterior talocrural joint mobilization after prolonged ankle immobilization: A preliminary study. *J Man Manip Ther*, 16, 100–105.

Magee, D. J. 1992. *Orthopedic Physical Assessment*. Philadelphia, PA: W.B. Saunders.

Maitland, C. 1977. *Peripheral Manipulation*, 2nd edn. Sydney, Australia: Butterworths.

Mcmillian, D. J., Moore, J. H., Hatler, B. S., & Taylor, D. C. 2006. Dynamic vs. static-stretching warm up: the effect on power and agility performance. *J Strength Cond Res*, 20, 492–499.

Mcpartland, J. M. 2004. Travell trigger points— molecular and osteopathic perspectives. *J Am Osteopath Assoc*, 104, 244–249.

Millis, D. L., Levine, D., & Taylor, R. A. 2004. *Canine Rehabilitation & Physical Therapy*. St Louis, MO: Saunders.

Norkin, C. C. & White, D. J. 1985. *Measurement of Joint Motion: A Guide to Goniometry*, 1st edn. Philadelphia, PA: Davis.

O'Sullivan, K., Murray, E., & Sainsbury, D. 2009. The effect of warm-up, static stretching and dynamic stretching on hamstring flexibility in previously injured subjects. *BMC Musculoskelet Disord*, 10, 37.

Poppendieck, W., Wegmann, M., Ferrauti, A., Kellman, M., Pfeiffer, M., & Meyer, T. 2016. Massage and performance recovery: A meta-analytical review. *Sports Med*, 46, 183–204.

Saavedra, F. J., Cordeiro, M. T., Alves, J. V., Fernandes, H., M., Reis, V. M., & Mont'Alverne, D. G. B. 2014. The influence of positional release therapy on the myofascial tension of the upper trapezius muscle. *Revista Brasileira de Cineantropometria e Desempenho Humano*, 16(2); doi: 10.5007/1980-0037.2014v16n2p191.

Salvo, S. G. 2012. *Massage Therapy: Principles and Practice*, 4th edn. St Louis, MO: Saunders.

Sefton, J. M., Yarar, C., Carpenter, D. M., & Berry, J. W. 2011. Physiological and clinical changes after therapeutic massage of the neck and shoulders. *Man Ther*, 16, 487–494.

Simons, D. G., Travell, J. G., & Simons, L. S. 1999. *Travell & Simons' Myofascial Pain and Dysfunction: The Trigger Point Manual*, 2nd edn. Baltimore, MD: Williams & Wilkins.

Sonkusale, J. T., Damke, U. S., & Bhave, S. M. 2016. Comparing the effectiveness of deep transverse friction massage on supraspinatus as an adjunct to PNF in idiopathic adhesive capsulitis of shoulder. *Indian Journal of Physiotherapy and Occupational Therapy – An International Journal*, 10(2), 114–120.

Speicher, T. 2016. *Clinical Guide to Positional Release Therapy*. Champaign, IL: Human Kinetics.

Speicher, T. & Draper, D. O. 2006. *Top-10 positional-release therapy techniques to break the chain of pain: Part 2*. Sacred Heart University Faculty Publications. November.

Travell, J. G. & Simons, D. G. 1983. *Myofascial Pain and Dysfunction, The Trigger Point Manual*. Baltimore, London, Los Angeles, Sydney: Williams & Wilkins.

Van Den Dolder, P., Ferreira, P., & Refshauge, K. 2010. Is soft tissue massage an effective treatment for mechanical shoulder pain? A study protocol. *J Man Manip Ther*, 18, 50–54.

Zusman, M. 2010. There's something about passive movement. *Med Hypotheses*, 75, 106–110.

Zusman, M. 2011. Mechanism of mobilization discussion paper; Curtin Univ, Perth, WA, Australia. *Phys Ther Rev*, 16, 233–236.

7
Rehabilitation Physical Modalities

Krista Niebaum, MPT, CCRT, Laurie McCauley, DVM, DACVSMR, CVC, CVA, CCRT, and Carolina Medina, DVM, DACVSMR, CVA, CVCH, CCRT

Summary

Physical modalities are tools that can be used to complement a patient's rehabilitation treatment plan through the use of thermal, sound, electrical, and light energy. They can be used to address pain, swelling, soft tissue restrictions, joint range of motion (ROM) limitations, and muscle weakness, as well as to promote tissue healing, thereby improving a patient's ability to participate in other aspects of rehabilitation therapy (e.g., therapeutic exercise, functional mobility retraining, etc.). A general overview of the physical modalities most commonly used in canine rehabilitation is presented, with a goal of assisting the therapist in determining if and when their use may improve treatment outcome. The modalities discussed are cryotherapy and superficial heating (superficial thermal agents), therapeutic ultrasound (TUS), neuromuscular electrical stimulation (NMES) and transcutaneous electrical nerve stimulation (TENS) (electrical stimulation modalities), low-level laser therapy (LLLT)/photobiomodulation, and extracorporeal shock wave therapy (ESWT). Patients affected by orthopedic and neurological injuries, working and sporting dogs, and the geriatric population can all benefit from use of physical modalities at some point during their rehabilitation program.

Introduction

The primary goal of any rehabilitation treatment plan is to maximize the patient's functional recovery. This may be achieved through a variety of methods including therapeutic exercises (Chapter 8), manual techniques (Chapter 6), functional mobility retraining, and use of assistive devices (Chapters 11 and 18). Physical modalities use thermal, sound, electrical, and light energy to impact the physiology of the target tissue. Physical modalities should be viewed as tools to *augment* and *complement* the treatment plan. Used with an understanding of the impact each has on different tissues, these tools can be effective toward reducing pain, supporting tissue healing, improving flexibility and joint ROM, and facilitating muscle strengthening,

---

Canine Sports Medicine and Rehabilitation, Second Edition. Edited by Chris Zink and Janet B. Van Dyke.
© 2018 John Wiley & Sons, Inc. Published 2018 by John Wiley & Sons, Inc.

thereby maximizing the patient's ability to participate in and benefit from other aspects of the treatment plan.

The decision to use any physical modality must be based on an in-depth understanding of the modality and a thorough assessment of the patient's status, both to determine which modality may be effective and its suitability for that specific patient. Frequent reassessment will help the therapist to further the use of a modality, transition between modalities, or discontinue use altogether at the appropriate time.

The scope of this chapter does not permit a detailed explanation of the physics of each modality, nor will it provide a comprehensive list of the research related to each. Textbooks dedicated to physical modality use in rehabilitation medicine are available and should be referenced for additional information (Cameron, 2013; Bellew et al., 2016). The reader might also review the current literature as the techniques and recommendations continue to evolve.

Superficial thermal agents: cold and heat

Superficial thermal agents are primarily used to reduce swelling and pain, but can also promote healing and improve mobility. Some evidence also indicates that their use can assist with muscle activation. Superficial thermal agents are convenient modalities as they are readily available, involve minimal expense, and are frequently safe to include as part of a home treatment program.

Superficial cold: cryotherapy

Cryotherapy is the use of cold with a goal of *removing* energy from tissues in the form of heat. Its application can result in tissue cooling 2–4 cm deep (Nadler et al., 2004). In canine rehabilitation, this energy transfer generally occurs through conduction as the cold source is placed in direct contact with the body. The initial physiological response is cutaneous vasoconstriction with a resultant reduction in blood flow to the area (Khoshnevis et al., 2015). Cryotherapy is therefore most often used in the acute phase of injury with the goals of reducing inflammation and pain. However, it may also be used in the

rehabilitation setting to decrease muscle spasm, lessen muscle spasticity, elicit stronger muscle contraction during functional movements, and limit post-exercise soreness.

Evidence supporting cryotherapy use

Therapeutic effects on pain

There is ample evidence supporting cryotherapy use when treating acute injuries involving muscles (Deal et al., 2002; Siqueira et al., 2017), tendons (Knobloch et al., 2007; Zhang et al., 2014; Haslerud et al., 2017), and joints (Cobbold & Lewis, 1956; Pan et al., 2015) to reduce local blood flow and subsequent development of inflammation and edema. This anti-inflammatory effect can in turn alleviate the pain associated with injury (Zhang & An, 2007). Combining compression with cryotherapy can provide additional benefit toward abatement of swelling and pain. In a 2016 meta-analysis, Song and colleagues found that patients who received compressive cryotherapy following knee surgery generally had less swelling and pain than those who had cryotherapy only, especially in the early stages of rehabilitation (Song et al., 2016). This may promote a more rapid progression into the active rehabilitation phase. While compressive cryotherapy units have been available for human patients for some time, units designed for the canine patient are now available as well (Figure 7.1). Drygas et al. (2011) found that dogs treated with compressive cryotherapy

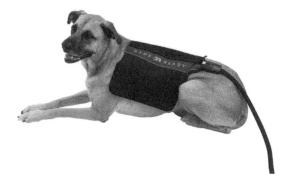

Figure 7.1   Example of a compressive cryotherapy unit designed for the canine patient. Source: Image courtesy of Game Ready. Reproduced with permission of Game Ready.

units post-tibial plateau leveling osteotomy (TPLO) had decreased pain, swelling, and lameness with increased passive range of motion when compared to sham-treated dogs.

In addition to reducing inflammation, cryotherapy may lessen pain through several other mechanisms. Decreased tissue temperatures have been shown to lower sensory nerve conduction velocities (Herrera et al., 2011) and increase both pain threshold and pain tolerance (Algafly & George, 2007; Park et al., 2014). Analgesia may also result via the gate control theory of pain, with overstimulation of cold receptors blocking the transmission of pain signals to higher centers. Pain reduction may also be attributable to the downregulation of pain-sensitizing inflammatory mediators (Zhang et al., 2014).

While efforts have been made to assess the ability of cryotherapy to address pain in animals (Downer, 1978; Sluka et al., 1999; Corti, 2014), these effects can be more easily measured in human patient populations. Indeed, its use has been shown to reduce the need for additional pain medications following orthopedic surgery (Ohkoshi et al., 1999; Barber, 2000; Kuyucu et al., 2015). Cryotherapy has been shown to be effective in reducing the discomfort associated with osteoarthritis (Guillot et al., 2017), muscle injury (Fonseca et al., 2016), fractures (Barca et al., 2016), rheumatoid arthritis (Księżopolska-Orłowska et al., 2016), and surgical wounds (Gatewood et al., 2017). Cryotherapy can also reduce painful muscle spasms (Nadler et al., 2004), possibly related to a decreased firing rate of muscle spindle and Golgi tendon organ receptors (Mense, 1978; Feys et al., 2005). A reduction in electromyogram (EMG) activity following cryotherapy has been demonstrated as well (Macedo Cde et al., 2016). Finally, cold therapy may limit development of post-exercise soreness (Brophy-Williams et al., 2011; Fonseca et al., 2016), helping to encourage patient participation and compliance.

Therapeutic effects on tissue protection and healing

Cold application after injury can reduce the risk of further tissue damage by decreasing cellular metabolism (Merrick et al., 1999), which, through decreased cellular oxygen demands, can diminish secondary hypoxic cellular injury (Merrick, 2002). In addition, Siqueira and colleagues found that performing three 30-minute cryotherapy sessions for the 3 days following muscle injury reduced the production of reactive oxygen species, indicating reduced oxidative stress (Siqueira et al., 2017).

Cold therapy offers clear protective and healing benefits at the tissue and organism levels as well. For example, temperature reduction has shown a protective effect on microcirculation in the area of injury (Schaser et al., 2007). Additionally, Oliveira and colleagues demonstrated that cryotherapy application immediately following muscle trauma resulted in a smaller area of damage as compared to untreated muscles (Oliveira et al., 2006). Cryotherapy may also decrease the risk of compartment syndrome often associated with skeletal muscle ischemic injury and closed soft tissue injuries (Wright et al., 1989; Schaser et al., 2007). Finally, cryotherapy can assist with overall healing of the patient as a decrease in pain alone can lead to earlier patient mobilization (Bleakley et al., 2006; Song et al., 2016).

Therapeutic effects on tissue flexibility and joint ROM

Regaining muscle flexibility and joint ROM is key to functional recovery. The therapist can employ several techniques toward improving both muscle flexibility and joint mobility (Chapters 5 and 6) but they may involve some discomfort for the patient. When working with human patients, the procedure can be explained, often resulting in better relaxation and subsequent outcome of the treatment. In canine rehabilitation, however, achieving and maintaining a relaxed patient during a potentially uncomfortable treatment may be more difficult. The therapist may experience greater success if cryotherapy is performed prior to these techniques. For example, Park and colleagues found that brief periods of local cryotherapy (3 minutes) reduced uncomfortable stretch sensations and increased the pressure pain threshold of tight muscles (Park et al., 2014). Larsen and colleagues showed that greater flexibility gains could be achieved with longer periods (20 minutes) of icing prior to stretch (Larsen et al., 2015). Lastly, cryotherapy may be effective prior to trigger point pressure release techniques (see Chapter 6) as well. In these ways, cryotherapy may promote greater cooperation from canine patients who experience discomfort with soft tissue techniques.

Cold application can also have positive effects on the mobility of patients with neurological injury through a temporary reduction of spasticity. A number of studies (Price *et al.*, 1993; Allison & Abraham, 2001) have demonstrated measurable decreases in spasticity with a resultant increase in active ROM and ease of movement. Lee and colleagues achieved 30–60 minutes of spasticity relief following cold therapy in rabbits affected by spastic paraplegia due to spinal cord transection (Lee *et al.*, 2002).

Therapeutic effects on muscle strength

Short periods of cryotherapy may promote muscle force production. A neurological rehabilitation technique developed by Rood and known as *quick icing* uses rapid movements of ice over the skin as a sensory stimulus to facilitate movement in individuals with decreased muscle tone or impaired motor control (Cameron, 2013). Cryotherapy can also be effective in counteracting the muscle inhibition often associated with peripheral joint swelling, such as quadriceps inhibition following stifle injury or surgery. Evidence suggests that, for human patients following anterior cruciate ligament (ACL) reconstruction, those who received focal knee joint cryotherapy prior to rehabilitation exercises experienced greater strength gains (Hart *et al.*, 2014). The therapist should be aware, however, that when muscle inhibition is not an issue, cooling a joint and the surrounding tissues can decrease muscle strength (Drinkwater & Behm, 2007; Hadler *et al.*, 2014) and joint proprioception (Torres *et al.*, 2016).

Considerations for clinical application

In the canine rehabilitation setting, cryotherapy is typically provided with cold packs or ice massage although devices that provide cold and compression together are also being used more. When determining which method to use, the size and accessibility of the body part should be considered as well as the patient's tolerance of straps, massage, and/or compression.

Reusable cold packs include gel packs of various sizes that can fit different body parts and often include a sleeve to protect the skin (Figure 7.2) as well as elastic straps to hold the pack in place. Cold packs designed to fit specific parts of the dog are also available (Figure 7.3).

Units that combine cold and compression are now available for the canine patient. These units often offer the ability to adjust several treatment parameters (temperature, pressure, time, etc.) and come with sleeves or wraps designed to fit different areas of the patient (Figure 7.4).

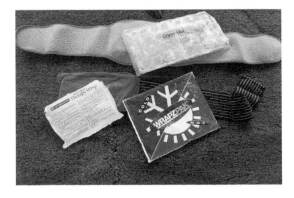

Figure 7.2 Cold packs are available in different sizes to promote better fit to the treatment site.

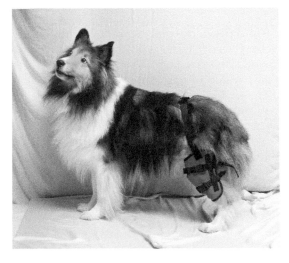

Figure 7.3 An example of a cold pack specifically designed to fit the canine patient. Source: Image courtesy of CanineIcer.com.

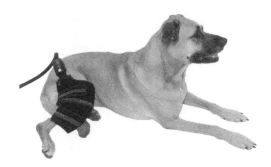

Figure 7.4   Compressive cryotherapy units offer different wraps to address treatment of various body parts. Game Ready wrap on a dog's stifle. Source: Image courtesy of Game Ready. Reproduced with permission of Game Ready.

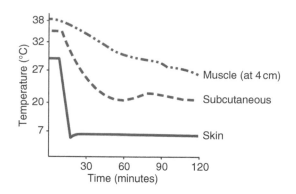

Figure 7.6   Rate of temperature change at different tissue depths during cryotherapy to the human calf. Source: Adapted from Bierman & Friedlander, 1940.

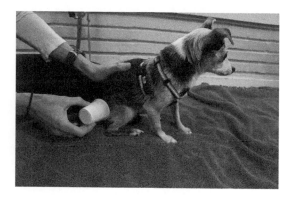

Figure 7.5   Water is frozen in a paper cup to provide ice massage cryotherapy to a smaller patient.

Cold packs can also be made in the clinic or at the patient's home with crushed ice or a slush created by freezing a combination of three parts water to one part alcohol in a sealable bag. A thin damp towel should be placed between the cold pack and the patient unless the hair coat is thick.

For smaller treatment areas or body parts that are not easily covered with a cold pack, or when working with smaller patients, ice massage is useful (Figure 7.5). It can be particularly effective prior to manual therapy techniques that may be uncomfortable. Freezing water in a paper cup provides an easy means for ice massage as the practitioner's hand is protected from the cold, and the paper can be torn away as the ice melts. Ice popsicles can also be made

by placing a handle, such as a tongue depressor, into the water before freezing.

The depth of the target tissue, ability of surrounding tissues to conduct heat (Bierman & Friedlander, 1940; Petrofsky & Laymon, 2009), and temperature of the cooling agent relative to the target tissue should be considered when determining the duration of cold application (Figure 7.6). Deeper tissues and animals with more adipose tissue, a poor conductor of heat, will require additional treatment time (Otte *et al.*, 2002; Merrick *et al.*, 2003a; Petrofsky & Laymon, 2009). Longer treatment time will also likely be required for dogs with thicker hair coats. The general recommendation for treatment duration of ice massage is 5 to 10 minutes (Sharma & Noohu, 2014). Cold pack treatment time can range from 10 to 60 minutes (Otte *et al.*, 2002), depending largely on the intensity of the cold modality as well as patient tolerance. In general, a minimum of 20 minutes of cold pack application time for target tissues at a depth of 1 cm or more has been recommended for canine patients (Akgun *et al.*, 2004; Millard *et al.*, 2013). Given the time required to achieve therapeutic cooling with a cold pack, the author (K.N.) frequently requests that clients with outpatients perform cryotherapy treatments in the car or at home rather than using in-clinic treatment time. This may vary, however, depending on the goal of the cryotherapy treatment or the rehabilitation practice setting (inpatient vs outpatient).

Precautions and contraindications

Caution should be used when applying cold over superficial nerves, areas of decreased sensation, or open wounds. Care should also be taken when working with very small dogs to avoid hypothermia. Cryotherapy should not be used over areas of compromised circulation or in patients with thermoregulatory disorders or cold sensitivities. Patients should be monitored for signs of nonfreezing cold injuries (Khoshnevis *et al.*, 2015, 2016) or other injuries such as frostbite (Rivlin *et al.*, 2014). Furthermore, areas previously affected by frostbite should not receive cryotherapy.

One final consideration: a cooled area can require an extended period of time to return to baseline temperature (Akgun *et al.*, 2004; Khoshnevis *et al.*, 2016). Cold can also increase joint stiffness (Uchio *et al.*, 2003) and tendon stiffness (Alegre *et al.*, 2016), and decrease proprioceptive awareness (Alexander *et al.*, 2016). This can be important when providing cryotherapy prior to therapeutic exercises, or when treating sporting or working dogs that will return to activity soon after treatment.

Superficial heat

Superficial heat is used in the rehabilitation setting to reduce pain, increase blood flow, improve connective tissue extensibility and joint mobility, and promote muscle relaxation. During the subacute and chronic stages of healing, heat application may also help alleviate remaining inflammation. As with cryotherapy, superficial heat is most frequently delivered through conduction, with the heating agent placed directly onto the body part. Superficial heating modalities are used to increase tissue temperature up to 3 cm below the skin's surface (Draper *et al.*, 1998) although the greatest effects occur in the first 1 to 2 cm. Depending on the treatment goal, the temperature of the target tissue must be increased by 1–4 °C to result in therapeutic effects (Draper & Ricard, 1995). A tissue temperature rise of 1 °C leads to an increase in metabolic rate, a 2–3 °C temperature increase helps to alleviate muscle spasm, pain, and chronic inflammation, and an increase of 4 °C promotes collagen extensibility (Lehmann *et al.* 1967a, 1967b; Draper, 2014).

Evidence supporting the use of superficial heat

Therapeutic effects on pain

Superficial heat has been shown to effectively reduce the perception of pain in human patients including those with chronic knee pain (Kim *et al.*, 2013; Petrofsky *et al.*, 2016a), wrist pain due to either soft tissue or joint involvement (Michlovitz *et al.*, 2004), and acute low back pain (Nadler *et al.*, 2003), with more rapid and sustained relief as compared to oral ibuprofen (Stark *et al.*, 2014) or cryotherapy (Dehghan & Farabod, 2014). Superficial heat therapy also shows positive results toward improving the discomfort associated with chronic musculoskeletal conditions in veterinary patients (Corti, 2014; Epstein *et al.*, 2015).

There are several mechanisms through which heat may reduce pain. With increased tissue temperature, cutaneous blood flow is augmented due to vasodilation (Baker & Bell, 1991; Okada *et al.*, 2005; Biyik Bayram & Caliskan, 2016). This may lead to pain relief if the source of discomfort is related to tissue ischemia from reduced blood flow (Ochiai *et al.*, 2014) or chemical mediators that stimulate nociceptors. Increased tissue temperatures have also been shown to increase pain thresholds, possibly related to the release of endorphins and/or an inhibition of afferent and efferent C fibers in the area (On *et al.*, 1997). Additionally, pain relief may occur due to a decrease in muscle activity in the area (Lewis *et al.*, 2012) and/or the resolution of muscle spasms, believed to be due to a reduction of muscle spindle firing rates (Mense, 1978). Finally, superficial heat may act as a counterirritant, reducing pain perception as described in the gate control theory of pain.

Therapeutic effects on tissue healing and protection

In the post-acute and chronic stages of healing, temperature elevation of injured superficial tissues can support continued recovery by augmenting the delivery of nutrients and oxygen through vasodilation (Nadler *et al.*, 2004). This effect has been shown when treating chronic wounds as well (Petrofsky *et al.*, 2007). More recently, Neff and colleagues demonstrated that superficial heating can even enhance blood flow into areas with compromised vasculature, such as tissues affected by peripheral artery disease (Neff *et al.*, 2016), by promoting capillary growth (Kuhlenhoelter *et al.*, 2016), further supporting healing.

Xia and colleagues demonstrated an increase in the metabolic activity with superficial heating as well as stimulation of cell proliferation of *in vitro* human skin fibroblasts, believed to represent a mechanism of improved wound healing *in vivo* (Xia *et al.*, 2000). Ito and colleagues noted similar findings using a therapeutic thermal environment (37 °C) to promote articular chondrocyte metabolism and cell proliferation (*in vitro*), information that may be important in the treatment of osteoarthritis (Ito *et al.*, 2014).

Therapeutic temperature elevation may also provide protection to damaged tissues during the healing process. Khan and colleagues found that providing 38 °C heating over skin graft donor site wounds led to the expected increase in local blood flow but also a significant increase in lymphocyte movement into the tissues, possibly indicating an enhancement of the immunity within the wound (Khan *et al.*, 2004). Furthermore, Ikeda and colleagues found that superficial heating increased subcutaneous oxygen tension, a measure that correlates strongly with resistance to infection as well as improved wound strength (Ikeda *et al.*, 1998).

Therapeutic effects on tissue flexibility and joint ROM

Heat increases the viscoelastic properties of connective tissues (Hardy & Woodall, 1998). Superficial heating can therefore promote improved flexibility and joint ROM (Petrofsky *et al.*, 2013) if the restricted ligament, tendon, or joint capsule is located within 2–3 cm of the surface. In humans, use of superficial heat combined with stretching is more effective than stretching alone (Funk *et al.*, 2001; Robertson *et al.*, 2005; Nakano *et al.*, 2012) although there is also some evidence that active heating through exercise may provide greater benefits toward

muscle flexibility (Rosario & Foletto, 2015). This is worth considering when designing rehabilitation treatment plans for both human and canine patients, especially if time is restricted. Including superficial heat therapy as part of the home exercise program (HEP) can also lead to significant increases in active ROM (Petrofsky *et al.*, 2016a). Finally, heat application can be helpful when stretching patients who have contractures and/or spasticity due to neurological injury, as shown with rats with spinal cord injuries (Iwasawa *et al.*, 2016).

Therapeutic effects on muscle strength

While superficial heat application has not been shown to have direct effects on muscle strength, a study by Petrofsky and colleagues showed that patients with chronic knee pain who used heat therapy prior to performance of a daily HEP (in combination with in-clinic therapy) had significantly enhanced strength gains as compared to the exercise-only group (Petrofsky *et al.*, 2016a), likely related to improved comfort and resulting increased compliance.

Considerations for clinical application

In canine rehabilitation, superficial heating is typically provided through application of a hot pack. This can include moist heat (hydrocollator) packs, gel packs warmed in hot water or a microwave, or clay packs (Figure 7.7). There is evidence that moist heat

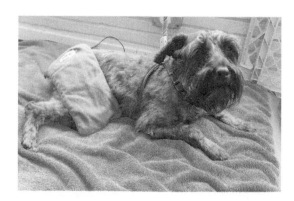

Figure 7.7 Patient receiving superficial heat therapy via clay pack over the hip, lateral thigh musculature, and stifle.

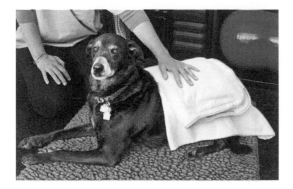

Figure 7.8   Patient receiving superficial heat therapy via hydrocollator pack in a relaxed position. Note the additional padding between the pack and the patient.

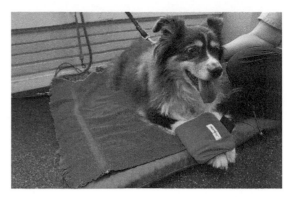

Figure 7.9   Patient receiving superficial heat therapy prior to carpal joint mobilization.

may be more effective than dry (Igaki *et al.*, 2014) although the impact of the canine patient's coat is unknown. When using a hot pack, the patient should be positioned to encourage relaxation while still permitting access to the treatment area (Figure 7.8). If needed, additional padding should be placed between the patient and the pack to prevent burns, and the skin should be checked frequently. Recommended treatment duration is 20–25 minutes (Lin, 2003), although Millard and colleagues found that 10-minute application was sufficient for heating up to 1.5 cm in depth and no additional tissue heating had occurred at 20 minutes (Millard *et al.*, 2013). Additional treatment time may be required when treating overweight patients as adipose tissue impairs heat transfer. However, there may also be an increased burn risk as skin temperature increases are greater in obese patients (Petrofsky & Laymon, 2009). In the canine rehabilitation setting, superficial heating is typically used before manual therapies (soft tissue mobilization, stretching, passive ROM, or joint mobilization—see Chapter 6) are performed (Figure 7.9), or prior to active exercise to improve ease of movement.

Precautions and contraindications

Caution should be used when heating over areas of decreased circulation or open wounds, in patients with inflammatory conditions, or when treating sedated animals or those with decreased sensation. Use of superficial heating

agents also carries a risk of burns or other thermal tissue injury (Jabir *et al.*, 2013; Cho *et al.*, 2015). Contraindications include acute inflammation, active bleeding, fever, and applying heat over a malignancy.

Therapeutic ultrasound

Therapeutic ultrasound (TUS) uses sound energy at frequencies greater than 20,000 Hz to affect biological tissues through both thermal and nonthermal mechanisms. Sound waves are produced via the reverse piezoelectric effect (compression and expansion of a piezoelectric crystal). These sound waves are essentially mechanical pressure waves and, as they move through tissues, absorbed energy is converted into kinetic energy. This causes a chain reaction of molecules vibrating and colliding into neighboring molecules. Absorption is greatest in tissues with high protein content.

Phonophoresis, a treatment that uses TUS energy in an effort to deliver medications transdermally, will not be discussed in this chapter. It is worth noting that many medications that are compounded with ultrasound gel may effectively block transmission of sound energy, resulting in a less effective treatment overall (Cage *et al.*, 2013). Therapists who use this treatment should ensure that medications are compatible with TUS. For additional information, the reader is referred to the physical modality textbooks previously noted (Cameron, 2013; Bellew *et al.*, 2016).

Therapeutic effects of TUS: thermal and nonthermal

TUS can provide heating benefits to tissues up to 5 cm deep without causing thermal damage to more superficial tissues. TUS can increase pain thresholds, blood flow, metabolic rate, and collagen extensibility. It can also decrease muscle guarding and spasm and reduce subacute and chronic inflammation.

The nonthermal, or mechanical, effects of TUS include microstreaming and cavitation. Microstreaming, or acoustic streaming, refers to small-grade, unidirectional pressure waves created in the fluids around cells. Cavitation is the compression and expansion of small gas bubbles in body fluids. Both may modify cellular function and membrane permeability, thus assisting with tissue repair and swelling reduction.

Parameters of treatment

Frequency, measured in megahertz (MHz), determines the depth of sound energy penetration. Most TUS units offer two frequencies: 1 MHz and 3 MHz. The 1 MHz option provides a deeper heating of up to 5 cm in depth; 3 MHz is selected when heating of more superficial tissue is desired, within 1–2.5 cm. The 3 MHz option is also used when TUS is applied around a bony prominence to avoid periosteal pain.

Intensity, measured in watts per centimeter squared (W/cm^2), affects the degree and rate of temperature increase. Higher intensities will cause greater and more rapid temperature elevations. A typical intensity range found on TUS units is 0.25–3.0 W/cm^2.

Two *modes* are generally available for providing TUS: continuous and pulsed. Continuous mode refers to a constant flow of energy. Pulsed mode has regular breaks in energy flow and is described by its duty cycle, the percentage of time that ultrasound is being emitted during one pulse period. Most TUS units provide duty cycles from 5% to 50%. Pulsed mode is usually chosen when only minimal heating or the nonthermal effects of TUS are desired, such as when treating an acute injury.

The *duration* of TUS treatments must be sufficient if the goal is to achieve therapeutic levels of tissue heating (an increase of 1 to 4 °C).

When TUS is part of a patient's treatment plan, all application parameters must be considered in combination with the depth of the target tissue, the size of the treatment area, the stage of healing, and the goal of treatment (Miller *et al.*, 2008). Especially when deeper heating is desired, in addition to using the correct frequency, sufficient intensity and duration is needed to achieve and then *maintain* the temperature elevation for an adequate time period in order for therapeutic effects to occur. Even small variations in dosage can have a large impact on temperature change (Demchak & Stone, 2008).

Evidence supporting the use of TUS

Therapeutic effects on pain

When providing thermal effects, TUS can reduce the discomfort associated with trigger points (Draper *et al.*, 2010; Benjaboonyanupap *et al.*, 2015), muscular soreness following an overuse injury (Aaron *et al.*, 2017), plantar fasciitis (Krukowska *et al.*, 2016), rotator cuff injury (Yildirim *et al.*, 2013), and myofascial pain (Ilter *et al.*, 2015; Rai *et al.*, 2016), with improvments often maintained for extended periods of time (Kavadar *et al.*, 2015). Furthermore, when combined with active therapeutic exercise, TUS provides benefits above those seen with exercise alone for patients with lumbar disc disease (Boyraz *et al.*, 2015) and spinal stenosis, such that use of analgesic medications is decreased (Goren *et al.*, 2010). TUS has also been shown to effectively reduce the pain associated with osteoarthritis (Zhang *et al.*, 2016; Yeğin *et al.*, 2017), a condition also seen frequently in the canine rehabilitation setting.

The nonthermal effects of TUS appear to offer pain-reducing benefits as well. Both a 2014 review by Zeng and colleagues and a 2015 randomized, placebo-controlled, double-blind study by Yildiz and colleagues found that continuous *and* pulsed TUS are effective in improving both pain status and functional mobility in the management of knee osteoarthritis (Zeng *et al.*, 2014; Yildiz *et al.*, 2015). This information could be useful if thermal modalities are contraindicated for a patient.

The mechanisms by which TUS reduces pain are likely similar to those of superficial heat—increased blood flow to the area may assist in removing pain mediators in the area, nerve conduction is impacted, and muscle spasm decreased. In addition, the mechanical effects of TUS may alter cell membrane permeability, leading to decreased inflammation and related discomfort (Kavadar et al., 2015; Rai et al., 2016). There is evidence that TUS may have a positive impact on the central pathways of pain processing as well (Hsieh, 2005).

Therapeutic effects on tissue healing and protection

Just as with superficial heating agents, the heating effects of TUS cause vasodilation (Noble et al., 2007) leading to increased local blood circulation and oxygenation (Morishita et al., 2014a; Chang et al., 2015). This promotes healing by delivering nutrients and removing waste products. When specifically treating tendons, TUS has been shown to improve the microcirculation (Chang et al., 2015) and tensile strength (Enwemeka, 1989; Ng, 2011) of injured tendons as compared to nontreated controls. Chang and colleagues then correlated these positive indicators of healing with improved tendon function following surgical repair of Achilles tendon tears (Chang et al., 2017). Similar findings with canine patients were noted in a study by Saini and colleagues in which TUS was employed in the treatment of surgically severed Achilles tendons in dogs (Saini et al., 2002). Also, Mueller and colleagues described two canine cases of partial gastrocnemius muscle avulsion (not surgically induced) that were treated conservatively with ultrasound and showed complete return to full activity (Mueller et al., 2009).

TUS also has angiogenic effects in tissues with compromised blood supply. Huang and colleagues and Lu and colleagues demonstrated that TUS can reverse peripheral ischemia in type 2 diabetic mice as evidenced by increased blood perfusion and capillary density (Huang et al., 2014; Lu et al., 2016a). In a subsequent study by Lu and colleagues, TUS was found to impart similar angiogenic benefits in rats with hypertensive peripheral arterial disease (Lu et al., 2016b).

The nonthermal effects of TUS benefit tissue healing as well, such as following tendon repair (Geetha et al., 2014) and when treating tenosynovitis (Sharma et al., 2015). In the treatment of wounds, especially in the inflammatory and proliferative phases of healing, pulsed TUS can promote angiogenesis and granulation tissue formation, and speed wound contraction (Fantinati et al., 2016) while also helping to control necrotic tissue by increasing the phagocytic capacity of macrophages (Korelo et al., 2016). Indeed, full-thickness wounds such as surgically created wounds (Mahran, 2014) and pressure ulcers (Polak et al., 2014) demonstrate more rapid healing when treated with pulsed ultrasound using lower intensities ($0.5\,W/cm^2$), strongly suggesting that the mechanical effects are involved with healing. Pulsed TUS also accelerates wound contraction through enhanced collagen production and density, especially in wounds with adequate blood supply (Altomare et al., 2009).

Pulsed TUS may also have protective effects for tissues surrounding an injury. Using pulsed TUS, Martins and colleagues demonstrated a reduction in the oxidative stress and secondary tissue damage often seen following a crushing injury of muscle (Martins et al., 2016).

Additionally, the nonthermal effects of TUS may enhance peripheral nerve regeneration. Mourad and colleagues found a more rapid return to full foot function when low-intensity ultrasound was applied 3 days per week for 30 days following sciatic nerve crush injury in rats (Mourad et al., 2001). A 2005 study demonstrated improved nerve fiber density and a greater number of Schwann cell nuclei in treated injured rat sciatic nerves as compared to those not treated (Raso et al., 2005), and Akhlaghi and colleagues showed 90% of full functional recovery after just 2 weeks of pulsed TUS following sciatic nerve crush injury (Akhlaghi et al., 2012).

Finally, both the thermal and nonthermal effects of TUS may promote healing and regeneration of articular cartilage. A 2012 study demonstrated an increase in the cartilage thickness in human patients with mild to moderate knee osteoarthritis following 24 sessions of pulsed TUS (Loyola-Sánchez et al., 2012). Nam and colleagues also found that both pulsed and continuous TUS increased chondrogenesis in rat tibial articular cartilage (Nam et al., 2014).

Therapeutic effects on tissue flexibility and joint ROM

TUS is often used to provide heating to deeper muscle (Levine *et al.*, 2001) (Figure 7.10), ligament (Leung *et al.*, 2006), or tendon (Montgomery *et al.*, 2013). When providing thermal effects, TUS can improve muscle flexibility (Knight *et al.*, 2001; Nakano *et al.*, 2012) and increase collagen extensibility (Lehmann *et al.*, 1970; Draper *et al.*, 1993). This can be used to improve ROM through relaxation of muscle tissue (Morishita *et al.*, 2014b) or noncontractile tissues such as periarticular tissue (Morrisette *et al.*, 2004) prior to joint mobilization (Draper, 2010).

Thermal effects may also reduce development of muscle contracture during joint immobilization as evidenced by continued longitudinal orientation of collagen fibrils and better joint ROM post-immobilization as compared to subjects that did not receive TUS (Okita *et al.*, 2009). This leads to a better functional outcome following injuries that require immobilization.

The nonthermal effects of TUS also promote increased joint ROM. Yildiz and colleagues investigated the effects of both pulsed and continuous TUS as compared to a control group in human subjects with knee osteoarthritis. All three groups were also instructed in a HEP. Both TUS groups were found to achieve significantly better knee ROM measurements by the conclusion of the study, and these gains were maintained at the 2-month follow-up (Yildiz *et al.*, 2015), suggesting that ROM benefits can still be imparted when other patient characteristics make nonthermal TUS the more appropriate choice.

Therapeutic effects on muscle strength

As with superficial heat, TUS has not been shown to have a direct effect on increasing muscle strength. However, a 2015 study by Norte and colleagues did find that treatment with nonthermal TUS improved muscular activity in patients with persistent quadriceps dysfunction associated with intra-articular knee injuries (Norte *et al.*, 2015). Additionally, Matsumoto and colleagues showed that pulsed TUS helps to inhibit the development of disuse muscle atrophy during joint immobilization through stimulation of satellite cells (Matsumoto *et al.*, 2014).

Considerations for clinical application

When using TUS on canine patients, it should be recalled that energy absorption is greatest in tissues with high protein content. Hair is made of the protein keratin. For this reason, the hair coat can significantly reduce the delivery of

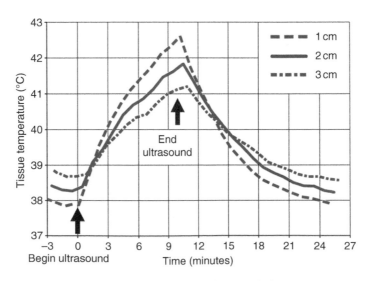

Figure 7.10   Rate of temperature change at various tissue depths during and after 3.3 MHz therapeutic ultrasound (TUS) of the caudal thigh muscle of the dog. Source: Adapted from Levine *et al.*, 2001.

sound energy to target tissues (Steiss & Adams, 1999) and should therefore be clipped in the treatment area.

Different tissues also heat at different rates. For example, the rate of heating in tendon is about three times faster than that of muscle (Draper, 2014). There is also evidence that patients with a higher body mass index may experience less effective outcomes due to poor transmission of TUS energy through adipose tissue (Muftic & Miladinovic, 2013).

Sound energy also does not transmit well through air; a coupling medium is required to deliver ultrasound energy into tissues. There are direct and indirect coupling methods. The technique selected is often based on the size and contours of the body part being treated. The direct method is used when the treatment area is relatively smooth and larger than the transducer head. Some TUS units are equipped with several sizes of transducer heads (Figure 7.11). A water-soluble gel is usually used as the coupling medium and is applied on the treatment area. The transducer head then maintains contact with the gel throughout treatment.

Indirect coupling methods may be selected when the treatment area is irregularly shaped, is smaller than the transducer head, or if the pressure of direct coupling will cause discomfort.

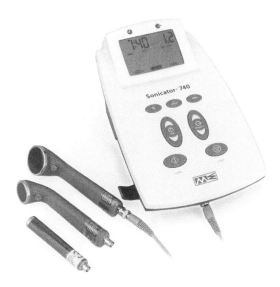

Figure 7.11 Example of a therapeutic ultrasound (TUS) unit with various sized transducer heads.

The most commonly used indirect method is submersion. The body part is placed into a container of water and the transducer head is held approximately 1–2 cm from the skin surface. It is important to note that with the submersion technique, heating is significantly less than with direct coupling techniques (Forrest & Rosen, 1989; Draper *et al.*, 1993).

To ensure adequate energy delivery, the treatment area should not exceed two to three times the size of the transducer head. Treatment duration of 5 to 10 minutes is generally recommended, but according to Draper, the depth of the target tissue, the intensity, and the treatment goal need to be considered to determine an appropriate duration. There are several methods mentioned in the literature for determining TUS dosage. Draper has established the rate of tissue heating per minute for both 1 MHz and 3 MHz frequencies using four different intensities. Based on this, proper treatment duration can be established when tissue heating is a goal (Draper, 2014). Another technique has been proposed by Watson in which the tissue depth, stage of healing, and the size of the treatment area are considered to help determine frequency, intensity, duty cycle, and duration (Watson, 2009). Regardless of how the therapist determines the treatment dosage, the patient's comfort must be a primary concern and parameters should be adjusted accordingly.

The speed of transducer head movement should also be considered. As the distribution of energy is not uniform under the transducer, maintaining it in one location can lead to development of hot spots and possible tissue damage. Moving the transducer head slowly and evenly (approximately 4 cm/s) leads to a better energy distribution. The need to move the transducer head more rapidly to avoid patient discomfort is often an indicator of a lower quality TUS unit. Ensuring the TUS unit has a low beam nonuniformity ratio (BNR) reduces the risk of development of hotspots under the transducer.

Finally, the transducer should be positioned directly over the target tissue and perpendicular to the skin. If the angle of delivery moves beyond 75°, the beam will travel along the skin rather than into the target tissue, rendering the treatment ineffective (Michlovitz & Nolan, 2005).

Of note, when using TUS to promote flexibility, some debate exists regarding the best time to apply a stretch force. In general, stretching should be performed during the final minutes of TUS and immediately following (Chan *et al.*, 1998; Knight *et al.*, 2001), although some studies suggest that the *stretching window* may last up to 15 minutes after the ultrasound treatment has been completed (Draper *et al.*, 1995; Rose *et al.*, 1996; Morishita *et al.*, 2014b).

As with any piece of therapeutic equipment, the quality of the TUS unit is important. As noted above, a lower BNR is desirable as this corresponds to a higher quality crystal and a more uniform ultrasound beam. A higher BNR may cause the patient more discomfort, leading to the inability to achieve a therapeutic effect. It is also important to note that there are studies demonstrating variation between manufacturers regarding the time needed to achieve the same level of tissue heating (Gange *et al.*, 2016) so it is important to become familiar with the performance of each unit (Geetha *et al.*, 2014). Regular calibration is vital for guaranteeing the intended treatment is indeed rendered. Artho and colleagues tested 83 TUS units being used in clinic settings. Of those, 39% were found to be outside the calibration standard for at least one output setting (Artho *et al.*, 2002).

Precautions and contraindications

Caution should be used when applying TUS over fractures, in areas of decreased circulation, over areas of decreased pain and/or temperature sensation, and on sedated or anesthetized animals.

TUS use should be avoided over cardiac pacemakers, thrombi, the lower trunk during pregnancy, the eyes or testes, open epiphyseal plates, or the spinal cord after laminectomy, as well as in areas of malignancy, infection, or bleeding. More recent evidence also cautions against the use of TUS in demyelinating conditions (Aydin *et al.*, 2016).

Finally, as with any heating modality, care should be taken to avoid tissue burns. These may occur when the selected intensity is too high, the treatment time is too long, or the transducer is held in place.

Electrical stimulation

The two forms of electrical stimulation (ES) most often used in canine rehabilitation are neuromuscular electrical stimulation (NMES) and transcutaneous electrical nerve stimulation (TENS).

Neuromuscular electrical stimulation (NMES)

NMES is primarily used to address muscular weakness associated with both orthopedic and neurological diagnoses. It causes a muscle contraction by depolarizing the motor nerve with an electrical current delivered via electrodes placed on the skin. There are two types of NMES units: portable, battery-operated units and electric line-powered units. For most canine rehabilitation applications, portable units provide sufficient output to achieve the desired therapeutic effect (Figure 7.12). Regardless of the type, most NMES units offer the same treatment parameters although the terms used to describe each may vary.

Parameters of treatment

Amplitude

Amplitude, or intensity, describes the total magnitude of the electrical wave and is measured in milliamperes (mA). Increased amplitude results in a stronger contraction as more

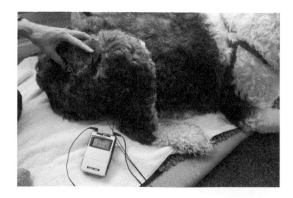

Figure 7.12   Patient receiving neuromuscular electrical stimulation (NMES) via a portable, battery-operated unit.

muscle fibers are recruited, but may also result in greater discomfort.

Pulse duration

Pulse duration, or pulse width, is the time of one pulse and is measured in microseconds (µs). Larger pulse durations can require less current amplitude to achieve muscle contraction but may also stimulate more pain fibers.

Frequency

Frequency, or pulse rate, is the number of pulses per second and is measured in hertz (Hz). Strong muscle contractions are often elicited with frequencies of 60 to 100 Hz. Higher frequencies may increase muscle fatigue (Gondin et al., 2010) and thus limit the patient's ability to participate in active exercise following NMES.

On/off cycle

The on/off cycle describes the time that current is being delivered and the time that current is stopped. Both are usually measured in seconds. The *duty cycle* is the ratio of on-time to the total cycle time. As the on-time lengthens, or if the off-time is insufficient to provide adequate rest between contractions, muscle fatigue becomes more likely.

Ramp

Ramp is the time during which the current is gradually increased or decreased to improve patient comfort. It is usually measured in seconds. A longer ramp time may be required for patients affected by spasticity, but sufficient time at peak intensity must be ensured to promote strength development.

Mode

Most NMES units have two channels and offer three treatment modes: constant, in which the current is delivered without breaks; simultaneous, in which the current is delivered according to the on/off settings for both channels concurrently; and alternating or reciprocal, in which current delivery is still based on on/off settings but the timing between channels can be adjusted.

Evidence supporting the use of NMES

Therapeutic effects on pain

There is evidence that NMES use can reduce pain, especially when the discomfort is related to orthopedic issues such as knee osteoarthritis (Laufer et al., 2014) and patellofemoral pain (Glaviano & Saliba, 2016). A 2015 study by Demircioglu and colleagues found that the addition of quadriceps NMES to a standard rehabilitation program following total knee arthroplasty resulted in significantly improved pain scores as compared to patients who received the rehabilitation program alone (Demircioglu et al., 2015). The exact mechanism of pain reduction is not entirely understood—short-term improvements may be related to concurrent stimulation of sensory nerves, or the immediate improvements in muscle activation and resultant better kinematics during functional activities (Glaviano et al., 2016). More lasting effects may also be due to increased muscle strength promoting more normal joint mechanics, thus reducing additional joint stress and further damage.

Therapeutic effects on tissue healing and protection

While many studies exist demonstrating the ability of electrical stimulation to promote tissue healing, the majority employ waveforms other than those typically used in NMES, such as high-voltage pulsed current (HVPC) and direct current (DC). These waveforms will not be covered in this chapter; the reader is again referred to other sources for further information (Ud-Din & Bayat, 2014; Hamm, 2015).

NMES can be used to promote healing of some tissue types, however, such as peripheral nerve. Willand and colleagues found that following tibial nerve transection and repair in rats, daily NMES of the gastrocnemius (via implanted, intramuscular electrodes) resulted in significantly greater numbers of re-innervated motor units as compared to untreated muscles (Willand et al., 2015).

In terms of tissue protection, NMES can be effective in the management of venous disease (Ravikumar et al., 2017; Williams et al., 2017), and there is increasing evidence toward its use in peripheral arterial disease (Williams *et al.*, 2017). By improving blood flow and reducing risk of edema development, the elicited muscle contractions help to decrease the development of wounds commonly seen with these diagnoses, even as effectively as intermittent pneumatic compression (Broderick *et al.*, 2014; Williams *et al.*, 2015).

Therapeutic effects on tissue flexibility and joint ROM

In a 2016 study by Yoshimura and colleagues, NMES was used to provide cyclic muscle twitch contraction to immobilized rat soleus muscle (accomplished through plaster casting for 4 weeks), resulting in substantially improved dorsiflexion ROM as compared to immobilized joints that did not receive NMES. Further examination of the muscle tissue revealed significant difference in the collagen composition of the perimysium and endomysium, suggesting that NMES use reduces the development of immobilization-induced muscle contracture (Yoshimura *et al.*, 2016).

NMES can also assist in improving mobility of limbs affected by spasticity following stroke, based on both decreased measures of spasticity (Modified Ashworth Scale) and increased joint ROM via goniometry (Stein *et al.*, 2015). Potentially more translatable to canine patients often seen in rehabilitation, similar results have been found when using NMES to address spasticity following spinal cord injury (Carty *et al.*, 2013).

Therapeutic effects on muscle strength

NMES is most commonly used to facilitate muscle strengthening and/or to slow disuse atrophy. Indeed, NMES has been used to promote muscle strength in human patients for decades (Ward & Shkuratova, 2002). Studies have shown NMES to be capable of promoting strength gains similar to those seen with resistance training in healthy individuals (Pantović *et al.*, 2015) and that it can enhance gains when combined with active exercise for patients with orthopedic diagnoses such as knee osteoarthritis (de Oliveira Melo *et al.*, 2016) or following orthopedic surgeries such as anterior cruciate ligament (ACL) reconstruction (Lepley *et al.*, 2015) or total knee replacement (Chughtai *et al.*,

2016). NMES can also lead to increased strength in patients with significant illnesses (Roxo *et al.*, 2016), such as chronic heart failure (Jones *et al.*, 2016), chronic obstructive pulmonary disease (COPD) (Coquart *et al.*, 2016), and in patients in the ICU following cardiothoracic surgery (Fischer *et al.*, 2016). There is some emerging evidence that NMES may promote muscle strengthening even in severely weakened individuals such as those with myotonic dystrophy, for whom there are otherwise very limited strengthening options (Cudia *et al.*, 2016).

NMES has also demonstrated efficacy in postural retraining. A 2016 study showed that trunk NMES combined with physical therapy (neurodevelopmental therapy) led to better improvements in upright posture and sitting balance of children with cerebral palsy as compared to patients who received Kinesio Taping® in combination with the same physical therapy intervention (Karabay *et al.*, 2016). Similar gains in postural control have been observed with trunk NMES use in adult patients following stroke (Ko *et al.*, 2016). Additionally, postural balance and control can be improved through NMES use in otherwise healthy elderly individuals through targeted treatment of distal musculature (plantarflexors) used in balance reactions. This study and others also show that NMES can positively impact the muscle weakness associated with aging (Benavent-Caballer *et al.*, 2014; Mignardot *et al.*, 2015).

Strength gains with NMES are also possible in patients who are unwilling or unable to actively contract target muscles (Karabay *et al.*, 2012, 2016). Many human and canine patients may not be able to maximally contract a muscle after injury or surgery. In these cases, an electrically induced muscle contraction can produce greater torque—and therefore greater strength gains—than if NMES were not used (Fitzgerald *et al.*, 2003). Clinically, there is evidence that NMES use following orthopedic surgery results in decreased muscle mass loss, increased muscle strength, and improved functional muscle use (Snyder-Mackler *et al.*, 1991).

NMES can also be used to improve motor control and timing (Kim *et al.*, 2016). This is especially useful when considering the canine patient, who is likely unable to follow specific verbal and tactile cues to contract a specific muscle at the appropriate time.

Finally, NMES has shown benefit for specific patient types, some of which may translate well to the canine patient. Elnaggar found improved shoulder function and bone mineralization when NMES was combined with weight-bearing exercises in children with obstetric brachial plexus injury (Elnaggar, 2016). NMES can also help maintain residual limb muscle strength following amputation while patients await arrival of their prostheses (Talbot *et al.*, 2017). Pan and colleagues showed that NMES improves the muscle dysfunction resulting from chronic intermittent hypoxia in rats (Pan *et al.*, 2016), potentially indicating a treatment for weakness in dogs with laryngeal paralysis. Finally, multiple studies have demonstrated the potential for muscular strength gains in patients following spinal cord injury (Bickel *et al.*, 2015; Gorgey *et al.*, 2016), resulting in improved functional mobility (Beaumont *et al.*, 2014).

Transcutaneous electrical nerve stimulation (TENS)

The form of ES most often used for pain relief is TENS. Conventional TENS is used to stimulate sensory nerves rather than motor nerves (Figure 7.13). This is believed to reduce pain perception through several possible mechanisms including the gate theory of pain inhibition (Melzack & Wall, 1965), activation of endogenous opioids, and/or suppression of spinal substance P and pro-inflammatory cytokines (Chen *et al.*, 2015). This enables patients who were limited by pain to participate more fully in their rehabilitation program. TENS may also benefit patients who are unable to tolerate pain medications.

Evidence supporting the use of TENS

Therapeutic effects on pain

TENS has been used for pain relief for decades, and recent research has provided additional evidence to support its use. There are now studies that promote TENS in addressing orthopedic pain (Valenza *et al.*, 2016; Son *et al.*, 2017), nerve pain (Upton *et al.*, 2017), acute pain (Johnson *et al.*, 2015), chronic pain (Gozani, 2016), myofascial pain (Azatcam *et al.*, 2017), postoperative pain (Chughtai *et al.*, 2016), complex regional pain syndrome (Bilgili *et al.*, 2016), and pain associated with cancer (Loh & Gulati, 2015). Several studies have found that TENS can decrease the need for pain medications (Pivec *et al.*, 2015; Gozani, 2016; Jauregui *et al.*, 2016).

TENS can also be effective in the management of pain associated with neurological diagnoses. In a review by Sawant and colleagues, evidence was found that TENS provides benefits toward management of central pain in patients with multiple sclerosis (Sawant *et al.*, 2015) and the neuropathic pain frequently experienced following spinal cord injury (Özkul *et al.*, 2015).

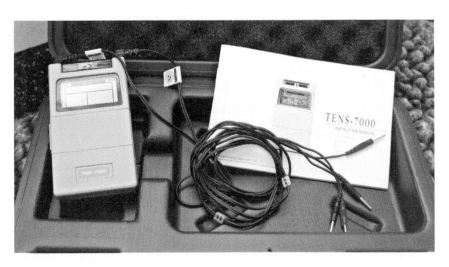

Figure 7.13   Example of a transcutaneous electrical nerve stimulation (TENS) unit.

Finally, TENS can be safely used for pain relief for an extended period of time without significant side effects (Cherian *et al.*, 2016).

Therapeutic effects on tissue healing and protection

TENS can have positive effects toward wound healing and tissue protection, possibly by affecting local blood flow through neural activation. Atalay and Yilmaz (2009) found that post-mastectomy skin flaps that were treated with TENS showed significantly less necrosis as compared to those that received standard postoperative care. TENS may also be effective in treating chronic wounds, even those that have failed to heal despite consistent routine care (Yarboro & Smith, 2014). Additionally, TENS can reduce tissue edema, including lower extremity lymphedema, potentially protecting against the progression to chronic lymphedema and possible development of cellulitis and chronic skin ulcers (Choi & Lee, 2016). Finally, Zotz and Paula (2015) found that the anti-inflammatory effects of TENS appear to reduce development of heterotopic ossification.

Therapeutic effects on tissue flexibility and joint ROM

When used in conjunction with a stretching program, TENS promotes greater muscle flexibility gains as compared to stretching alone (Karasuno *et al.*, 2016). Studies have also demonstrated that subjects with myofascial pain in the upper trapezius muscle who received TENS in addition to the standard care program had greater cervical spine ROM improvements when compared to those who received standard care only (Azatcam *et al.*, 2017; Dissanayaka *et al.*, 2016). TENS can have immediate positive effects on joint ROM, especially if limitations are related to pain (Valenza *et al.*, 2016).

Patients with spasticity can also gain mobility with TENS treatment due to spasticity reduction (Fernández-Tenorio *et al.*, 2016), leading to improved function (Karakoyun *et al.*, 2015; Laddha *et al.*, 2016). Of note, a review by Mills and Dossa (2016) showed better spasticity reduction may occur when TENS treatment is combined with active therapy.

Therapeutic effects on muscle strength

There are some studies that indicate sensory level TENS may have beneficial effects toward muscle function. However, the results may be more from facilitation rather than direct strengthening. For example, a literature review by Harkey and colleagues found that TENS was significantly more effective than NMES, cryotherapy, or manual therapy in addressing the quadriceps muscle inhibition often seen with knee injuries. In the studies reviewed, TENS was applied to the knee joint rather than the quadriceps muscle but was hypothesized to still have a positive effect on muscle contraction by targeting the presynaptic reflex inhibitory mechanisms that are believed to cause quadriceps dysfunction (Iles, 1996; Harkey *et al.*, 2014). A more recent study has supported these findings (Son *et al.*, 2016) and followed with an additional study to demonstrate direct translation of improved quadriceps function to better quality gait (Son *et al.*, 2017).

There is evidence that TENS may promote improved muscle function in neurologically involved patients as well. Jung and colleagues demonstrated improved trunk muscle activation and improved motor control in patients with stroke when TENS was added to conventional physical therapy treatment (Jung *et al.*, 2016), especially when treatment included task-related training (Chan *et al.*, 2015).

Considerations for clinical application

To ensure safety, muzzling may be recommended, at least for the first ES treatment, to allow assessment of the patient's tolerance for the modality. However, one author (K.N.) has not found a need for additional restraint if ES is introduced slowly and the patient's response to the initial sensation is monitored closely. It is the author's opinion that if a patient appears to be distressed by the sensation of ES, the treatment should be discontinued and a different therapeutic technique pursued.

The general procedure for providing NMES is to place the electrodes over the muscle to be stimulated (Figure 7.14). A coupling medium is needed to transmit the current from the electrode to the skin. Some electrodes are coated

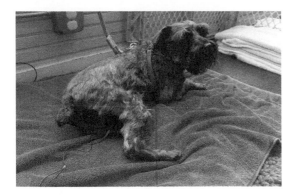

Figure 7.14   Patient receiving neuromuscular electrical stimulation (NMES) to the hamstring muscle group.

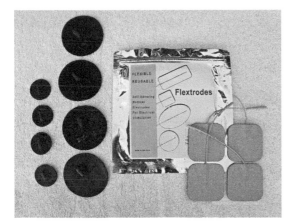

Figure 7.15   Examples of various electrical stimulation (ES) electrodes.

with a conductive polymer, while carbon silicone-rubber electrodes are used with an aqueous gel. Especially in dogs with thicker coats, the hair may need to be clipped to improve transmission, but the author has found that additional gel is typically sufficient to provide a route for the current to travel from the electrode through the hair to the skin.

The size of the electrodes should fit the target muscle. Small electrodes are available to accommodate smaller patients and/or treatment areas (Figure 7.15), but can cause discomfort with higher amplitudes due to the greater current density. The electrodes selected should be as large as possible to maximize comfort but not so large that overflow of current to other adjacent muscles occurs. The electrodes should also not contact each other, nor should their coupling medium, as this will result in the

current flowing directly from one electrode to the other instead of into the patient's tissues. There does need to be sufficient distance between the electrodes, however, as this impacts the resulting strength of the muscle contraction regardless of the stimulation intensity (Vieira *et al.*, 2016).

During initial treatments with NMES, the patient may be more receptive in a relaxed position. The author recommends using the constant or continuous output mode (no off-time) while slowly increasing the intensity/amplitude until the desired muscle contraction is obtained, then switching to the desired mode for the remainder of the treatment. As the dog becomes more familiar with the sensation, using NMES in a functional position (e.g., standing) may result in improved motor learning (Jochumsen *et al.*, 2016) (Figure 7.16).

Recommended NMES parameters for muscle strengthening are as follows (Millis *et al.*, 1997):

- Frequency between 25 and 50 Hz.
- Pulse duration between 100 and 400 μs.
- Ramp up and down of 2 to 4 s.

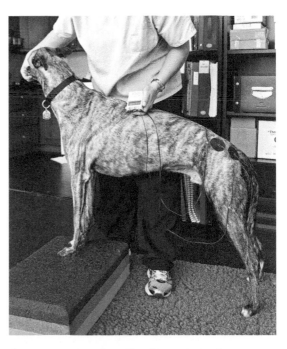

Figure 7.16   Neuromuscular electrical stimulation (NMES) with the patient in a functional position.

- On/off time ratio of 1:3 to 1:5 (a larger ratio is used with weaker muscles to avoid fatigue).
- Amplitude sufficient to cause a strong contraction is required to produce strength gains (Snyder-Mackler *et al.*, 1994).
- Frequency of treatment of 3 to 7 sessions per week.

For TENS treatments, the electrodes are often placed over the area of pain, over the peripheral nerve or spinal nerve roots that innervate the painful area, or over acupuncture points (Montenegro *et al.*, 2016). Various electrode placements may be trialed to determine the best effect for each patient.

When using TENS for improving flexibility, the general recommendations are to apply the stretch force after using TENS to reduce discomfort when treating orthopedic diagnoses. When addressing spasticity in neurological patients, the stretching force should be applied during or immediately after TENS treatment of the antagonist muscle (Karasuno *et al.*, 2016).

Recommended parameters for TENS are as follows (Nolan, 2005):

- Frequency between 30 and 150 Hz.
- Pulse duration between 50 and 100 μs.
- Amplitude to elicit a comfortable sensory response—sufficient amplitude is required to achieve an analgesic response (Moran *et al.*, 2011) and may need to be increased within each treatment (Pantaleão *et al.*, 2011).

- Duration of treatment varies according to the activity.

For both NMES and TENS, the therapist should be prepared to adjust treatment parameters in order to achieve the best outcome (Glaviano & Saliba, 2016).

Precautions and contraindications for ES

Precautions for ES include treatment over areas of decreased sensation, directly over wounds or skin irritation, in patients with osteoporosis (because of fracture risk), and in patients with obesity (because fat is a poor conductor of current).

Contraindications include stimulation directly over the heart, in areas of infection or cancer, over the trunk during pregnancy, over areas of thrombosis or thrombophlebitis, over the carotid sinus or pharyngeal area, in patients with seizure disorders, or any time active movement of the body part is contraindicated. The presence of a cardiac pacemaker is a relative contraindication as recent evidence has shown that ES is safe if the muscle stimulated is a sufficient distance from the pacemaker (Kamiya *et al.*, 2016) and only patients that are stable enough to tolerate the treatment are selected (Cenik *et al.*, 2016).

Finally, the therapist must monitor the tissues under electrodes as burns (Ford *et al.*, 2005) and other skin irritations (Naderi Nabi *et al.*, 2015) may occur.

Case Study 7.1   Post-TPLO rehabilitation—physical modalities

Signalment: 4 y.o. M/N Boxer.

Presenting complaint/history: Left TPLO to address cranial cruciate rupture. Began rehabilitation 5 days post-surgery.

Initial evaluation findings:

- Gait (walk): left pelvic limb toe-touch weight bearing with lack of hip/stifle extension at end-stance.
- Left stifle ROM: flexion 50% of normal, extension 75%.
- Muscle atrophy: moderate atrophy L hamstrings and quadriceps groups.

- Flexibility: L sartorius and iliopsoas moderately tight.
- Palpation: significant swelling, moderate warmth around the L stifle (no signs of infection).

Assessment: 5 days post-op L TPLO, expected deficits.

Goals: Regain normal postures, transfers, and gait quality within 9–10 weeks.

Treatment plan: In addition to manual therapies, therapeutic exercises, and continual instruction in appropriate home exercises, the following physical modalities were included in the treatment plan:

- TENS around L stifle (frequency: 50 Hz; pulse duration: 75 µs; amplitude to patient tolerance for 15 minutes). Used to improve tolerance for manual therapies. Discontinued when patient tolerated manual work without significant discomfort.
- NMES, L quadriceps and hamstrings (frequency: 35 Hz; pulse duration: 100 µs; 2 s ramp; 10 s on, 30 s off; amplitude to patient tolerance for 10 min). Performed with the patient in supported standing as tolerated. Discontinued when patient was able to produce strong voluntary muscle contractions.
- TUS, L sartorius—area already shaved (mode: continuous; frequency: 3 MHz; intensity: 1.0 W/cm²; duration: 7 min), gentle stretch applied during the last 2 minutes. Discontinued when muscle guarding resolved, flexibility regained.
- Cryotherapy, L stifle, 15 min at end of sessions—patient day-boarding at clinic. Cryotherapy used throughout rehab course to decrease inflammation and minimize post-exercise discomfort.
- Low-level laser therapy (LLLT), stifle joint line, 4 J/cm², increasing to 6 J/cm² as therapy progressed. Also used for muscle trigger points (R teres major, L iliopsoas) as noted, 6 J/cm². LLLT used throughout rehab course to promote healing.

At 10 weeks post-surgery, the patient had regained full range of motion, near-symmetrical muscle mass, and near-symmetrical gait mechanics at a walk and controlled trot.

Low-level laser therapy (LLLT)/photobiomodulation

LASER is an acronym for "light amplification by stimulated emission of radiation." Laser application is also referred to as photobiomodulation. Lasers produce electromagnetic radiation that is monochromatic, coherent, and collimated. These qualities allow laser light to penetrate tissues. Photons can be reflected (not penetrate the tissue), transmitted (pass through the tissue), or refracted (pass through the tissue but in an altered direction), the last two of which result in physiological changes at the molecular, cellular, and gross level. Light energy is absorbed by chromophores (light-absorbing molecules found in the tissue) causing a number of biological effects (Yadav & Gupta, 2016).

Classes of lasers

Lasers are classified according to their power, maximum permissible exposure (MPE), and wavelength. Power, measured in watts (joules/s), is the rate of energy production. Dosage, the amount of energy delivered to the tissue, is determined by multiplying power by time. The dose required to treat the tissue is dependent upon wavelength, power density, type of tissue, condition of tissue, acuity of the problem, pigmentation, depth of target tissue, and treatment technique (scanning vs point-to-point).

Doses that are too low are not effective and doses that are too high can be biosuppressive. The energy provided can then be determined in power density (W/cm²) or energy density (J/cm²). The wavelength of laser light determines the depth of penetration (Chung et al., 2012). Except for the 970–980 nm wavelength, where there is a peak in water absorption, longer wavelengths provide deeper penetration (Hudson et al., 2013). There is evidence that wavelengths of 810–830 nm penetrate the skin most effectively (Passarella & Karu, 2014), while 780–950 nm wavelengths are better for deeper tissues (Chung et al., 2012).

Other sources report that wavelengths of 600–700 nm are best for treating superficial tissues as the photons are absorbed at this layer rather than passing through to the deeper tissue. A direct comparison of energy and penetration showed 50% more penetration with a 808 nm wavelength compared to 980 nm (Hudson et al., 2013).

Lasers are also categorized based on their potential for causing harm. Therapeutic lasers fall into class 3R, class 3B, and class 4. Class 3R lasers have 1–5 mW of power. Class 3B lasers have 5–500 mW of power, are commonly used in rehabilitation, and produce nonvisible light that is not damaging to the eye when reflected off matte surfaces. Protective eyewear should be used when in close proximity to these lasers. Class 4 lasers have greater than 500 mW of power, and include both therapy and surgical lasers. Surgical lasers range from 15 to 40 W

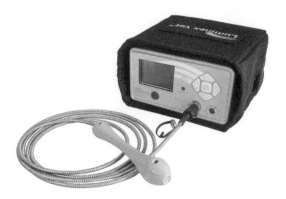

Figure 7.17   Example of a low-level laser therapy (LLLT) unit. Source: Courtesy of Respond Systems. Reproduced with permission of Respond Systems.

with the intent of heating and evaporating to cut the tissue and to control bleeding and pain by cauterizing the blood vessels and nerves along the incision line. Class 4 therapeutic lasers can be classified into heating and non-heating lasers. Use of nonheating lasers is known as low-level laser therapy (LLLT). LLLT influences cellular processes through photobio-modulation (Figure 7.17). Heating lasers are therapeutic lasers that create heat in the tissue quickly if not moved constantly during a therapy session.

Evidence supporting the use of LLLT

Therapeutic effects on pain

Light energy is absorbed by chromophores (light-absorbing molecules found in the cell) causing a number of biological effects including oxygen production, changes in cell calcium ion balance, ATP production, changes in cell membrane permeability (Passarella *et al.*, 1984; Karu, 1988; Nasu *et al.*, 1989), and reduction in inflammation by reducing production of cytokines—cyclooxygenase 2 (COX2), tumor necrosis factor α (TNFα), interleukin 1 (IL-1), and IL-6 (Sakurai *et al.*, 2000; Alves *et al.*, 2013b). LLLT may also facilitate collagen synthesis (Abergel *et al.*, 1984), growth factor release (Yu *et al.*, 1994), and stimulation of fibroblast development (Pourreau-Schneider *et al.*, 1990), all promoting tissue repair. LLLT may increase angiogenesis and therefore the formation of new capillaries in injured tissues (Corazza *et al.*, 2007). Indeed, evidence has

been found that LLLT can lead to more rapid closure (Hopkins *et al.*, 2004), increased tensile strength (Vasilenko *et al.*, 2010), and greater collagen content during wound healing (Medrado *et al.*, 2003). LLLT has also shown an ability to affect the healing of nerves (Gigo-Benato *et al.*, 2004), connective tissues, such as ligament (Fung *et al.*, 2002), and may have positive effects on injured cartilage (Guzzardella *et al.*, 2001; Guzzardella *et al.*, 2002).

Additionally, LLLT may assist in pain reduction through increased metabolism of endogenous opiates, or a change in the conduction latencies of nerves (Snyder-Mackler & Bork, 1988; Lowe *et al.*, 1994).

There are numerous studies supporting the use of LLLT to address both acute and chronic pain related to orthopedic and neurological diagnoses. For example, a 2016 study by Ojea and colleagues found that human patients who received postoperative LLLT experienced less incisional pain as compared to a sham group (Ojea *et al.*, 2016); this is likely meaningful for postoperative canine patients as well. LLLT has also been shown to reduce the pain associated with chronic orthopedic conditions such as ankylosing spondylitis (Stasinopoulos *et al.*, 2016), temporomandibular joint (TMJ) pain (Cavalcanti *et al.*, 2016), and knee osteoarthritis (Assis *et al.*, 2015; Bjordal, *et al.*, 2003). Indeed, in a study by Ip (2015), patients with knee osteoarthritis who received LLLT in addition to conventional physical therapy were significantly less likely to require joint replacement surgery as compared to patients who received physical therapy alone. This outcome remained true even 6 years after treatment was completed (Ip, 2015).

LLLT can be effective in decreasing neuropathic pain (de Oliveira Martins *et al.*, 2013; Janzadeh *et al.*, 2016). Kobiela Ketz and colleagues used a peripheral nerve injury model in rats with resulting pain as assessed by mechanical hypersensitivity. Subjects treated with LLLT every other day (initiated 7 days after injury) showed improvements in pain status after just two treatments, and were returned to baseline mechanical hypersensitivity levels within 10 treatments (Kobiela Ketz *et al.*, 2017). A 2016 literature review also supported the positive effect of LLLT in the treatment of neuropathic pain (de Andrade *et al.*, 2016).

The literature also supports using LLLT to address myofascial pain (Rayegani *et al.*, 2011; Taheri *et al.*, 2016), neck pain (Chow *et al.*, 2009), low back pain (Huang *et al.*, 2015), osteoarthritis (Youssef *et al.*, 2016), and rheumatoid arthritis (Alves *et al.*, 2013a). Several studies noted reduced need for analgesic medications following treatment with LLLT (Cavalcanti *et al.*, 2016; Khalighi *et al.*, 2016). LLLT has also been shown to reduce discomfort through stimulation of acupuncture or muscle trigger points (Snyder-Mackler *et al.*, 1989; Al Rashoud *et al.*, 2014; Erthal *et al.*, 2016).

While the mechanisms by which LLLT affects pain are still not fully understood, it is believed that LLLT application may cause enhancement of peripheral endogenous opioid production (Hagiwara *et al.*, 2007), an inhibition of action potentials by the peripheral nerve endings of nociceptors (Cotler *et al.*, 2015), and a reduction of nociceptor activation at the spinal level (Nadur-Andrade *et al.*, 2016).

It is important to note that the effects of LLLT are dependent on multiple factors including dose, wavelength, single versus combination of wavelength, depth of target tissue, and frequency of treatment. There are laser studies that do not have satisfactory outcomes on healing or pain management with laser therapy, but when closely examined, these studies may not have appropriate parameters.

Therapeutic effects on tissue healing and protection

The absorption of light energy by chromophores causes a number of biological effects including increased ATP production and changes in cell membrane permeability (Karu, 1988; Karu *et al.*, 1995; Vartika *et al.*, 2015), promoting improved cellular function. LLLT has been shown to facilitate collagen synthesis (Tatmatsu-Rocha *et al.*, 2016) with a greater collagen content observed in treated wounds (Guerra Fda *et al.*, 2013; Ranjbar & Takhtfooladi, 2016). Increased growth factor release (Saygun *et al.*, 2012; Martignago *et al.*, 2015) and stimulation of fibroblast development (Frozanfar *et al.*, 2013; Rathnakar *et al.*, 2016) also occurs, with a resultant increase in wound tensile strength (Vasilenko *et al.*, 2010; Suzuki & Takakuda, 2016). Additionally, LLLT increases angiogenesis

(de Medeiros *et al.*, 2017) leading to the formation of new capillaries in injured tissues (Ihsan, 2005; Corazza *et al.*, 2007; Wagner *et al.*, 2016), and more rapid wound healing in general (Hopkins *et al.*, 2004; da Silva *et al.*, 2010; Lima *et al.*, 2017). A 2016 study by Mathur and colleagues demonstrated that, even in challenging wound environments such as diabetic foot ulcers, the addition of LLLT to conventional therapy promotes a more rapid reduction in wound size and higher amounts of granulation tissue in as little as 2 weeks compared with patients who received conventional wound care only (Mathur *et al.*, 2017). Furthermore, LLLT may be useful in the treatment of infected wounds as shown by a significant reduction in bacterial growth (Ranjbar & Takhtfooladi, 2016).

When considering specific tissue types, LLLT has shown positive effect toward the healing of connective tissues, such as ligament (Fung *et al.*, 2002) and tendon (de Jesus *et al.*, 2014) as well as skin. A 2016 study showed that LLLT promotes healing of tendinopathy as evidenced by increased production of collagen (Marques *et al.*, 2016). It can also accelerate skeletal muscle repair (Assis *et al.*, 2016; De Marchi *et al.*, 2017), assist in the recovery of articular tissues following injury (Alves *et al.*, 2014; Lemos *et al.*, 2016), improve cartilage thickness in patients with osteoarthritis (OA) (S *et al.*, 2016), protect articular cartilage (Bublitz *et al.*, 2014; Assis *et al.*, 2016; Tomazoni *et al.*, 2017), hasten the formation of new bone tissue (de Almeida *et al.*, 2016; Tim *et al.*, 2016), promote better bone health in animals with spinal cord injury (Medalha *et al.*, 2016), and promote functional recovery of nerves (Gigo-Benato *et al.*, 2004; Rochkind *et al.*, 2009; Takhtfooladi *et al.*, 2015; Ziago *et al.*, 2017). Indeed, there is evidence that LLLT reduces inflammation and promotes functional recovery following spinal cord injury in a rat model (Veronez *et al.*, 2017). Specific to the canine patient, LLLT may promote CNS healing as demonstrated by a more rapid return to ambulatory status following hemilaminectomy to address intervertebral disc disease (IVDD) (Draper *et al.*, 2012).

Therapeutic effects on tissue flexibility and joint ROM

Likely through a combination of pain reduction and decreased inflammation, LLLT can increase joint ROM. A 2016 study by Youssef and colleagues compared patients with knee osteoarthritis who participated in an exercise program with or without LLLT treatment. While all subjects demonstrated improved pain levels and knee ROM, those subjects who received LLLT demonstrated significantly greater improvements in both areas (Youssef *et al.*, 2016). Similar findings were noted for OA in joints of the hand (Baltzer *et al.*, 2016) with improvement in all aspects (pain, swelling, and joint mobility) following LLLT treatment.

When working with neurological patients, LLLT may be able to improve mobility by reducing spasticity, although the effects may be temporary. Children with cerebral palsy are often affected by spasticity, including in the muscles of the jaw, which limits the ability to open the mouth. Santos and colleagues delivered LLLT to the masseter and anterior temporal muscles for six treatments over 3 weeks. Up to 6 weeks after treatments were completed, the LLLT subjects continued to show increased amplitude of mouth opening. By the sixth week, however, measurements returned to baseline (Santos *et al.*, 2016). This reduction in spasticity may provide the therapist with time to perform more effective stretching, thereby achieving more permanent results.

Therapeutic effects on muscle strength

Emerging research is showing that LLLT can assist in reducing muscle fatigue. In a 2015 review, Leal-Junior and colleagues found that pre-exercise LLLT led to reduced muscle fatigue based on the subjects' ability to perform increased number of repetitions as compared to controls (Leal-Junior *et al.*, 2015). In a progressive intensity running study the use of LLLT before exercise increased exercise performance (as measured by $VO2_{max}$ and time to exhaustion) and decreased oxidative stress and muscle damage. The latter was evaluated by measuring levels of superoxide dismutase (SOD), creatine kinase (CK), and lactate dehydrogenase (LDH) (De Marchi *et al.*, 2012).

LLLT may also result in enhanced strength gains. Vanin and colleagues found that healthy volunteer subjects who received LLLT prior to each training session over a 12-week course achieved significantly greater measurements of maximum voluntary contraction and weight lifted in 1-repetition maximum as compared to subjects who did not receive LLLT (Vanin *et al.*, 2016). Similar results have been noted in older healthy adults. Toma and colleagues found that, when combined with strength training, LLLT promoted greater strength gains in elderly women (Toma *et al.*, 2016).

Considerations for clinical application

When using LLLT with canine patients, recommendations include clipping or parting the hair to maximize skin contact with the probe in patients with thick, long coats. If using a heating laser this may be necessary in most patients. More frequent movement of the probe is indicated when treating over dark-colored hair or skin if using a high-powered laser due to the absorption of photon energy by melanin. The absorption of the photons at a superficial level is considered *attenuation* or loss of penetration due to superficial absorption. This attenuation requires a slightly higher total amount of energy to create the full effect of the laser at deeper target tissue. This energy has to be distributed slower to prevent injury to the tissue from overheating. Laser photons are also absorbed by the ink in tattoos causing them to heat faster than pigmented tissue. For this reason, applying laser over a tattoo should only be done when the benefit outweighs the risk, and again, the energy needs to be delivered slowly to prevent overheating the skin. Topical medications should be washed off, and the clinician, patient, and everyone in the room should wear protective eyewear. Cryotherapy before LLLT may provide additional benefit (Haslerud *et al.*, 2017) due to vasoconstriction decreasing water and hemoglobin in the tissue, two of the major laser-absorbing chromophores, allowing deeper penetration secondary to less attenuation. Joints to be treated should be placed in the open or loose-packed position and, when possible, have traction applied to maximize energy delivery to the joint capsule and cartilage surfaces (Figure 7.18). As inflammatory mediators are deposited into the joint from the synovial capsule, treating this structure is important when the goal is reducing or preventing inflammation. LLLT is considered safe to use over

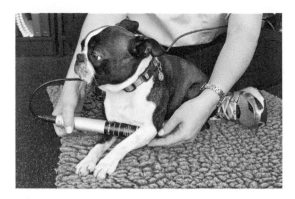

Figure 7.18   Patient receiving low-level laser therapy (LLLT) of the elbow joint.

plastic, metal and/or cement implants, though low doses should be delivered if a heating laser is used over implants. Finally, aseptic technique should be used when treating wounds by either applying clear plastic wrap over the probe or by maintaining a small space over the wound surface.

Multiple techniques are commonly described for delivering LLLT. One technique, *gridding* or *point-to-point*, is achieved by holding the probe in one place for a duration of time to deliver a specific dose and then moving the probe to the next spot to be treated. The benefit of this treatment is that photons of energy saturate or *photo-bleach* the tissue, allowing deeper penetration of the beam. Depending on the unit involved, these treatment spots may be the size of the probe or the distance between the probe locations may be centimeters apart. Space is needed due to refraction. Some laser probes adjust for this by having a large probe with only a small diode. Other companies have multiple diodes inside the probe, close to the edges, requiring further probe placement on the tissue. A second technique, *surround*, is primarily used with wounds; the periphery of the wound is treated with a higher dose of energy than the area directly over the wound. The granulation tissue requires less energy as there is no melanin to attenuate the photon beam. Angiogenesis is desired at the area of the granulation tissue as is reduction of bacteria. Deep penetration is not needed, reducing the need for higher doses. *Scanning*, or continuously moving the probe, is another method of treating the tissue. This is essential when using a heating laser to prevent

thermal damage. When using a nonheating laser, scanning can also be used to treat tissue. Scanning allows lower doses of energy to be applied to the tissue multiple times rather than one larger dose. In this author's (L.M.) experience, scanning works better for muscle issues and wounds whereas point-to-point is more effective on deep tissue, joints, and when pain control is the goal.

Mode of operation of the laser may be continuous, pulsed wave, or combined depending on the unit, each with different biological effects. Pulsed wave may be more beneficial in treating deeper tissues (Keshri *et al.*, 2016), wound healing, and post-stroke management. Continuous wave may be more efficacious in the treatment of nerve regeneration. Further research is needed to delineate the benefits of each mode.

When considering dosage, specific recommendations have not been fully established. The effects of LLLT are believed to be biphasic in that low doses appear to stimulate healing while higher doses may inhibit it (Huang *et al.*, 2009; Gagnon *et al.*, 2016). The authors recommend referring to the manufacturer's recommendations for each unit. Information can also be found on the World Association of Laser Therapy (WALT) website.

Precautions and contraindications

LLLT is not recommended for use in patients with epilepsy that can be triggered by a photosensitivity. Lasers that cause tissue to heat should not be used over open epiphyseal plates, over the gonads, or in proximity to surgical implants. Precautions should be considered when using laser over an area of skin that has a tattoo as skin heating can occur, and over the injection site of long-acting steroids as a pain response has been noted (Laurie McCauley, unpublished finding, 2017). Contraindications include treatment over the cornea, over the endocrine glands, in areas of active bleeding, over the pregnant uterus, and over neoplasia. Laser may be used in areas of neoplasia as a palliative form of pain control, with the understanding that tumor growth may escalate with the laser therapy, as long as there is clear, written, informed consent.

Case Study 7.2   Hip dysplasia—physical modalities

Signalment: 11 y.o. F/S Golden Retriever.

Presenting complaint/history: Referred for pain and weakness associated with bilateral (B) hip dysplasia and severe DJD. Receiving NSAID. Tolerating two 10-minute walks per day; difficulty negotiating stairs at home.

Initial evaluation:

- Gait (walk): lack of hip extension at end-stance, narrow-based pelvic limbs, increased weight shifted onto thoracic limbs.
- Hip ROM: B extension 70% of normal.
- Muscle atrophy: significant atrophy of B hamstring and gluteal groups.
- Flexibility/palpation: B iliopsoas, B deep gluteals, B piriformis muscles tight and tender.

Assessment: Significant ROM, strength, flexibility restrictions associated with chronic hip DJD, resulting in functional deficits.

Goals: Improve joint and muscular comfort to promote increased ROM, strength, flexibility and overall mobility to allow continued leashed-walks with client and to negotiate the stairs in the home 3× per day in 10–12 weeks.

Treatment plan: In addition to manual therapies, therapeutic exercises, and continual instruction in appropriate home exercises, the following physical modalities were included in the treatment plan:

- NMES, B gluteals and hamstrings (frequency: 25 Hz; pulse duration: 150 μs; 2 s ramp; 10 s on, 30 s off; amplitude to patient tolerance for 10 min). Used throughout rehabilitation in progressively more functional positions (sternal, standing, during sit-to-stand transfer, etc.).
- Hot packs, B hips during NMES before active exercise, 10 min. Patient's skin checked every 3 minutes.
- TUS, B iliopsoas—area shaved before treatment (mode: continuous; frequency: 1 MHz; intensity: 1.0 W/cm^2: duration: 10 min), gentle stretch applied during last 2 minutes. Discontinued when flexibility and comfort sufficiently improved.
- Cryotherapy, B hips, 20 min during ride home from session (second client in backseat with patient). Used throughout rehabilitation course to decrease pain and inflammation.
- LLLT, bilateral hips, 7 J/cm^2, increasing to 9 J/cm^2 as therapy progressed. B iliopsoas 6 J/cm^2. Used throughout rehabilitation course for pain control.

With 12 weeks of therapy, the patient regained functional hip extension range, increased muscle mass, improved active hip extension and control during gait, and was able to easily complete two 30-minute walks per day and negotiate the stairs at home.

Extracorporeal shock wave therapy (ESWT)

Extracorporeal shock wave therapy (ESWT), also known as high-energy focused sound wave therapy, was first introduced in the early 1980s as a noninvasive method for treating kidney stones (Sems *et al.*, 2006). Shock waves are single pulsed sound waves that dissipate mechanical energy at the interface of substances with different acoustic impedance. Shock waves produce approximately 1000 times the pressure magnitude of ultrasound waves and deliver energy at a controlled focal volume. The mechanical energy transferred to tissues following ESWT causes various biological responses at the cellular level. This modality has been increasingly used to treat a variety of musculoskeletal conditions in humans and veterinary patients (Rompe *et al.*, 1996; Schaden *et al.*, 2001; Laverty and McClure, 2002; Dahlberg *et al.*, 2005; Sems *et al.*, 2006; Mueller *et al.*, 2007). Benefits of ESWT include: increased bone, tendon, and ligament healing, accelerated wound healing, antibacterial properties, and pain relief (Rompe *et al.*, 1996; Laverty & McClure, 2002; Sems *et al.*, 2006). The exact mechanism of action of ESWT has yet to be fully elucidated; however, the mechanical stimulation of cells is hypothesized to result in increased expression of cytokines and growth factors leading to decreased inflammation, neovascularization, and cellular proliferation (Wang *et al.*, 2002, 2003, 2005; Sems *et al.*, 2006). ESWT has also been demonstrated to speed healing and increase quality of healing in soft tissue and bone, protect chondrocytes, disintegrate calcifications, and recruit stem cells to the treatment site (Schaden *et al.*, 2001; Gerdesmeyer *et al.*, 2003; Wang *et al.*, 2005; Aicher *et al.*, 2006; Moretti *et al.*, 2008). The mechanism behind the pain-relieving function of ESWT is thought to be due to increased serotonin activity in the dorsal horn, and descending inhibition of pain signals (Rompe *et al.*, 1996; Sems *et al.*, 2006). ESWT has been used clinically for the treatment of chronic musculoskeletal conditions such as osteoarthritis and tendinopathies, delayed and nonunion fractures, and chronic wounds (Rompe *et al.*, 1996; Schaden *et al.*, 2001; Laverty & McClure, 2002; Dahlberg *et al.*, 2005; Sems *et al.*, 2006; Mueller *et al.*, 2007).

Mueller and colleagues (2007) conducted a study to evaluate the effects of ESWT on the pelvic limb function of dogs suffering from coxofemoral osteoarthritis. Twenty-four client-owned dogs with coxofemoral osteoarthritis were investigated; 18 of them received radial shock wave therapy and six were left untreated as controls. Force plate analysis on a treadmill was used to assess the dogs' pelvic limb function before treatment and 4 weeks after the last treatment. The ESWT dogs were re-evaluated 3 and 6 months after treatment. In the ESWT dogs, differences between the ground reaction forces exerted by the right and left pelvic limbs disappeared 4 weeks after treatment; whereas in the control dogs only the peak vertical force distribution changed significantly. The significant improvement in the ESWT dogs was confirmed by changes in the symmetry indices. Significant improvements in vertical impulse and peak vertical force were observed 3 months after treatment. Researchers concluded that ESWT is an effective treatment modality for dogs with coxofemoral osteoarthritis (Mueller *et al.*, 2007).

Kieves and colleagues (2015) evaluated the influence of ESWT on radiographic evidence of bone healing after tibial plateau leveling osteotomy (TPLO). Forty-two dogs (50 stifles) that underwent a TPLO were randomly assigned to receive either ESWT or sham. Treatments were delivered to the osteotomy site immediately postoperatively and a second treatment was done 2 weeks later. Radiographs were evaluated by blinded radiologists 8 weeks postoperatively. Based on 5-point and 10-point bone healing scales, the mean healing scores were significantly greater in the ESWT group than the sham group. The researchers determined that ESWT led to more advanced bone healing after a TPLO.

Gallagher and colleagues (2012) conducted a study to determine if ESWT after TPLO has a beneficial effect on patellar ligament inflammation assessed by thickening of the ligament and ligament fiber disruption. Thirty dogs that had TPLO had the affected stifle examined by radiographs and ultrasonography preoperatively and 4, 6, and 8 weeks after TPLO. At 4 and 6 weeks, dogs in the treatment group were anesthetized and treated with ESWT. Patellar ligament thickness on a lateral radiographic projection was measured at ¼, ½, and ¾ of the distance from origin to insertion. Ultrasound images were evaluated for patellar ligament disruption and periligament edema. A significant radiographic difference between groups was reached at 6 and 8 weeks postoperatively. No significant ultrasonographic differences were found. Researchers determined that ESWT decreases the radiographic signs of patellar ligament desmitis.

Becker and colleagues (2015) performed a retrospective study reviewing medical records of 15 dogs with shoulder lameness that failed previous conservative management. ESWT was administered every 3–4 weeks for a total of three treatments. Short-term, in-hospital subjective lameness evaluation revealed resolution of lameness in 3 of 9 dogs, and reduced lameness in 6 of 9 dogs available for evaluation 3–4 weeks following the last treatment. Long-term lameness score via telephone interview was either improved or normal in 7 of 11 dogs (64%). Researchers proposed that ESWT may result in improved function based on subjective patient evaluation and did not have any negative side effects in dogs with lameness attributable to instability, calcifying, and inflammatory conditions of the shoulder.

Webliography

Watson, T. 2009. Ultrasound treatment dose calculations. Available at: http://faculty.mu.edu.sa/public/uploads/1334234703.029US%20dose%20chart%20jan%202009%20(2).pdf (accessed October 26, 2017).

World Association of Laser Therapy. 2010. Recommended treatment doses for low level laser therapy, 904nm. Available at: http://waltza.co.za/wp-content/uploads/2012/08/Dose_table_904nm_for_Low_Level_Laser_Therapy_WALT-2010.pdf (accessed October 26, 2017).

World Association of Laser Therapy. 2010. Recommended treatment doses for low level laser therapy, 780–860 nm. Available at: http://waltza.co.za/wp-content/uploads/2012/08/Dose_table_780-860nm_for_Low_Level_Laser_Therapy_WALT-2010.pdf (accessed October 26, 2017).

References

Aaron, S. E., Delgado-Diaz, D. C., & Kostek, M. C. 2017. Continuous ultrasound decreases pain perception and increases pain threshold in damaged skeletal muscle. *Clin J Sport Med*, 27, 271–277.

Abergel, R. P., Meeker, C. A., Dwyer, R. M., Lesavoy, M. A., & Uitto, J. 1984. Nonthermal effects of ND:YAG laser on biological functions of human skin fibroblasts in culture. *Lasers Surg Med*, 3(4), 279–284.

Aicher, A., Heeschen, C., Sasaki, K., Urbich, C., Zeiher, A. M., & Dimmeler, S. 2006. Low-energy shock wave for enhancing recruitment of endothelial progenitor cells. *Circulation*, 114, 2823–2830.

Akgun, K., Korpinar, M. A., Kalkan, M. T., Akarirmak, U., Tuzun, S. & Tuzun, F. 2004. Temperature changes in superficial and deep tissue layers with respect to time of cold gel pack application in dogs. *Yonsie Med J*, 45, 711–718.

Akhlaghi, Z., Mobarakeh, J. I., Mokhtari, M., Behnam, H., Rahimi, A. A., Khajeh Hosseini, M. S., & Samiee, F. 2012. The effects of altered ultrasound parameters on the recovery of sciatic nerve injury. *Iran Biomed*, 16, 107–112.

Alegre, L. M., Hasler, M., Wenger, S., Nachbauer, W., & Csapo, R. 2016. Does knee joint cooling change in vivo patellar tendon mechanical properties? *Eur J Appl Physiol*, 116, 1921–1929.

Alexander, J., Selfe, J., Oliver, B., Mee, D., Carter, A., Scott, M., *et al.* 2016. An exploratory study into the effects of a 20 minute crushed ice application on knee joint position sense during a small knee bend. *Phys Ther Sport*, 18, 21–26.

Algafly, A. A. & George, K. P. 2007. The effect of cryotherapy on nerve conduction velocity, pain threshold and pain tolerance. *Br J Sports Med*, 41, 365–369.

Allison, S. C. & Abraham, L. D. 2001. Sensitivity of qualitative and quantitative spasticity measures to clinical treatment with cryotherapy. *Int J Rehabil Res*, 24, 15–24.

Al Rashoud, A. S., Abboud, R. J., Wang, W., & Wigderowitz, C. 2014. Efficacy of low-level laser therapy applied at acupuncture points in knee osteoarthritis: a randomised double-blind comparative trial. *Physiotherapy*, 100, 242–248.

Altomare, M., Nascimento, A. P., Romana-Souza, B., Amadeu, T. P., & Monte-Alto-Costa, A. 2009. Ultrasound accelerates healing of normal wounds but not of ischemic ones. *Wound Repair Regen*, 17, 825–831.

Alves, A. C., De Carvalho, P. T., Parente, M., Xavier, M., Frigo, L., Aimbire, F., *et al.* 2013a. Low-level laser therapy in different stages of rheumatoid arthritis: a histological study. *Lasers Med Sci*, 28, 529–536.

Alves, A. C., Vieira, R., Leal-Junior, E., Dos Santo, S. S., Ligeiro, A. P., Albertini, R., *et al.* 2013b. Effect of low-level laser therapy on the expression of inflammatory mediators and on neutrophils and macrophages in acute joint inflammation. *Arthritis Res Ther*, 15(5), R116.

Alves, A. C., Albertini, R., Dos Santos, S. A., Leal-Junior, E. C., Santana, E., Serra, A. J., *et al.* 2014. Effect of low-level laser therapy on metalloproteinase MMP-2 and MMP-9 production and percentage of collagen types I and III in a papain cartilage injury model. *Lasers Med Sci*, 29, 911–919.

Artho, P. A., Thyne, J. G., Warring, B. P., Willis, C. D., Brismée, J. M., & Latman, N. S. 2002. A calibration study of therapeutic ultrasound units. *Phys Ther*, 82, 257–263.

Assis, L., Almeida, T., Milares, L. P., Dos Passos, N., Araujo, B., Bublitz, C., *et al.* 2015. Musculoskeletal atrophy in an experimental model of knee osteoarthritis: the effects of exercise training and low-level laser therapy. *Am J Phys Med Rehabil*, 94, 609–616.

Assis, L., Manis, C., Fernandes, K. R., Cabral, D., Magri, A., Veronez, S., & Renno, A. C. 2016. Investigation of the comparative effects of red and infrared laser therapy on skeletal muscle repair in diabetic rats. *Am J Phys Med Rehabil*, 95, 525–534.

Atalay, C. & Yilmaz, K. B. 2009. The effects of transcutaneous electrical nerve stimulation on postmastectomy skin flap necrosis. *Breast Cancer Res Treat*, 117, 611–614.

Aydin, E., Tastaban, E., Omurlu, I. K., Turan, Y., & Şendur, Ö. F. 2016. Effects of deep heating provided by therapeutic ultrasound on demyelinating nerves. *J Phys Ther Sci*, 28, 1278–1283.

Azatcam, G., Atalay, N. S., Akkaya, N., Sahin, F., Aksoy, S., Zincir, O., & Topuz, O. 2017. Comparison of effectiveness of transcutaneous electrical nerve stimulation and Kinesio taping added to exercises in patients with myofascial pain syndrome. *J Back Musculoskelet Rehabil*, 30, 291–298.

Baker, R. J. & Bell, G. W. 1991. The effect of therapeutic modalities on blood flow in the human calf. *J Ortho Sports Phys Ther*, 13, 23–27.

Baltzer, A. W., Ostapczuk, M. S., & Stosch, D. 2016. Positive effects of low level laser therapy (LLLT) on Bouchard's and Heberden's osteoarthritis. *Lasers Surg Med*, 48, 498–504.

Barber, F. A. 2000. A comparison of crushed ice and continuous flow cold therapy. *Am J Knee Surg*, 13, 97–101.

Barca, I., Colangeli, W., Cristofaro, M. G., Giudice, A., Giofrè, E., Varano, A., & Giudice, M. 2016. Effects of cold therapy in the treatment of mandibular angle fractures: hilotherm system vs ice bag. *Ann Ital Chir*, 87, 411–416.

Beaumont, E., Guevara, E., Dubeau, S., Lesage, F., Nagai, M., & Popovic, M. 2014. Functional electrical stimulation post-spinal cord injury improves locomotion and increases afferent input into the central nervous system in rats. *J Spinal Cord Med*, 37, 93–100.

Becker, W., Kowaleski, M. P., Mccarthy, R. J., & Blake, C. 2015. Extracorporeal shockwave therapy for shoulder lameness in dogs. *Am Anim Hosp Assoc*, 51, 15–19.

Bellew, J. W., Michlovitz, S. L., & Nolan, T. P. 2016. *Michlovitz's Modalities for Therapeutic Interventions*, 6th edn. Philadelphia, PA: F.A. Davis Co.

Benavent-Caballer, V., Rosado-Calatayud, P., Segura-Ortí, E., Amer-Cuenca, J. J., & Lisón, J. F. 2014. Effects of three different low-intensity exercise interventions on physical performance, muscle CSA and activities of daily living: a randomized controlled trial. *Exp Gerontol*, 58, 159–165.

Benjaboonyanupap, D., Paungmali, A., & Pirunsan, U. 2015. Effect of therapeutic sequence of hot pack and ultrasound on physiological response over trigger point of upper trapezius. *Asian J Sports Med*, 6(3), e23806.

Bickel, C. S., Yarar-Fischer, C., Mahoney, E. T., & Mccully, K. K. 2015. Neuromuscular electrical stimulation-induced resistance training after SCI: a review of the Dudley protocol. *Top Spinal Cord Inj Rehabil*, 21, 294–302.

Bierman, W. & Friedlander, M. 1940. The penetrative effect of cold. *Arch Phys Ther*, 21, 585–593.

Bilgili, A., Çakir, T., Doğan, Ş., K., Erçalik, T., Filiz, M. B., & Toraman, F. 2016. The effectiveness of transcutaneous electrical nerve stimulation in the management of patients with complex regional pain syndrome: a randomized, double-blinded, placebo-controlled prospective study. *J Back Musculoskelet Rehabil*, 29, 661–671.

Biyik Bayram, S. & Caliskan, N. 2016. Effects of local heat application before intravenous catheter insertion in chemotherapy patients. *J Clin Nurs*, 25, 1740–1747.

Bjordal, J. M., Couppé, C., Chow, R., Tunér, J., & Ljunggren, E. A. 2003. A systematic review of low level laser therapy with location-specific doses for pain from chronic joint disorders *Aust J Physiother*, 49, 107–116.

Bleakley, C. M., Mcdonough, S. M., Macauley, D. C., & Bjordal, J. 2006. Cryotherapy for acute ankle sprains: a randomised controlled study of two different icing protocols. *Br J Sports Med*, 40, 700–705.

Boyraz, I., Yildiz, A., Koc, B., & Sarman, H. 2015. Comparison of high-intensity laser therapy and ultrasound treatment in the patients with lumbar discopathy. *Biomed Res Int*, 2015, Art. ID 304328.

Broderick, B. J., O'connell, S., Moloney, S., O'halloran, K., Sheehan, J., Quondamatteo, F., *et al.* 2014. Comparative lower limb hemodynamics using neuromuscular electrical stimulation (NMES) versus intermittent pneumatic compression (IPC). *Physiol Meas*, 35, 1849–1859.

Brophy-Williams, N., Landers, G., & Wallman, K. 2011. Effect of immediate and delayed cold water immersion after a high intensity exercise session on subsequent run performance. *J Sports Sci Med*, 10, 665–670.

Bublitz, C., Medalha, C., Oliveira, P., Assis, L., Milares, L. P., Fernandes, K. R., *et al.* 2014. Low-level laser therapy prevents degenerative morphological changes in an experimental model of anterior cruciate ligament transection in rats. *Lasers Med Sci*, 29, 1669–1678.

Cage, S. A., Rupp, K. A., Castel, J. C., Saliba, E. N., Hertel, J., & Saliba, S. A. 2013. Relative acoustic transmission of topical preparations used with therapeutic ultrasound. *Arch Phys Med Rehabil*, 94, 2126–2130.

Cameron, M. H. 2013. *Physical Agents In Rehabilitation: From Research To Practice*, 4th edn. St Louis, MO: Elsevier Saunders.

Carty, A., Mccormack, K., Coughlan, G. F., Crowe, L., & Caulfield, B. 2013. Alterations in body composition and spasticity following subtetanic neuromuscular electrical stimulation training in spinal cord injury. *J Rehabil Res Dev*, 50, 193–202.

Cavalcanti, M. F., Silva, U. H., Leal-Junior, E. C., Lopes-Martins, R. A., Marcos, R. L., Pallotta, R. C., *et al.* 2016. Comparative study of the physiotherapeutic and drug protocol and low-level laser irradiation in the treatment of pain associated with temporomandibular dysfunction. *Photomed Laser Surg*, 34, 652–656.

Cenik, F., Schoberwalter, D., Keilani, M., Maehr, B., Wolzt, M., Marhold, M., & Crevenna, R. 2016. Neuromuscular electrical stimulation of the thighs in cardiac patients with implantable cardioverter defibrillators. *Wien Klin Wochenschr*, 128, 802–808.

Chan, A. K., Myrer, J. W., Measom, G. J., & Draper, D. O. 1998. Temperature changes in human patellar tendon in response to therapeutic ultrasound. *J Athl Train*, 33, 130–135.

Chan, B. K., Ng, S. S., & Ng, G. Y. 2015. A home-based program of transcutaneous electrical nerve stimulation and task-related trunk training improves trunk control in patients with stroke: a randomized controlled clinic trial. *Neurorehabil Neural Repair*, 29, 70–79.

Chang, Y. P., Chiang, H., Shih K. S., Ma, H. L., Lin, L. C., Hsu, W. L., *et al.* 2015. Effects of therapeutic physical agents on achilles tendon microcirculation. *J Orthop Sports Phys Ther*, 45, 563–569.

Chang, Y. P., Shih, K. S., Chiang, H., Ma, H. L., Lin, L. C., Peng, W. C., et al. 2017. Characteristics of intratendinous microcirculation shortly after an achilles rupture and subsequent treatment outcomes. *PMR*, 9, 32–39.

Chen, Y. W., Tzeng, J. I., Lin, M. F., Hung, C. H., & Wang, J. J. 2015. Transcutaneous electrical nerve stimulation attenuates postsurgical allodynia and suppresses spinal substance P and proinflammatory cytokine release in rats. *Phys Ther*, 95, 76–85.

Cherian, J. J., Harrison, P. E., Benjamin, S. A., Bhave, A., Harwin, S. F., & Mont, M. A. 2016. Do the effects of transcutaneous electrical nerve stimulation on knee osteoarthritis pain and function last? *J Knee Surg*, 29, 497–501.

Cho, Y. S., Choi, Y. H., Yoon, C., & You, J. S. 2015. Factors affecting the depth of burns occuring in medical institutions. *Burns*, 41, 604–608.

Choi, Y. D. & Lee, J. H. 2016. Edema and pain reduction using transcutaneous electrical nerve stimulation treatment. *J Phys Ther Sci*, 28, 3084–3087.

Chow, R. T., Johnson, M. I., Lopes-Martins, R. A., & Bjordal, J. M. 2009. Efficacy of low-level laser therapy in the management of neck pain: a systematic review and meta-analysis of randomized placebo or active-treatment controlled trials. *Lancet*, 374, 1897–1908.

Chughtai, M., Elmallah, R. D., Mistry, J. B., Bhave, A., Cherian, J. J., Mcginn, T. L., *et al.* 2016. Nonpharmacologic pain management and muscle strengthening following total knee arthroplasty. *J Knee Surg*, 29, 194–200.

Chung, H., Dai, T. Sharma, S. K., Huang, Y. Y., Carroll, J. D., & Hamblin, M. R. 2012. The nuts and bolts of low-level laser (light) therapy. *Ann Biomed Eng*, 40, 516–533.

Cobbold, A. F. & Lewis, O. J. 1956. Blood flow to the knee joint of the dog; effect of heating, cooling and adrenaline. *J Physiol*, 132, 379–383.

Coquart, J. B., Grosbois, J. M. Olivier, C., Bart, F., Castres, I., & Wallaert, B. 2016. Home-based neuromuscular electrical stimulation improves exercise tolerance and health-related quality of life in patients with COPD. *Int J Chron Obstruct Pulmon Dis*, 11, 1189–1197.

Corazza, A. V., Jorge, J., Kurachi, C., & Bagnato, V. S. 2007. Photobiomodulation on the angiogenesis of skin wounds in rats using different light sources. *Photomed Laser Surg*, 25, 102–106.

Corti, L. 2014. Nonpharmaceutical approaches to pain management. *Top Companion Anim Med*, 29, 24–28.

Cotler, H. B., Chow, R. T., Hamblin, M. R., & Carroll, J. 2015. The use of low level laser therapy (LLLT) for musculoskeletal pain. *MOJ Orthop Rheumatol*, 2, 00068.

Cudia, P., Weis, L., Baba, A., Kiper, P., Marcante, A. Rossi, S., *et al.* 2016. Effects of functional electrical stimulation lower extremity training in myotonic dystrophy type I: a pilot controlled study. *Am J Phys Med Rehabil*, 95, 809–817.

Dahlberg, J., Fitch, G., Evans, R. B., Mcclure, S. R., & Conzemius, M. 2005. The evaluation of extracorporeal shockwave therapy in naturally occurring osteoarthritis of the stifle joint in dogs. *Vet Comp Orthop Traumatol*, 18, 147–152.

da Silva, J. P., da Silva, M. A., Almeida, A. P., Lombardi Junior, I., & Matos, A. P. 2010. Laser therapy in the tissue repair process: a literature review. *Photomed Laser Surg*, 28, 17–21.

Deal, D. N., Tipton, J., Rosencrance, E., Curl, W. W. & Smith T. L. 2002. Ice reduces edema. *A study of microvascular permeability in rats. J Bone Joint Surg Am*, 84-A, 1573–8.

de Almeida, J. M., de Moraes, R. O., Gusman, D. J., Faleiros, P. L., Nagata, M. J., Garcia, V. G., *et al.* 2016. Influence of low-level laser therapy on the healing process of autogenous bone block grafts in the jaws of systemically nicotine-modified rats: a histomorphometric study. *Arch Oral Biol*, 75, 21–30.

de Andrade, A. L., Bossini, P. S., & Parizotto, N. A. 2016. Use of low level laser therapy to control neuropathic pain: a systematic review. *J Photochem Photobiol B*, 164, 36–42.

Dehghan, M. & Farahbod, F. 2014. The efficacy of thermotherapy and cryotherapy on pain relief in patients with acute low back pain, a clinical trial study. *J Clin Diagn Res*, 8(9), LC01–4.

de Jesus, J. F., Spadacci-Morena, D. D., Rabelo, N. D., Pinfildi, C. E., Fukuda, T. Y., & Plapler, H. 2014. Low-level laser therapy on tissue repair of partially injured achilles tendon in rats. *Photomed Laser Surg*, 32, 345–50.

De Marchi, T., Leal Junior, E.C., Bortoli, C., Tomazoni, S.S., Lopes-Martins, R.A., & Salvador, M. 2012. Low-level laser therapy (LLLT) in human progressive-intensity running: effects on exercise performance, skeletal muscle status, and oxidative stress. *Lasers Med Sci*, 27(1), 231–236.

De Marchi, T., Schmitt, V. M., Machado, G. P., de Sene, J. S., de Col, C. D., Tairova, O., *et al.* 2017. Does photobiomodulation therapy is better than cryotherapy in muscle recovery after a high-intensity exercise? A randomized double-blind, placebo-controlled clinical trial. *Lasers Med Sci*, 32, 429–437.

Demchak, T. J. & Stone, M. B. 2008. Effectiveness of clinical ultrasound parameters on changing intramuscular temperature. *J Sports Rehabil*, 17, 220–9.

de Medeiros, M. L., Araújo-Filho, I., da Silva, E. M., de Sousa Queiroz, W. S., Soares, C. D., de Carvalho, M. G., & Maciel, M. A. 2017. Effect of low-level laser therapy on angiogenesis and matrix metalloproteinase-2 immunoexpression in wound repair. *Lasers Med Sci*, 32, 35–43.

Demircioglu, D. T., Paker, N., Erbil, E., Bugdayci, D., & Emre, T. Y. 2015. The effects of neuromuscular electrical stimulation on functional status and quality of life after knee arthroplasty: a randomized controlled study. *J Phys Ther Sci*, 27, 2501–2506.

de Oliveira Martins, D., Martinez dos SANTOS, F., Evany de OLIVEIRA, M., de Britto, L. R. G., Benedito DIAS LEMOS, J., & Chacur, M. 2013. Laser therapy and pain-related behavior after injury of the inferior alveolar nerve: possible involvement of neurotrophins. *J Neurotrauma*, 30, 480–486.

de Oliveira Melo, M., Pompeo, K. D., Baroni, B. M., & Vaz, M. A. 2016. Effects of neuromuscular electrical stimulation and low-level laser therapy on neuromuscular parameters and health status in elderly women with knee osteoarthritis: a randomized trial. *J Rehabil Med*, 48, 293–299.

Dissanayaka, T. D., Pallegama, R. W., Suraweera, H. J., Johnson, M. I., & Kariyawasam, A. P. 2016. Comparison of the effectiveness of transcutaneous electrical nerve stimulation and interferential therapy on the upper trapezius in myofascial pain syndrome: a randomized controlled study. *Am J Phys Med Rehabil*, 95, 663–672.

Downer, A. 1978. Cryotherapy for animals. *Mod Vet Pract*, 59, 659–662.

Draper, D. O. 2010. Ultrasound and joint mobilizations for achieving normal wrist range of motion after injury or surgery: a case series. *J Athl Train*, 45, 486–491.

Draper, D. O. 2014. Facts and misfits in ultrasound therapy: steps to improve your treatment outcomes. *Eur J Phys Rehabil Med*, 50, 209–216.

Draper, D. O. & Ricard, M. D. 1995. Rate of temperature decay in human muscle following 3 MHz ultrasound: the stretching window revealed. *J Athl Train*, 30, 304–307.

Draper, D. O., Sunderland, S., Kirkendall, D. T., & Ricard, M. 1993. A comparison of temperature rise in human calf muscles following applications of underwater and topical gel ultrasound. *J Orthop Sports Phys Ther*, 17, 247–251.

Draper, D. O., Castel, J. C., & Castel, D. 1995. Rate of temperature increase in human muscle during 1 MHz and 3 MHz continuous ultrasound. *J Orthop Sports Phys Ther*, 22, 142–150.

Draper, D. O., Harris, S. T., Schulthies, S., Durrant, E., Knight, K. L., & Ricard, M. 1998. Hot-pack and 1-MHz ultrasound treatments have an additive effect on muscle temperature increase. *J Athl Train*, 33, 21–24.

Draper, D. O., Mahaffey, C., Kaiser, D., Eggett, D., & Jarmin, J. 2010. Thermal ultrasound decreases tissue stiffness of trigger points in upper trapezius muscles. *Physiother Theory Pract*, 26, 167–172.

Draper, W. E., Schubert, T. A., Clemmons, R. M., & Miles, S. A. 2012. Low-level laser therapy reduces time to ambulation in dogs after hemilaminectomy: a preliminary study. *J Small Anim Pract*, 53, 465–469.

Drinkwater, E. J. & Behm, D. G. 2007. Effects of 22 degrees C muscle temperature on voluntary and evoked muscle properties during and after high-intensity exercise. *Appl Physiol Nutr Metab*, 32, 1043–1051.

Drygas, K.A., Mcclure, S.R., Goring, R.L., Pozzi, A., Robertson, S.A., & Wang, C. 2011. Effect of cold compression therapy on postoperative pain, swelling, range of motion, and lameness after tibial plateau leveling osteotomy in dogs. *J Am Vet Med Assoc*, 238(10),1284–1291.

Elnaggar, R. K. 2016. Shoulder function and bone mineralization in children with obstetric brachial plexus injury after neuromuscular electrical stimulation during weight-bearing exercises. *Am J Phys Med Rehabil*, 95, 239–247.

Enwemeka, C. S. 1989. The effects of therapeutic ultrasound on tendon healing. A biomechanical study. *Am J Phys Med Rehabil*, 68, 283–287.

Epstein, M. E., Rodanm, I., Griffenhagan, G., Kadrlik, J., Petty, M. C., Robertson, S. A., & Simpson, W. 2015. 2015 AAHA/AAFP pain management guidelines for dogs and cats. *J Feline Med Surg*, 17, 251–272.

Erthal, V., Marta-Ferreira, D., Werner, M. F., Baggio, C. H., & Nohama, P. 2016. Anti-inflammatory effect of laser acupuncture in ST36 (Zusanli) acupoint in mouse paw edema. *Lasers Med Sci*, 31, 315–322.

Fantinati, M. S., Mendonça, D. E., Fantinati, A. M., Santos, B. F., Reis, J. C., Afonso, C. L., et al. 2016. Low intensity ultrasound therapy induces angiogenesis and persistent inflammation in the chronic phase of the healing process of third degree burn wounds experimentally induced in diabetic and non-diabetic rats. *Acta Cir Bras*, 31, 463–471.

Fernández-Tenorio, E., Serrano-Muñoz, D., Avendaño-Coy, J., & Gómez-Soriano, J. 2016. Transcutaneous electrical nerve stimulation for spasticity: a systemic review. *Neurologia*, July 26.

Feys, P., Helsen, W., Liu, X., Mooren, D., Albrecht, H., Nuttin, B., & Ketelaer, P. 2005. Effects of peripheral cooling on intention tremor in multiple sclerosis. *J Neurol Neurosurg Psychiatry*, 76, 373–379.

Fischer, A., Spiegl, M., Altmann, K., Winkler, A., Salamon, A., Themessl-Huber, M., *et al.* 2016. Muscle mass, strength and functional outcomes in critically ill patients after cardiothoracic surgery: does neuromuscular electrical stimulation help? The Catastim 2 randomized controlled trial. *Crit Care,* 20, 30.

Fitzgerald, G. K., Piva, S. R., & Irrgang, J. J. 2003. A modified neuromuscular electrical stimulation protocol for quadriceps strength training following anterior cruciate ligament reconstruction. *J Orthop Sports Phys Ther,* 33, 492–501.

Fonseca, L. B., Brito, C. J., Silva, R. J., Silva-Grigoletto, M. E., da Silva, W. M. Jr, & Franchini, E. 2016. Use of cold-water immersion to reduce muscle damage and delayed-onset muscle soreness and preserve muscle power in jiu-jitsu athletes. *J Athl Train,* 51, 540–549.

Ford, K. S., Shrader, M. W., Smith, J., Mclean, T. J. & Dahm, D. L. 2005. Full-thickness burn formation after the use of electrical stimulation for rehabiltia-tion of unicompartmental knee arthroplasty. *J Arthroplasty,* 20, 950–953.

Forrest, G. & Rosen, K. 1989. Ultrasound: effective-ness of treatments given under water. *Arch Phys Med Rehabil,* 70, 28–29.

Frozanfar, A., Ramezani, M., Rahpeyma, A., Khajehahmadi, S., & Arbab, H. R. 2013. The effects of low level laser therapy on the expression of collagen type I gene and proliferation of human gingival fibroblasts (Hgf3-Pi 53): in vitro study. *Iran J Basic Med Sci,* 16, 1071–1074.

Fung, D. T., Ng, G. Y., Leung, M. C., & Tay, D. K. 2002. Therapeutic low energy laser improves the mechanical strength of repairing medial collateral ligament. *Lasers Surg Med,* 31, 91–96.

Funk, D., Swank, A. M., Adams, K. J., & Treolo, D. 2001. Efficacy of moist heat pack application over static stretching on hamstring flexibility. *J Strength Cond Res,* 15, 123–126.

Gagnon, D., Gibson, T. W. G., Singh, A., Zur Linden, A. R., Kazienko, J. E., & Lamarre, J. 2016. An in vitro method to test the safety and efficacy of low-level laser therapy (LLLT) in the healing of a canine skin model. *BMC Vet Res.* 12, 73.

Gallagher, A., Cross, A.R., & Sepulveda, G., 2012. The effect of shock wave therapy on patellar ligament desmitis after tibial plateau leveling osteotomy. *Vet Surg,* 41, 482–485.

Gange, K. N., Kjellerson, M. C., & Berdan, C. J. 2016. The Dynatron Solaris® Ultrasound Machine heats slower than textbook recommendations at 3 MHz, 1.0 W/cm(2). *J Sports Rehabil,* 1-23. doi: 10.1123/jsr.2016-0173 [Epub ahead of print].

Gatewood, C. T., Tran, A. A., & Dragoo, J. L. 2017. The efficacy of post-operative devices following knee arthroscopic surgery: a systematic review. *Knee Surg Sports Traumatol Arthrosc,* 25, 501–516.

Geetha, K., Hariharan, N. C., & Mohar, J. 2014. Early ultrasound therapy for rehabilitation after zone II flexor tendon repair. *Indian J Plast Surg,* 47, 85–91.

Gerdesmeyer, L., Wagenpfeil, S., Haake, M., Maier, M., Loew, M., Wortler, K., *et al.* 2003. Extracorporeal shock wave therapy for the treatment of chronic calcifying tendonitis of the rotator cuff. *J Am Med Assoc,* 290, 2573–2580.

Gigo-Benato, D., Geuna, S., de Castro Rodrigues, A., Tos, P., Fornaro, M., Boux, E., *et al.* 2004. Low-power laser biostimulation enhances nerve repair after end-to-side neurorrhaphy: a double-blind randomized study in the rat median nerve model. *Lasers Med Sci,* 19, 57–65.

Glaviano, N. R. & Saliba, S. A. 2016. Immediate effect of patterned electrical neuromuscular stimulation on pain and muscle activation in individuals with patellofemoral pain. *J Athl Train,* 51, 118–128.

Glaviano, N. R., Huntsman, S., Dembeck, A., Hart, J. M., & Saliba, S. A. 2016. Improvements in kine-matics, muscle activity and pain during functional tasks in females with patellofemoral pain follow-ing a single patterned electrical stimulation treat-ment. *Clin Biomech,* 32, 20–27.

Gondin, J., Giannesini, B., Vilmen, C., Dalmasso, C., Le Fur, Y., Cozzone, P. J. & Bendahan, D. 2010. Effects of stimulation frequency and pulse dura-tion on fatigue and metabolic cost during a single bout of neuromuscular electrical stimulation. *Muscle Nerve,* 41, 667–678.

Goren, A., Yildiz, N., Topuz, O., Findikoglu, G., & Ardic, F. 2010. Efficacy of exercise and ultrasound in patients with lumbar spinal stenosis: a prospec-tive randomized controlled trial. *Clin Rehabil,* 24, 623–631.

Gorgey, A. S., Caudill, C., & Khalil, R. E. 2016. Effects of once weekly NMES training on knee extensors fatigue and body composition in a person with spinal cord injury. *J Spinal Cord Med,* 39, 99–102.

Gozani, S. N. 2016. Fixed-site high-frequency trans-cutaneous electrical nerve stimulation for treat-ment of chronic low back and lower extremity pain. *J Pain Res,* 9, 469–479.

Guerra Fda, R., Vieira, C. P., Almeida, M. S., OLIVEIRA, L. P., de Aro, A. A., & Pimentel, E. R. 2013. LLLT improves tendon healing through increase of MMP activity and collagen synthesis. *Lasers Med Sci,* 28, 1281–1288.

Guillot, X., Tordi, N., Prati, C., Verhoeven, F., Pazart, L., & Wendling, D. 2017. Cryotherapy decreases synovial Doppler activity and pain in knee arthritis: A randomized-controlled trial. *Joint Bone Spine,* 84, 477–483.

Guzzardella, G.A., Torricelli, P., Nicoli Aldini, N., & Giardino, R. 2001. Laser technology in orthopedics: preliminary study on low power laser therapy to improve the bone-biomaterial interface. *Int J Artif Organs*, 24(12), 898–902.

Guzzardella, G.A., Fini, M., Torricelli, P., Giavaresi, G., & Giardino, R. 2002. Laser stimulation on bone defect healing: an in vitro study. *Lasers Med Sci*, 17(3), 216–220.

Hadler, A., Gao, C., & Miller, M. 2014. Effects of cooling on ankle muscle strength, electromyography, and gait ground reaction forces. *J Sports Med*, 2014, Art. ID 520124.

Hagiwara, S., Iwasaka, H., Okuda, K., & Noguchi, T. 2007. GaIAIs (830 nm) low-level laser enhances peripheral endogenous opioid analgesia in rats. *Lasers Surg Med*, 39, 797–802.

Hamm, R. L. 2015. *Text and Atlas of Wound Diagnosis and Treatment*. New York, NY: McGraw-Hill Education.

Hardy, M. & Woodall, W. 1998. Therapeutic effects of heat, cold, and stretch on connective tissue. *J Hand Ther*, 11, 148–156.

Harkey, M. S., Gribble, P. A., & Pietrosimone, B. G. 2014. Disinhibitory interventions and voluntary quadriceps activation: a systematic review. *J Athl Train*, 49, 411–421.

Hart, J. M., Kuenze, C. M., Diduch, D. R., & Ingersoll, C. D. 2014. Quadriceps muscle function after rehabilitation with cryotherapy in patients with anterior cruciate ligament reconstruction. *J Athl Train*, 49, 733–739.

Haslerud, S., Lopes-Martins, R. A., Frigo, L., Bjordal, J. M., Marcos, R. L., Naterstad, I. F., *et al.* 2017. Low-level laser therapy and cryotherapy as mono- and adjunctive therapies for achilles tendinopathy in rats. *Photomed Laser Surg*, 35, 32–42.

Herrera, E., Sandoval, M. C., Camargo, D. M., & Salvini, T. F. 2011. Effect of walking and resting after three cryotherapy modalities on the recovery of sensory and motor nerve conduction velocity in healthy subjects. *Rev Bras Fisioter*, 15, 233–240.

Hopkins, J. T., Mcloda, T. A., Seegmiller, J. G., & David Baxter, G. 2004. Low-level laser therapy facilitates superficial wound healing in humans: a triple-blind, sham-controlled study. *J Athl Train*, 39, 223–229.

Hsieh, Y. L. 2005. Reduction in induced pain by ultrasound may be caused by altered expression of spinal neuronal nitric oxide synthase-producing neurons. *Arch Phys Med Rehabil*, 86, 1311–1317.

Huang, J. J., Shi, Y. Q., Li, R. L., Hu, A., Zhou, H. S., Cheng, Q., *et al.* 2014. Angiogenesis effect of therapeutic ultrasound on ischemic hind limb in mice. *Am J Transl Res*, 6, 703–713.

Huang, Y. Y., Chen, A. C., Carroll, J. D., & Hamblin, M. R. 2009. Biphasic dose response in low level light therapy. *Dose Response*, 7, 358–383.

Huang, Z., Ma, J., Chen, J., Shen, B., Pei, F., & Kraus, V. B. 2015. The effectiveness of low-level laser therapy for nonspecific chronic low back pain: a systematic review and meta-analysis. *Arthritis Res Ther*, 17, 360.

Hudson, D. E., Hudson, D. O., Wininger, J. M., & Richardson, B. D. 2013. Penetration of laser light at 808nm and 980nm in bovine tissue samples. *Photomed Laser Surg*, 31, 163–168.

Igaki, M., Higashi, T., Hamamoto, S., Kodama, S., Naito, S., & Tokuhara, S. 2014. A study of the behavior and mechanism of thermal conduction in the skin under moist and dry heat conditions. *Skin Res Technol*, 20, 43–49.

Ihsan, F. R. 2005. Low-level laser therapy accelerates collateral circulation and enhances microcirculation. *Photomed Laser Surg*, 23, 289–294.

Ikeda, T., Tayefeh, F., Sessler, D. I., Kurz, A., Plattner, O., Petschnigg, B., *et al.* 1998. Local radiant heating increases subcutaneous oxygen tension. *Am J Surg*, 175, 33–37.

Iles, J. F. 1996. Evidence for cutaneous and corticospinal modulation of presynaptic inhibition of Ia afferents from the human lower limb. *J Physiol*, 491, 197–207.

Ilter, L., Dilek, B., Batmaz, I., Ulu, M. A., Sariyildiz, M. A., Nas, K., & Cevik, R. 2015. Efficacy of pulsed and continuous therapeutic ultrasound in myofascial pain syndrome: a randomized controlled study. *Am J Phys Med Rehabil*, 94, 547–554.

Ip, D. 2015. Does addition of low-level laser therapy (LLLT) in conservative care of knee arthritis successfully postpone the need for joint replacement? *Lasers Med Sci*, 30, 2335–2339.

Ito, A., Aoyama, T., Tajino, J., Nagai, M., Yamaguchi, S., Iijima, H., *et al.* 2014. Effects of the thermal environment on articular chondrocyte metabolism: a fundamental study to facilitate establishment of an effective thermotherapy for osteoarthritis. *J Jpn Phys Ther Assoc*, 17, 14–21.

Iwasawa, H., Nomura, M., Sakitani, N., Watanabe, K., & Moriyama, H. 2016. Stretching after heat but not after cold decreases contractures after spinal cord injury in rats. *Clin Orthop Relat Res*, 474, 2692–2701.

Jabir, S., Frew, Q., Griffiths, M., & Dziewulski, P. 2013. Burn injury to a reconstructed breast via a hot water bottle. *J Plast Reconstr Aesthet Surg*, 66(11), e334–335.

Janzadeh, A., Nasirinezhad, F., Masoumipoor, M., Jameie, S. B., & Hayat, P. 2016. Photobiomodulation therapy reduces apoptotic factors and increases glutathione levels in a neuropathic pain model. *Lasers Med Sci*, 31, 1863–1869.

Jauregui, J. J., Cherian, J. J., Gwam, C. U., Chughtai, M., Mistry, J. B., Elmallah, R. K., *et al.* 2016. A meta-analysis of transcutaneous electrical nerve stimulation for chronic low back pain. *Surg Technol Int*, 28, 296–302.

Jochumsen, M., Niazi, I. K., Signal, N., Nedergaard, R. W., Holt, K., Haavik, H., & Taylor, D. 2016. Pairing voluntary movement and muscle-located electrical stimulation increases cortical excitability. *Front Hum Neurosci.* 10, 482.

Johnson, M. I., Paley, C. A., Howe, T. E., & Sluka, K. A. 2015. Transcutaneous electrical nerve stimulation for acute pain. *Cochrane Database Syst Rev*, (6), CD006142. doi: 10.1002/14651858.CD006142.pub3

Jones, S., Man, W. D., Gao, W., Higginson, I. J., Wilcock, A., & Maddocks, M. 2016. Neuromuscular electrical stimulation for muscle weakness in adults with advanced disease. *Cochrane Database Syst Rev*, (1), DC009419. doi: 10.1002/14651858. CD009419.pub2

Jung, K. S., Jng, J. H., In, T. S., & Cho, H. Y. 2016. Effects of weight-shifting exercises combined with transcutaneous electrical nerve stimulation on muscle activity and trunk control in patients with stroke. *Occup Ther Int*, 23, 436–443.

Kamiya, K., Satoh, A., Niwano, S., Tanaka, S., Miida, K., Hamazaki, N., *et al.* 2016. Safety of neuromuscular electrical stimulation in patients implanted with cardioverter defibrillators. *J Electrocardiol*, 49, 99–101.

Karabay, İ., Doğan, A., Arslan, M. D., Dost, G., & Ozgirgin, N. 2012. Effects of functional electrical stimulation on trunk control in children with diplegic cerebral palsy. *Disabil Rehabil*, 34, 965–970.

Karabay, İ., Doğan, A., Ekiz, T., KÖseoğlu, B. F., & Ersöz, M. 2016. Training postural control and sitting in children with cerebral palsy: Kinesio taping vs. neuromuscular electrical stimulation. *Complement Ther Clin Pract*, 24, 67–72.

Karakoyun, A., Boyraz, I., Gunduz, R., Karamercan, A., & Ozgirgin, N. 2015. Electrophysiological and clinical evaluation of the effects of transcutaneous electrical nerve stimulation on the spasticity in the hemiplegic stroke patients. *J Phys Ther Sci*, 27, 3407–3411.

Karasuno, H., Ogihara, H., Morishita, K., Yokoi, Y., Fujiwara, T., Ogoma, Y., & Abe, K. 2016. The combined effects of transcutaneous electrical nerve stimulation (TENS) and stretching on muscle hardness and pressure pain threshold. *J Phys Ther Sci*, 28, 1124–1130.

Karu, T. 1988. Molecular mechanism of the therapeutic effects of low intensity laser radiation. *Lasers in the Life Sciences*, 2, 53–74.

Karu, T., Pyatibrat, L., & Kalendo, G. 1995. Irradiation with He-Ne laser increases ATP level in cells cultivated in vitro. *J Photochem Photobiol B*, 27, 219–223.

Kavadar, G., Çağlar, N., Özen, Ş., & Demircioğlu, D. 2015. Efficacy of conventional ultrasound therapy on myofascial pain syndrome: a placebo controlled study. *Agri*, 27, 190–196.

Keshri, G. K., Gupta, A., Yadav, A., Sharma, S. K., & Singh, S. B. 2016. Photobiomodulation with pulsed and continuous wave near-infrared laser (810 nm, AI-Ga-Az) augments dermal wound healing in immunosuppressed rats. *PLoS One*, 11, e0166705.

Khalighi, H. R., Mortazavi, H., Mojahedi, S. M., Azari-Marhabi, S., & Moradi Abbasabadi, F. 2016. Low level laser therapy versus pharmacotherapy in improving myofascial pain disorder syndrome. *J Lasers Med Sci*, 7, 45–50.

Khan, A. A., Banwell, P. E., Bakker, M. C., Gillespie, P. G., Mcgrouther, D. A. & Roberts, A. H. 2004. Topical radiant heating in wound healing: an experimental study in a donor site wound model. *Int Wound J*, 1, 233–240.

Khoshnevis, S., Craik, N. K., & Diller, K. R. 2015. Cold-induced vasoconstriction may persist long after cooling ends: an evaluation of multiple cryotherapy units. *Knee Surg Sports Traumatol Arthrosc*, 23, 2475–2483.

Khoshnevis, S., Craik, N.K., Matthew Brothers, R., & Diller, K.R. 2016. Cryotherapy-induced persistent vasoconstriction after cutaneous cooling: hysteresis between skin temperature and blood perfusion. *J Biomech Eng*, 138(3), 4032126.

Kieves, N.R., Mackay, C.S., Adducci, K., Rao, S., Goh, C., Palmer, R.H., & Duerr, F.M. 2015. High energy focused shock wave therapy accelerates bone healing: A blinded, prospective, randomized, canine clinical trial. *Veterinary and Comparative Orthopaedics Traumatology*, 28, 425–432.

Kim, H., Suzuki, T., Saito, K., Kim, M. Kojima, N., Ishizaki, T., *et al.* 2013. Effectiveness of exercise with or without thermal therapy for community-dwelling elderly Japanese women with non-specific knee pain: a randomized controlled trial. *Arch Gerontol Geriatr*, 57, 352–359.

Kim, S. Y., Kim, J. H., Jung, G. S., Baek, S. O., Jones, R., & Ahn, S. H. 2016. The effects of transcutaneous neuromuscular electrical stimulation on the activation of deep lumbar stabilizing muscles of patients with lumbar degenerative kyphosis. *J Phys Ther Sci*, 28, 399–406.

Knight, C. A., Rutledge, C. R., Cox, M. E., Acosta, M., & Hall, S. J. 2001. Effect of superficial heat, deep heat, and active exercise warm-up on the extensibility of the plantar flexors. *Phys Ther*, 81, 1206–1214.

Knobloch, K., Grasemann, R., Spies, M., & Vogt, P. M. 2007. Intermittent KoldBlue cryotherapy of 3 × 10 min changes mid-portion Achilles tendon microcirculation. *Br J Sports Med*, 41, e4.

Ko, E. J., Chun, M. H., Kim, D. Y., Yi, J. H., Kim, W., & Hong, J. 2016. The additive effects of core muscle strengthening and trunk NMES on trunk balance in stroke patients. *Ann Rehabil Med*, 40, 142–151.

Kobiela Ketz, A., Byrnes, K. R., Grunberg, N. E., Kasper, C. E., Osborne, L., Pryor, B., *et al.* 2017. Characterization of macrophage/microglial activation and effect of photobiomodulation in the spared nerve injury model of neuropathic pain. *Pain Med*, 18, 932–946.

Korelo, R. I., Krycsyk, M., Garcia, C., Naliwaiko, K., & Fernandes, L. C. 2016. Wound healing treatment by high frequency ultrasound, microcurrent, and combined therapy modifies the immune response in rats. *Braz J Phys Ther*, 20, 133–141.

Krukowska, J., Wrona, J., Sienkiewicz, M., & Czernicki, J. 2016. A comparative analysis of analgesic efficacy of ultrasound and shock wave therapy in the treatment of patients with inflammation of the attachment of the plantar fascia in the course of calcaneal spurs. *Arch Orthop Trauma Surg*, 136, 1289–1296.

Księżopolska-Orłowska, K., Pacholec, A., Jędryka-Góral, A., Bugajska, J., Sadura-Sieklucka, T., Kowalik, K., *et al.* 2016. Complex rehabilitation and the clinical condition of working rheumatoid arthritis patients: does cryotherapy always overtop traditional rehabiltiation? *Disabil Rehabil*, 38, 1034–1040.

Kuhlenhoelter, A.M., Kim, K., Neff, D., Nie, Y., Blaize, A.N., Wong, B.J., *et al.* 2016. Heat therapy promotes the expression of angiogenic regulators in human skeletal muscle. *Am J Physiol Regul Integr Comp Physiol*, 311(2), R377–391.

Kuyucu, E., Bülbül, M., Kara, A., Koçyiğit, F., & Erdil, M. 2015. Is cold therapy really efficient after knee arthroplasty? *Ann Med Surg (Lond)*, 4, 475–478.

Laddha, D., Ganesh, G. S., Pattnaik, M., Mohanty, P., & Mishra, C. 2016. Effect of transcutaneous electrical nerve stimulation on plantar flexor muscle spasticity and walking speed in stroke patients. *Physiother Res Int*, 21, 247–256.

Larsen, C. C., Troiano, J. M., Ramirez, R. J., Miller, M. G., & Holcomb, W. R. 2015. Effects of crushed ice and wetted ice on hamstring flexibility. *J Strength Cond Res*, 29, 483–488.

Laufer, Y., Shtraker, H., & Elboim Gabyzon, M. 2014. The effects of exercise and neuromuscular electrical stimulation in subjects with knee osteoarthritis: a 3-month follow-up study. *Clin Interv Aging*, 9, 1153–1561.

Laverty, P. & Mcclure, S. 2002. Initial experience with extracorporeal shock wave therapy in six dogs—part 1. *Vet Comp Orthop Traumatol* 15, 177–183.

Leal-Junior, E. C., Vanin, A. A., Miranda, E. F., de Carvalho Pde, T., Dal Corso, S., & Bjordal, J. M. 2015. Effect of phototherapy (low-level laser therapy and light-emitting diode therapy) on exercise performance and markers of exercise recovery: a systematic review with meta-analysis. *Lasers Med Sci*, 30, 925–939.

Lee, S. U., Bang, M. S., & Han, T. R. 2002. Effect of cold air therapy in relieving spasticity: applied to spinalized rabbits. *Spinal Cord*, 40, 167–173.

Lehmann, J. F., Delateur, B. J., Stonebridge, J. B., & Warren, C. G. 1967a. Therapeutic temperature distribution produced by ultrasound as modified by dosage and volume of tissue exposed. *Arch Phys Med Rehabil*, 48, 662–666.

Lehmann, J. F., Delateur, B. J., Warren, C. G., & Stonebridge, J. B. 1967b. Heating produced by ultrasound in bone and soft tissue. *Arch Phys Med Rehabil*, 48, 397–401.

Lehmann, J. F., Masock, A. J., Warren C. G., & Koblanski, J. N. 1970. Effect of therapeutic temperatures on tendon extensibility. *Arch Phys Med Rehabil*, 51, 481–487.

Lemos, G. A., Rissi, R., de Souza Pires, I. L., de Oliveira, L. P., deE Aro, A. A., Pimentel, E. R., & Palomari, E. T. 2016. Low-level laser therapy stimulates tissue repair and reduces the extracellular matrix degradation in rats with induced arthritis in the temporomandibular joint. *Lasers Med Sci*, 31, 1051–1059.

Lepley, L. K., Wojtys, E. M., & Palmieri-Smith, R. M. 2015. Combination of eccentric exercise and neuromuscular electrical stimulation to improve biomechanical limb symmetry after anterior cruciate ligament reconstruction. *Clin Biomech (Bristol, Avon)*, 30, 738–747.

Leung, M. C., Ng, G. Y., & Yip, K. K. 2006. Therapeutic ultrasound enhances medial collateral ligament repair in rats. *Ultrasound Med Biol*, 32, 449–452.

Levine, D., Millis, D. L., & Mynatt, T. 2001. Effects of 3.3-MHz ultrasound on caudal thigh muscle temperature in dogs. *Vet Surg*, 30, 170–174.

Lewis, S. E., Holmes, P. S., Woby, S. R., Hindle, J., & Fowler, N. E. 2012. Short-term effect of superficial heat treatment to paraspinal muscle activity, stature recovery, and psychological factors in patients with chronic low back pain. *Arch Phys Med Rehabil*, 93, 367–372.

Lima, A. C., Fernandes, G. A., de Barros Araújo, R., Gonzaga, I. C., de Oliveira, R. A., & Nicolau, R. A. 2017. Photobiomodulation (laser and LED) on sternotomy healing in hyperglycemic and normoglycemic patients who underwent coronary bypass surgery with internal mammary artery grafts: a randomized, double-blind study with follow-up. *Photomed Laser Surg*, 35, 24–31.

Lin, Y. H. 2003. Effects of thermal therapy in improving the passive range of knee motion: comparison of cold and superficial heat application. *Clin Rehabil*, 17, 618–623.

Loh, J. & Gulati, A. 2015. The use of transcutaneous electrical nerve stimulation (TENS) in a major cancer center for the treatment of severe cancer-related pain and associated disability. *Pain Med*, 16, 1204–1210.

Lowe, A.S., Baxter, G.D., Walsh, D.M., & Allen, J.M. 1994. Effect of low intensity laser (830 nm) irradiation on skin temperature and antidromic conduction latencies in the human median nerve: relevance of radiant exposure. *Lasers Surg Med*, 14(1), 40–46.

Loyola-Sánchez, A., Richardson, J., Beattie, K. A., Otero-Fuentes, C., Adachi, J. D., & Macintyre, N. J. 2012. Effect of low-intensity pulsed ultrasound on the cartilage repair in people with mild to moderate knee osteoarthritis: a double-blinded, randomized, placebo-controlled pilot study. *Arch Phys Med Rehabil*, 93, 35–42.

Lu, Z. Y., Li, R. L., Zhou, H. S., Huang, J. J., Su, Z. X., Qi, J., *et al.* 2016a. Therapeutic ultrasound reverses peripheral ischemia in type 2 diabetic mice through PI3K-Akt-eNOS pathway. *Am J Transl Res*, 8, 3666–3667.

Lu, Z. Y., Li, R. L., Zhou, H. S., Huang, J. J., Qi, J., Su, Z. X., *et al.* 2016b. Rescue of hypertension-related impairment of angiogenesis by therapeutic ultrasound. *Am J Transl Res*, 8, 3087–3096.

Macedo Cde, S., Vicente, R. C., Cesário, M. D., & Guirro, R. R. 2016. Cold-water immersion alters muscle recruitment and balance of basketball players during vertical jump landing. *J Sports Sci*, 34, 348–357.

Mahran, H. G. 2014. Influence of contact ultrasonic with different power densities on full-thickness wounds healing: an experimental study. *Int J Physiother Res*, 2, 567–576.

Marques, A. C., Albertini, R., Serra, A. J., da Silva, E. A., de Oliveira, V. L., Silva, L. M., *et al.* 2016. Photobiomodulation therapy on collagen type I and III, vascular endothelial growth factor, and metalloproteinase in experimentally induced tendinopathy in aged rats. *Lasers Med Sci*, 31, 1915–1923.

Martignago, C. C., Oliveira, R. F., Pires-Oliveira, D. A., Oliveira, P. D., Pacheco Soares, C., Monzani, P. S., & Poli-Frederico, R. C. 2015. Effect of low-level laser therapy on gene expression of collagen and vascular endothelial growth factor in a culture of fibroblast cells in mice. *Lasers Med Sci*, 30, 203–208.

Martins, C. N., Moraes, M. B., Hauck, M., Guerreiro, L. F., Rossato, D. D., Varela, A. S. Jr, *et al.* 2016. Effects of cryotherapy combined with therapeutic ultrasound on oxidative stress and tissue damage after musculoskeletal contusion in rats. *Physiotherapy*, 102, 377–383.

Mathur, R. K., Sahu, K., Saraf, S., Patheja, P., Khan, F., & Gupta, P. K. 2017. Low-level laser therapy as an adjunct to conventional therapy in the treatment of diabetic foot ulcers. *Lasers Med Sci*, 32, 275–282.

Matsumoto, Y., Nakano, J., Oga, S., Kataoka, H., Honda, Y., Sakamoto, J., & Okita, M. 2014. The non-thermal effects of pulsed ultrasound irradiation on the development of disuse muscle atorphy in rat gastrocnemius muscle. *Ultrasound Med Biol*, 40, 1578–1586.

Medalha, C. C., Santos, A. L., Veronez Sde, O., Fernandes, K. R., Magri, A. M., & Renno, A. C. 2016. Low level laser therapy accelerates bone healing in spinal cord injured rats. *J Photochem Photobiol B*, 159, 179–185.

Medrado, A. R., Pugliese, L. S., Reis, S. R., & Andrade, Z. A. 2003. Influence of low level laser therapy on wound healing and its biological action upon myofibroblasts. *Lasers Surg Med*, 32(3), 239–244.

Melzack, R. & Wall, P. D. 1965. Pain mechanisms: a new theory. *Science*, 150, 971–979.

Mense, S. 1978. Effects of temperature on the discharges of muscle spindles and tendon organs. *Pflugers Arch*, 374, 159–166.

Merrick, M. A. 2002. Secondary injury after musculoskeletal trauma: a review and update. *J Athl Train*, 37, 209–217.

Merrick, M. A., Rankin, J. M., Andres, F. A., & Hinman, C. L. 1999. A preliminary examination of cryotherapy and secondary injury in skeletal muscle. *Med Sci Sports Exerc*, 31, 1516–1521.

Merrick, M. A., Jutte, L. S., & Smith, M. E. 2003a. Cold modalities with different thermodynamic properties produce different surface and intramuscular temperatures. *J Athl Train*, 38, 28–33.

Merrick, M. A., Bernard, K. D., Devor, S. T., & Williams, M. J. 2003b. Identical 3-MHz ultrasound treatments with different devices produce different intramuscular temperatures. *J Orthop Sports Phys Ther*, 33, 379–385.

Michlovitz, S. L. & Nolan, T. 2005. *Modalities forTherapeutic Intervention*. Philadelphia, PA: F.A. Davis Co.

Michlovitz, S., Hun, L., Erasala, G. N., Hengehold, D. A., & Weingand, K. W. 2004. Continuous low-level heat wrap therapy is effective for treating wrist pain. *Arch Phys Med Rehabil*, 85, 1409–1416.

Mignardot, J. B., Deschamps, T., Le Goff, C. G., Roumier, F. X., Duclay, J., Martin, A., *et al.* 2015. Neuromuscular electrical stimulation leads to physiological gains enhancing postural balance in the pre-frail elderly. *Physiol Rep*, 3, 312471.

Millard, R. P., Towle-Millard H. A., Rankin D. C., & Roush J. K. 2013. Effects of cold compress application on tissue temperature in healthy dogs. *Am J Vet Res*, 74, 443–447.

Miller, M. G., Longoria, J. R., Cheatham, C. C., Baker, R. J., & Michael, T. J. 2008. Intramuscular temperature difference between the mid-point and peripheral effective radiating area with ultrasound. *J Sports Sci Med*, 7, 286–291.

Millis, D., Levine, D., Brumlow, M., & Weigel, J. 1997. A preliminary study of early physical therapy following surgery for cranial cruciate ligament rupture in dogs. In: Scientific Presentation Abstracts: The Seventh Annual American College of Veterinary Surgeons Symposium October 1997, Orland, FL. *Vet Surg*, 26(5), 434.

Mills, P. B. & Dossa, F. 2016. Transcutaneous electrical nerve stimulation for management of limb spasticity: a systematic review. *Am J Phys Med Rehabil*, 95, 309–318.

Montenegro, E. J., Guimarães de Alencar, G., Rocha de Siqueira, G., Guerino, M. R., Maia, J. N., & Araújo De Oliveira, D. 2016. Effect of low frequency transcutaneous electrical nerve stimulation of TE5 (waiguan) and PC6 (neiguan) acupoints on cold-induced pain. *J Phys Ther Sci*, 28, 76–81.

Montgomery, L., Elliott, S. B., & Adair, H. S. 2013. Muscle and tendon heating rates with therapeutic ultrasound in horses. *Vet Surg*, 42, 243–249.

Moran, F., Leonard, T., Hawthorne, S., Hughes, C. M., Mccrum-Gardner, E., Johnson, M. I., *et al.* 2011. Hypoalgesia in response to transcutaneous electrical nerve stimulation (TENS) depends on stimulation intensity. *J Pain*, 12, 929–935.

Moretti, B., Florenzo, I., Notarnicola, A., Lapadula, G., Moretti, L., Patella, V., & Garofalo, R., 2008. Extracorporeal shock waves down-regulate the expression of interleukin-10 and tumor necrosis factor-alpha in osteoarthritic chondrocytes. *BMC Musculoskelet Disord*, 9, 16.

Morishita, K., Karasuno, H., Yokoi, Y., Morozumi, K., Ogihara, H., Ito, T., *et al.* 2014a. Effects of therapeutic ultrasound on intramuscular blood circulation and oxygen dynamics. *J Jpn Phys Ther Assoc*, 17, 1–7.

Morishita, K., Karasuno, H., Yokia, Y., Morozumi, K., Ogihara, H., Ito, T., *et al.* 2014b. Effects of therapeutic ultrasound on range of motion and stretch pain. *J Phys Ther Sci*, 26, 711–715.

Morrisette, D. C., Brown, D., & Saladin, M. E. 2004. Temperature change in lumbar periarticular tissue with continuous ultrasound. *J Orthop Sports Phys Ther*, 34, 754–760.

Mourad, P. D., Lazar, D. A., Curra, F. P., Mohr, B. C., Andrus, K. C., Avellino, A. M., *et al.* 2001. Ultrasound accelerates functional recovery after peripheral nerve damage. *Neurosurgery*, 48, 1136–1140.

Mueller, M., Bockstahler, B., Skalicky, M., Mlacnik, E., & Lorinson, D. 2007. Effects of radial shockwave therapy on the limb function of dogs with hip osteoarthritis. *Vet Rec*, 160, 762–765.

Mueller, M. C., Gradner, G., Hittmair, K. M., Dupre, G., & Bockstahler, B. A. 2009. Conservative treatment of partial gastrocnemius muscle avulsions in dogs using therapeutic ultrasound – a force plate study. *Vet Comp Orthop Traumatol*, 22, 243–248.

Muftic, M. & Miladinovic, K. 2013. Therapeutic ultrasound and pain in degenerative diseases of musculoskeletal system. *Acta Inform Med*, 21, 170–172.

Naderi Nabi, B., Sedighinejad, A., Haghighi, M., Biazar, G., Hashemi, M., Haddadi, S., & Fathi, A. 2015. Comparison of transcutaneous electrical nerve stimulation and pulsed radiofrequency sympathectomy for treating painful diabetic neuropathy. *Anesth Pain Med*, 5, e29280.

Nadler, S. F., Steiner, D. J., Petty, S. R., Erasala, G. N., Hengehold, D. A., & Weingand, K. W. 2003. Overnight use of continuous low-level heatwrap therapy for the relief of low back pain. *Arch Phys Med Rehabil*, 84, 335–342.

Nadler, S. F., Weingand, K., & Kruse, R. J. 2004. The physiologic basis and clinical applications of cryotherapy and thermotherapy for the pain practitioner. *Pain Physician*, 7, 395–399.

Nadur-Andrade, N., Dale, C. S., Oliveira, V. R., Toniolo, E. F., Feliciano, R. D., da Silva, J. A. Jr, & Samuner, S. R. 2016. Analgesic effect of photobiomodulation on Bothrops Moojeni venom-induced hyperalgesia: a mechanism dependent on neuronal inhibition, cytokines and kinin receptors modulation. *PLoS Negl Trop Dis*. 10, 30004998.

Nakano, J., Yamabayashi, C., Scott, A. & Reid, W. D. 2012. The effect of heat applied with stretch to increase range of motion: a systematic review. *Phys Ther Sport*, 13, 180–188.

Nam, K. W., Seo, D. Y., & Kim, M. H. 2014. Pulsed and continuous ultrasound increase chondrogenesis through the increase of heat shock protein 70 expression in rat articular cartilage. *J Phys Ther Sci*, 26, 647–650.

Nasu, F., Tomiyasu, K., Inomata, K., & Calderhead, R. G. 1989. Cytochemical effects of gaalas diode laser radiation on rat saphenous artery calcium ion dependent adenosine triphosphatase activity. *Laser Therapy*, 1(2), 89–92

Neff, D., Kuhlenhoelter, A. M., Lin, C., Wong, B.J., Motaganahalli, R. L., & Roseguini, B. T. 2016. Thermotherapy reduces blood pressure and circulating endothelin-1 concentration and enhances leg blood flow in patients with symptomatic peripheral artery disease. *Am J Physiol Regul Integr Comp Physiol*, 311(2), R392–400

Ng, G. Y. 2011. Comparing therapeutic ultrasound with microamperage stimulation therapy for improving the strength of Achilles tendon repair. *Connect Tissue Res*, 52, 178–182.

Noble, J. G., Lee, V., & Griffith-Noble, F. 2007. Therapeutic ultrasound: the effects upon cutaneous blood flow in humans. *Ultrasound Med Biol*, 33, 279–285.

Nolan, T. 2005. Electrotherapeutic modalities: electrotherapy and iontophoresis. In: Michlovitz, S. L. & Nolan, T. P. (eds), *Modalities for Therapeutic*

Intervention, 4th edn. Philadelphia, PA: F.A. Davis Co., pp. 97–122.

Norte, G. E., Saliba, S. A., & Hart, J. M. 2015. Immediate effects of therapuetic ultrasound on quadriceps spinal reflex excitability in patients with knee injury. *Arch Phys Med Rehabil*, 96, 1591–1598.

Ochiai, S., Watanabe, A., Oda, H., & Ikeda, H. 2014. Effectiveness of thermotherapy using a heat and steam generating sheet for cartilage in knee osteoarthritis. *J Phys Ther Sci*, 26, 281–284.

Ohkoshi, Y., Ohkoshi, M., Nagasaki, S., Ono, A., Hashimoto, T., & Yamane, S. 1999. The effect of cryotherapy on intraarticular temperature and postoperative care after anterior cruciate ligament reconstruction. *Am J Sports Med*, 27, 357–362.

Ojea, A. R., Madi, O., Neto, R. M., Lima, S. E., de Carvalho, B. T., Ojea, M. J., et al. 2016. Beneficial effects of applying low-level laser therapy to surgical wounds after bariatric surgery. *Photomed Laser Surg*, 34, 580–584.

Okada, K., Yamaguchi, T., Minowa, K., & Inoue, N. 2005. The influence of hot pack therapy on the blood flow in masseter muscles. *J Oral Rehabil*, 32, 480–486.

Okita, M., Nakano, J., Kataoka, H., Sakamoto, J., Origuchi, T., & Yoshimura, T. 2009. Effects of therapeutic ultrasound on joint mobility and collagen fibril arrangement in the endomysium of immobilized rat soleus muscle. *Ultrasound Med Biol*, 35, 237–244.

Oliveira, N. M., Rainero, E., & Salvini, T. F. 2006. Three intermittent sessions of cryotherapy reduce the secondary muscle injury in skeletal muscle of rat. *J Sports Sci Med*, 5, 228–234.

On, A. Y., Colakoglu, S., Hepguler, S., & Aksit, R. 1997. Local heat effect on sympathetic skin responses after pain of electrical stimulus. *Arch Phys Med Rehabl*, 78, 1196–1199.

Otte, J. W., Merrick, M. A., Ingersoll, C. D., & Cordova, M. L. 2002. Subcutaneous adipose tissue thickness alters cooling time during cryotherapy. *Arch Phys Med Rehabil*, 83, 1501–1505.

Özkul, Ç., Kilinç, M., Yildirim, S. A., Topçuoğlu, E. Y., & Akyüz, M. 2015. Effects of visual illusion and transcutaneous electrical nerve stimulation on neuropathic pain in patients with spinal cord injury: a randomised controlled cross-over trial. *J Back Musculoskelet Rehabil*, 28, 709–719.

Pan, L., Hou, D., Liang, W., Fei, J., & Hong, Z. 2015. Comparison of the effects of pressurized salt ice packs with water ice packs on patients following total knee arthroplasty. *Int J Clin Exp Med*, 8, 18179–18184.

Pan, L. L., Ke, J. Q., Zhao, C. C., Huang, S. Y., Shen, J., Jiang, X. X., & Wang, X. T. 2016. Electrical stimulation improves rat muscle dysfunction caused by chronic intermittent hypoxia-hypercapnia via regulation of miRNA-related signaling pathways. *PLoS One*, 11, e0152525.

Pantaleão, M. A., Laurino, M. F., Gallego, N. L., Cabral, C. M., Rakel, B., Vance, C., et al. 2011. Adjusting pulse amplitude during transcutaneous electrical nerve stimulation (TENS) application produces greater hypoalgesia. *J Pain*, 12, 581–590.

Pantović, M., Popović, B., Madić, D., & Obradović, J. 2015. Effects of neuromuscular electrical stimulation and resistance training on knee extensor/flexor muscles. *Coll Antropol*, 39, 153–157.

Park, K. N., Kwon, O. Y., Weon, J. H., Choung, S. D., & Kim S. H. 2014. Comparison of the effects of local cryotherapy and passive cross-body stretch on extensibility in subjects with posterior shoulder tightness. *J Sports Sci Med*, 13, 84–90.

Passarella, S. & Karu, T. 2014. Absorption of monochromatic and narrow band radiation in the visible and near IR by both mitochondrial and non-mitochondrial photoacceptors results in photobiomodulation. *J Photochem Photobiol B*, 140, 344–358.

Passarella, S., Casamassima, E., Molinari, S., Pastore, D., Quagliariello, E., Catalano, I. M., & Cingolani, A. 1984. Increase of proton electrochemical potential and ATP synthesis in rat liver mitochondria irradiated in vitro by helium-neon laser. *FEBS Lett*, 175(1), 95–99.

Petrofsky, J. S. & Laymon, M. 2009. Heat transfer to deep tissue: the effect of body fat and heating modality. *J Med Eng Technol*, 33, 337–348.

Petrofsky, J. S., Lawson, D., Suh, H. J., Rossi, C., Zapata, K., Broadwell, E., & Littleton, L. 2007. The influence of local versus global heat on the healing of chronic wounds in patients with diabetes. *Diabetes Technol Ther*, 9, 535–544.

Petrofsky, J. S., Laymon, M., & Lee, H. 2013. Effect of heat and cold on tendon flexibility and force to flex the human knee. *Med Sci Monit*, 19, 661–667.

Petrofsky, J.S., Laymon, M.S., Alshammari F.S., & Lee, H. 2016a. Use of low level of continuous heat as an adjunct to physical therapy improves knee pain recovery and the compliance for home exercise in patients with chronic knee pain: a randomized controlled trial. *J Strength Cond Res*, 30(11), 3107–3115.

Petrofsky, J., Berk, L., Bains, G., Khowailed, I. A., Lee, H., & Laymon, M. 2016b. The efficacy of sustained heat treatment on delayed-onset muscle soreness. *Clin J Sport Med*, 27, 329–337.

Pivec, R., Minshall, M. E., Mistry, J. B., Chughtai, M., Elmallah, R. K., & Mont, M. A. 2015. Decreased opioid utilization and cost at one year in chronic low back pain patients treated with transcutaneous electric nerve stimulation (TENS). *Surg Technol Int*, 27, 268–274.

Polak, A., Franek, A., Blaszczak, E., Nawrat-Szoltysik, A., Taradaj, J., Weircigroch, L., *et al.* 2014. A prospective, randomized, controlled, clinic study to evaluate the efficacy of high-frequency ultrasound in the treatment of stage II and stage III pressure ulcers in geriatric patients. *Ostomy Wound Manage*, 60, 16–28.

Pourreau-Schneider, N., Ahmed, A, Soudry, M., Jacquemier, J., Kopp, F., Franquin, J.C., & Martin, P. M. 1990. Helium-neon laser treatment transforms fibroblasts into myofibroblasts. *Am J Pathol*, 137(1), 171–178.

Price, R., Lehmann, J. F., Boswell-Bessette, S., Burleigh, A., & Delateur, B. J. 1993. Influence of cryotherapy on spasticity at the human ankle. *Arch Phys Med Rehabil*, 74, 300–304.

Rai, S., Ranjan, V., Misra, D., & Panjwani, S. 2016. Management of myofascial pain by therapeutic ultrasound and transcutaneous electrical nerve stimulation: a comparative study. *Eur J Dent*, 10, 46–53.

Ranjbar, R. & Takhtfooladi, M. A. 2016. The effects of low level laser therapy on Staphylococcus aureus infected third-degree burns in diabetic rats. *Acta Cir Bras*, 31, 250–255.

Raso, V. V., Barbieri, C. H., Mazzer, N., & Fasan, V. S. 2005. Can therapeutic ultrasound influence the regeneration of peripheral nerves? *J Neurosci Methods*, 142, 185–192.

Rathnakar, B., Rao, B. S., Prabhu, V., Chandra, S., Rai, S., Rao, A. C., *et al.* 2016. Photo-biomodulatory response of low-power laser irradiation on burn tissue repair in mice. *Lasers Med Sci*, 31, 1741–1750.

Ravikumar, R., Williams, K. J., Babber, A., Lane, T. R., Moore, H. M., & Davies, A. H. 2017. Randomized controlled trial: potential benefits of a footplate neuromuscular electrical stimulation device in patients with chronic venous disease. *Eur J Vasm Endovasc Surg*, 53, 114–121.

Rayegani, S., Bahrami, M., Samadi, B., Sedighipour, L., Mokjtarirad, M., & Eliaspoor, D. 2011. Comparison of the effects of low energy laser and ultrasound in treatment of shoulder myofascial pain syndrome: a randomized single-blinded clinical trial. *Eur J Phys Rehabil Med*, 47, 381–389.

Rivlin, M., King, M., Kruse, R., & Ilyas, A. M. 2014. Frostbite in an adolescent football player: a case report. *J Athl Train*, 49, 97–101.

Robertson, V. J., Ward, A. R., & Jung, P. 2005. The effect of heat on tissue extensibility: a comparison of deep and superficial heating. *Arch Phys Med Rehabil*, 86, 819–825.

Rochkind, S., Geuna, S., & Shainberg, A. 2009. Phototherapy in peripheral nerve injury: effects on muscle preservation and nerve regeneration. *Int Rev Neurobiol*, 87, 445–464.

Rompe, J. D., Hope, C., Kullmer, K., Heine, J., & Burger, R. 1996. Analgesic effect of extracorporeal shock-wave therapy on chronic tennis elbow. *J Bone Joint Surg Br*, 78, 233–237.

Rosario, J. L. & Foletto, Á. 2015. Comparative study of stretching modalities in healthy women: heating and application time. *J Bodyw Mov Ther*, 19, 3–7.

Rose, S., Draper, D. O., Schulthies, S. S., & Durrant, E. 1996. The stretching window part two: rate of thermal decay in deep muscle following 1-Mhz ultrasound. *J Athl Train*, 31, 139–143.

Roxo, R. S., Xavier, V. B., Miorin, L. A., Magalhães, A. O., Sens, Y. A., & Alves, V. L. 2016. Impact of neuromuscular electrical stimulation on functional capacity of patients with chronic kidney disease on hemodialysis. *J Bras Nefrol*, 38, 344–350.

S, G. N., Kamal, W., George, J., & Manssor, E. 2016. Radiological and biochemical effects (CTX-II, MMP-3, 8 and 13) of low-level laser therapy (LLLT) in chronic osteoarthritis in Al-Kharj, Saudi Arabia. *Lasers Med Sci*. 32(2), 297–303.

Saini, N. S., Roy, K. S., Bansal, P. S., Singh, B., & Simran, P. S. 2002. A preliminary study on the effect of ultrasound therapy on the healing of surgically severed achilles tendons in five dogs. *J Vet Med A Physiol Pathol Clin Med*, 49, 321–328.

Santos, M. T., Diniz, M. B., Gouw-Soares, S. C., Lopes-Martins, R. A., Frigo, L., & Baeder, F. M. 2016. Evaluation of low-level laser therapy in the treatment of masticatory muscles spasticity in children with cerebral palsy. *J Biomed Opt*, 21, 28001.

Sakurai, Y., Yamaguchi, M., & Abiko, Y. 2000. Inhibitory effect of low-level laser irradiation on LPS-stimulated prostaglandin E production and cyclooxygenase-2 in human gingival fibroblasts. *Eur J Oral Sci* 108, 29–34.

Sawant, A., Dadurka, K., Overend, T., & Kremenchutzky, M. 2015. Systematic review of efficacy of TENS for management of central pain in people with multiple sclerosis. *Mult Scler Relat Disord*, 4, 219–227.

Saygun, I., Nizam, N., Serdar, M. A., Avcu, F., & Tözüm, T. F. 2012. Low-level laser irradiation affects the release of basic fibroblast growth factor (bFGF), insulin-like growth factor-I (IGF-I), and receptor of IGF-I (IGFBP3) from osteoblasts. *Photomed Laser Surg*, 30, 149–154.

Schaden, W., Fischer, A., & Sailler, A. 2001. Extracorporeal shock wave therapy of nonunion or delayed osseous union. *Clin Orthop Relat Res*, 387, 90–94.

Schaser, K. D., Disch, A. C., Stover, J. F., Lauffer, A., Bail, H. J., & Mittlmeier, T. 2007. Prolonged superficial local cryotherapy attenuates microcirculatory impairment, regional inflammation, and muscle necrosis after closed soft tissue injury in rats. *Am J Sports Med*, 35, 93–102.

Sems, A., Dimeff, R., & Iannotti, J. P. 2006. Extra-corporeal shock wave therapy in the treatment of chronic tendinopathies. *J Am Acad Orthop Surg*, 14, 195–204.

Sharma, G. & Noohu, M. M. 2014. Effect of ice massage on lower extremity functional performance and weight discrimination ability in collegiate footballers. *Asian J Sports Med*, 5(3), e23184.

Sharma, R., Aggarwal, A. N., Bhatt, S., Kumar, S., & Bhargava, S. K. 2015. Outcome of low level lasers versus ultrasonic therapy in de Quervain's tenosynovitis. *Indian J Orthop*, 49, 542–548.

Siqueira, A. F., Vieira, A., Ramos, G. V., Marqueti, R. C., Salvini, T. F., Puntel, G. O. & Durigan, J. L. 2017. Multiple cryotherapy applications attenuate oxidative stress following skeletal muscle injury. *Redox Rep*, 22, 323–329.

Sluka, K. A., Christy, M. R., Peterson, W. L., Rudd, S. L., & Troy, S. M. 1999. Reduction of pain-related behaviors with either cold or heat treatment in an animal model of actue arthritis. *Arch Phys Med Rehabil*, 80, 313–317.

Snyder-Mackler, L. & Bork, C. E. 1988. Effect of helium-neon laser irradiation on peripheral sensory nerve latency. *Phys Ther*, 68, 223–225.

Snyder-Mackler, L., Barry, A. J., Perkins, A. I., & Soucek, M. D. 1989. Effects of helium-neon laser irradiation on skin resistance and pain in patients with trigger points in the neck or back. *Phys Ther*, 69, 336–341.

Snyder-Mackler, L., Ladin, Z., Schepsis, A. A., & Young, J. C. 1991. Electrical stimulation of the thigh muscles after reconstruction of the anterior cruciate ligament. *Effects of electrically elicited contraction of the quadriceps femoris and hamstring muscles on gait and on strength of the thigh muscles. J Bone Joint Surg Am*, 73, 1025–1036.

Snyder-Mackler, L., Delitto, A., Stralka, S. W., & Bailey, S. L. 1994. Use of electrical stimulation to enhance recovery of quadriceps femoris muscle force production in patients following anterior cruciate ligament reconstruction. *Phys Ther*, 74, 901–907.

Son, S. J., Kim, H., Seeley, M. K., Feland, J. B., & Hopkins, J. T. 2016. Effects of transcutaneous electrical nerve stimulation on quadriceps function in individuals with experimental knee pain. *Scand J Med Sci Sports*, 26, 1080–1090.

Son, S. J., Kim, H., Seeley, M. K., & Hopkins, J. T. 2017. Efficacy of sensory transcutaneous electrical nerve stimulation on perceived pain and gait patterns in individuals with experimental knee pain. *Arch Phys Med Rehabil*, 98, 25–35.

Song, M., Sun, X., Tian, X., Zhang, X., Shi, T., Sun, R., & Dai, W. 2016. Compressive cryotherapy versus cryotherapy alone in patients undergoing knee surgery: a meta-analysis. *Springerplus*, 5(1), 1074.

Stark, J., Petrofsky, J., Berk, L., Bains, G., Chen, S. & Doyle, G. 2014. Continuous low-level heatwrap therapy relieves low back pain and reduces muscle stiffness. *Phys Sportsmed*, 42, 39–48.

Stasinopoulos, D., Papdopoulos, K., Lamnisos, D., & Stergioulas, A. 2016. LLLT for the management of patients with ankylosing spondylitis. *Lasers Med Sci*, 31, 459–469.

Stein, C., Fritsch, C. G., Robinson, C., Sbruzzi, G., & Plentz, R. D. 2015. Effects of electrical stimulation in spastic muscles after stroke: systematic review and meta-analysis of randomized controlled trials. *Stroke*, 46, 2197–2205.

Steiss, J. E. & Adams, C. C. 1999. Effect of coat on rate of temperature increase in muscle during ultrasound treatment of dogs. *Am J Vet Res*, 60, 76–80.

Suzuki, R. & Takakuda, K. 2016. Wound healing efficacy of a 660-nm diode laser in a rat incisional wound model. *Lasers Med Sci*, 31, 1683–1689.

Taheri, P., Vahdatpour, B., & Andalib, S. 2016. Comparative study of shock wave therapy and laser therapy effect in elimination of symptoms among patients with myofascial pain syndrome in upper trapezius. *Adv Biomed Res*, 5, 138.

Takhtfooladi, M. A., Jahanbakhsh, F., Takhtfooladi, H. A., Yousefi, K., & Allahverdi, A. 2015. Effect of low-level laser therapy (685 nm, 3 J/cm^2) on functional recovery of the sciatic nerve in rats following crushing lesion. *Lasers Med Sci*, 30, 1047–1052.

Talbot, L. A., Breded, E., & Metter, E. J. 2017. Effects of adding neuromuscular electrical stimulation to traditional military amputee rehabilitation. *Mil Med*, 182, e1529–e1535.

Tatmatsu-Rocha, J. C., Ferraresi, C., Hamblin, M. R., Damasceno Maia, F., do Nascimento, N. R., Driusso, P., & Parizotto, N. A. 2016. Low-level laser therapy (904 nm) can increase collagen and reduce oxidative and nitrosative stress in diabetic wounded mouse skin. *J Photochem Photobiol B*, 164, 96–102.

Tim, C. R., Bossini, P. S., Kido, H. W., Malavazi, I., Von Zeska Kress, M. R., Carazzolle, M. F., *et al.* 2016. Effects of low level laser therapy on inflammatory and angiogenic gene expression during the process of bone healing: a microarray analysis. *J Photochem Photobiol B*, 154, 8–15.

Toma, R. L., Vassão, P. G., Assis, L., Antunes, H. K., & Renno, A. C. 2016. Low level laser therapy associated with a strength training program on muscle performance in elderly women: a randomized double blind control study. *Lasers Med Sci*, 31, 1219–1229.

Tomazoni, S. S., Leal-Junior, E. C., Pallotta, R. C., Teixeira, S., de Almeida, P., & Lopes-Martins, R. Á. 2017. Effects of photobiomodulation therapy, pharmacological therapy, and physical exercise as single and/or combined treatment on the inflammatory response induced by experimental osteoarthritis. *Lasers Med Sci*, 32, 101–108.

Torres, R., Silva, F., Pedrosa, V., Ferreira, J., & Lopes, A. 2016. The acute effect of cryotherapy on muscle strength and shoulder proprioception. *J Sport Rehabil*, 11, 1–24.

Uchio, Y., Ochi, M., Fujihara, A., Adachi, N., Iwasa, J., & Sakai, Y. 2003. Cryotherapy influences joint laxity and position sense of the healthy knee joint. *Arch Phys Med Rehabil*, 84, 131–135.

Ud-Din, S. & Bayat, A. 2014. Electrical stimulation and cutaneous wound healing: a review of clinical evidence. *Healthcare (Basel)*, 2, 445–467.

Upton, G. A., Tinley, P., Al-Aubaidy, H., & Crawford, R. 2017. The influence of transcutaneous electrical nerve stimulation parameters on the level of pain perceived by participants with painful diabetic neuropathy: a crossover study. *Diabetes Metab Syndr*, 11, 113–118.

Valenza, M. C., Torres-Sánchez, I., Cabrera-Martos, I., Valenza-Demet, G., & Cano-Cappellacci, M. 2016. Acute effects of contract-relax stretching vs. TENS in young subjects with anterior knee pain: a randomized controlled trial. *J Strength Cond Res*, 30, 2271–2278.

Vanin, A. A., Miranda, E. F., Machado, C. S., de Paiva, P. R., Albuquerque-Pontes, G. M., Casalechi, H. L., et al. 2016. What is the best moment to apply phototherapy when associated to a strength training program? A randomized, double-blinded, placebo-controlled trial: phototherapy in association to strength training. *Lasers Med Sci*, 31, 1555–1564.

Vartika, K., Jatinder, K. D., & Gauri, K. 2015. Low level laser therapy: a panacea for oral maladies. *Laser Ther*, 24, 215–223.

Vasilenko, T., Slezak, M., Kovac, I., Bottkova, Z., Jakubco, J., Kostelnikova, M., et al. 2010. The effect of equal daily dose achieved by different power densities of low-level laser therapy at 635 and 670 nm on wound tensile strength in rats: a short report. *Photomed Laser Surg*, 28, 281–283.

Veronez, S., Assis, L., Del Campo, P., de Oliveira, F., de Castro, G., Renno, A. C. & Medalha, C. C. 2017. Effects of different fluences of low-level laser therapy in an experimental model of spinal cord injury in rats. *Lasers Med Sci*. 32(2), 343–349.

Vieira, T. M., Potenzi, P., Gastaldi, L., & Botter, A. 2016. Electrode position markedly affects knee torque in tetanic, stimulated contractions. *Eur J Appl Physiol*, 116, 335–342.

Wagner, V. P., Curra, M., Webber L. P., Nör, C., Matte, U., Meurer, L., & Martins, M. D. 2016. Photobiomodulation regulates cytokine release and new blood vessel formation during oral wound healing in rats. *Lasers Med Sci*, 31, 665–671.

Wang, F.S., Yang, K.D., Chen, R.F., Wang, C.J., & Sheen-Chen, S.M. 2002. Extracorporeal shock wave promotes growth and differentiation of bone-marrow stromal cells towards osteoprogeni-tors associated with induction of TGF-beta1. *J Bone Joint Surg Br*, 84(3), 457–461.

Wang, F. S., Yang, K. D., Kuo, Y. R., Wang, C. J., Sheen-Chen, S. M., Huang, H. C., & Chen, Y. J. 2003. Temporal and spatial expression of bone morphogenetic proteins in extracorporeal shock wave-promoted healing of segmental defect. *Bone*, 32(4), 387–396.

Wang, C.J., Wang, F.S., Huang, C.C., Yang, K.D., Weng, L.H., & Huang, H.Y. 2005. Treatment for osteonecrosis of the femoral head: comparison of extracorporeal shock waves with core decompression and bone-grafting. *J Bone Joint Surg Am*, 87(11), 2380–2387.

Ward, A. R. & Shkuratova, N. 2002. Russian electrical stimulation: the early experiments. *Phys Ther*, 82, 1019–1030.

Willand, M. P., Chiang, C. D., Zhang, J. J., Kemp, S. W., Borschel, G. H., & Gordon, T. 2015. Daily electrical muscle stimulation enhances functional recovery following nerve transection and repair in rats. *Neurorehabil Neural Repair*, 29, 690–700.

Williams, K. J., Moore, H. M., & Davies, A. H. 2015. Haemodynamic changes with the use of neuromuscular electrical stimulation compared to intermittent pnuematic compression. *Phlebology*, 30, 365–372.

Williams, K. J., Ravikumar, R., Gaweesh, A. S., Moore, H. M., Lifsitz, A. D., Lane, T. R., et al. 2017. A review of the evidence to support neuromuscular electrical stimulation in the prevention and management of venous disease. *Adv Exp Med Biol*, 906, 377–386.

Wright, J. G., Araki, C. T., Belkin, M., & Hobsom, R. W. 1989. Postischemic hypothermia diminishes skeletal muscle reperfusion edema. *J Surg Res*, 47, 389–396.

Xia, Z., Sato, A., Hughes, M. A., & Cherry, G. W. 2000. Stimulation of fibroblast growth in vitro by intermittent radiant warming. *Wound Repair Regen*, 8, 138–144.

Yadav, A. & Gupta, A. 2017. Non-invasive red and near-infrared wavelength-induced photobiomodulation: promoting impaired cutaneous wound healing. *Photodermatol Photoimmunol Photomed*, 33(1), 4–13.

Yarboro, D. D. & Smith, R. 2014. Transcutaneous electrical nerve stimulation to manage a lower extremity wound complicated by peripheral arterial disease: a case report. *Ostomy Wound Manage*, 60, 40–45.

Yeğin, T., Altan, L., & Kasapoğlu Aksoy, M. 2017. The effect of therapeutic ultrasound on pain and physical function in patients with knee osteoarthritis. *Ultrasound Med Biol*, 43, 187–194.

Yildirim, M. A., Ones, K,. & Celik, E. C. 2013. Comparison of ultrasound therapy of various durations in the treatment of subacromial impingement syndrome. *J Phys Ther Sci*, 25, 1151–1154.

Yildiz, S. K., Özkan, F. Ü., Aktaş, I., Silte, A. D., Kaysin, M. Y., & Badur, N. B. 2015. The effectiveness of ultrasound treatment for the management of knee osteoarthritis: a randomized, placebo-controlled, double-blind study. *Turk J Med Sci*, 45, 1187–1191.

Yoshimura, A., Sakamoto, J., Honda, Y., Kataoka, H., Nakano, J., & Okita, M. 2016. Cyclic muscle twitch contraction inhibits immobilization-induced muscle contracture and fibrosis in rats. *Connect Tissue Res*, 58, 487–495.

Youssef, E. F., Muaidi, Q. I., & Shanb, A. A. 2016. Effect of laser therapy on chronic osteoarthritis of the knee in older subjects. *J Lasers Med Sci*, 7, 112–119.

Yu, W., Naim, J.O., & Lanzafame, R.J. 1994. Expression of growth factors in early wound healing in rat skin. *Lasers Surg Med*, 15(3), 281–289.

Zeng, C., Li, H., Yang, T., Deng, Z. H., Yang, Y., Zhang, Y., Ding, X., & Lei, G. H. 2014. Effectiveness of continuous and pulsed ultrasound for the management of knee osteoarthritis: a systematic review and network meta-analysis. *Osteoarthritis Cartilage*, 22, 1090–1099.

Zhang, C., Xie, Y., Luo, X., Ji, Q., Lu, C., He, C., & Wang, P. 2016. Effects of therapeutic ultrasound on pain, physical functions and safety outcomes in patients with knee osteoarthrits: a systematic review and meta-analysis. *Clin Rehabil*, 30, 960–971.

Zhang, J. M. & An, J. 2007. Cytokines, inflammation and pain. *Int Anesthesiol Clin*, 45, 27–37.

Zhang, J., Pan, T., & Wang, J. H. 2014. Cryotherapy suppresses tendon inflammation in an animal model. *J Orthop Translat*, 2, 75–81.

Ziago, E. K., Fazan, V. P., Lyomasa, M. M., Sousa, L. G., Yamauchi, P. Y., da Silva, E. A., *et al.* 2017. Analysis of the variation in low-level laser energy density on the crushed sciatic nerves of rats: a morphological, quantitative, and morphometric study. *Lasers Med Sci*, 32, 369–378.

Zotz, T. G. & Paula, J. B. 2015. Influence of transcutaneous electrical stimulation on heterotopic ossification: an experimental study in wistar rats. *Braz J Med Biol Res*, 48, 1055–1062.

8 Therapeutic Exercise

Laurie McCauley, DVM, DACVSMR, CVC, CVA, CCRT, and
Janet B. Van Dyke, DVM, DACVSMR, CCRT

Summary

Therapeutic exercises can benefit the postoperative patient, the geriatric OA patient, and the elite athlete with the goal of peak performance. Therapeutic exercise programs address proprioception, balance, muscle strengthening, endurance, and gait retraining. Patient evaluation is vital as program design depends upon the current status as well as expectations for return to work and/or sport. This evaluation directs the therapist to create short-, medium-, and long-term goals, which are reassessed at each visit. Therapeutic exercise programs should contain five variables: frequency, intensity, duration, environment, and impact. It is important to train the client how to perform the exercises in the home exercise program (HEP). Common therapeutic exercise equipment includes physioballs, cavaletti rails, balance blocks and discs, weights, tunnels, rocker boards, wobble boards, and treadmills. Many other materials can be used to create exercises to strengthen specific muscles or muscle groups, and to change balance, gait, posture, or neurological function. The imagination of the therapist is the only limitation on the materials used and the exercises created. Patient considerations such as motivation, footing, assistive devices, and leash/harness control should be assessed prior to beginning any exercise program, and therapist/client body mechanics should also be taken into consideration to prevent injury. Before creating any exercise program, the therapist should evaluate stance, transitions (stand to sit, sit to down, down to sit, and sit to stand) and gait. After the patient is taught each exercise, these should be re-evaluated. If there is improvement, the exercise should be beneficial. If there is no change, the exercise might be beneficial. If there is a negative change, the exercise is either unsuited to the dog, was done incorrectly, or too many reps were done.

Exercises are designed to address specific impairments. For each exercise, the client is provided with a goal, a detailed technique, and a progression. The therapist should be prepared to choose from a variety of exercises, environments, and equipment to main-

---

Canine Sports Medicine and Rehabilitation, Second Edition. Edited by Chris Zink and Janet B. Van Dyke.
© 2018 John Wiley & Sons, Inc. Published 2018 by John Wiley & Sons, Inc.

tain client and patient motivation. The progression of the exercises depends upon the patient response, which is evaluated during each session. Categories of exercises include proprioception, balance, speed, endurance, focal strength, pelvic limb-specific, thoracic limb-specific, neurorehabilitation, and land treadmill endurance training.

Overview

The principles of exercise physiology have been well described in Chapter 3. The goal of this chapter is to introduce the concepts of therapeutic exercise as applied to the injured patient as well as to the canine athlete needing to refine fitness. Once the patient is discharged from the therapeutic exercise program, it will progress to a conditioning and/or retraining program as described in Chapter 10. Therapeutic exercise programs for dogs initially borrowed from human therapeutic exercise research and applied these principles to dogs. The field is now describing how these techniques have provided canine patients with successful return to independence, competition, and work. In addition to improving general conditioning for any patient in a rehabilitation practice, the employment of therapeutic exercise programs also provides the often-overlooked benefit of strengthening the human-animal bond (Westgarth *et al.*, 2014).

The basic principle that pain leads to muscle, tendon, and ligament atrophy, which in turn, causes instability of the joints with progressive pain is well understood. What are the techniques that can be applied to the aging or debilitated canine patient to prevent or reverse this cycle? A Canadian study in humans found that moderate exercise does not lead to acceleration of knee arthritis whether or not there is pre-existing disease. Exercise improved physical function and reduced pain, and was considered an underused modality in the management of osteoarthritis pain (Selten *et al.*, 2016).

Therapeutic exercise programs focus on proprioception and balance, weight shifting, muscle strengthening, re-education of normal posture, and gait training. Proprioception and balance work is important for puppies, athletes, and for the neurologically impaired patient. Weight shift training is used post-injury or postoperatively, initially training the patient to use the affected limb, and later encouraging appropriate weight distribution during activities of daily living (Saunders, 2007). Strengthening can focus on an isolated muscle, limb, or body region. Posture re-education addresses the static postures (stand, sit, down) as well as the transitions between these postures. Gait retraining addresses the patient who does not properly use one or more limbs or who has developed an abnormal gait behavior or pattern.

When planning a therapeutic exercise program, it is important to be aware of the differences between two types of muscles: those that tend to stabilize joints and those that create motion. Stabilizing muscles tend to be shorter bellied muscles that are situated closer to the bone than mobilizing muscles, and they insert closer to the joint. Stabilizers have more type I fibers, and have a relatively short excursion length. Type I muscle fibers are more readily affected by disuse than type II muscle fibers.

Mobilizing muscles are more superficial, generally with longer bellies and tendons, creating a longer lever arm and excursion, and they have more type II fibers. Type II muscle fibers atrophy in the geriatric dog by up to 25%, simply as an aging change.

Stabilizer muscles are less commonly diagnosed with strain injuries than their mobilizer counterparts (Newsholme *et al.*, 1988; Latorre *et al.*, 1993) but in the author's (L.M.) experience, they are more likely to have myofascial trigger points leading to diminished function and altered active range of motion. A lack of harmony between the stabilizers and the mobilizers can result in muscle imbalances and injury.

Need for exercise

All healthy working dogs, including competitive sporting, hunting, and service dogs, need regular exercise to maintain optimal health. Even conformation dogs need regular controlled exercise for success in the show ring (Wakshlag & Shmalberg, 2014). Noncompetitive pet dogs can benefit from regular, focused exercise programs for general as well as emotional health. This is particularly true for geriatric dogs, which can benefit from a daily routine of gentle exercise to prevent disuse atrophy and progressive loss of independence.

In addition to the commonly recognized use of therapeutic exercise for orthopedic and neurological disorders, therapeutic exercise is routinely recommended for patients that may not show overt musculoskeletal abnormalities. These include dogs with nonclinical (or not-yet clinical) musculoskeletal disorders such as hip laxity, and those with nonorthopedic disorders such as diabetes, hypothyroidism, and heart disease.

Evaluation

In addition to assessing the patient for specific areas of weakness, the rehabilitation therapist should evaluate the patient's emotional and intellectual abilities. Is this patient able to follow commands? Are they able to focus long enough to learn new skills? Are they willing to please or are they obstinate/aggressive? Finally, what is the patient's job or sport?

In addition, the client should be assessed. What is their ability to understand the patient's issues and our goals? The therapist should assess the client's ability to commit the time required to complete a planned program. Their physical strength must match the home exercise plan for the patient (Millis, 2015). What is their level of experience and skills? Is this a trained professional with experience (athletic trainer, physical therapy professional) or a well-meaning layperson? Finally, what are the client's expectations for return to function?

Evaluating the athlete is particularly challenging for the rehabilitation therapist, because in addition to overt injury, canine athletes often present with very subtle impairments that have led to diminished performance. Evaluation of these dogs requires tests that are specific and sensitive enough to detect weaknesses in otherwise very fit individuals (Steiss, 2002). The authors often find certain patterns of impairments in this group of patients including evidence of overtraining, residual impairments from previous injuries,

fatigue or poor conditioning of paraspinal muscles, and poor balance.

Setting goals

The rehabilitation therapist should have both short- and long-term goals for each patient, based upon the patient's age, life stage, and progress since injury, as well as the client's commitment to the program (Price, 2014). If the expectation for complete recovery seems unrealistic, short- and intermediate-term goals should be set, with progress reassessed at each visit.

Goals should be set for each component of the program. Proprioception goals range from decreasing ataxia in the neurological patient to increasing body awareness in the immature athlete in an effort to prevent injuries. Strength goals for an athlete might be to carry a dumbbell over a jump, while those for the geriatric patient might be to climb stairs and get on the bed. Endurance goals for a hunting dog might be to complete five 150-yard retrieves in water, while the endurance goal for an IPO-3 dog might be to run 5 miles. For a pet dog, an appropriate goal might be to walk around the block with the client. Examples of gait training goals include eliminating a crabbing gait in the conformation dog, correcting persistent pelvic limb circumduction in the dog whose lumbosacral pain has been resolved, and increasing stride length in the racing or agility dog.

In the human clinical setting, care plans are often developed on functional progressions, including SAID (specific adaptations to imposed demands), and manipulating workout variables—FITTR (frequency, intensity, time/duration, type/mode, and rate of progression)—(Chu & Shiner, 2007). Progression from rehabilitation to performance conditioning for the injured canine athlete should be no different.

Variables

Each therapeutic exercise program described in this chapter will have five variable parameters:

(1) Frequency of working (daily, multiple times per day, weekly).
(2) Speed/intensity (rate of completing a repetition while maintaining proper form).

(3) Duration of work (time or distance traveled).
(4) Environment (terrain, footing, substrate).
(5) Impact (no impact, low impact, high impact).

The effectiveness of a workout should not be measured by patient fatigue. It should focus on the quality of the movements. The exercise-to-fatigue approach may lead to overtraining, exercise-related pain, and even overuse injuries.

Getting started

The rehabilitation therapist should coach the client and the patient simultaneously when initiating any new exercise that will be applied to the home exercise program (HEP). It is most effective to train the patient how to do an exercise before training the client how to perform the exercise with the patient. The client is then asked to attempt the exercise with the patient (Sharp, 2010). The exercise may be modified during the training session to best fit the abilities of the patient and/or the client, whose available time and likely compliance are considered when creating the HEP.

The patient's willingness to work with both the rehabilitation therapist and the client should be assessed. Dogs are smart enough to find many ways to avoid doing difficult exercises correctly. The rehabilitation therapist should be aware of the common avenues for evading work so that they can be prepared for the behavior and correct or prevent it.

For example, a common exercise used to strengthen the gluteal, adductor, and hamstring muscles involves training the dog to do a sit-to-stand movement on a hill, facing perpendicular to the slope. This activity isolates and strengthens the muscles in the downhill leg. The patient will frequently evade by positioning itself more parallel to the slope with the thoracic limbs downhill. This allows the patient to use gravity to assist the thoracic limbs to pull itself into a standing position rather than using the pelvic limbs to push off into a standing position. To prevent this, the rehabilitation therapist should stand uphill of the dog in a position that discourages this behavior, by giving a "heel" command or by keeping a hand on the patient's collar or harness.

Rules

There are several rules that can aid in achieving success with therapeutic exercise programs:

(1) Always start within the animal's comfort zone, gradually increasing each of the variables until the goals are met. If the goal is to complete 10 repetitions (reps) of an activity with good form, the therapist might start with three to four reps. As the patient approaches the ability to complete 10 good reps, the exercise is made more difficult. This might involve changing to a more challenging movement or doing the same movement in a more challenging environment (Drum *et al.*, 2015).
(2) Strength work is generally done three to five times per week, alternating training days with days off. It is important to maintain the dog's motivation to carry out the exercises, and overtraining can quickly lead to a loss of motivation.
(3) Some clients will insist on working their dogs every day despite clear instructions. For this group, exercises focus upon the thoracic limb one day, the core the next day, the pelvic limb the next day, and so on to prevent overtraining and allow muscles time to repair.
(4) Daily stretching routines are advised (see Chapter 6).

Tools of the trade

This section describes commonly used equipment in a canine rehabilitation practice. The temptation is to find the least expensive option for each of these pieces of equipment. Instead, the emphasis should be on establishing safety for the patient as well as the client. Each piece of equipment will be described below, with clinical applications explained later in the chapter.

Physioballs

Also known as Swiss balls or exercise balls, physioballs come in a variety of shapes and sizes. A peanut ball is shaped like a peanut, and has two points of contact with the ground eliminating side-to-side motion (Figure 8.1). This is the most stable ball, so it is used for most new patients. A physio roll is similarly stable to the peanut, but does not have a gutter in the middle to help support the patient. Egg-shaped balls have some side-to-side motion making exercises on them more difficult than on the peanut or roll. The most challenging shape is the round ball, which moves equally in all directions.

Regardless of the shape of the ball, all physioball work should be initiated with the ball less inflated to create more contact area and friction with the ground (Sekendiz *et al.*, 2010). This makes the ball more stable. As the patient becomes stronger, air can be added to the ball, making it less stable. This is followed by progressing to more challenging shapes of balls. Patients who are afraid of the ball can be calmed by gently bouncing the patient on the ball. This should be used only during the initial session with the ball. Once the patient is confident that the ball will not hurt him, the instability of the ball helps to strengthen muscles. Dogs can stand with all four feet balancing on the ball or while walking the ball to the side in both directions or walking it forward and backward. The front feet can be placed on the ball with the rear feet on the floor walking the ball forward and backward or the rear feet on the ball walking it forward and backward. In addition, the dog can perform transitions such as sit-to-stand on

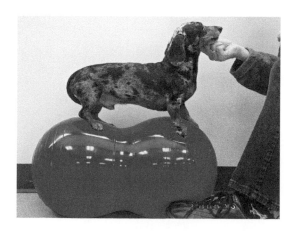

Figure 8.1 The patient is asked to balance on the peanut ball with varied amounts of stabilization support. It can be placed next to the wall for added support. Source: Photo by Whitney Rupp.

the ball as well as sitting up and begging while maintaining control of the ball.

Cavaletti

Cavaletti poles have been used for equine exercises for many years (Clayton, 2016). Patients are asked to step over cavaletti poles without touching them for enhancing balance and proprioception, improving weight bearing on previously injured limbs, strengthening flexors, and elongating stride length. Poles can be spaced evenly as well as in more challenging patterns (Figure 8.2). Cavaletti poles used for canine therapeutic exercise are commonly made of PVC pipe or wood. The author (L.M.) uses 2×2″, 2×4″, and 2×6″ planks in 3-foot lengths that fit into a standard home hallway, or 3-foot long PVC pipe sections that can be supported on small jump standards or on gently crushed aluminum cans. When the patient requires higher cavaletti poles, traffic cones with holes drilled at 2″ intervals can be used to support the poles. Cones can also be used to create obstacles courses (weave poles and figure-8s). These objects can be used to train weight shifting, balance, and unilateral side strengthening.

Planks

Planks in sections of 2×8″ and 2×10″ in 10-foot lengths can be placed on cinder construction blocks (Figure 8.3). Patients work on balance and proprioception by walking along these elevated platforms. To make plank walking more difficult, dogs can work on warped planks, narrower planks, or planks at a higher elevation, and can practice stepping over or on objects placed on the plank.

Blocks

Blocks have a 4×6″ nonslip surface area, and are 2, 4, or 6 inches tall. Smaller or weaker patients start on the lower blocks. Blocks can be used for the easiest form of diagonal leg lifts to strengthen trunk muscles in patients who are too weak for more active strength work (Figure 8.4). This exercise emphasizes stabilizer

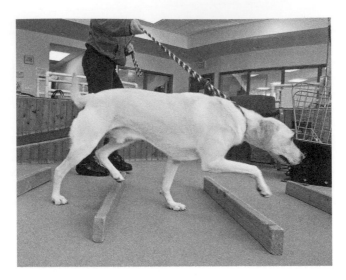

Figure 8.2 The cavaletti poles are spaced so that each foot steps only once in each space. The height of the pole dictates how much flexion will be needed to get through the poles cleanly. Source: Photo by Whitney Rupp.

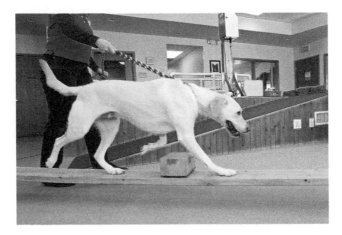

Figure 8.3 This patient walks on a 2 × 8 × 10″ plank working on his balance. He is then challenged, having to step over blocks while walking on the plank. The last challenge is to use a warped board to make it wobble while he is walking. Source: Photo by Whitney Rupp.

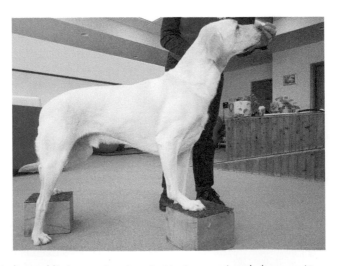

Figure 8.4 The patient's diagonal limbs are placed on the blocks to work on balance and improve trunk strength. Source: Photo by Whitney Rupp.

muscles. Many variations are possible including placing different height blocks under front and rear feet or placing only the diagonal feet on the blocks.

Land treadmill

When shopping for a treadmill, belt length is a key component. Human treadmill belts are generally 4 to 5 feet long. This length is acceptable for small dogs, but large dogs require a 6-foot or longer belt—these can be found only on dog-specific treadmills (Figure 8.5). One downside to the canine treadmills is that the belt is generally narrower, so the therapist cannot walk on the belt with the patient. Incline and or decline capability is important. The ability to move in reverse is nice, but not essential as the dog can be placed on the belt facing the opposite direction or the machine turned 180° to replicate the belt moving in reverse. The belt should start with a simple one-button push or turn, rather than the patient having to start walking before settings can be altered, and it should have a starting speed less than 0.4 miles per hour. The speed control must be such that the patient cannot increase the speed of the belt by running faster.

Balance discs

Inflatable discs are used as low, unstable surfaces. The patient is asked to balance with one or more feet on the disc. Discs are used for balance and stabilizer muscle strengthening, and are easier than standing on a ball. The patient who is able to stand with his front feet elevated on a chair can progress to doing this while his rear feet are on the disc (Figure 8.6). This can be made more difficult by having front feet on an unstable surface and rear feet on a disc while the therapist gently lifts one pelvic or thoracic limb off the supporting surface for short periods of time.

Tunnels

Tunnels can be created using children's tunnels, agility tunnels, a line of chairs, or cavaletti poles attached to adjacent cones. Tunnels are used to encourage the patient to crouch or crawl, strengthening the thoracic limbs, trunk, and pelvic limbs primarily through eccentric contractions (Figure 8.7).

Air mattress

An air mattresses can be used to enhance proprioception and balance. Initial work is done with the patient standing on the mattress while it is fully inflated. Difficulty increases as air is removed until the patient can begin to make contact with the floor. To further increase the difficulty, the patient can be encouraged to walk on this unstable surface or someone can walk on the unstable surface next to the patient.

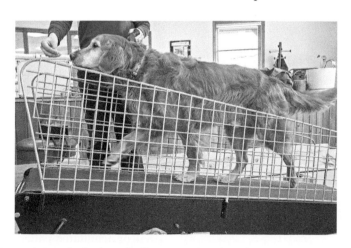

Figure 8.5   Healthy dog trotting on the land treadmill. Source: Photo by Whitney Rupp.

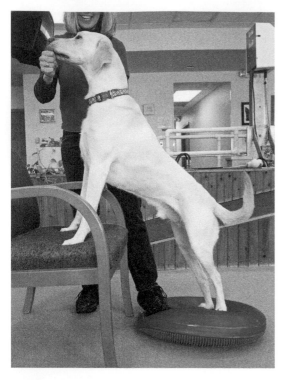

Figure 8.6   Patient is standing with his front feet on a chair and his rear feet on a disc. This, in contrast to the rear feet on the ground and the front feet on the ball, uses the same body posture, but requires greater effort enhancing stability at the pelvic limbs. Source: Photo by Whitney Rupp.

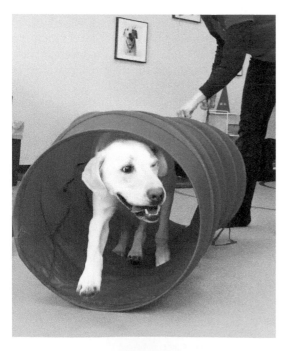

Figure 8.7   A children's tunnel can be used to have a patient crawl before they are strong enough to crouch all the way to the floor. Source: Photo by Whitney Rupp.

Weights

Weights are most often used to create an annoyance on one limb, encouraging weight shifting to the contralateral limb. Weights can be anywhere from 2 ounces to 1 pound depending upon the size of the patient (Figure 8.8). The lowest weight that brings about the desired effect should be used.

Rocker boards and wobble boards

Rocker boards and wobble boards differ in that a rocker board offers unidirectional movement over a rail (Figure 8.9) while a wobble board sits atop a hemisphere, creating multidirectional movement. Rocker boards are best used for strengthening the muscles of the limb while wobble boards are more appropriate for enhancing balance of the patient. To make this exercise more difficult, the patient might have two limbs on one board and the other two limbs elevated or on another unstable surface.

Patient considerations

Fatigue

A key concern when using therapeutic exercises on dogs is their tendency to hide fatigue (Drum *et al.*, 2015). The rehabilitation therapist should watch carefully for signs of fatigue including excessive panting, spade-shaped tongue (Figure 8.10), elevated heart rate, drooping tail and or ears, trembling muscles, gait changes (shortened stride in one or more limbs or change from a trot to an amble or pace), or refusal to continue. When a patient refuses to continue, the rehabilitation therapist should consider asking for one more rep to prevent the patient from developing an avoidance behavior. Finally, the patient should be assessed the next day. If the patient is stiff or sore, this is noted in the record, and the intensity and/or duration of the program is decreased in the following session.

Footing

Weak or debilitated patients require special surface considerations. Flooring should be nonslip and the surface should be soft to prevent injury

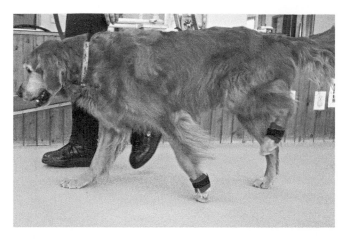

Figure 8.8 Weights can be used to entice a patient to lift the weighted limb higher than normal to exaggerate movement of the limb and extend weight-bearing times on the contralateral limb. Source: Photo by Whitney Rupp.

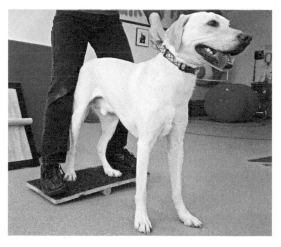

Figure 8.9 The patient stands with rear feet on the rocker board. The therapist stands with her legs on either side of the feet but does not allow the patient to touch or lean on her legs. The motion should be irregular and the therapist should have control of the patient via the collar or harness. Source: Photo by Whitney Rupp.

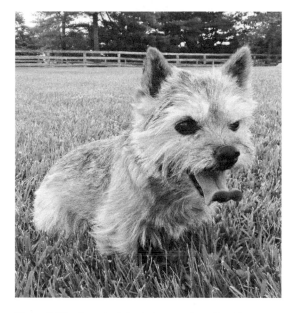

Figure 8.10 As a dog's body temperature rises the tongue widens and curls to create more surface area for evaporation and cooling.

if falls occur. Regular hospital flooring can be modified using yoga mats or horse stall mats. The home environment can be modified using nonslip throw rugs or, if weather permits, the exercises can be performed outdoors on a grass surface (Drum *et al.*, 2015).

Control

For the safety of the patient, the rehabilitation therapist should always control the patient with a leash and/or harness. Harnesses should be nonrestrictive to shoulder motion. A 6-foot or longer leash can be wrapped in a way to create dog reins (Figure 8.11) or a *suitcase harness* (Figure 8.12). Dog reins are used for patients that pull when walking. As in a horse, a gentle pull back on the chest plate area communicates to the patient that pulling forward is not the desired behavior. For the suitcase harness the handler stands beside the patient with the cranial hand holding the leash just above

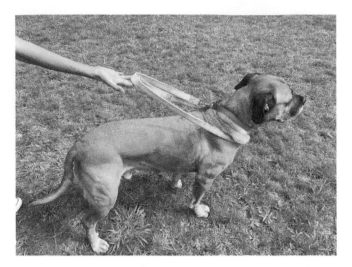

Figure 8.11   Reins are used to prevent the patient from pulling. The leash must come across the chest plate not touching the shoulders or throat.

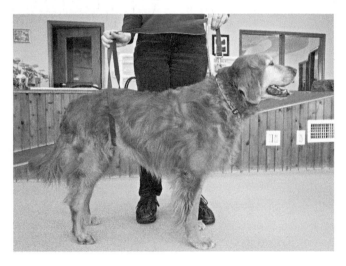

Figure 8.12   The suitcase harness helps maintain control of both the front and rear quarters of the dog, and can aid in balance or weight support if needed. Source: Photo by Whitney Rupp.

the collar. The rest of the leash extends caudally and is looped around the patient's caudal abdomen, supported by the therapist's caudal hand, being careful not to have it cross the penis in male dogs. This gives the handler the ability to drive the patient forward, sideways, or backward without their being able to spin away. The collar is used as a form of communication with the patient allowing the rehabilitation therapist to gently direct the patient's movement by subtle hand motions.

Supportive and assistive devices

Wide slings can be used for support allowing for proper posture in the patient who is incapable of supporting full weight. Boots can be used to prevent scuffing of the feet of ataxic or nonambulatory patients, or to prevent slipping in the weak patient or self-mutilation in patients with dysesthesias. Many harnesses are available to assist the therapist and nursing staff to support the weak or minimally ambulatory patient (Davies, 2017). These can also be used as a form of communication with the patient during exercises.

Patient motivation

Most dogs are very treat-motivated, but the rehabilitation therapist should have especially high-value treats such as cheese or peanut butter available to motivate the patient to work. As with human patients, canine patients can become tired of certain motivators (Goldberg, 2016). Timing of delivery of the treat is critical. This should be done immediately upon the patient demonstrating the correct behavior. Initially, each correct behavior is rewarded. Gradually, treats can be given less often and randomly as the patient masters the new skill. Small individual treats are used during the training phase. For some exercises, where constant attention is desired, a frozen peanut butter mug can be employed. Peanut butter is smeared around the insides of a container such as a mug, which is an appropriate size for the patient's muzzle. The container lined with peanut butter is stored in the freezer. When the dog is working, the container is held so that the patient can lick the inside, working continuously for the reward during an exercise such as standing on a physioball. A variety of sizes of peanut butter containers can be kept in the freezer so that they are readily available for the next patient (Figure 8.13).

Therapist body mechanics

The rehabilitation therapist should maintain correct body posture to protect against work-related injuries (Milhem *et al.*, 2016). It is also important to demonstrate correct body mechanics as an example for the client correcting their posture as needed when they practice the exercises with their pet. Proper body mechanics include keeping the elbows close to the body, avoiding full flexion or extension of any joint including the spine, and might include using tools to prevent excessive spinal flexion/extension or side bending. Personal body posture may go unnoticed as the client focuses on the challenge of the exercise, so it is important for

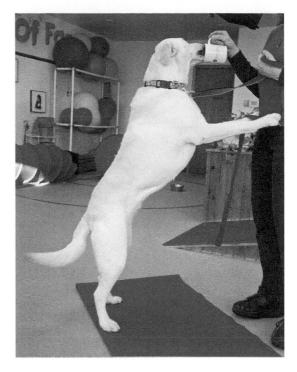

Figure 8.13   Peanut butter slathered on the inside of a mug and frozen makes a long-lasting treat for dogs that need to have their head moved into a specific position or just to distract a dog while it stays in a certain position. Source: Photo by Whitney Rupp.

the rehabilitation therapist to point out any dangerous or inappropriate posture throughout the exercise.

Creating a treatment calendar

A treatment calendar should be created that provides the client with very specific details regarding which exercises to do each day of the week. Clients have time constraints that should be discussed and accommodated. For individuals with a tight work schedule, assignments are limited to the key exercises that will keep the patient progressing appropriately. For the client with a lot of available time, boundaries should be set to prevent potential overtraining. Some clients are weekend warriors, wanting to accomplish all treatments in two consecutive days. For these individuals, splitting the workout into body zones will prevent excessive soreness in any muscle group.

Except for the stretching routine, patients start with three to four repetitions of each exercise if they are able, with the goal of working up to 10 quality repetitions. Once the patient can complete 10 repetitions with ease, the exercise is made more difficult. Strength exercises are undertaken 3 to 5 days per week. For the 3-day program, training is done every other day. For the 5-day program, the two days off should not be consecutive. Proprioception work, weight shift exercises (isometrics), balance work, and stretching can be performed daily. Endurance and cardiopulmonary work, when indicated, are generally done every other day, alternating with strength work. The high-end athlete can do some endurance work daily, but cross training is suggested.

When to progress

A decision whether to advance the therapeutic exercise program should made at each assessment of the patient. The frequency of assessments depends upon the individual patient.

Neurorehabilitation patients might make daily progress while in the hospital, and then be reassessed at each return visit. The postoperative orthopedic patient will generally be reassessed every 2 to 4 weeks (Connell, 2010). The high-end athlete might take months to move to the next level.

When it is clear that the current level of work is not difficult for the patient, the exercise should be made more demanding. The patient may be tired when he gets done, but if he is ready to play 30 minutes later, the therapist can likely increase his activities. If the patient seems tired during the rest of the day, the current level of work should be maintained or slightly decreased. If the patient is stiff or sore the next day, or hesitant to work, the intensity of the exercise should be halved and then slowly advanced. Immediately after an exercise, the patient's posture and transitions should be the same or better than they were before the exercise. If performing the exercise creates a decline in posture, ability, or transitions, the repetitions or frequency of the exercise should be reduced or a less challenging exercise prescribed.

Case Study 8.1   Cranial cruciate ligament insufficiency

Signalment: 3 y.o. M/I Pitbull. Presented 4 days post TTA, right.

Clinical findings: Significant swelling with heat/inflammation and restricted flexion, stifle; restricted flexion, tarsus; 2 cm discrepancy in muscle mass with right thigh smaller; feather weight-bearing stance, right.

Goals: Eliminate swelling, normal ROM stifle and tarsus, even muscle mass, full weight-bearing right pelvic limb.

Therapy: Cryotherapy and PROM used to attain first two goals. Therapeutic exercises used to attain last two goals. Changes in status are noted.

Week 1—leash walks in yard to eliminate q.i.d.
Week 2—Toe touch weight bearing; 3–5-minute walks b.i.d to q.i.d. with leashed activity in yard to eliminate.
Week 3—Increased weight bearing; added 1–2 sit-to-stand exercises to each leash walk, diagonal leg left weight-shifting exercises, and rocker board: 3 sets of 30 seconds b.i.d.

Week 4—Walks of 0.2 to 0.3 miles, with a sit-to-stand every tenth of a mile; three sets of 45 seconds on rocker board.
Week 5—Walks of 0.4 miles, with 2 sit-to-stand exercises every tenth of a mile, continued rocker board, added cavaletti pole exercises (2 × 2″ planks).
Week 6—Walks of 20 minutes b.i.d., with 3 sit-to-stand exercises every tenth of a mile, cavaletti poles (2 × 4″ planks), and weave poles 30″ apart.
Week 8—Walks of 30 minutes b.i.d.; front feet on chair, rear feet on cushion (with perturbations) 4 reps of 1 minute, 5 sit-to-stand exercises each side of the street, weave poles 24″ apart, continue cavaletti poles, add 3 feet on wobble board and right rear stabilizing balance (3 reps of 45 seconds).
Week 10—Continue walks, weaves, sit-to-stands, wobble board, and cavaletti poles; front feet on ball controlling ball position 3 reps of 1 minute.
Week 12—Normal range of motion, even muscle girth, no visible lameness, normal postures and transitions. Discharged from rehabilitation.

Specific exercises

In this section, specific exercises are described; each one includes a goal, a technique, and a progression.

Walking

For the patient who is post-injury or postoperative, initiating proper walk training is the most important and the easiest first step to take.

Goal: Maintain a correct gait pattern throughout the exercise.

Technique: The patient with concurrent cardiac disease may simply go out to sniff and meander for a set period of time, while the metabolically healthy patient may be asked to maintain a speed-walking pace. Progression would involve changing the terrain (ramps and hills) or the substrate (sand or gravel). Increasing the speed is also a form of progression. The patient that has had surgery for CCL insufficiency is started with short toileting leash walks b.i.d. to t.i.d. for the first week, then the exercise is made more difficult by adding one block (approximately 0.1 mile) for each week after surgery for up to 6 to 8 weeks.

Proprioception

For the healthy canine athlete, proprioceptive exercises can enhance neuromuscular control and functional joint stability, thus decreasing the risk of injury. For the injured canine patient, proprioception work is vital to ward off repeat injury. For this reason, it is imperative that the rehabilitation therapist be well versed in the science of proprioception. Sherrington described the proprioceptive system as "afferent information from proprioceptors (mechanoreceptors) located in the proprioceptive field that contributes to conscious sensations, total posture, and segmental posture" (Sherrington, 1906; Lephart et al., 2000). Hewett and colleagues (2002) expanded the definition to include the complex interaction between the afferent and efferent systems. Dynamic joint stability is the result of neuromuscular control and proprioception while postural control requires the integration of visual, vestibular, and proprioceptive inputs (Ghez, 1991; Shumway-Cook & Woollacott, 1995). Any disruption in mechanoreceptor input

that affects proprioception will negatively affect dynamic joint stability and therefore posture.

Mechanoreceptors

Mechanoreceptors (articular, cutaneous, and muscle receptors) are located in connective tissues throughout the body. Golgi tendon organ-like receptors are the largest of the articular mechanoreceptors. They are slow to respond to stimuli, have a high activation threshold, and are active only during dynamic joint states, thus sensing the extremes of the joint's normal movement range (Zimny, 1988). The role of cutaneous receptors in initiating reflexive responses, such as the flexion withdrawal reflex in response to potentially harmful stimuli, is well established (Hulliger et al., 1979). The muscle spindle and the Golgi tendon organ (GTO) are the two primary types of muscle receptors (Hulliger et al., 1979). Sensory output from the muscle spindle detects joint position throughout the range of motion (Matthews, 1981; Caraffa et al., 1996). GTOs are located at musculotendinous junctions. During a muscle contraction this junction is stretched, distorting the receptor endings of the GTO afferent neurons. Activation of the GTO afferents leads to inhibition of the motor neurons to the stretched muscles and excitation of the motor nerves to the antagonistic muscles. This feedback loop is referred to as the inverse myotactic reflex.

In human sports medicine, several proprioceptive training programs have been shown to be effective in reducing injury rates (Caraffa et al., 1996; Hewett et al., 1999; Wedderkopp et al., 1999; Heidt et al., 2000; Myklebust et al., 2003). These programs incorporate several steps to retraining the injured athlete, as described by Caraffa and colleagues (1996). Their perturbation training program for nonsurgical anterior cruciate ligament (ACL) patients involves an early phase, exposing the athlete to perturbations in all directions with the goal of eliciting an appropriate muscular response to applied perturbations (no rigid co-contraction). The middle phase introduces light sport-specific activity during perturbation techniques, with the goal of improving athlete accuracy in matching muscle responses to perturbation intensity, direction, and speed. The late phase involves increased intensity of perturbations by using sport-specific stances. The goal is to obtain accurate, selective muscular responses to perturbations in any direction and of any intensity, magnitude, or speed.

Proprioception training exercises

The authors have four basic proprioception retraining exercises. The goal of each is to stimulate mechanoreceptors at all three levels (articular, cutaneous, and muscle).

Cavaletti poles in designs

Goal: Navigate an obstacle course without touching the poles.

Technique: First the patient is taught the game. They must walk over poles without touching any pole. They are given a treat for each positive result. Once they understand the game, the therapist creates designs and patterns for the patient to navigate (Figure 8.14).

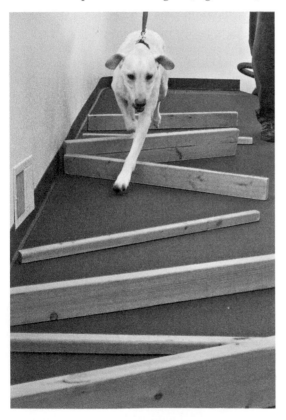

Figure 8.14 Cavaletti poles on a hill, in a pattern, and with differently sized boards, are very mentally and physically challenging exercises. The closer the boards are together, the harder it is for the patient, as they must decide the spaces in which to step to avoid knocking the boards. Source: Photo by Whitney Rupp.

Progression: Move the poles closer together so that the patient needs to decide whether to step between or over two poles. Next create patterns on a hill, then patterns on a hill with the poles at different heights.

Zigzag walking on a hill

Goal: Walk across the slope of a hill in both directions while maintaining a coordinated gait. This exercise challenges the proprioceptive system by having the patient lift contralateral feet higher on the slope in each direction (Figure 8.15).

Technique: Traverse the hill at a 10- to 80-deree angle to the slope. Turn every two to eight strides maintaining the same angle to the slope but walking in the opposite direction.

Progression: Change directions more frequently and with a steeper slope.

Rocker/wobble board

Rocker board goal: Patient should be able to maintain balance while the rehabilitation therapist applies nonrhythmic perturbations to the board.

Rocker board technique: Starting with the patient's thoracic or pelvic limbs on the ground and the other two limbs on the board, the rehabilitation therapist controls the board. The motion applied to the board should be nonrhythmic to prevent the patient from anticipating the board's motions.

Rocker board progression: A higher board can be used. More sudden movements can be applied. The stable feet can be placed on a surface above the board. The front and rear feet can both be on unstable surfaces.

Wobble board goal: The patient should be able to maintain balance while the rehabilitation therapist applies nonrhythmic perturbations to the board.

Wobble board technique: The wobble board is designed to move in all directions whereas the rocker board moves in just one plane. Because the wobble board forces more engagement of the proprioceptive system; it is particularly advantageous for patients with early neurological disease and for puppies.

Wobble board goal: The patient should be able to maintain balance while the rehabilitation therapist applies nonrhythmic perturbations to the board.

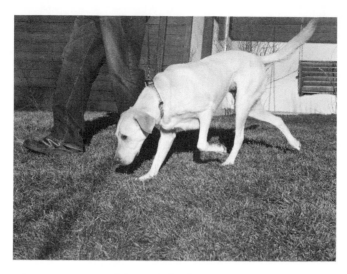

Figure 8.15 Trotting in a zigzag pattern up and down a hill enhances proprioception as each step is at a different height. Source: Photo by Whitney Rupp.

Wobble board technique: Place the weakest legs on the board, whether the thoracic or pelvic limbs or, in small to medium sized patients, all four limbs. The rehabilitation therapist can control the patient using a harness if needed and should try not to let the dog lean on them for support. The rehabilitation therapist applies nonrhythmic movements to the board, forcing the patient to react to maintain balance.

Wobble board progression: Feet that are not on the board can be placed on an elevated and/ or unstable surface (disc or noodle), shifting the weight onto the weak limbs on the board. This increases the difficulty from simple balance to balance accompanied by strength. When multiple reps of this exercise are too easy, the patient is moved to a more challenging unstable surface such as a ball or to more difficult land exercises.

Weaves

Goal: Walk through the pattern of poles in a coordinated manner (good body posture) and make a tight pivot turn at each end of the pattern.

Technique: Use a minimum of six traffic cones set 18 to 48 inches apart, depending upon the patient's size and current level of ability (more closely placed cones are more difficult). The patient should walk alternately to the right and the left of the cones with the handler staying outside of the pattern. The patient should pivot tightly around each end pole to work on

balance while making sharp turns. To improve flexibility or proprioception on one side of the patient, use an odd number of cones. This causes the patient to have to turn in the same direction around each end pole. Agility dogs should not do this exercise because it might interfere with their performance of the weave poles by training a similar but different skill that should be performed more slowly than is required in competition.

Progression: More tightly spaced cones, stepping over poles when walking beside the cones, faster reps.

Proprioception

Progression: Once the patient can navigate each of the proprioceptive activities, proprioception can be further improved by having the dog perform multiple different exercises in a circuit. This can be further advanced by having the dog perform multiple repetitions of the entire circuit.

Balance and weight shifting

Goal: Improve balance and isometric contraction.

Balance beam

Technique: Using the planks described above, the patient is asked to walk along a plank without stepping off.

Progression: The patient is asked to walk on a narrower plank, then on a warped plank, and finally to step on or over obstacles on the plank.

Balance blocks

Technique: Start with each foot standing on one of four blocks in an appropriate standing position. The patient is asked to hold this posture for gradually longer periods of time.

Progression: The blocks are brought closer to the midline, creating a narrow-based stance, until both thoracic limbs are standing on one block and both pelvic limbs are standing on the other (Figure 8.16). Then the thoracic limb block is moved closer to the pelvic limb block until all four feet are on one block.

To make this exercise more difficult, the rehabilitation therapist can add rhythmic stabilization perturbations to the patient (see below).

Trampoline, air mattress, soft cushions

Technique: After introducing the patient to this unstable surface, the rehabilitation therapist gradually increases the challenge to the patient's balance by having the patient sit or stand while the surface is moved, or having the patient move around on the surface with or without the therapist manipulating it. Soft foam cushions offer the least amount of challenge followed by discs, air mattresses, and trampolines.

Progression: Starting with two feet on the unstable surface and two feet on a stable surface, the rehabilitation therapist allows the patient to find their own balance. Once this is achieved, the patient is asked to stand on the surface with all four feet. Next, perturbations of the unstable surface are added. This exercise can be made more difficult by placing the patient's thoracic limbs on one unstable surface and the pelvic limbs on another, with perturbations added when appropriate. For the athlete working on high-end balance, the patient can stand with rear feet on a balance disc and front feet on a physioball; increasing the height difference between thoracic and pelvic limbs increases the difficulty. To strengthen the trunk and improve balance, the patient can also be asked to perform sit-to-beg on each surface.

Speed work

Goal: Improve the patient's stride length, efficiency, and burst speed.

Cavaletti poles for stride length

Technique: Starting with the poles separated by a distance equal to the patient's height at the greater tubercle, and monitoring the patient's comfort (discomfort is indicated by stutter-stepping or stepping over more than one pole), the patient is trotted through a set of six to

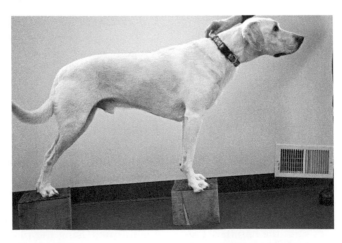

Figure 8.16 The patient's limbs are placed on two blocks to enhance balance and proprioception. Source: Photo by Whitney Rupp.

eight poles. The height of the poles should be approximately half the height from the ground to the dog's accessory carpal pad throughout this exercise.

Progression: The distance between the poles is slowly increased, encouraging the patient to increase thoracic limb reach and pelvic limb drive. This is done until the patient is incapable of taking longer strides as indicated by taking two steps between each pair of poles.

Burst exercises (intervals)

Technique: The patient is first warmed up by walking and then trotting appropriate to their level of fitness. Sprints are added. These may involve chasing a ball or other rapid acceleration activity. Two to ten repetitions are completed, followed by a slight cool down, and then more sprints. The number of intervals and length of each exertion period is increased based upon the patient's ability. Patients generally start with two to three intervals of two to five bursts. The high-end athlete should be able to complete five sets of 10 repetitions. The therapist should monitor for signs of fatigue or sore muscles after this work.

When working with the high-end athlete that is training for competition, the goal is to replicate the movements they will do in competition. When working with a new athlete, skills are trained once or twice per week. For the seasoned athlete, training should focus on sprints and endurance, with minimal attention paid to skill training unless an injury has interrupted training for more than 3 to 4 weeks, in which case skill training needs to be reviewed before competition.

Endurance work

Walking, running, and swimming are used to condition patients whose jobs require long duration running and/or trotting.

Goal: Increase the duration and intensity of training as the patient's fitness improves. A conditioned police dog may run on the treadmill with the incline at near maximum levels for up to 60 minutes. Retrievers may practice five to six water retrieves of up to 150 yards or sprint work involving 30 to 50 ball retrieves. The rehabilitation therapist should emphasize cross training on all endurance skills to prevent overtraining injury as well as boredom and frustration for the patient.

The stabilizer muscles also require training that increases stamina, and the physioball can be very helpful with this. The first technique is termed walking-forward-with-the-ball. The patient's front feet are placed on a peanut ball, with the patient in control of the ball. As the rehabilitation therapist encourages the patient to move forward, the patient's rear feet walk forward while the front feet must step backward to keep the ball in control and rolling forward. This exercise progresses to backward-walking-with-the-ball. With the patient in the same position on the ball, the therapist rolls the ball encouraging the patient to walk backward with the rear feet. This requires that the patient step forward with the front feet on the ball. The next level of difficulty is to have the patient circle the ball while keeping the front feet on the ball. The pelvic limbs walk in a clockwise or counterclockwise direction around the ball. These three ball exercises work the abductors, adductors, and joint stabilizers of all four limbs and the trunk.

Unilateral or focal strengthening

Goal: Increase weight bearing on the affected limb to increase strength on that side. These exercises are for the patient who is already fully and appropriately walking on the limb, but who requires unilateral exercise to attain symmetry.

Hill walking perpendicular to the slope

This exercises the uphill limbs, as this side has to push off and resist gravity to a greater extent than the downhill limbs. This exercise requires the rehabilitation therapist to walk across the hill so that the affected limb is consistently working harder than the contralateral limb. If the patient appears to use the uninjured limb more than the affected limb, the patient is reassessed and, if needed, treated for pain before increasing the difficulty of the exercise.

Hill sit-to-stand or push-ups

Technique: The patient is oriented perpendicular to the slope with the affected limb downhill. Initially, the patient is asked to maintain a square sit, resisting the tendency to slip downhill, for 30 seconds.

Progression: The patient is then asked to perform repetitive sit-to-stand exercises for pelvic limb strengthening or push-ups (down-to-sits) for thoracic limb strengthening.

Three legs on a wobble board

This technique is used to strengthen the limb that is not on the board without creating any shear force on the joints.

Progression: The rehabilitation therapist adds more jerky perturbations to the board and/or uses wobble board progression as discussed earlier.

Three leg stands

Technique: The therapist lifts one leg, holding it for 3 to 10 seconds, forcing the patient to balance on the other three limbs. Once the first limb is gently placed on the ground the next limb is lifted. Lifting each of the four limbs constitutes one repetition.

Hemi-stand and hemi-walk

Technique: The therapist lifts two of the patient's legs, and asks him to stand or walk on two limbs. Standing is usually done by picking up ipsilateral limbs and shifting weight to the contralateral side. Walking is usually performed by picking up either the thoracic limbs or pelvic limbs and pushing, not pulling, the patient to encourage them to take steps with the limbs that are on the ground.

Leg lifts

Technique: While the dog is standing square, the therapist tickles the toes on the limb that requires strengthening to induce the patient to move the limb in the desired direction, creating either adduction, abduction, full limb flexion, or upper joint extension with flexion of the two distal joints.

Therapy band

Technique: The band is positioned around the affected limb with the dog standing square. Tension is applied in the direction opposite the action of the muscle that is to be strengthened.

Exercises for orthopedic disorders

Spinal/neurological impairments

Stand with ball support

Purpose: Engage limb muscles before the patient is able to support full weight.

Goal: Minimize atrophy and stimulate strong contractions.

Technique: Patients that are unable to support full weight can be placed over a round or peanut ball with their weight supported through their chest on the ball. This allows the patient to contract the limb muscles through rocking and perturbations. The patient will reach out for support, causing muscle contractions in the limbs.

Progression: The patient can progress to standing on their own. The next step is to have them support themselves with either the thoracic or pelvic limbs on a cushion.

Ball or cushion work

Purpose 1: Strengthen stabilizer muscles of the limbs.

Goal: Strong contractions of the limb and trunk muscles.

Technique: Ataxic patients are placed on a cushion. This encourages the patient to work to maintain balance. Once the patient is stronger, the therapist can cause perturbations of the cushion.

Purpose 2: To strengthen neck muscles. This exercise is referred to as head-in-a-box.

Goal: Increase the length of time that the patient is able to move its head and change its center of gravity while maintaining balance with the front feet on a chair or ball.

Technique: The patient stands with front feet on a cushion, ball, or chair while the therapist moves a cookie around the patient's head to get him to move his head in all directions. The name of the exercise implies the imagery of the patient's head surrounded by a box. The cookie is moved to all areas of the box, causing the patient to fully use the neck muscles in active range of motion. No resistance is used at this point (Figure 8.17).

Rhythmic stabilization

Rhythmic stabilization, as explained in Chapter 5, is alternating isometric contractions of opposing (agonist and antagonist) muscles.

Purpose: To strengthen the stabilizer muscles of the limbs and trunk.

Goal: The muscles of the trunk are engaged without the patient taking a step.

Technique: This exercise can be made progressive for the neuro patient as follows: For the patient that is unable to support its weight but can lie in sternal recumbency, gentle perturbations are applied while encouraging the patient to maintain this position. Once the patient is able to support itself in a sit position, it is asked to sit tall (Figure 8.18) while gentle perturbations are applied. Next, with the patient standing squarely, the movements are repeated, finally progressing to having the patient perform the exercise while standing on an unstable surface.

Sit-up-and-beg and beg-to-stand

Purpose: Strengthen core and pelvic limb musculature.

Goal: Complete multiple reps of the exercise without falling. Swaying is OK.

Technique: The patient is encouraged to sit squarely to prevent putting abnormal stress on the stifles. The therapist asks the patient to sit up. For the patient that is unstable, the therapist can assist by supporting one foot. Holding the foot higher gives more support to the patient. As the patient grows stronger, the foot can be lowered, encouraging the patient to hold the

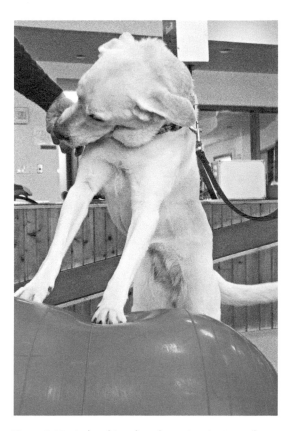

Figure 8.17 In head-in-a-box the patient is tempted with food to place their head in all possible positions to strengthen the neck muscles. This exercise also strengthens thoracic limbs, pelvic limbs, and trunk by maintaining balance while constantly shifting weight. Source: Photo by Whitney Rupp.

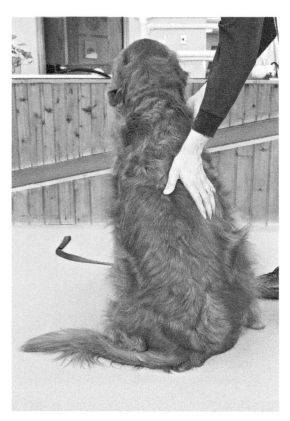

Figure 8.18 The tall sit can be made more challenging by adding perturbations. Source: Photo by Whitney Rupp.

beg position alone. Patients with strong legs and weak cores will attempt to stand up on their pelvic limbs rather than holding the beg position.

Progression: To strengthen core and pelvic limb musculature, the dog is started in the beg position (Figure 8.19) and then encouraged to stand up on the pelvic limbs, gradually returning to the beg position without allowing the front feet to touch the floor. The standing exercise involves concentric contractions, so is relatively easy for the patient, whereas the return to beg position requires eccentric contractions that are significantly more challenging.

Dance

Purpose: Strengthen the pelvic limb and trunk muscles.

Goal: Strong contractions of the muscles of the core and pelvic limbs without the patient

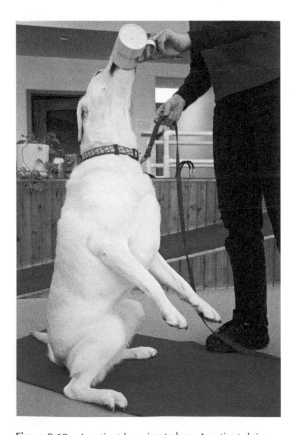

Figure 8.19 A patient learning to beg. A patient doing sit-up-and-beg needs to sit squarely with their body-weight almost entirely over the pelvic limbs. Source: Photo by Whitney Rupp.

pulling forward to support the majority of weight on the thoracic limbs and without thoracolumbar flexion.

Technique: The patient is encouraged to stand on the pelvic limbs with the front feet on an elevated surface high enough for the thoracic limbs to be extended, the thoracolumbar spine maintained in a neutral position, and the hips comfortably extended (Figure 8.20A,B). As the patient gains strength and confidence in the exercise, the surface under the front feet can be raised.

Progression: Front or rear feet are placed on an unstable surface such as a cushion, progressing to a ball.

Snoopy exercises

Purpose: Strengthen the trunk muscles without causing any compression or loading to the spine.

Goal: The patient engages the core musculature to the point of starting to sway.

Technique: With the patient standing squarely on all four feet, one front foot is lifted and placed on a block. Next, the diagonal rear foot is lifted, placing it on a similar sized block.

Note: The limbs should be elevated in a straight anterior/posterior direction rather than allowing abduction of the limbs leading to spinal rotation. The patient is observed for any trunk sway, indicating that the exercise is challenging. If the patient does not sway, the difficulty of the exercise is increased by having the dog stand with elevated legs on higher blocks, with the height of the blocks never exceeding the height of the patient's stifle. Next, the therapist lifts the limbs at the carpal and tarsal joints with minimal support, using two fingers, rather than the entire hand. The legs are lifted to the height of the carpus, gradually increasing the extension of each limb until sway is observed (Figure 8.21).

Final progression: Add rhythmic stabilization while maintaining full limb extension.

Goosing

Purpose: Strengthen abdominal musculature in patients with lordosis. This is contraindicated in patients with kyphosis.

Goal: Visibly lift the thoracolumbar spine.

Technique: With the patient standing squarely, the therapist tickles the ventral chest,

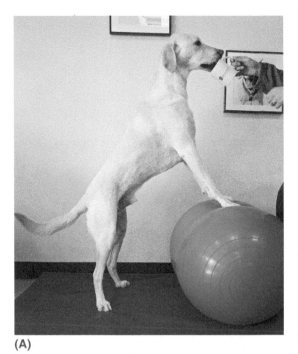

(A)

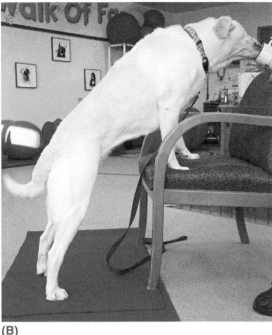

(B)

Figure 8.20   (A) The patient's thoracic limbs are placed on the ball with the weight shifted to the pelvic limbs. The patient must use all four limbs and trunk muscles to maintain balance and control of the ball. Peanut butter is a great training tool. (B) Incorrect position. This patient is leaning forward, placing too much weight on the thoracic limbs and stressing the trunk. The position can be adjusted by moving the peanut butter mug to shift the dog's weight toward its pelvic limbs. Source: Photos by Whitney Rupp.

ventral abdomen, or caudal thigh area to create contraction of the abdominal musculature leading to thoracolumbar flexion. This position is maintained for 3 to 20 seconds depending on the patient's ability. Within 3 to 5 weeks of daily work, a significant improvement is expected in the topline.

Cookie stretches

Purpose: Stretch the paraspinal muscles. This exercise is also used to assess spinal flexibility and pain in the associated musculature.

Goal: Full cervical and thoracic lateral spinal flexion with or without lumbar lateral spinal flexion; full cervical and thoracic ventroflexion with or without lumbar spinal flexion; full cervical, thoracic, and lumbar extension; and moderate cervical and thoracic rotation.

Technique: The therapist should find a treat of significantly high value to make the patient wish to comply with this exercise. In addition, the treat must be durable enough for the patient to nibble on it throughout the entire exercise.

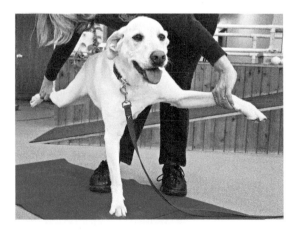

Figure 8.21   Snoopies, or diagonal leg lifts, can be done with blocks or by lifting the limbs, making certain not to let the patient abduct the legs or lean on the therapist to support their balance. Source: Photo by Whitney Rupp.

With the patient standing squarely, the therapist stands at the rear of the patient facing perpendicular to the direction of the patient's spine with the patient's caudal thighs touching the therapist's leg (Figure 8.22). This prevents

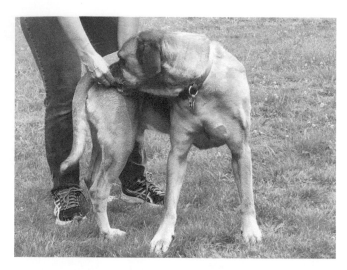

Figure 8.22   Lateral flexion of the spine and thoracic stretching are achieved by having the dog follow a cookie placed at the shoulder then moved along the body wall from the shoulder to the hip.

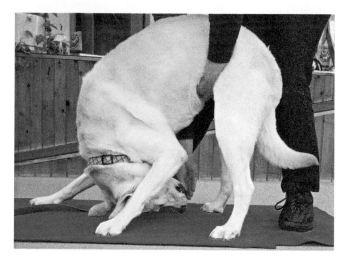

Figure 8.23   Ventral flexion of the spine is achieved by placing a cookie at the manubrium, then moving it to the floor between the feet and gradually moving the cookie caudally along the floor until the patient's head is parallel to the floor. Source: Photo by Whitney Rupp.

the dog from stepping aside to avoid completing the stretches. A cookie is first placed in front of the patient's nose, then moved to the point of one shoulder to initiate cervical lateral flexion as the patient's head follows the cookie. Next, the cookie is moved slowly along the body wall in a straight line from the shoulder to the hip to encourage thoracic stretching. Some patients can reach their nose to their tuber ischium. Next, the cookie is moved distally along the pelvic limb to the rear foot to engage spinal rotation.

The second stretch begins with the cookie at the manubrium. It is then moved to the floor between the front feet, gradually moving caudally along the floor with the goal of reaching a point where the top of the patient's head is parallel to the floor (Figure 8.23) .

For the third exercise, the patient's front feet should be on a surface elevated at least as high as the dorsal rim of the patient's scapula. The cookie is held above the patient's eyes, encouraging the nose to be held perpendicular to the floor creating cervical, thoracic, and lumbar spinal extension as indicated by thoraco-lumbar concavity.

Pelvic limb exercise

Side stepping

Purpose: Strengthen the thoracic and pelvic limb abductor and adductor muscles, particularly the gluteal, pectineus, and pectoralis muscles.

Goal: Full abduction and adduction with the feet crossing over once the patient is strong enough to do so.

Technique: With the patient standing perpendicular to the therapist's path, the collar is held in one hand while the other hand is placed 1–2″ from the opposite hip. The second hand is there so that if the patient tries to twist out of position, the hand gently reminds them that it is not an acceptable alternative to straight side stepping. Alternatively, one can use the suitcase harness described earlier, as this gives the handler the ability to drive the patient sideways without the patient being able to spin away. The therapist steps forward taking equidistant steps to keep the pelvis square so as not to stress the therapist's lower back, encouraging the patient to step sideways away from the therapist.

Progression: Have the patient side step over poles, up and down hills, and on a peanut ball. The patient that is able to perform side steps on hills or inclines should perform equal reps moving up and down the hill as well as to the left and to the right.

Sit-to-stand

Purpose: Strengthen the hamstring and gluteal muscles.

Goal: Sit squarely and use only pelvic limbs in transitioning to stand.

Technique: The patient is asked to sit squarely from a square stance. While holding the collar to prevent the patient from stepping forward, the therapist tickles the abdomen to encourage the patient to stand by extending only the pelvic limbs. If the patient places a pelvic limb laterally, the therapist tickles the foot to encourage its return to a square position. The therapist should not move the foot for the patient, as this will not change the behavior. To

strengthen one side more than the other, when asking the patient to rise, the therapist gently moves the collar to the affected side. Though this is a simple exercise, like human sit-ups or push-ups, many repetitions can quickly lead to increased strength.

Progression: This exercise can be performed on progressively more unstable surfaces or facing up an incline, but not down as this would allow the dog to overuse the thoracic limbs instead of the pelvic limbs.

Backwards walking

Purpose: Strengthen hamstring, gluteal, and triceps muscles.

Goal: Step back with full extension of hip, stifle, tarsus, and elbow rather than squatting or hopping.

Technique 1: With the patient standing squarely, a cookie is held to the thoracic inlet while the therapist walks toward the patient's front, encouraging him to back up.

Technique 2: With the patient standing parallel to a wall and the therapist standing at his side, one hand is used to prevent the patient from stepping away from the wall, while the other gently guides the patient to step backward.

Technique 3: Using the suitcase harness with equal pressure in each hand, guide the patient backward.

Technique 4 (for the obedience-trained dog): With the patient standing in heel position, the therapist walks backward quickly enough to prevent the patient from sitting or crouching with the pelvic limbs.

Sitting on a hill

Purpose: Strengthen the gluteal and hamstring muscles.

Goal: Maintain the patient's body perpendicular or parallel to the slope while facing up hill.

Technique: With the patient facing perpendicular to the slope, the therapist asks for a square sit, not allowing the hips to slide downhill or the front feet to point downhill. With the patient facing uphill, the therapist asks for a square sit without the patient pulling weight forward onto his thoracic limbs or letting his hips slide downhill. The patient will attempt to face downhill to evade the effort required.

Progression: Move to a steeper incline or perform more repetitions of sit-to-stands on the hill.

Thoracic limb exercises

Wheelbarrow

Purpose: Strengthen the thoracic limb and core musculature.

Goal: Full contractions of thoracic limb and trunk muscles.

Technique: Using a rear end sling or hands under the abdomen, the therapist lifts the patient by the caudal abdomen until the pelvic limbs are one inch off the ground, being certain that there is no thoracolumbar spinal extension or carpal hyperextension. The therapist observes for contractions of trunk and/or thoracic limb muscles. This can be a stationary exercise, or the patient can be asked to walk forward on the thoracic limbs. The therapist must be careful not to apply direct pressure to the penis.

Contraindications: Carpal hyperextension, shoulder impairment, or pain on spinal extension.

Push-ups

Purpose: Strengthen the thoracic limb muscles.

Goal: Controlled movement throughout, using the thoracic limbs rather than the core muscles.

Technique: With the patient in a square sit, the therapist holds a cookie in front of the patient's nose and lowers it slowly until it is close to the floor before slowly sweeping the cookie forward, encouraging the patient to take very small steps with the thoracic limbs as he transitions into a sphinx position. The therapist uses the cookie in the reverse direction to encourage small thoracic limb steps back into a square sit.

Crawling

Purpose: Strengthen thoracic limb, trunk, and pelvic limb musculature.

Goal: Patient is able to reach and push with all four limbs keeping the trunk close to the floor.

Technique: On a nonslip, nonabrasive surface, a tunnel is created using cavaletti poles inserted into cones or using a line of chairs. The higher the tunnel's ceiling the easier this exercise is for the patient. The patient lies down in front of the tunnel and treats are placed at intervals throughout, encouraging the patient to crawl through the tunnel (Figure 8.24). Verbal cues are given during the crawl. Once the patient has learned this command, the exercise can be completed without the tunnel by simply holding the treat close to the ground in a way that forces the patient to reach forward with his nose, giving the verbal cue to crawl while the cookie is advanced.

Progression: Crawl in a pattern (figure 8s or through weave poles), up and down hills, and/or backward.

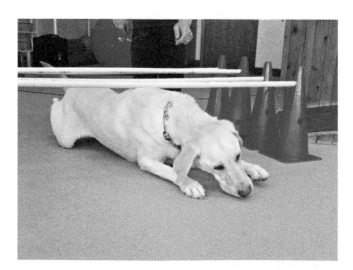

Figure 8.24   This patient is learning to crawl by using cones and PVC poles. Initially, treats are placed under the poles to make this a fun game. Source: Photo by Whitney Rupp.

High fives

Purpose: Strengthen muscles of shoulder extension, abduction, and adduction as well as thoracic limb advancement.

Goal: The patient touches one front foot to the therapist's *correct* hand. The patient must learn that his right foot must reach for the therapist's left hand no matter where the hand is placed.

Technique: The therapist shakes a cookie in a closed hand until the patient paws at the hand, the hand opens and the patient is rewarded. Next, the patient is rewarded only when he uses the correct foot. Once the patient understands the game, the cookie is no longer needed, and the therapist can place their hand in any position, encouraging extension, abduction, or adduction, and encouraging the patient to reach with the appropriate foot to complete the exercise (Figure 8.25).

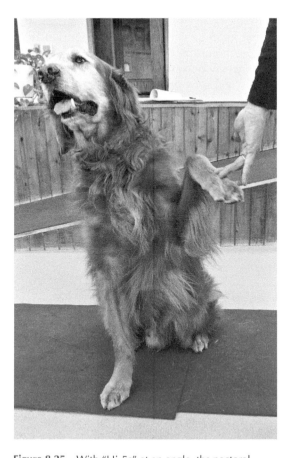

Figure 8.25 With "Hi-5s" at an angle, the pectoral, rhomboideus, and trapezius muscles are strengthened along with the supraspinatus and biceps brachii. Source: Photo by Whitney Rupp.

Neurological rehabilitation

The goal with patients with neurological disease is to challenge them, pushing them to their limits but ending on a positive note with lots of praise and encouragement. For the patient that is unable to support his weight, gentle joint compressions (described in Chapter 6) are used initially.

Purpose: Stimulate proprioceptive fibers; encourage joint fluid circulation; and enhance circulation to adjacent tissues. This can be accomplished in multiple positions for each joint.

Tickling

Purpose: Minimize atrophy of flexors and extensors of the limbs.

Goal: Cause flexion of entire limb by stimulating the toes. In the pelvic limb, stimulate sufficiently to cause not only flexion, but also a secondary kicking of the limb into extension.

Technique: The therapist tickles or pinches toes, pads, or fur between the pads until desired effect is obtained.

Sphinx lying

This is a transitional posture between lateral recumbency and sitting. Patients with neurological disease may present with restrictions in multiple joints and spasticity or weakness. Patients with cervical neurological disease often present with thoracic limb extension and weakness in shoulder flexors.

Purpose: Encourage appropriate posture early in neurological rehabilitation to allow for more normal transitions as function returns.

Goal: Achieve a posture with elbows caudal to shoulders and full hip, stifle, and tarsal flexion.

Technique: The patient is positioned in this posture, supporting him as needed.

Progression: Add rhythmic stabilization.

Tall sits

Purpose: Strengthen the core musculature.

Goal: Achieve a normal postured sit with carpi under shoulders, feet appropriately positioned on the floor, and spine and trunk in a normal orientation (not leaning in either direction and showing no kyphosis).

Technique: The patient is positioned into a square sit with carpi directly under the shoulders, not allowing the feet to slide forward or to collapse into carpal flexion. The patient is encouraged to hold this posture for as long as possible (Figure 8.26A,B).

Progression: Add rhythmic stabilization.

Standing

Purpose: Re-educate normal posture.

Goal: Stand in square position, supporting full weight independently.

Technique: With the patient in a square stand, muscle groups that appear weak are stimulated. For instance, if the patient has lordosis, the abdomen is goosed; if leaning, the side is tickled; if collapsing a joint, the extensors are stimulated.

Progression: Add rhythmic stabilization.

Transitions

Purpose: Re-education of movements from lateral recumbency to a standing position.

Goal: Independent and appropriate transitions.

Technique: Once the patient can hold a posture, the transition movement into this posture is trained. *Lateral to sphinx:* With the patient in lateral recumbency, a cookie is moved toward the shoulder to encourage lifting the head. The toes of the down thoracic limb are pinched to encourage shoulder and elbow flexion. The toes of both pelvic limbs are then pinched to create flexion in both pelvic limbs, while tickling the chest and body wall on the down side to encourage lifting away from the floor.

Progression: For the patient that can hold the sphinx position, transition from sphinx to tall sit. While an assistant kneels behind the patient to prevent slipping back or falling to one side, the therapist holds a cookie to the patient's nose, lifting it over the nose while pinching the front toes to encourage stepping backward until a proper sitting position is attained. The carpal joints may need to be supported once this position is reached.

Progression to stand: With the patient in a tall sit, the therapist moves a cookie forward from

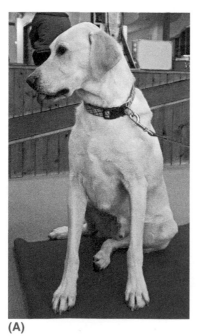
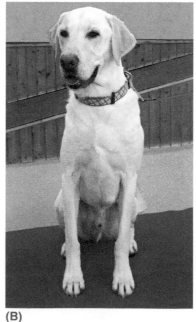

(A)   (B)

Figure 8.26   (A) An unbalanced sit puts abnormal stresses on the joints of the pelvic limbs as well as the pelvis and spine. (B) A square sit is maintained by having the hips, stifles, and tarsi in a straight line with the shoulders over the carpal joints. The spine should be straight as well. The tall sit can be made more challenging by adding perturbations. Source: Photos by Whitney Rupp.

the nose while tickling the pubic bone area to encourage hip, stifle, and tarsal extension. In the beginning, this exercise is usually done with two people.

Weight shifting for balance

Purpose: Strengthen the stabilizer muscles to improve posture during ambulation.

Goal: Achieve proper balance while standing on two to three limbs.

Technique: The therapist lifts each limb just off the ground using two fingers to minimize assistance, observing for trunk muscle contraction. Swaying indicates challenge. The foot is lowered when fatigue is evident. Rotate through all four feet.

Progression: Lift two feet (diagonal or ipsilateral), and repeat as above.

Isometrics

Purpose: Strengthen postural muscles.

Goal: Patient is able to resist loading over the scapulae or pelvis without collapsing.

Technique: With the patient in a square stand, the therapist places a palm over the scapulae or pelvis, applying gentle downward pressure with even distribution left to right. During pelvis work, the abdomen is tickled so the patient does not think they are required to sit.

Wobble board

Purpose: Strengthen stabilizer muscles, and enhance balance and proprioception.

Goal: Patient is able to maintain balance while therapist applies nonrhythmic perturbations to the board.

Technique: See previous discussion in this chapter.

Patterning

This is the last exercise done in a progression of exercises before ambulation is attempted in a patient with ataxia or paresis. The overall goal is to first work on transition from lateral to sternal recumbency, sternal recumbency to a tall sit, and a tall sit to stand using reps of sit-to-stand to "turn on" the pelvic limb muscles, work on balance by stimulating the muscles of the trunk (isometrics and weight shifting as above), pat-

terning to remind the body of the progression of steps, and then assisted ambulation. When the patterning step is eliminated, the ambulation is noticeably less coordinated and the progression is hampered.

Purpose: Helping the patient with neurological disease, who has initiated the progression through transitions from lateral recumbency to stand, to develop an appropriate gait pattern as well as balance and transitions in dynamic movement.

Goal: Normal or close to normal ambulation. Gait patterning is a manner of moving the feet and the pattern of footsteps at various speeds.

Technique: With the patient standing, the therapist moves each foot through the full stride, incorporating the stance and swing phases. The proper footfall for walk is one pelvic limb followed by the ipsilateral thoracic limb, then the other pelvic limb followed by the ipsilateral thoracic limb. The patient may be supported with an assistive device, allowing weight shifting away from and stimulation of the next limb to move.

Most patients with neurological disease have increased tone in the adductors, which may lead to adduction and tripping or stumbling during ambulation. If this is present, the patient is asked to stand and the caudomedial aspect of the foot is stimulated by the therapist to cause contraction of the abductor muscles. A finger is placed on the gluteal and biceps femoris muscles to confirm contraction during the adductor stimulation. After 10 repetitions, ambulation is again attempted and the outcome should be no or significantly less crossing over. This exercise is performed before doing any ambulation work in patients that do not yet have an appropriate gait pattern.

Progression: Speed is increased to the appropriate speed for walking, and assistance is decreased. One way to stimulate ambulation and give mild assistance is to support the dog by holding the base of the tail at up to a 45° angle to the floor; this does not cause discomfort or affect the spine. As the dog's balance improves, hand placement on the tail can gradually move caudally until just the hair on the tip of the tail is held for minor balance support.

Once the patient can rise and walk independently the next step is to add weaves (from gentle to tight), hills (straight up and down, adding

Case Study 8.2 Hemilaminectomy

Signalment: 5 y.o. F/S Dachshund. Immediate P.O. L2-3 hemilaminectomy with fenestrations, cranial and caudal.

Clinical findings: Left pelvic limb: No conscious proprioception (CP), diminished deep pain, intact superficial pain, minimal voluntary motion. Right pelvic limb: No CP, present deep and superficial pain, diminished voluntary motion. No ROM, joint, or muscle abnormalities found.

Goal: Normal neurological status and ambulation

Therapy: Throughout therapy: massage of the muscles, PROM, and joint compressions were done. Exercises performed in a certain order to turn on the nervous and musculoskeletal systems, with ambulation at the conclusion.

Initial exercises, done while patient needed assistance rising and ambulating, started with transitions from lateral recumbency to sternal to sit-to-stand, with facilitation used on whichever muscle groups were not firing appropriately. Square sit-to-stand exercises, weight shifting to the left rear foot by diagonal and then contralateral leg lifts, standing alone,

followed by standing with rhythmic stabilizations, patterning of each limb in the proper order (10 reps), and finally ambulation exercises making sure each foot stepped appropriately in sequence and bore weight correctly.

Once patient could rise unassisted and ambulate, but with moderate ataxia and frequent falling, different exercises, again in a specific order, to work on balance and trunk strength, were initiated. Sit-to-stands; standing with rhythmic stabilization; single pelvic limb elevation to make patient balance on one pelvic limb at a time; rear feet on rocker board; front feet on pool noodle; low cavaletti poles 1.5 × patient's body length apart; hill walking; widely spaced weave poles; 3″-high steps.

As patient progressed to mild ataxia, exercise regime included circuit course of cavaletti poles in increasingly difficult patterns and, later, patterns on a hill; front feet on peanut ball walking forward and backward; standing on peanut ball; tightly spaced weaves; 3″ steps; balance beam. As patient progressed, small obstacles were placed on beam for her to step over.

Goal was successfully attained.

---

zigzags to challenge proprioception), and stepping over cavaletti poles. *Note:* Each time the patient is worked, the therapist should use multiple exercises that challenge transitions, then balance, then pattern, finally putting it all together in ambulation. Different exercises can be used each time to keep the work fresh for the patient, always focusing upon where the patient is weak. As the dog progresses, avoid any area where there might be pain as a result of previous exercise.

Land treadmill

The land treadmill can be used for patients with neurological disease, any patient needing endurance work, patients requiring pelvic limb strengthening and weight shifting to the rear, and especially patients after pelvic limb surgery, who tend to habitually transfer weight to the thoracic limbs. The treadmill encourages rebalancing during ambulation. It can be used

in reverse or on an incline for specific patients where the focus is on hamstring and/or gluteal strength. Lauer and colleagues (2009) found that a 5% incline increased the electromyographic activity of the hamstring muscle group in dogs walking on treadmills.

The treadmill should be placed so that it faces something that the patient would like to walk toward, rather than a wall. If using a human treadmill, a sidewall is needed on each side, or the treadmill can be placed against a wall on one side, to prevent patients from stepping off to the side.

Getting started

Training the patient to use the treadmill is simple if a few important steps are followed. A harness and or a nonchoke collar with a leash are used, with the handler holding the harness or leash so that the patient has approximately 1 foot of play forward and backward. The patient

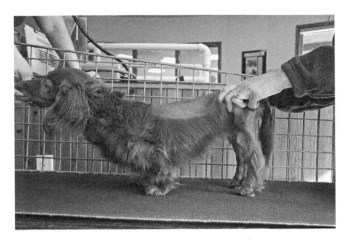

Figure 8.27   Hand position is important when assisting a patient to ambulate on the treadmill. The therapist must assist without impeding motion and stimulate the motions that the patient has the hardest time performing. Source: Photo by Whitney Rupp.

is walked over the tread three times from back to front. Each time the patient completes this action he is given lots of praise and a treat as positive reinforcement. On the third pass, the patient is asked to sit or lie down on the belt, then get off for the reward. On the fourth pass, with the patient standing, the tread is started, getting it to the appropriate walk speed for this patient within 1–2 seconds. If this is done too slowly, it is confusing for the patient. Done too quickly, the patient will panic and crouch onto the tread, risking falling off the back of the belt. The handler must have a cookie available at all times to encourage the patient to rise if he is starting to crouch.

Goal: The patient should move in a proper walk, amble, or trot, not a pace (see Chapters 2 and 10 for more details). If the patient paces at what should be a trot speed, the handler should tug gently to the side on the collar, causing a brief moment of imbalance, which will generally create a transition to the trot.

Belt speed

Patients with neurological disease are generally started using a slow belt speed of 0.1–0.5 miles per hour (0.16–0.8 kilometers per hour)—just fast enough to encourage a walk. If a treadmill is not available, the therapist can lean over the patient while walking forward and move the

feet in a proper pattern (Figure 8.27). For neurologically intact patients, the speed should allow for a comfortable walk with no pauses in footfalls. As the speed increases, the patient will go through an amble (fast walk) to the trot. The appropriate trotting speed is a function of the patient's body type. A Dachshund may trot well at 1.2 to 1.5 miles per hour (1.9–2.4 kilometers per hour) while a Golden Retriever will trot at closer to 4 to 5 miles per hour (6.4–8 kilometers per hour). Border Collies are often not comfortable at a walk and may trot at slower than expected speeds.

Endurance exercise

Endurance exercise on a treadmill should not begin before the patient has reached skeletal maturity. Additionally, warm-up and cooldown periods of 2–5 minutes each should be incorporated into any endurance work on the treadmill. Exercises start within comfortable parameters for the patient. For an athlete, the dog can be walked at a fast speed at the highest incline, usually 11° on most canine treadmills.

The exercise period might start with three sets of 3- to 5-minute sessions, progressing to two sets of 10 to 15 minutes, then to one set of 20 to 30 minutes. When the patient can work at this pace and incline for 20 to 30 minutes, the progression includes adding two to three sets of 1 to 2 minutes at a working trot. Progression is based upon the patient's reaction on getting off the treadmill as well as tongue shape, facial expression, and tail posture during the exercise.

Heart rate monitors can be used to mirror interval training in human patients. An athlete can do this exercise three to five times per week. Progression ends when the patient can spend 30 minutes on the treadmill, doing a 2-minute warm up, a fast trot for 26 minutes, and a 2-minute cool down. To keep the patient challenged, the therapist or client can add reverse walking, gradually increasing this to 6 to 8 minutes of walking backward. As always, the therapist should be prepared with plans to change the exercise duration, environment, or equipment as needed to keep the patient/athlete motivated and progressing toward short- and long-term goals.

References

Caraffa, A., Cerulli, G., Projetti, M., Aisa, G., & Rizzo, A. 1996. Prevention of anterior cruciate ligament injuries in soccer. A prospective controlled study of proprioceptive training. *Knee Surg Sports Traumatol Arthrosc*, 4, 19–21.

Chu, D. A. & Shiner, J. 2007. Plyometrics in rehabilitation. In: Donatelli, R. (ed.), *Sports-Specific Rehabilitation*. St Louis, MO: Churchill Livingstone-Elsevier, p. 233.

Clayton, H. M. 2016. Core training and rehabilitation in horses. *Vet Clin Equine*, 32(2), 49–71.

Connell, L. 2010. Small animal post-operative orthopaedic rehabilitation. *The Veterinary Nurse*, 1(1), 12–21.

Davies, W. L. 2017. Managing assistive devices in the rehabilitation practice. In: *Proceedings Western Veterinary Conference*, Las Vegas, pp. 1–4.

Drum, M. G., Marcellin-Little, D. J., & Davis, M. S. 2015. Principles and applications of therapeutic exercises for small animals. *Vet Clin Small Anim*, 45(1), 73–90.

Ghez, C. 1991. Posture. In: Kandel, E., Schwartz, J., & Jessell, T. (eds), *Principles of Neural Science*. New York, NY: Elsevier, pp. 533–547.

Goldberg, M. E. 2016. Getting started in physical rehabilitation. *Today's Veterinary Technician*, Mar/April, pp. 54–59.

Heidt, R. S., Jr Sweeterman, L. M., Carlonas, R. L., Traub, J. A., & Tekulve, F. X. 2000. Avoidance of soccer injuries with preseason conditioning. *Am J Sports Med*, 28, 659–662.

Hewett, T. E., Lindenfeld, T. N., Riccobene, J. V., & Noyes, F. R. 1999. The effect of neuromuscular training on the incidence of knee injury in female athletes. A prospective study. *Am J Sports Med*, 27, 699–706.

Hewett, T. E., Paterno, M. V., & Myer, G. D. 2002. Strategies for enhancing proprioception and neuromuscular control of the knee. *Clin Orthop Relat Res*, 402, 76–94.

Hulliger, M., Nordh, E., Thelin, A. E., & Vallbo, A. B. 1979. The responses of afferent fibres from the glabrous skin of the hand during voluntary finger movements in man. *J Physiol*, 291, 233–249.

Latorre, R., Gil, F., Vazquez, J. M., Moreno, F., Mascarello, F., & Ramirez, G. 1993. Skeletal muscle fibre types in the dog. *J Anat*, 182, 329–337.

Lauer, S. K., Hillman, R. B., Li, L., & Hosgood, G. L. 2009. Effects of treadmill inclination on electromyographic activity and hind limb kinematics in healthy hounds at a walk. *Am J Vet Res*, 70, 658–664.

Lephart, S., Reimann, B., & Fu, F. 2000. *Proprioception and Neuromuscular Control in Joint Stability*, 1st edn. Champaign, IL: Human Kinetics.

Matthews, P. B. 1981. Evolving views on the internal operation and functional role of the muscle spindle. *J Physiol*, 320, 1–30.

Milhem, M., Kalichman, L., Ezra, D., & Alperovitch-Najenson, D. 2016. Work-related musculoskeletal disorders among physical therapists: A comprehensive narrative review. *Int J Occup Med Environ Health*, 29(5), 735–747.

Millis, D. L. 2015: Physical therapy and rehabilitation in dogs.In: Gaynor, J. S. & Muir, W. W. III (eds), *Handbook of Veterinary Pain Management*, 3rd edn. St Louis, MO: Elsevier/Mosby, pp. 383–421.

Myklebust, G., Engebretsen, L., Braekken, I. H., Skjolberg, A., Olsen, O. E., & Bahr, R. 2003. Prevention of anterior cruciate ligament injuries in female team handball players: a prospective intervention study over three seasons. *Clin J Sport Med*, 13, 71–78.

Newsholme, S. J., Lexell, J., & Downham, D. Y. 1988. Distribution of fibre types and fibre sizes in the tibialis cranialis muscle of beagle dogs. *J Anat*, 160, 1–8.

Price, H. 2014. Introduction to veterinary physiotherapy. *Companion Animal*, 19(3), 130–133.

Saunders, D. G. 2007. Therapeutic exercise. *Clin Tech Small Anim Pract*, 22, 155–159.

Sekendiz, B., Cug, M., & Korkusuz, F. 2010. Effects of swiss-ball core strength training on strength, endurance, flexibility, and balance in sedentary women. *J Strength Cond Res*, 24(11), 3032–3040.

Selten, E. M., Vriezekolk, J. E., Geenen, R., van der Laan, W. H., van der Meulen-dilling, R. G., Nijhof, M. W., *et al.* 2016. Reasons for treatment choices in knee and hip osteoarthritis: a qualitative study. *Arthritis Care Res*, 68(9), 1260–1267.

Sharp, B. 2010. Physiotherapy and physical rehabilitation. In: Lindley, S. & Watson, P. (eds), *BSAVA Manual of Canine and Feline Rehabilitation, Supportive and Palliative Care.* Gloucester, UK: British Small Animal Veterinary Association, pp. 90–113.

Sherrington, C. S. 1906. *The Integrative Action of the Nervous System.* New Haven, CT: Yale University Press.

Shumway-Cook, A. & Woollacott, M. 1995. *Motor Control: Theory and Practical Applications.* Baltimore, MD: Williams & Wilkins.

Steiss, J. E. 2002. Muscle disorders and rehabilitation in canine athletes. *Vet Clin North Am Small Anim Pract*, 32(1), 267–285.

Wakshlag, J. & Shmalberg, J. 2014. Nutrition for working and service dogs. *Vet Clin North Am Small Anim Pract*, 44(4), 719–740.

Wedderkopp, N., Kaltoft, M., Lundgaard, B., Rosendahl, M., & Froberg, K. 1999. Prevention of injuries in young female players in European team handball. A prospective intervention study. *Scand J Med Sci Sports*, 9, 41–47.

Westgarth, C., Christley, R. M., & Christian, H. E. 2014. How might we increase physical activity through dog walking?: A comprehensive review of dog walking correlates. *Int J Behav Nutr Phys Act*, 20(11), 83.

Zimny, M. L. 1988. Mechanoreceptors in articular tissues. *Am J Anat*, 182, 16–32.

9 Aquatic Therapy

Jody Chiquoine, MSN, FNP, CCRT, Ellen Martens, MsPT, MT, CCRT,
Laurie McCauley, DVM, DACVSMR, CVC, CVA, CCRT,
and Janet B. Van Dyke, DVM, DACVSMR, CCRT

Summary

Aquatic therapy encompasses any exercise or manual therapy completed in an aquatic environment. The benefits of aquatic therapy include the ability to offer prescriptive exercise that is functional without being painful. Balance exercises can be completed safely in an aquatic environment well before they can be attempted on land. Elevated metabolism resulting from the resistance provided by water helps to speed weight loss while increasing muscle strength. Underwater treadmill (UWTM) work adds the benefits of gradually increased weight bearing while giving the therapist the option to quickly change tread speed as needed. The inherent properties of water, including buoyancy, hydrostatic pressure, viscosity, fluid dynamics, and resistance make aquatic training efficient for achieving rehabilitation and maintaining total fitness. There is a substantial difference between *swimming* as an exercise and *aquatic therapy*, which encompasses all therapeutic work done in the water. Aquatic therapy programs are designed using the same system of short-, middle-, and long-term goals described in Chapter 8. Swim sets are interspersed with rest sets during which manual therapies can be applied. Program goals include improving flexibility, strength, balance, coordination, postural awareness, speed, and endurance. Reassessment visits determine the rate of progression of each program. Equipment used in aquatic therapy includes life vests, harnesses, slings, balance equipment, leg weights, resistance mitts, balloons, and pool noodles. Assistive and resistive techniques are employed as well as gait patterning, tail work, and facilitation. There are some breed-related swimming and UWTM characteristics about which the therapist should be aware before initiating a training session, and there also are precautions specific to the injury or surgical procedure being rehabilitated. UWTM variables include water temperature, tread speed, water depth, resistance, and duration.

Canine Sports Medicine and Rehabilitation, Second Edition. Edited by Chris Zink and Janet B. Van Dyke.
© 2018 John Wiley & Sons, Inc. Published 2018 by John Wiley & Sons, Inc.

Introduction

Benefits

Today, therapists, sports coaches and trainers understand the many benefits of aquatic therapy. Scientific research regarding the physiology of human immersion in water and applying the knowledge of water properties to aquatic treatment has revolutionized sports medicine (Thein & McNamara, 1992; Ruoti et al., 1997).

Pain is a central and consistent symptom for many canine patients and contributes to the cycle of disuse atrophy and progressive disability. Water-based therapies help to make movement more comfortable, offering prescriptive exercise that is functional, mechanically correct, and muscularly challenging without being painful (Chauvet et al., 2011). A warm water environment (86–94 °F/30–34.5 °C) offers muscle relaxation that is soothing for many conditions. This is enhanced by hydrostatic pressure causing a swaddling effect on immersed body parts (Thein & McNamara, 1992; Ruoti et al., 1997; Jadelis et al., 2001).

Aquatic therapy challenges balance and coordination. Balance exercises can be attempted earlier and more safely in water than on land, providing early opportunities for limb, trunk, and postural training, resulting in improved strength, balance, and coordination (Ruoti et al., 1997; Jadelis et al., 2001; Stager & Tanner, 2004).

Aquatic therapy raises metabolism and can help with weight loss, decreasing fat, strengthening muscles, and reducing the deconditioning effects of immobility (Ruoti et al., 1997; Lavoie & Montpetit, 1986). In humans slow, steady swimming burns a higher percentage of fat than fast swimming. Fast swimming uses carbohydrates and burns 500–700 calories per hour. Swimming, whether slow or fast, can benefit patients seeking weight loss or muscle gain (Stager & Tanner, 2004).

Swimming uses the body's muscles more completely than other activities such as running. Heredity influences the distribution of muscle fiber types, making some breeds great sprinters and others slow, steady swimmers (Stager & Tanner, 2004). The therapist should design a combined aquatic therapy program that focuses on the patient's specific needs and targets the appropriate muscle fibers. Human studies demonstrate improvement in lean body mass (especially lean leg mass), decreased body fat and reduced waist to hip ratio when using an underwater treadmill (UWTM) rather than a land treadmill (Greene et al., 2009).

Passive range of motion in humans is improved in water compared to on land (Ruoti et al., 1997). Marsolais and colleagues. (2003) reported that the active range of motion, especially in the pelvic limbs, is greater with swimming and with water walking than with land-walking.

Precautions

Sutures and staples are generally removed prior to initiating aquatic therapy. Occasionally, with the surgeon's approval, the advantages of early therapy outweigh the risks of aquatic therapy prior to suture removal (Tomlinson, 2013). When early aquatic therapy is recommended, and sutures or staples are in place, transparent film dressings such as Tegaderm™ can be applied if the surface of the skin is flat and shaved. A precautionary treatment plan should be devised for patients with respiratory problems, such as laryngeal paralysis or exertional dyspnea, and those with behavioral issues, such as mild aggression or dislike of water. It is recommended that a therapist be in the pool with the patients that may have breathing difficulties while exercising in a water environment (Carver, 2016). Aggressive dogs can frequently be handled more easily in the water as their confidence is reduced. Swimming during pregnancy can be offered if discussed with the primary veterinarian, and can be designed so that the level of exertion is appropriate. Swimming is not recommended for dogs in the first 6 weeks post tibial plateau leveling osteotomy (TPLO) or tibial tuberosity advancement (TTA) due to the increased forces that kicking places on the patellar tendon (Monk, 2016). Patients with medially luxating patellas can have difficulties with swimming as the pelvic limbs tend to abduct and externally rotate at the hip, causing increased medial drag on the patella. The therapist should be aware of this, and use manual techniques to prevent the abduction and rotation. The underwater tread-mill is preferable to swimming during early rehabilitation for patients that have had total hip replacement as swimming can cause excess strain on the soft tissues of the coxofemoral joint. Dogs with muscle/tendon injuries should avoid swimming as this can cause excessive strain on healing soft tissues. Patients with wobblers or cervical disc disease should not swim as they tend to extend their cervical spine excessively. UWTM therapy is an option for this group. Toy breed puppies and seniors should be kept warm throughout the session. During cold weather clients are asked to start and warm their car when the dog comes out of the pool so that by the time the patient is dry, the car is warm.

Physical properties of water relevant to canine sports medicine

The inherent properties of water make aquatic training efficient for achieving rehabilitation and maintaining total fitness (Bishop *et al.*, 1989; Thein & McNamara, 1992).

Buoyancy

Archimedes' principle states that when a body is wholly or partially immersed in a fluid, it experiences an upward thrust equal to the weight of the displaced fluid. As water depth increases, weight bearing decreases, thus reducing the compressive forces on joints (Bates & Hanson, 1992).

Hydrostatic pressure

Pascal's law states that fluid pressure is exerted equally on all surfaces of an immersed body at rest at a given depth; this pressure increases with the density of the fluid and depth of sub-mersion. Hydrostatic pressure reduces limb edema and pooling of fluid and blood in super-ficial and deep tissues thereby encouraging healing and reducing complication rates. Hydrostatic pressure causes a decrease in noci-ceptor sensitivity resulting in pain reduction (Bates & Hanson, 1992; Ruoti *et al.*, 1997).

The hydrostatic effects on the cardiopulmo-nary system result in a central shift of the peripheral blood volume (Arborelius *et al.*, 1972). This results in increased diuresis so patients may urinate large quantities shortly after swimming. Due to hydrostatic pressure, dogs with chest expansion problems related to congestive heart failure or pulmonary disease need careful monitoring. The hydrostatic pressure properties of aquatic therapy can be used to strengthen intercostal muscles as a mild resistance exercise.

Viscosity

Viscosity is the frictional resistance created by the cohesiveness of fluid molecules. Water is 15 times more viscous than air thus requiring more effort to move through it. Water walking for humans, with the water at shoulder height, requires 65% more effort than walking on land (Greene *et al.*, 2009). Working against viscosity increases muscle strength, tone, and cardiac fit-ness (Ruoti *et al.*, 1997). Viscosity helps weak canine patients to stand and walk before they can do so on land.

Fluid dynamics

Hydrodynamic forces impact any object in water. These forces include laminal flow, fron-tal resistance, and drag. Laminal and turbulent flow affect effort. Laminal flow is the straight flow of water particles moving at one speed and in one direction. Resistance to movement increases with the velocity of flow. Turbulent flow is the interrupted flow of water particles in all directions, creating more dramatic pressure differentials. Here, resistance increases expo-nentially with velocity. These fluid dynamic principles have clinical application when designing swimming or UWTM programs (Ruoti *et al.*, 1997).

While swimming, friction and turbulence are the dominant resistive factors (Hall *et al.*, 1990; Ruoti *et al.*, 1997). Faster swimming or water walking creates greater turbulence, resistance, and friction and therefore increases exertion (Figure 9.1). This is advantageous for patients needing an intense workout but

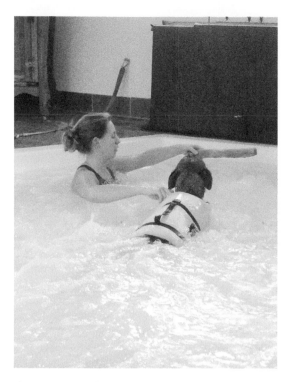

Figure 9.1 Turbulence using resistance jets increases strength training and cardiopulmonary fitness.

disadvantageous for patients that are anxious, thrashing, or deconditioned. Swimming or UWTM sessions will vary based on patient aptitude, comfort level, condition, fitness, and even coat length as longer hair increases resistance and drag.

When applying these fluid dynamic principles to dogs as they swim, the hydrodynamic forces create a pressure differential between the thoracic (high pressure) and pelvic (low pressure) limbs. Resulting eddies create tail suction, skin friction, and drag on the pelvic limbs. The pelvic limbs should respond with powerful kicking or they will sink. When a dog uses the pelvic limbs correctly the topline is at the water's surface. When the thoracic limbs, back, and tail are all fully under water, it is an indication that the pelvic limbs might be being used, but not fully. When the pelvic limbs are not used, the back is fully submerged and the thoracic limbs break the surface causing splashing (Catavitello *et al.*, 2015).

Pressure differentials and turbulence challenge the postural muscles and balance

mechanisms. This is advantageous for patients with balance and coordination impairments or those needing paraspinal and abdominal muscle strengthening.

Resistance

Resistance is controlled by speed, but surface area and equipment can also contribute (Abidin *et al.*, 1988; Bates & Hanson, 1992; Ruoti *et al.*, 1997). The speed of water flow is controlled with resistance jets (pool) or tread speed (UWTM). Surface area is controlled by water depth and equipment such as life vests, resistance mitts, balloons, and leg weights. Increased speed maximizes the plane effect when swimming, decreasing surface area in the water, and therefore decreasing resistance.

Therapeutic swimming

Muscles are used differently when swimming than when weight bearing on land (Bates & Hanson, 1992). The authors have observed greater active range of motion of canine shoulders and elbows in swimming when compared to land walking. Aquatic therapy increases the comprehensive challenge to coordination, balance, and kinesthetic movement mechanisms (Bates & Hanson, 1992). Stimulating neuroreceptors with swimming enhances early land walking in human patients (Bates & Hanson, 1992; Grosee, 2009). The authors believe that these kinesthetic movement mechanisms also apply to dogs. Tetraparetic dogs can stand in water with minimal assistance or can swim using multiple limbs before they are able to stand or walk on land.

Designing an aquatic conditioning program for the canine athlete

Canine athletes use swimming for effective rehabilitation treatment after injury or surgery and for cross training (Zink, 1997; Millis & Levine, 2013). Service dogs, search and rescue dogs, and K-9 corps members benefit from the physical and psychological advantages of swimming, and conformation dogs benefit with improved muscle tone and better endurance.

The following is a list of advantages of cross training for canine athletes (Zink, 1997)

- Engages commonly used performance muscle in a different way.
- Increases use of muscles that are used minimally on land.
- Increases joint flexibility due to greater passive range of motion (PROM)/active range of motion (AROM).
- Eliminates concussive forces to reduce joint compression/stress.
- Maximizes cardiac output and pulmonary conditioning.
- Provides a mental/psychological break from land training.
- Maintains high training levels off season.
- Allows return to performance sport with minimal training time.
- Reduces injury risk at early season competitions.
- Allows for intense exercise during warm, humid weather with no risk of overheating.

Getting started

The canine rehabilitation professional should first obtain a complete history that includes the patient's comfort in water. The medical, surgical, and sports injury history, including comorbidities, medications, and supplements, is obtained from the referring veterinarian. The objective findings are listed during physical evaluation. All subjective and objective information is integrated to formulate a clinical assessment and aquatic therapy plan. Measurable outcome goals are established with the client. Overall condition and body condition score are noted. The duration of disability and degree of muscle atrophy should also be considered. The client's ability to transport the dog to sessions is also factored into the equation. Each therapeutic program should be individualized, and should not be standardized or pre-formulated. Documentation of all aquatic therapy sessions is essential. Figure 9.2 shows an example of a system used by one author (E.M.) to record each aquatic therapy session.

Harness :

Life vest :

Swim diaper :

Toys :   yes / no

Treats :

Strength :

ROM :

Manual stimulation / motivation :

Air dry :   yes / no   Power :

Shampoo :   yes / no

	Date	Total time	Min + reps	Rest	Speed	Water height	Slope	Aids	Swimming	Jets / stimulation	Spa	Reaction to treatment
1												
2												
3												
4												
5												
6												
7												
8												
9												
10												

Figure 9.2   An example of an aquatic therapy record entry.

Program progression

Preoperative planning

Preoperative swimming allows the patient to become familiar with the pool and aquatic environment, reducing the incidence of postoperative mishaps at pool entry or exit, thrashing while swimming, and inability to rest quietly between sessions. The preoperative visit allows for client education and the opportunity to observe the progress of other patients with similar conditions (Lindley & Smith, 2010).

Factors to consider

Aquatic therapy is started conservatively, and increased according to the patient's comfort and ability. Most patients initially need body contact with the therapist in the pool. The amount of physical contact and bonding depends on the patient's comfort level and can be gradually reduced. Client's can be poolside to offer encouragement. Teaching pool commands such as "Rest" enhances responsiveness.

Swimming for 1 minute in a therapeutic pool, with current (resistance and turbulence) and a warm water environment (88–90 °F) is strenuous. A cool water pool with no resistance jets will allow for longer swim sets while a warm water therapeutic pool with varying current requires shorter swim sets due to greater effort and likely fatigue (Bates & Hanson, 1992). Vital signs are monitored by checking pulse, tongue color, size, and shape, ear temperature, and facial expression as well as alterations in swimming speed and emotional state (Table 9.1).

Table 9.1 Assessment of anxiety and fatigue when swimming

Anxiety	Fatigue
Anxious facial expression	Tired body posture
Rapid breathing/pulse	Deep or irregular breathing
Thrashing thoracic limbs	Slowed swim pace
Inability to rest	Reluctance to swim
Attempting to exit the pool	Change in tongue color/shape

During a 30-minute treatment, swim sets include multiple swim/rest cycles. As confidence and stamina increase, the swimming duration is lengthened and intensified and rest periods are shortened. During rest cycles the therapist provides treatments such as massage, standing exercises, joint mobilizations, bodywork, and PROM.

Program goals, principles, and exercises

Aquatic therapy programs use the same rehabilitation principles and goals as land-based programs. The pool becomes the gym so a myriad of exercises is offered. The primary goals for aquatic exercises are: flexibility, strength, balance, coordination, postural awareness, movement, speed, and endurance (Bates & Hanson, 1992; Grosee, 2009).

Flexibility

Flexibility is improved with stretching and joint mobilization provided during rest periods. Traction is also effectively applied.

Massage to release paraspinal trigger points and tail-pulls in water improves spinal mobility. Active exercises that improve flexibility include using food lures for lateral cervical and thoracolumbar stretching while standing or luring the dog to swim in tight circles, zigzags, or serpentine patterns.

Strength

Strength is improved with exercises that initially consist of slow swimming sets with low or no current. Circle swimming creates a differential workout for the legs on the outside and inside of the circle. Resistance can be applied by holding the harness or life vest while the dog swims. Standing exercises such as rhythmic stabilization, and cross-leg or three-leg standing can be effectively done in water. Dancing is performed with the patient standing on the pelvic limbs while the thoracic limbs rest on the pool edge or stair. This can be done safely in water before attempting the same exercise on land.

As strength improves, games are added, including multiple rapid ball-chasing sprints. Quick repetition of swimming into high current is excellent for increasing the difficulty of strength training. Throwing a ball off a backdrop encourages treading water, and is an intense strengthening work out. These games are good strength-training exercises for the rehabilitating canine athlete when vigorous land exercise or training are otherwise restricted. They also assist in preparing for returning to sports that require quick responsiveness, rapid acceleration, and speed while running and jumping. Leg weights and swim mitts (see "Equipment used in aquatic therapy") can be added to increase resistance.

Balance

Balance is improved, especially for the neurologically impaired patient, with water standing exercises. Swimming, especially in current (turbulence), requires body stabilization, which improves balance. Patients under 40 pounds (18 kg) can stand on a floating kick board (see "Equipment used in aquatic therapy") to improve balance.

Coordination

Coordination is improved with stationary and swimming exercises. Early limb movement from swimming helps to speed and improve gait sequencing on land in humans but has not been studied in canine patients (Lavoie & Montpetit, 1986; Bishop *et al.*, 1989). Backward walking or lateral stepping is performed on the bench or stair to enhance coordination (Figure 9.3). Shaking water from the coat after swimming helps to improve balance and coordination during early neurological recovery.

Postural awareness

Postural awareness is improved during early neurological recovery with exercises such as pendulum swings (supporting the dog under the axillae and gently swaying the dog through the water side to side), turning or circling on the bench, or sit-to-stand exercises performed while on the step or bench. Many of the proprioceptive neuromuscular facilitation (PNF) exercises that are performed on land can be safely completed during aquatic therapy sessions. During swimming, especially with turbulent current, the trunk and core muscles work to stabilize posture. Swimming in tight circles, figure eights, and zigzags further increase postural challenges.

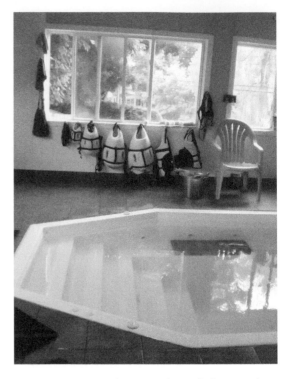

Figure 9.3 Using wide stairs in the pool allows a safe entry and exit.

Speed

As conditioning improves, the swimming speed increases with enthusiastic coaxing and the addition of lures and games. Water speed, such as with resistance jets, is also slowly increased to add the challenges of turbulence and resistance.

Endurance

Endurance improves via increased duration of swimming sets. Initially, swimming sets may be as short as 1 minute. Each set is followed by a rest period and the cycle is repeated, perhaps four to six times, depending on tolerance. The therapist monitors progress and steadily increases the duration of swimming time, reducing rest periods. Physical and emotional factors are considered including pulse, respiration, and evidence of anxiety. Progressively lengthened sets are especially beneficial for dogs returning to endurance sports that involve long-distance running or sustained activities.

Assessment of progress

Frequent review with the client identifies progress throughout the phases of aquatic therapy with the treatment plan and goals adjusted accordingly. Written progress notes, including functional status, muscle circumference, PROM, gait status, body condition score (BCS), treatment summary, adjusted goals and plan, are sent to the referring veterinarian monthly.

An aquatic therapy maintenance program can be started once aquatic rehabilitation is completed, or can be used for cross training exercise. Maintenance programs are generally provided by a therapist but some facilities offer self-swim programs for patients. Clients with performance dogs often desire self-swim programs.

Equipment used in aquatic therapy

Specific aquatic equipment is used to improve swimming and facilitate accomplishment of rehabilitation goals (Levine et al., 2014).

Life vests

A life vest provides control, improves leveling, and builds patient confidence. The life vest should be nonrestrictive to allow for complete motion of the shoulders and hips, and it should be easy to don and doff.

Harnesses

Harnesses are used on canine athletes that have prior pool experience and dogs that no longer need a life vest. Harnesses should exhibit the same qualities as the life vest.

Slings

Slings are used for safe transitions into and out of the pool. The sling reduces potential injury from slipping or struggling at the pool stairs. Once the patient is comfortable with transitions into and out of the pool, sling use can be discontinued.

Head wraps

Head wraps or snoods reduce the amount of head shaking by preventing water from entering the ears (Figure 9.4). Lamb's wool (not cotton) contains lanolin and repels water. The wool can be applied to the ear canal and secured with the head wrap.

Balance equipment

Balance equipment use increases coordination, balance, and muscle strength (Abidin et al., 1988; Bates & Hanson, 1992; Ruoti et al., 1997). A floating foam kick board is used on the water to accomplish effects similar to those of a wobble board on land (Figure 9.5). This floating balance board has advantages over land-based

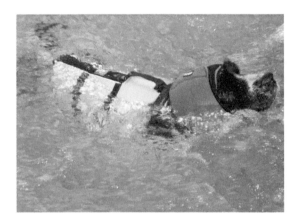

Figure 9.4 A water snood prevents water entering the ears and is helpful in reducing head shaking.

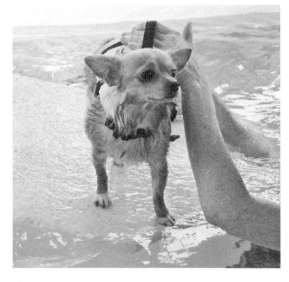

Figure 9.5 A floating balance board in the pool increases limb and core strength.

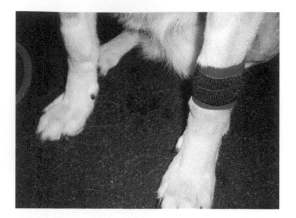

Figure 9.6   Leg weights used while swimming increase affected limb strength.

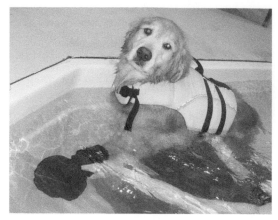

Figure 9.7   Swim mitts increase resistance at the pull phase of the stroke and improve limb strength.

balance equipment, as it can be used sooner in therapy and, should the patient fall off, they fall safely into water. These boards can be used for dogs that weigh 40 pounds (18 kg) or less.

Leg weights

Leg weights are effective for building muscle and can increase proprioceptive input (Figure 9.6). Leg weights are used once pain has resolved. Initially, the weight is used during 15–30% of the swim session. If there is no soreness, the duration of leg weight use is slowly increased. The amount of weight is determined by patient size and degree of disability, beginning with a small weight and slowly increasing as strength improves. Wet hair is slippery and hydrostatic pressure compresses the tissue so the wrap should be snuggly applied while the dog is dry.

Resistance swim mitts

Resistance swim mitts can be used in aquatic rehabilitation to build muscle and exaggerate range of motion (Figure 9.7) (Abidin *et al.*, 1988; Bates & Hanson, 1992; Ruoti *et al.*, 1997). Mitts are effective for thoracic limb issues because they increase resistance during the pull phase of the stroke. The work of the carpal flexors and extensors is increased due to resistance and viscosity. The mitt is initially used for 15–30% of the swim session. If there is no pain or soreness, the duration of mitt use is gradually increased.

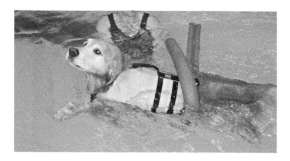

Figure 9.8   A pool noodle helps patients to maintain buoyancy until they are able to do so unassisted.

Foam pool noodles

A foam pool noodle can be placed under the belly to assist buoyancy (Figure 9.8). This helps the patient become level again when the pelvic limbs sink. Once the patient learns to swim properly, the noodle is removed.

Toys

Toys offer chasing games that encourage swimming. These games also provide fun physical and mental activity when vigorous land play is restricted. Assorted sizes, shapes, and textures of objects are provided. Toys with long loops of rope should not be used because the thoracic limbs can get caught in the loop. Toys should be checked regularly to prevent aspiration of broken pieces. Intense swimmers should use balls or decoys with center holes to allow the patient to breathe more easily while swimming with the object in the mouth. Patients that readily destroy toys often enjoy a stick with the bark removed, a plastic water-ski tow rope handle, or 12–18 inches of garden hose with wooden plugs in the ends.

Food

Food is used only if toys and voice encouragement are not sufficient to motivate swimming. Treats such as oyster crackers are best as they float and are readily eaten.

Therapeutic pool guidelines

Written guidelines should be reviewed annually with staff. Guidelines include emergency policies and procedures, a protocol for safe pool entry and exit, a guideline for assessment of anxiety and fatigue, a policy for monitoring vital signs while in the pool, a protocol for pool treatment for vomit or feces, and a daily pool chemical checklist.

Policies and procedures for pool emergencies include the procedure for dealing with dog and/or human injuries that are pool-related. Examples include: falls, bites, lacerations, chemical spills/splashes, and cardiac arrest. Emergency phone numbers should be posted clearly in the treatment areas.

The protocol for pool entry and exit includes safe techniques for using slings or lifts and expectations of staff during pool transfers (Prankel, 2008). Pools without stairs require a mechanical lift. Knowledge of this equipment and its proper use and maintenance is imperative. Staff should be trained and periodically reminded how to use proper body mechanics during transfers. Staff should know that many patients need encouragement before stepping onto submerged stairs; colored markings on stairs are helpful to increase visible contrast, and some heavy-coated patients need time to shed the weight of coat water in the partial antigravity environment of stairs because the weight of water (8 lb/gallon) adds to the effort of exiting.

A guideline for the assessment of anxiety and fatigue increases client assurance as well as staff awareness that patient anxiety is reduced

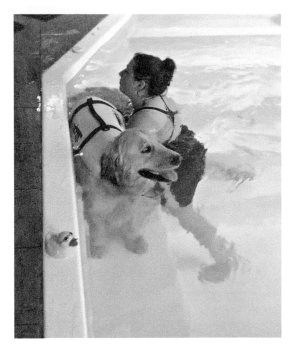

Figure 9.9 When fatigue is identified, the therapist must immediately alter the treatment session by reducing the swim time per set, increasing the rest time, and decreasing the intensity.

by increased physical contact with the therapist. It should explain that multiple short swim sets decrease anxiety and quickly build confidence and muscle. When fatigue is identified, the therapist should alter the treatment session by reducing the swim time per set, increasing the rest time, and decreasing the intensity (Figure 9.9).

A policy for monitoring vital signs while in the pool should indicate the frequency at which vital signs are taken, especially for high-risk patients. Respirations are monitored for quality and rate.

A protocol for pool treatment for vomit or feces is required (Centers for Disease Control and Prevention, 2016) Vomiting rarely occurs if food is withheld at least 3 hours prior to therapy. Excessive drinking of pool water can cause vomiting. When this occurs, the patient is removed from the pool and assessed. Particulate matter is quickly removed with the skimmer. If the vomiting is copious, the pool is treated with a quick-acting oxidizing shock and vacuumed. No patient can return to the pool for at least 20 minutes.

Patients with fecal incontinence may defecate in the pool. Anxiety contributes to defecation by incontinent patients. Swim diapers help to prevent defecation and contain stool. If defecation occurs, the patient should immediately be removed from the pool. Solid stool can be removed with a skimmer, and any particulate waste vacuumed. An oxidizing shock must be applied to the water. During the shock period, therapy can continue on land.

A daily pool chemical checklist includes recording the free chlorine, bromine, or saline levels, pH, total alkalinity, total hardness, and cyanuric acid. The checklist helps to identify trends in chemical variations and serves as a public health record should documentation be required.

Breed characteristics related to swimming

While each dog is an individual, there are some breed-related swimming characteristics. Labrador Retrievers and Spaniels like games based on repetitive ball retrieving and are high-energy swimmers. Golden Retrievers like toys and slow swimming, and can be timid in high currents.

Pointer types may not initially like toy games. Later, they play but become bored with repetition. Varying the game facilitates their swimming. German Shepherds and Belgian Tervurens and Malinois like swimming against the highest current and being lured with large sticks using a release command. Games should be fast but controlled.

Sighthounds are not motivated to retrieve or lure in water, and do best swimming in place toward their owner. Whippets tend to be anxious initially but become excellent swimmers and like games. Nonswimming working breeds (i.e., Great Pyrenees, Malamutes) become excellent swimmers. Their pace is slow and steady, and they prefer low current. Newfoundlands are often exceptional swimmers, using a slow, steady pace in low or high current.

Border Collies and Jack Russell Terriers have exceedingly high energy in all currents. They love fast fetch and lure games. Imposed short rest periods are imperative as they can swim to exhaustion. Vital signs in these patients should be regularly monitored. Toy and small breeds are superb swimmers but can easily become chilled. Vital signs and evidence of shivering should be monitored. They do best in low current or on the floating balance board.

Pit Bull types are excellent swimmers although some become anxious in water. When anxious, frenetic behavior manifests. Due to their high prey drive, caution should be used when employing toys and luring games.

Pool types

Aquatic therapy pools vary widely and a complete description is beyond the scope of this text. In warm regions, large in-ground (fiberglass or concrete) or above-ground (nylon) outdoor swimming pools are commonly used. In cold regions, smaller indoor resistance pools are used. Small indoor pools are advantageous because of the constraints for space, heating, dehumidification, and ventilation. Large indoor facilities often provide above-ground pools for nontherapeutic/fun swimming, but these are cost prohibitive to heat to therapeutic treatment levels.

Smaller (500–900 gallon/1900–3400 L) pools can be customized. Many large pools (3000+ gallons) are designed for therapy and feature whirlpool components, benches for resting, multiple levels of current, in-pool treadmill, and adjustable water depth. Therapeutic canine pools are sanitized with bromine or chlorine and use larger than normal filters (Bates & Hanson, 1992). One author (J.C.) finds that the best filters are diatomaceous earth or sand.

Any pool can be converted to salt water. These pools need careful monitoring of sodium and cyanuric acid levels to assure that the water is sanitized. Thorough sanitation may be an issue in high-volume centers. All pools, regardless of type, need careful attention to daily management. The amounts of fur, skin oils, and coat dirt create management challenges that are dramatically different than pool management for humans. In the authors' experience, a conservative estimate is that the impact of one dog is equal to that of 25–30 people in a pool.

Case Study 9.1   Hydrotherapy for fibrocartilaginous embolism (FCE) with complications

Signalment: 7 y.o. M/N retired racing Greyhound.

History: Diagnosed with cervical FCE. Family unable to provide physical care as patient tetraparetic and incontinent. Requested in-patient rehabilitation with aquatic therapy.

Examination: Left lateralizing tetraparetic, laterally recumbent, unable to independently turn or change/hold positions. CP deficits all limbs. Evidence of neurogenic atrophy and decreased superficial pain sensation all four limbs, worse on left. Mild urine scald and stage two decubitus left shoulder.

Primary goals: Improve limb muscle strength, especially left; improve trunk and core strength; improve proprioception and enhance position awareness; assure skin integrity with turning schedules and pressure-relief mattress; add diaper system to wick urine from skin; provide decubitus care.

Aquatic treatment and outcome: Initially treated in pool four times per week for 20–30 minutes (Figure 9.10). Sessions included six 45-second to 1-minute swim sets interspersed with four 3–5-minute rest periods. Therapy during rest periods included whirlpool, PROM, spinal mobilizations, traction, massage with trigger point release, PNF patterns, and assisted sit-to-stand. Patient moved all four limbs in water, although left thoracic limb and pelvic limbs weaker than right, and sequencing of pelvic limbs to thoracic limbs poor. Sequencing and strength steadily improved.

Over 4 weeks, swimming reduced to three times per week with increased duration and intensity. Sessions included four 5-minute swim sets interspersed with four 2-minute rest periods. Rest periods included more advanced exercises including independent position transitions from sit-to-stand and sphinx lie to stand on pool stairs or backing up on pool bench. The decubiti healed completely within 14 days. Ability to participate with land exercises was expedited due to early swimming and aquatic therapy. For example, patient could perform sit-to-stand 3 weeks sooner in water than on land.

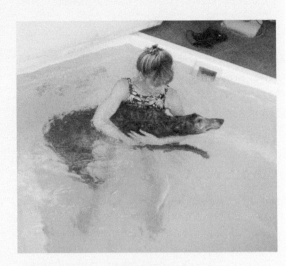

Figure 9.10   Early pool work consisted of six 45-second to 1-minute swim sets interspersed with four 3- to 5-minute rest periods.

Pool versus underwater treadmill (UWTM)

There are advantages for both the UWTM and swimming as aquatic treatment modalities (Table 9.2). Whenever possible, the therapist selects the best modality or combines these modalities based on the client's needs. The remainder of this chapter will focus on the UWTM.

The UWTM can help to eliminate the fear that some dogs show in being totally immersed in a swimming pool. Wolf's law suggests that weight bearing on the treadmill encourages increased bone strength over swimming alone. (Teichthal *et al.*, 2015) When working with canine athletes,

the therapist can change the level of the workout by increasing or decreasing the water height, and by altering the level of incline and/or tread speed. Small to medium patients can be cross-trained as both swimming and treadmill work can be accomplished in one unit.

Use of the UWTM assists or speeds gait retraining and sequencing, especially in neurologically impaired patients. A large percentage of one author's (L.M.) neurologically impaired patients will walk in water before they will on land. Work on the UWTM improves active ROM because of increased step height (Jackson *et al.*, 2002). It also allows for careful exercise of overweight patients with respiratory issues as the water is cooling, the buoyancy diminishes

Table 9.2   Comparison between swimming and underwater treadmills

Swimming in therapeutic pool	Underwater treadmill
Totally NWB	60% NWB
Maximum AROM of joints	Improved AROM compared to land
Nonambulatory patients with paraparesis/paralysis	Proprioceptive gait training
Improved core and trunk strength	Improved balance while walking
Cardiopulmonary conditioning	Cautious fracture loading
Endurance for cross training	Builds lean muscle in limbs
Fun for swimming patients	Helps non-swimmers get started
Facilitates PROM/all body work	Speeds gait retraining

AROM, active range of motion; NWB, non-weight bearing; PROM, passive range of motion.

the effort required, and unlike swimming, the UWTM gives the handler rapid control over the situation, allowing the patient to rest as needed.

The UWTM is advantageous over the land treadmill in that increasing water levels will reduce weight bearing on painful limbs. The amount of reduction in weight bearing has been documented for mesomorphic dogs (Levine *et al.*, 2010).

UWTM variables

Temperature

All dogs working on a UWTM at temperatures ranging from 30 to 34.4 °C (86–94 °F) had gradual increases in heart and respiratory rates, rectal temperature, and perceived exertional score, but there were no differences between dogs working at different temperatures (Utter *et al.*, 2002; Dunning *et al.*, 2003). Therefore, any temperature between 86 and 94 °F is considered safe for working with canine patients. The authors prefer using warmer temperatures in the winter and cooler temperatures in the summer, as it is more comfortable for the patients and the therapists.

Water depth

Carpal height water causes increased flexion of all joints without the resistance of water (Figure 9.11). This height is also used for those patients who prefer to float (lifting their legs to avoid working). Elbow height water is used for patients who are athletes, as there is minimal buoyancy advantage at this height. Just above-shoulder (or greater trochanter) height water provides for maximal buoyancy without altering the gait pattern. Water levels higher than this lead to a stilted gait, as the patient will take short strides with extended limbs to keep the nose above water (Figure 9.12) (Levine *et al.*, 2014).

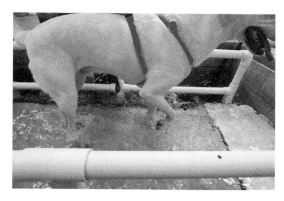

Figure 9.11   Water at carpal height enhances carpal flexion but diminishes resistance as most of the motion is done outside of the water.

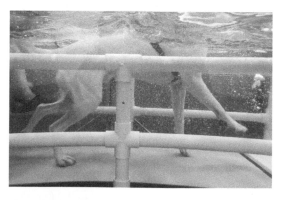

Figure 9.12   When the water is too high, above the shoulder joint, the gait is stilted and range of motion and flexion are greatly reduced. With the water at the level halfway between the elbow and the shoulder, a good workout with significantly decreased joint load, can be achieved.

Patients with minimal to moderate degenerative joint disease (DJD) are worked with the water midway between the shoulder and elbow, providing some buoyancy. As they become stronger the level can be lowered for a workout with resistance (controlled by speed) and diminished buoyancy. More profoundly arthritic patients initially start with water levels just over shoulder height. As the patient becomes stronger, the water may be lowered to halfway between shoulder and elbow, the speed and time can be increased, and jets or surface area resistance can be added.

Speed

Calibration of speed in UWTMs is not consistent. Two UWTMs from the same manufacturer may move at different speeds, despite the monitor reading "1.0 mph." If more than one UWTM will be used for the same patient, the therapist should calibrate the belt laps per minute. Patients with neurological disease are started at the slowest available speeds (usually 0.1–0.4 mph) to give them time to place their feet. For all other patients, the belt should start at a comfortable walk speed. If the belt moves too slowly, it is confusing for the patient. Short-legged patients, such as Dachshunds, require slow initial belt speeds (0.5–0.8 mph). Average size patients start at approximately 1.2–1.5 mph, while giant breeds can start at 2.2–2.5 mph for a comfortable walk. Trot speeds average as follows: small breeds 2.0–2.2 mph; medium breeds 2.5–5.3 mph; large breeds 6.0–9.0 mph. Patients may avoid breaking into a trot. If they attempt to pace, the therapist should cause a brief perturbation, such as a quick forward tug on the leash causing them to break into a trot.

Duration

The authors use the following plan with all patients. Patients are started at a walk with two to three reps of set periods of time. An older patient may start with two to three 45-second reps with 2-minute breaks. An athlete can start with three 3-minute reps with 2-minute breaks.

Progression involves gradually working up to fewer, longer reps. Breaks are always 2 minutes. Once the patient can do one solid interval of 25 minutes at a fast walk, short speed intervals are added. This starts with the patient undertaking two to three sets of trotting for 1 minute. The fast walk speed is maintained for the first and final 2 minutes to create a warm-up and cool-down period, and the remaining minutes are gradually moved up to a trot. The patient's perceived exertion during the exercise and after its completion is evaluated, and this is used to determine the level of work for the next session.

Resistance techniques

Tread speed can be used to increase resistance due to higher viscosity. Jets can also be used for resistance through turbulence. The therapist can adjust the velocity of water flow and the amount of air moving through the jets. Some treadmills allow the therapist to choose between jets positioned at different heights. Manual techniques can also be used to apply resistance, targeting specific muscle actions.

Starting the new patient

Preparation

Patients with urinary incontinence must be expressed prior to going into the UWTM. Patients who are fecally incontinent, but with anal tone, can be stimulated to defecate with a cotton swab. Patients with poor anal tone and those with diarrhea in the past 24 hours are not allowed in the UWTM.

Motivation

Food such as peanut butter smeared inside a cup or frozen yogurt in a small plastic cup works well to motivate most patients. Treats can be stacked in front of the patient where they can see them, rewarding their effort every 30 to 60 seconds. Some patients like to bite splashing water, so the assistant or client can splash the water gently. Retrievers will often be less anxious if they are given a ball, toy, or bumper when in the water. These should be sanitized between patients. Having a stuffed or real animal in front of a pet aggressive dog, can spur motivation.

Breed tendencies

Large, overweight, trusting breeds such as Golden Retrievers tend to float rather than walk on the tread. These patients are started with carpus-height water. The assistant can tug on the harness, providing verbal praise. Dobermans and Great Danes tend to abduct their limbs to stand on the stationary edges. The assistant places hands on the patient's pelvis and/or shoulder to control this. For very large patients, two people may be needed on the first visit. Shelties and Collies in their first visit tend to fall forward into the water as the tread pulls their feet behind them. Before they can fall, the assistant pulls the harness vertically and back, stimulating the forelimbs to move. Some patients want to ride to the back of the tread. If the assistant pulls on the harness, the patient will act like a donkey, leaning into the harness. This is corrected using gentle tugs on the harness with lots of verbal encouragement. Some dogs (especially working dogs) do not like having anyone behind them. The assistant or client should stand beside the tank, asking the patient to heel, or stand in front, encouraging them to come forward.

Assistive and resistive devices

Balloons

Balloons can be attached to the limbs to increase resistance due to increased surface area (Figure 9.13). The long, tubular balloon, not fully inflated, is tied off, squeezed, and twisted once in the middle, then bent into a circle with the knot end tied to the nipple at the balloon's tip. It must be tight enough to fit snugly on the patient's leg so it will not float up to circle the thigh. Balloons can be doubled on large patients for added resistance. The balloon also causes increased buoyancy, requiring more muscular

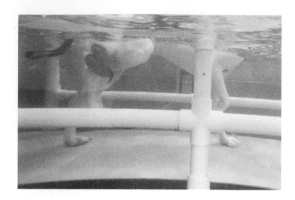

Figure 9.13   Clown balloons make great tools as they increase surface area, increasing resistance, and increase limb buoyancy, which enhances flexion of the stifle.

effort to get the foot down to the tread after the swing phase of the stride. When used just above the tarsus, stifle flexion increases due to added buoyancy at the initial swing phase.

Flippers

One author (L.M.) uses a device to create tarsal flexion with digital extension for patients too weak to accomplish this movement. A hook-and-loop strap with four holes is placed around the patient's limb just proximal to the tarsus. Two to four rubber bands run from the holes to encircle one to two toes each (Figure 9.14). If this works for the patient, a more durable device can be used long-term, weaning off its use as the patient gains strength. This type of device should not be left on for long periods of time as it can put a stretch/strain on the digital flexors causing discomfort and a reluctance to ambulate.

Hair bands

Hair bands can be used to increase proprioceptive input for patients who knuckle, drag, or slide their feet. The type of band, from tiny soft bands to large fluffy ones, is determined by the size of the patient and degree of desired skin contact. Bands can be placed above the foot, twisted into a figure 8 with the smaller ring around middle two toes, or the pads can be incorporated, so the band is between the toe pads and central pad (Figure 9.15) or above the

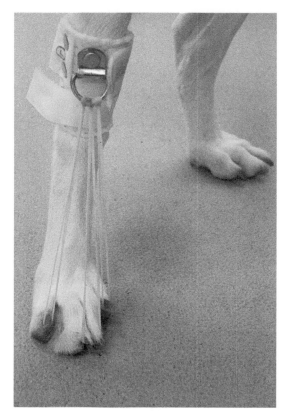

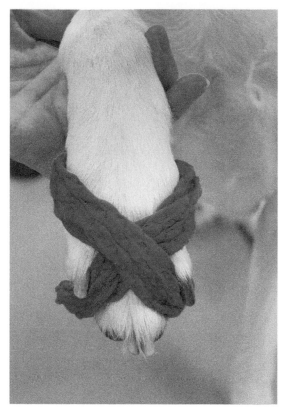

Figure 9.14 Flippers are devices used as tarsal flexion assistance devices. As they put strain on the toe flexor muscle and tendons, the rubber bands should come off the toes when the flippers are not being used. The tarsus piece can stay on the patient between exercises.

Figure 9.15 To enhance proprioception when just an elastic band around the foot is not enough, the band can be placed over the foot, twisted into a figure 8, and wrapped around the two middle toes.

central pad. If the patient grows accustomed to the band, a new configuration is used.

Harnesses

Almost all patients wear harnesses in the UWTM for control without putting tension on the neck. Patients that like to lean forward can be pulled straight back, forcing them to increase the use of their pelvic limbs (Figure 9.16). For patients that lag back, a leash or bungee cord can be attached to front of the harness.

Reins

A leash can be draped across the thoracic inlet and held like reins in two hands to prevent the

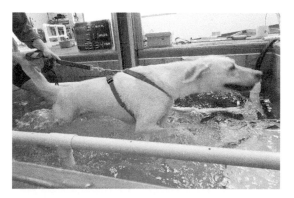

Figure 9.16 This patient is trotting in the water at 5.4 mph at elbow height. Maximal resistance with minimal buoyancy creates a truly athletic workout.

patient lunging and pulling. A gentle tug back as the patient starts to lunge discourages the action and decreases the chance they will attempt it again.

Assistive techniques

Patterning

Patients with neurological disease who have difficulty walking or who need to relearn the pattern of walking can be assisted by the use of patterning as described in Chapter 8. This is best done with the patient standing in water to provide buoyancy and balance. The therapist moves the feet through the proper motion of a step in the natural sequence of steps for the walk, repeating this pattern 10 times before turning on the treadmill.

Tail work

For patients who are not yet using their pelvic limbs optimally, the authors have found that tail work is quite beneficial. It is believed that stimulating the nerves of the tail causes stimulation of central pattern generators in the spine (see Chapter 17). The therapist uses a thumb to apply firm pressure to the top of the tail in a circular pattern, starting approximately one-third of the way down the tail looking for a spot that will initiate or improve motion of the pelvic limbs. If there is no response, the thumb moves distally and the process is repeated until a response is achieved (Figure 9.17). The tail can also be stroked with a hand circling the entire tail, and stroking from top to bottom. If this is not successful, the direction of stroking can be reversed, possibly increasing stimulation to the piloerector muscles. Finally, scratching the sides of the tail generates movement in some

patients. The therapist should avoid scratching the ventral surface of the tail as this can stimulate defecation.

Facilitation

The authors' application of stimulatory techniques to encourage motor function is based upon the concepts of facilitation, which is the enhancement or reinforcement of a reflex or other nerve activity by the arrival of other excitatory impulses at the reflex center. The following techniques are used, with the patient in the UWTM, at the terminal stance phase of the stride to initiate a proper stepping action in that leg. The therapist stimulates the foot from the lateral side to the area between the central pad and toe pads, stimulating until foot lift occurs (Figure 9.18). The calcanean tendon can be quickly rolled between the thumb and fingers to initiate withdrawal and foot lift at the terminal contact phase of the stride. Stroking the cranial tibial muscle belly from ventral to dorsal at terminal stance initiates tarsal flexion and foot lift. For patients that tend to adduct the pelvic limbs, the therapist can tap the superficial gluteal muscles at terminal stance to encourage abduction. Some patients respond well to the same stimulus on subsequent days, others require that the therapist change the stimulus. Some patients struggle with trunk strength and tend to move with the spine curved to one side. Here, the therapist can stimulate the trunk: on the convex side, stimulating the paraspinal and abdominal muscles encourages them to fire. This can be done at any time in the gait cycle.

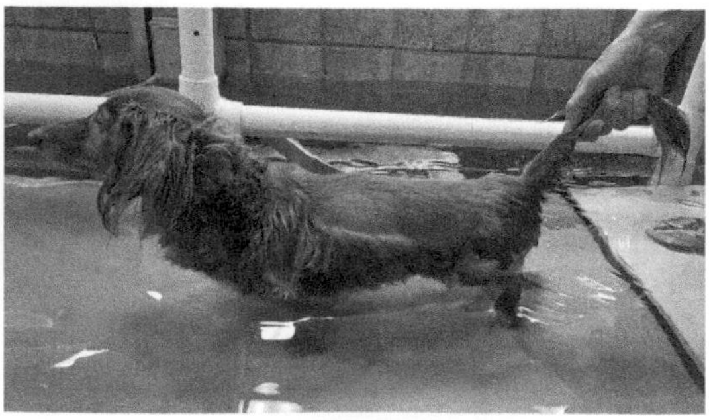

Figure 9.17   Tail work is applied to the proximal tail, moving distally until the desired effect is achieved.

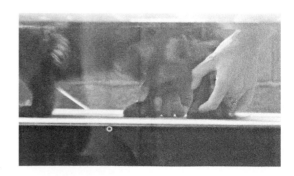

Figure 9.18   The therapist can stimulate the foot from the lateral side to the area between the central pad and toe pads, stimulating until foot lift occurs.

> **Case Study 9.2**   UWTM for postoperative medial patellar luxation (MPL)
>
> **Signalment:** 4 y.o. F/S Toy Poodle. Presented 4 weeks post MPL repair.
>
> **Clinical findings:** Patient NWB right pelvic limb (RPL) at all gaits. PROM is normal, patella location is normal, no pain on palpation.
>
> **Goal:** Normal weight bearing, ambulation, and transitions using right pelvic limb.
>
> **Therapy:** Therapeutic exercises and UWTM (q3d). Before starting treadmill work each visit, joint compressions performed on right pelvic limb joints,
>
> weight-shift training done to shift weight onto right pelvic limb, followed by gait patterning. With water at shoulder height and a fast-paced walk speed initiated, patient toe touches as treadmill starts, slowly, as other limbs become tired, patient progressively uses right pelvic limb. Carryover RPL weight bearing lasted longer after each session. By the eighth session, patient used RPL on all surfaces except occasionally when walking in wet grass. Verbal cues used to remind patient to "Use that leg" worked well. By the 12th session client reported patient using the limb consistently in all situations. Patient discharged from therapy with long-term HEP.

Massage

The authors recommend completing the UWTM workout with a 2- to 5-minute vigorous massage, using jets as well as manual techniques. This is done while the patient is still in the warm water. Patients and clients express gratitude for this positive final note to the workout.

Webliography

Centers for Disease Control. Fecal Incident Response. Recommendations for Aquatic Staff. Available at: https://www.cdc.gov/healthywater/swimming/pdf/fecal-incident-response-guidelines.pdf (accessed November 10, 2017).

References

Abidin, M. R., Thacker, J. G., Becker, D. G., Saunders, J. C., Nayak, S., Bacchetta, S. F., & Edlich, R. F. 1988. Hydrofitness devices for strengthening upper extremity muscles. *J Burn Care Rehabil*, 9, 199–202.

Arborelius, M. Jr, Ballidin, U. I., Lilja, B., & Lundgren, C. E. 1972. Hemodynamic changes in man during immersion with the head above water. *Aerosp Med*, 43, 592–598.

Bates, A. & Hanson, N. 1992. *Aquatic Exercise Therapy*. Philadelphia, PA: W.B. Saunders Company.

Bishop, P. A., Frazier, S., & Smith, J. 1989. Physiologic responses to treadmill and water running. *Physician Sports Medicine*, 17, 87–94.

Carver, D. 2016. Hydrotherapy. In: *Practical Physiotherapy for the Veterinary Nurse*. Chichester, UK: John Wiley & Sons, Ltd, pp. 168–181.

Catavitello, G., Ivanenko, Y. P., & Lacquaniti, F. 2015. Planar covariation of hindlimb and forelimb elevation angles during terrestrial and aquatic locomotion of dogs. *PLoS ONE*, 10(7), 1–26.

Chauvet, A., Laclair, J., Elliot, D. A., & German, A. J. 2011. Incorporation of exercise using an underwater treadmill and active client education into a weight management program for obese dogs. *Can Vet J*, 52, 491–495.

Dunning, D., Mccauley, L., & Knap, K. 2003. Effect of water temperature on heart and respiration rate, rectal temp and perceived exertional score in dogs exercising on an UWTM. In: *Proceedings of the 3rd International Symposium on Rehabilitation and Physical Therapy in Veterinary Medicine*. Raleigh, NC, p. 217.

Greene, N. P., Lambert, B. S., Greene, E. S., Carbuhn, A. F., Green, J. S., & Crouse, S. F. 2009. Comparative efficacy of water and land treadmill training for overweight or obese adults. *Med Sci Sports Exerc*, 41, 1808–1815.

Grosee, S. J. 2009. Aquatic progressions: The buoyancy of water facilitates balance and gait. *Rehab Management*, April, p. 25.

Hall, J., Bisson, D., & O'Hare, P. 1990. The physiology of immersion. *Physiotherapy*, 76, 517–521.

Jackson, A. M., Millis, D. L., Stevens, M., & Barnett, S. 2002. Joint kinematics of dogs walking on ground and aquatic treadmills. In: *Proceedings of the 2nd International Symposium on Rehabilitation and Physical Therapy in Veterinary Medicine*. Knoxville, TN, p. 191.

Jadelis, K., Miller, M. E., Ettinger, W. H. Jr, & Messier, S. P. 2001. Strength, balance, and the modifying effects of obesity and knee pain: results from the Observational Arthritis Study in Seniors (OASIS). *J Am Geriatr Soc*, 49, 884–891.

Lavoie, J. M. & Montpetit, R. R. 1986. Applied physiology of swimming. *Sports Med*, 3, 165–189.

Levine, D., Marcellin-little, D. J., Millis, D. L., Tragauer, V., & Osborne, J. A. 2010. Effects of partial immersion in water on vertical ground reaction forces and weight distribution in dogs. *Am J Vet Res*, 71, 1413–1416.

Levine, D., Millis, D. L., Flocker, J., & Macguire, L. 2014. Aquatic therapy. In: Millis, D. & Levine, D. (eds), *Canine Rehabilitation and Physical Therapy*, 2nd edn. Philadelphia, PA: Saunders/Elsevier, pp. 526–542.

Lindley, S. & Smith, H. 2010. Hydrotherapy. In: Lindley, S. & Watson, P. (eds), *BSAVA Manual of Canine and Feline Rehabilitation, Supportive and Palliative Care: Case Studies in Patient Management*. Gloucester, UK: British Small Animal Veterinary Association, pp. 114–122.

Marsolais, G. S., Mclean, S., Derrick, T., & Conzemius, M. G. 2003. Kinematic analysis of the hind limb during swimming and walking in healthy dogs and dogs with surgically corrected cranial cruciate ligament rupture. *J Am Vet Med Assoc*, 222, 739–743.

Millis, D., & Levine, D. 2013. *Canine Rehabilitation and Physical Therapy*, 2nd edn. St Louis, MO: Saunders.

Monk, M. 2016. Aquatic therapy. In: McGowan, C. M. & Goff, L. (eds), *Animal Physiotherapy: Assessment, Treatment and Rehabilitation of Animals*, 2nd edn. Chichester, UK: John Wiley & Sons, Ltd, pp. 225–237.

Prankel, S. 2008. Hydrotherapy in practice. *In Practice*, 30, 272–277.

Ruoti, R. G., Morris, D. M., & Cole A. J. 1997. *Aquatic Rehabilitation*. Philadelphia, PA: Lippincott-Raven Publishers, pp. 211–225.

Stager, J. M. & Tanner, D. A. 2004. *Swimming: Handbook of Sports Medicine and Science*. Oxford, UK: Blackwell Science.

Teichtahl, A. J., Wluka, A. E., Wijethilake, P., Wang, Y., Ghasem-zadeh, A., & Cicuttini, F. M. 2015. Wolff's law in action: a mechanism for early knee osteoarthritis. *Arthritis Res Ther*, 17, 207.

Thein, L. & Mcnamara, C. 1992. Aquatic exercise in rehabilitation and training. *Orthopedics of Physical Therapy Clinics of North America*, 1, 191–205.

Tomlinson, R. 2013. Use of canine hydrotherapy as part of a rehabilitation programme. *The Veterinary Nurse*, 3(10), 624–629.

Utter, A. C., Robertson, R. J., Nieman, D. C., & Kang, J. 2002. Children's OMNI Scale of Perceived Exertion: walking/running evaluation. *Med Sci Sports Exerc*, 34, 139–144.

Zink, C. 1997. *Peak Performance: Coaching the Canine Athlete*. Baltimore, MD: United Book Press.

10 Conditioning and Retraining the Canine Athlete

Chris Zink, DVM, PhD, DACVP, DACVSMR, CCRT, CVSMT, CVA, and Brittany Jean Carr, DVM, CCRT

Summary

Exercise has significant physical and psychological benefits for dogs. One of the most important is extension of health span, the length of time that a dog remains healthy and active. Rehabilitation professionals are frequently asked to design tailored conditioning programs for young dogs before starting athletic training and for adult canine athletes that need a more comprehensive and sports-specific conditioning program. In addition, active dogs that, having reached pet level fitness during a rehabilitation program after an injury or surgery, need a fitness program to allow them to return to athletic condition in preparation for an active lifestyle, re-entering sports competitions, or for a working dog role while at the same time preventing re-injury and compensatory overuse. These conditioning programs are distinct from therapeutic exercises (see Chapter 8) that are designed to regain function after injuries or surgery.

To design an appropriate conditioning program, the rehabilitation professional must first evaluate the dog's structure and gait (see Chapters 1 and 2), and identify the dog's structural strengths and weaknesses and current fitness level so that the conditioning program can target specific areas that need improvement.

A balanced exercise program includes strength (anaerobic/resistance) training that targets the thoracic limbs, pelvic limbs, and/or core body muscles, endurance (aerobic) training, proprioception and balance exercises, preparation and recovery plans (stretching and flexibility exercises), and appropriate skill training. The program should balance duration, frequency, and intensity of training while avoiding overtraining.

A sports retraining program requires that the rehabilitation professional has an understanding of the training requirements for the sport(s) in which the dog participates and provides specific guidance to the client as to what exercises and activities should be trained, and in what order and on what time schedule so that the dog is gradually and safely prepared for future extensive activity.

Benefits of conditioning

There are two broad categories for the benefits of conditioning. The first comprises the benefits provided by improvement of health span. Exercise has proven to have both physical and psychological benefits in people, including the extension not only of life span, but also of health span, or the length of time that an individual remains healthy and active (Maitland, 2012; Mason & Holt, 2012; Vina *et al.*, 2012). In fact, the psychological effects of exercise are so powerful that at least one study suggests that exercise should be considered a psychoactive drug (Vina *et al.*, 2012). Because of the similarities in the musculoskeletal, cardiovascular, and nervous systems of dogs and humans, the same benefits of exercise are afforded to dogs. Dogs that exercise have better body condition scores and cardiovascular function than more sedentary dogs, and experience the same psychological benefits (Menor-Campos *et al.*, 2011; Warren *et al.*, 2011; Bauer & Moritz, 2012; Raichlen *et al.*, 2012).

The second benefit is that appropriately conditioned performance and working dogs perform better and are less likely to suffer injuries. When injuries do occur, they tend to be less severe, and recovery is faster. In addition, fit working dogs suffer less stress, which translates to greater stamina and longevity as working dogs—a win-win situation for both dog and client.

Most of the conditioning that a canine athlete experiences is provided at home by the client, rather than in the clinic. The rehabilitation professional can have a significant impact on a canine athlete's career by providing the client with specific guidance regarding the most appropriate exercise program for his or her dog. There are several points in a canine athlete's career at which experienced rehabilitation professionals may be consulted regarding conditioning programs:

Three types of conditioning programs

(1) **Athletic readiness conditioning.** Clients will frequently ask rehabilitation professionals who understand canine structure and the requirements of the various canine performance events or working activities to evaluate their young dog's structure and provide them with a tailored exercise program. They know that an appropriate conditioning program for a young dog will yield benefits in better performance and reduced likelihood of injuries once the dog is old enough to compete.

(2) **Comprehensive athletic conditioning program.** Rehabilitation professionals often are consulted by clients with actively competing canine athletes or working dogs to develop a comprehensive conditioning program for the active adult dog to ensure that the dog is best prepared for its various activities and to help prevent or reduce the severity of injuries.

(3) **Athletic retraining.** Canine athletes and working dogs that have achieved pet-level fitness (able to easily and repeatedly sit and lie down, climb a flight of stairs, and walk on leash for at least 30 minutes) through rehabilitation therapy and therapeutic exercises still require a conditioning and retraining program that will move them to a state of appropriate fitness for the specifics of their athletic competitions or jobs. Much of this work will be in the hands of the client, who needs and wants to follow a detailed conditioning program to reach the goals. This pattern parallels the retraining programs of injured human athletes, who are provided a detailed program for regaining the specific physical requirements of the sport. This previously unrecognized type of exercise program is essential if the competitive or active dog is to regain full function without re-injury or compensatory injuries.

Communication with the client is key. It cannot be overemphasized how important it is to spend time providing the specific details that will allow the client to apply the conditioning program optimally. In general, this type of rehabilitation appointment takes 1 to 1½ hours and might include several follow-up appointments to monitor the client's activity and the response of the canine athlete to the exercises, and to modify the prescribed exercises accordingly. To develop a sports-specific conditioning program, it is essential that the rehabilitation professional understands the requirements of the sports or working functions in which the dog participates (see Chapter 1).

Components of an athletic readiness evaluation

Clinical examination

Before establishing a conditioning program for a canine athlete or working dog, or a dog destined to become one, the dog should be given a full clinical examination including complete blood count, serum chemistry screen, and urinalysis. This provides baseline information to keep on record and identifies any potential subclinical issues that need to be pursued and/or monitored.

Structural evaluation

The dog should be evaluated structurally (see Chapter 1) and its structural strengths and weaknesses for the specific planned athletic activities discussed with the client. This is important so that a conditioning and/or retraining program can be designed that takes advantage of the dog's strengths and mitigates its weaknesses.

For example, German Shepherd Dogs generally have abundant pelvic limb angulation. This gives them a very long stride, allowing them to jump high and long, which can be an advantage in protection and police work. On the other hand, the same laxity of tendons and ligaments that results in such abundant pelvic limb angulation also means that dogs of this breed have a higher incidence of hip dysplasia and frequently experience hyperextension/hyperflexion of various joints, particularly the coxofemoral joints, the tarsi, the carpi, and the toes. They frequently experience trauma to their tarsi, for example, because the plantar aspect of the metatarsals contacts the ground when the dog is running and jumping.

In contrast, Belgian Malinois, another frequently used police/military breed, tend to have straighter thoracic and pelvic limb assemblies with reduced angles at the shoulder, elbow, stifle, and tarsus. This provides these dogs with tremendous agility—they are known for their rapid acceleration and ability to turn sharply. They tend to suffer a different subset of injuries such as soft tissue injuries of the shoulder due to experiencing excessive load during eccentric contraction when landing on the thoracic limbs. These differences in structure and their potential effects on the dog's performance and longevity as an athlete or working dog should be accounted for when developing a conditioning program and should be discussed with the client. Developing a conditioning program that is specific to the dog's structure, the sports in which it competes, or the jobs that it must perform, and the client's abilities are discussed in this chapter.

Gait analysis

Every performance or working dog should be encouraged to have a baseline objective gait analysis (see Chapter 2) performed prior to training and performing. This provides data for reference in the event of an injury or change in performance. This is particularly important given individual and breed-related variation in gait characteristics. Further, if a pre-existing orthopedic condition is suspected, objective gait analysis can help identify and quantitate any lameness or abnormalities, which can then be addressed.

Fitness evaluation

The dog should be evaluated for overall muscle fitness. One of the best ways to evaluate general fitness is to palpate the size and tone of the core (paraspinal, ventral abdominal, and lateral abdominal), shoulder muscles (supraspinatus, infraspinatus, triceps), and pelvic limb muscles (gluteals, hamstrings, and quadriceps). The size of the muscles is partly breed-associated—compare the muscle sizes of an American Staffordshire Terrier or Greyhound with those of a Shetland Sheepdog or Tervuren—and partly related to long-term exercise. Muscle tone and definition, on the other hand, is related to the amount of resistance (strength) exercise the dog has experienced in the previous several weeks.

With experience in palpating the muscle size and tone of a variety of dogs of various breeds and various levels of fitness, it is relatively simple to record a semi-quantitative assessment of the size and tone of each of the six muscle groups (shoulder, paraspinal, lateral abdominal, ventral abdominal, quadriceps, and hamstrings) where the 50th percentile represents the average sedentary pet dog, greater than that represents increasing degrees of fitness, and less than that represents various degrees of muscle atrophy.

Over time, it becomes clear that many dogs have significant imbalances in musculature. For example, some dogs have large, well-toned quadriceps and weak, even atrophied hamstrings, while others have the reverse. Likewise, many dogs have imbalances between the size and fitness of the paraspinal and abdominal musculature. The value of this kind of assessment is that specific muscle groups that are atrophied or even just lacking size and tone compared to their antagonistic muscle groups can be targeted with specific strength training exercises.

The core body muscles are important for coordination of spinal and limb movements and are critical when immediate responses of the limbs are necessary. Since the thoracic limbs generally bear 60% of the dog's weight and all the weight of the dog plus the effects of gravity when a dog is jumping, cantering, or galloping, the thoracic limbs get more exercise than the pelvic limbs during routine daily activities and performance training/competition. As a result, canine rehabilitation professionals working with canine athletes, particularly those that are continuing to compete after their prime years, should place special emphasis on exercises to keep the pelvic limb and core muscles toned.

Body fat

A large proportion of dogs in North America are overweight or obese (German, 2006). Dogs are generally considered overweight when their weight is greater than 15% above ideal, and are obese when their weight is greater than 30% of ideal (Gosselin *et al.*, 2007), although these criteria have not been confirmed by rigorous epidemiological studies in dogs. Surprisingly many active dogs, competition dogs, and even working dogs are overweight, though it is less common for them to be obese. Interestingly, recent studies have shown that there can be a genetic predisposition to obesity in certain breeds of dogs (Miyabe *et al.*, 2015; Davison *et al.*, 2017).

There is strong evidence that people who are overweight have an increased risk of cancer and other systemic diseases as well as early death, though the evidence basis in dogs is not as rigorous (Cowey & Hardy, 2006; Martin *et al.*, 2006; Bach *et al.*, 2007; Zou & Shao, 2008). The increased prevalence of orthopedic disease in obese humans suggests that obese dogs are likely equally predisposed. Certainly, keeping an animal in optimal to slightly lean body condition has been shown to decrease the risk of development of osteoarthritis (OA) (Budsberg & Bartges, 2006).

While many veterinarians use visual body condition scores in which dogs' body condition ranges from 1 (very thin) to 5 or 9 (very overweight) to determine whether dogs are at a correct weight, these systems have significant limitations. They are not as helpful in coated dogs, in which the coat can make a dog look deceptively overweight, or in dogs such as sighthounds that naturally have obvious ribs and pelvic bones. A more important limitation is the fact that visual scores do not adequately differentiate between increased body size due to fat versus muscle. In fact, a study sponsored by Purina showed that the percentage fat in dogs with a body condition score of 5 varied from 13 to 22% (Brian Zanghi, 2017, personal communication).

One way to assess whether dogs have excess body fat is to palpate the thickness of the subcutaneous fat. This is easily done in the area of the dorsocaudal ribs, just ventral to the edge of the latissimus dorsi muscle (Figure 10.1). In that area, there is just a layer of skin and a layer of subcutaneous fat overlying the ribs. When the mobile skin and subcutaneous tissues in that area are pinched and pulled away from the body, the layer of subcutaneous fat slips through the fingers first (Figure 10.2). In an active dog, canine athlete, or working dog, that layer should be as thin as tissue paper. There is no advantage for an active, working dog (with the possible exception of immediately pre-race long-distance mushing dogs) to be carrying extra subcutaneous fat.

This skin-pinch system helps to determine whether the dog is carrying excess fat on its body, allowing for evaluation of body fat separately from muscle. With experience, the canine sports medicine/rehabilitation professional can closely estimate the thickness of the layer of subcutaneous fat and add that to the dog's clinical records.

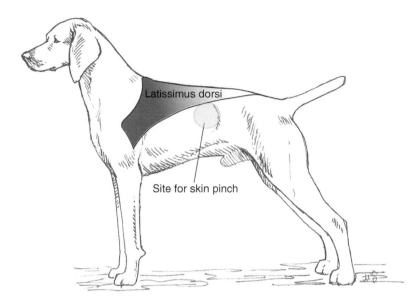

Figure 10.1 To palpate the layer of subcutaneous fat, pinch the tissues in the area of the dorsocaudal ribs, just ventral to the latissimus dorsi muscle. In that area, there is just skin and subcutaneous fat overlying the ribs.

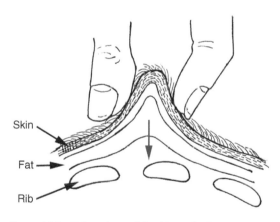

Figure 10.2 When the mobile skin and subcutaneous tissues over the dorsocaudal ribcage are pinched and pulled away from the ribs, the layer of subcutaneous fat slips through the fingers first (red arrow).

Health screening

Every performance and working dog should be screened for common genetic and developmental problems. For example, all dogs should be screened for hip dysplasia, since this condition is common and can occur even in very small breeds. All dogs over 30 lb (11 kg) and all dogs of chondrodystrophic breeds should be screened for elbow dysplasia, which can significantly affect the performance of working dogs. Elbow dysplasia or incongruities can occur even in purebred dogs with several generations of ancestors that have been tested free of the condition by radiographic evaluation, due to the lack of sensitivity and specificity of evaluation of elbow radiographs (Kunst *et al.*, 2014). In addition, dogs should be screened for breed-specific disorders that can affect performance, including musculoskeletal, cardiovascular, hematological, and ocular disorders.

Nutrition and supplementation

The veterinary sports medicine/rehabilitation professional should inquire as to what foods the client is feeding to ensure that adequate nutrition, particularly appropriate amounts of highly digestible protein and fats, is being supplied to meet the requirements not only for performance but also for healing and repair after exercise (see Chapter 4). It can be difficult to keep track of the most popular dog foods used by clients. One way to deal with this is to search the manufacturer's website each time a client mentions what food they are feeding, and store the information, including the nutritional content and ingredients list, in a file that can be referred to with subsequent clients. Information on supplements can be kept in a similar way.

Frequently canine athletes are administered numerous supplements, many of which have minimal scientific evidence of efficacy. Supplements often have high levels of inexpensive ingredients such as calcium, sometimes disguised as healthy-sounding ingredients such as organic abalone shells. These have the potential to create imbalances in important nutritional components such as the calcium:phosphorus ratio. As a result, it is important that the canine sports medicine/rehabilitation professional inquires about all supplements that their patients are receiving, not just at the first visit but at every visit.

Nonetheless, there is significant evidence that canine athletes and working dogs can benefit from being supplemented with omega-3 fatty acids for their anti-inflammatory activity (Xu et al., 2015), probiotics for their immune benefits (Marsella et al., 2012; Kumar et al., 2017), and joint protective nutraceuticals (Gupta et al., 2012; Martí-Angulo et al., 2014). These three supplements are recommended by many veterinarians who work with active dogs, canine athletes, and working dogs.

Five components of a balanced exercise program

Imagine a soccer player who practiced playing the game with his team, but never lifted weights to increase his strength or did any aerobic exercise to increase his cardiovascular system's ability to oxygenate his blood. It is unlikely that he would make it to the top of his game. Many clients spend the majority, if not all, of their training time practicing the skills of their chosen sport(s) with their dogs. However, many do not have a comprehensive conditioning program that provides targeted strength, endurance, balance, body awareness, and flexibility training. It is important to explain to clients that to maximize performance and minimize the likelihood and severity of injuries, they should have a long-term plan for overall conditioning that includes all components of a balanced regimen.

Strength (anaerobic) training

The most common form of strength-building activity is resistance training. In resistance training, the dog's muscular effort is performed against an opposing force. In other words, the movement of a body part is opposed and made more difficult by a force generated by some additional stressor such as accelerating upward against gravity, moving against inertia, braking against momentum, or pushing against friction or an elastic band that will contract to a relaxed state. Resistance exercise is used to develop the strength and size of skeletal muscles. When properly performed, resistance training can provide significant functional benefits and improvement in overall health and well-being. Strength is closely linked to speed (compare the speeds of runners executing the 100 m dash vs marathon runners). Explaining this to clients who participate in speed-related sports can help convince them of the importance of these exercises.

Strength-building exercises are *isometric* if a body part is holding still against the force of muscle contraction. In isometric exercise, the joint angle and muscle length do not change during contraction. Isometric exercises are opposed by a force equal to the force output of the muscle, and there is no net movement.

Strength exercises are *isotonic* if a body part is moving because of muscular contraction. Isotonic exercises strengthen the muscle throughout the entire range of motion of the exercise used. Isotonic contraction is *concentric* if the muscle shortens during contraction, and *eccentric* if the muscle lengthens.

There are three concepts to consider when prescribing a strength exercise: specificity, overload, and concussion. *Specificity* refers to the ability of an exercise to affect specific group(s) of muscles that might require the exercise due to weakness or muscle imbalance. *Overload* refers to carefully and gradually performing exercises with higher resistance so that muscles will hypertrophy and strength will increase. *Concussion* should be avoided as much as possible to avoid stressing the already active canine body.

The goal of resistance training is to *gradually* and *progressively* increase the work done by the musculoskeletal system so that it gets stronger (Fisher *et al.*, 2016). Compared with low-intensity exercise, moderate and high-intensity resistance exercises are potent stimuli for increases in muscle protein synthesis (MacDougall *et al.*, 1995; Phillips *et al.*, 1997), satellite cell activity (Hawke & Garry, 2001; Harridge, 2007) and decreases in proteolysis (Louis *et al.*, 2007).

The basic principle of strength training to achieve momentary overload involves a manipulation of the types of exercises, the resistance against which the muscles move, the number of repetitions of a given exercise, the number of sets (each set consisting of a number of repetitions), and the tempo, or how quickly the exercise is performed.

Whereas humans can lift free weights or use resistance machines, dogs most often use their bodies as the weight and build strength by moving their bodies over short distances with bursts of muscular energy. Strength can also be built by having a dog pull an object over the ground (dragged against friction) or push against an elastic band such as a Thera-Band® (Thera-Band, Akron, OH).

Strength training exercise is primarily anaerobic (Zatsiorsky & Kraemer, 2006). Even while training at a lower intensity, anaerobic glycolysis is still the major source of power, although aerobic metabolism makes a small contribution (Knuttgen, 2003). The aerobic contribution of strength exercise is perhaps even more significant in dogs than in humans, because in dogs type IIX (more oxidative) muscle fibers replace the IIB glycolytic fibers seen in humans (Maxwell *et al.*, 1977; Braund *et al.*, 1978; Latorre *et al.*, 1993; Acevedo & Rivera, 2006).

It is helpful to categorize the different canine strength exercises as targeting the thoracic limbs, pelvic limbs, or core body muscles, although many exercises target more than one area to varying degrees (Table 10.1). Conveniently, many excellent strength exercises can be performed in very small spaces indoors in air-conditioned comfort with minimal physical effort on the part of the client. Clients with canine athletes are proficient at training dogs to perform various physical activities, so their dogs will be capable of being trained to perform a very wide variety of strength exercises. Further, these clients have significant financial and time investments in the patient and most are strongly committed to gaining and maintaining their dog's strength,

Table 10.1   Strength (resistance) exercises

Indoors				Outdoors	
Main target				Main target	
Whole body	Forelimbs	Core muscles	Pelvic limbs	Whole body	Pelvic limbs
Rolling a peanut ball	Wave	Beg Beg while perturbing balance Beg on progressively softer surfaces	Beg-stand-beg while perturbing balance Beg-stand-beg on progressively softer surfaces	Hiking over varied terrain	Running up hills (straight or angled ascent)
Backing up stairs	High nines	Diagonal leg lifts	Circling with thoracic limbs on perch	Jump chutes	Sledding (on snow or land)
Sit-to-stand while elevating front feet	Wheelbarrow	One side leg lifts	Pulling forward against a therapy band or stretchy leash	Retrieving over short distances on land or water	Weight-pulling Cart-pulling
Stand/ down/stand	Handstand	Roll over		Trotting over cavaletti	
				Plyometrics	
Tugging	Circling with pelvic limbs on perch	Wobble board			
Digging					
Crawl					

understanding that it means health, longevity, and athletic success. The following is not an exhaustive list of exercises by any means, but should provide a variety of targeted exercises to prevent boredom on the part of the client or the dog.

One more point: strength training needs to be fun for both the person and the dog, but especially for the dog. If a dog does not enjoy the activity that it is being asked to perform, its focus will drift, and its movements will cease to be purposeful. Strength-building activities should be used that take advantage of activities for which the dog is predisposed by genetics (like retrieving) or for which the dog shows clear signs of excitement, even if that is just the excitement of receiving treats.

Indoor strength exercises

Whole body strength exercises

Rolling a peanut ball. A peanut-shaped physioball that is about elbow height is placed with the long side perpendicular to the dog and the client, who are facing each other (Figure 10.3). The dog then places its front feet on the peanut ball and rolls it towards the client, who uses their foot to control the speed of the ball's movement. Once the dog is proficient, a larger peanut ball can be used and the dog can move it both forward and backward.

Backing up stairs. The dog is taught first to back up on level ground (a good proprioceptive exercise) and gradually to back up hills and eventually to back up a flight of stairs (Figure 10.4). This is an especially good exercise for the stabilizers of the thoracic limbs.

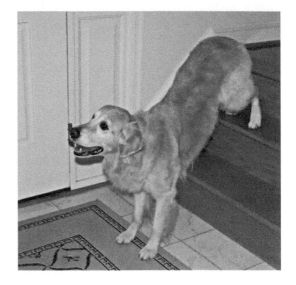

Figure 10.4 Backing up stairs. The client can start by having the dog back up on a level surface, then hills, then progressing to stairs. This is an excellent exercise for the stabilizers of the thoracic limbs and proprioception of the pelvic limbs.

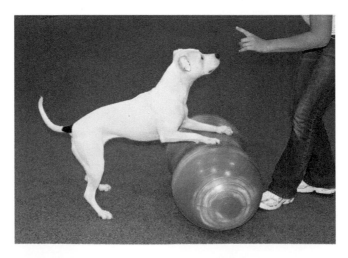

Figure 10.3 Dog standing with front feet on a peanut-shaped physioball. The dog will roll the ball forward and eventually backward for an excellent pelvic limb and core exercise.

Sit-to-stand with front feet elevated. The client has the dog stand square with front feet slightly elevated, for example on a 2 × 4″ piece of wood (Figure 10.5). The dog then sits without moving its front feet from their position. This requires the dog to bring its pelvic limbs forward, ventroflexing the spine and tucking its ischium down on top of the flexed pelvic limbs, rather than rocking backward into a sit. The dog is then asked to stand, again without moving the front feet. The dog can be encouraged to stand up by tickling the caudal abdomen. Once the dog can perform this easily 10 times, the front feet can be gradually elevated to greater heights until the front feet are approximately at elbow height off the ground.

Stand/down/stand. The dog is placed in a square stand with the front and rear feet beside each other, then is asked to lie down and stand back up without moving the feet (Figure 10.6). This exercise is hardest for dogs with abundant pelvic limb angulation and/or straight thoracic limb angulation because of their instability in the rear and often reduced strength of the thoracic limbs.

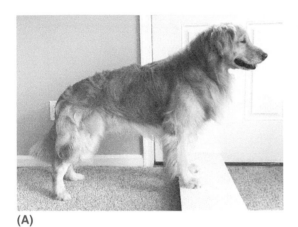
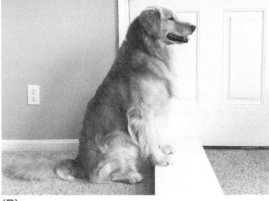

(A)   **(B)**

Figure 10.5   The client has the dog stand square with front feet slightly elevated as shown (**A**), and later using more elevated blocks. The dog should then move from a stand to a sit and back again without moving the front feet from their position (**B**).

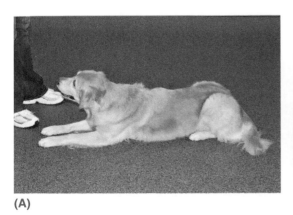
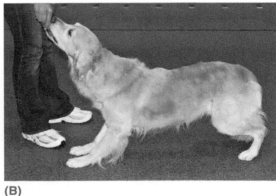

(A)   **(B)**

Figure 10.6   (**A**) Dog demonstrating the down-stand-down. (**B**) The dog transitions between the stand and down without moving its feet.

Tugging. Playing tug is a favorite activity of many performance dogs (Figure 10.7). When the client holds the tug object low, the dog pushes backward with the front feet. This exercise strengthens the stabilizer muscles of the thoracic limbs. When the client holds the tug object higher, the pelvic limbs are engaged more. Both heights work the core musculature

Digging. Any dog can be trained to dig by hiding a plastic bag with treats in it (making small slits to let the scent diffuse from the bag) a few inches below loose dirt, sand, or mulch (Figure 10.8). The dog is then encouraged to find the treats. Over time the treats can be buried deeper and deeper. This exercise not only strengthens the thoracic limbs, but also the core and pelvic limbs.

Crawl. Dogs can be taught to crawl by first having them crawl under a chair (Figure 10.9), and then a low table such as a coffee table. They can then be transitioned to crawling under a set of elevated poles. Gradually the poles can be lowered, then the center poles can be removed so the dog just needs the end poles.

Thoracic limb strengthening exercises

Wave. The dog is taught to wave each front foot separately, holding the foot higher than the head for as long as possible, preferably

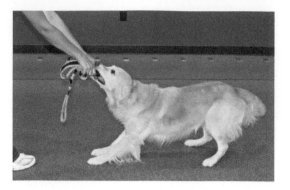

Figure 10.7   Tugging. When the client holds the tug object low, the exercise strengthens the stabilizer muscles of the thoracic limbs. With the tug object held higher the pelvic limbs work harder. Both heights work the core musculature.

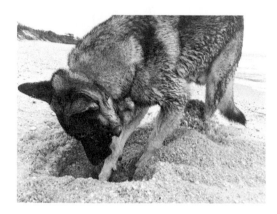

Figure 10.8   A dog can be trained to dig by searching for a plastic bag containing treats hidden in loose dirt or sand. This exercise not only strengthens the thoracic limbs, but also the core and pelvic limbs. Source: Photo by Roseann Baars.

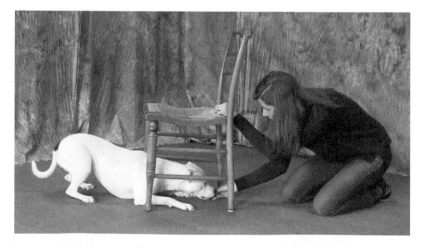

Figure 10.9   Dogs can be taught to crawl by initially having them crawl under a chair, eventually graduating to a set of elevated poles.

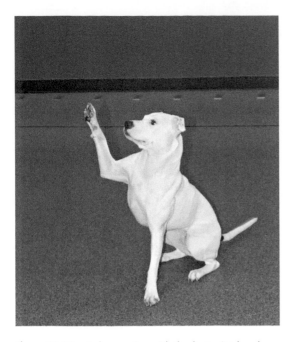

Figure 10.10 A dog waving with the foot raised and held above head level.

more than 5 seconds (Figure 10.10). One way to get a dog to initiate this movement is to take a piece of sticky tape such as duct tape or packing tape and make it into a roll with the sticky side out. Place the tape roll on the dog's eyebrow, and wait until the dog lifts its foot to rub the tape off, at which time the dog is praised effusively and immediately given a treat. With repetition, the dog will start to lift its foot before the tape is placed. At this point, the reward can be delayed a little bit at a time until the dog lifts its foot higher and higher. This exercise not only strengthens the flexor muscles of the thoracic limb that is being raised but also the stabilizer muscles of the thoracic limb that is supporting the dog.

High-nines. The client places their hand randomly at nine locations: three at head level (one to each side, and one centered on the dog), three at chest level, and three at carpus level (Figure 10.11A). The dog then places each foot firmly on the client's hand at each of the various locations (Figure 10.11B), thus adducting or abducting

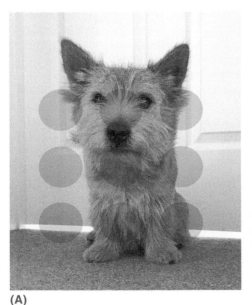

(A)

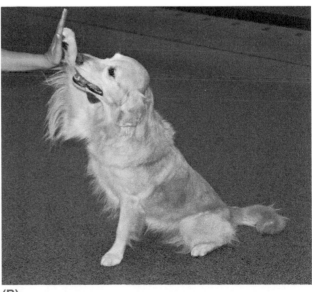

(B)

Figure 10.11 "High-nines." The client should imagine nine locations in front of the dog: three at head level (one to each side, and one centered on the dog), three at chest level, and three at carpus level **(A)**. The dog then places each foot firmly on the client's hand at each of the various locations randomly **(B)**, thus adducting or abducting the thoracic limbs, depending on which muscles are being targeted.

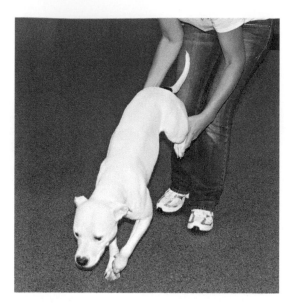

Figure 10.12   A dog practicing the wheelbarrow. The client holds the pelvic limbs flexed and elevated. The higher the pelvic limbs are elevated, the more weight is shifted to the thoracic limbs and the harder the exercise is. The dog can be walked forward and turned to the right and left. To increase difficulty, the dog can be walked over the rungs of a ladder, up an incline, and eventually up stairs.

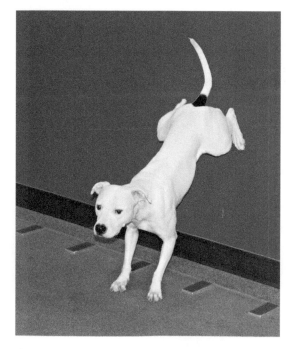

Figure 10.13   Dog demonstrating the handstand.

each of the thoracic limbs, depending on which muscles are being targeted.

Wheelbarrow. The dog's pelvic limbs are grasped gently at the tarsus and the rear is raised off the ground, flexing the legs at the pelvis, stifle, and tarsus (Figure 10.12). The higher the rear is raised, the more the weight is shifted to the thoracic limbs and the more difficult the exercise. The dog can be walked forward and turned to the right and left. To increase difficulty, the dog can be walked over the rungs of a ladder, up an incline, and eventually up a flight of stairs.

Handstand. The dog is trained to back up a ramp that is angled against a wall at progressively steeper angles. Eventually the dog will stand on the thoracic limbs and use its pelvic limbs to back up a wall into a handstand (Figure 10.13). The dog can then be taught to move sideways to the right and left along the wall and ultimately to step over poles oriented perpendicular to the wall. This exercise strengthens the muscle groups that are used when agility dogs land from jumps and when they stop with two feet on the ground and two feet on the contact obstacles, a position referred to as a "2-on, 2-off contact."

Pelvic limbs on perch. The dog places its pelvic limbs on an elevated perch. This can be a box that is raised 3–4″ off the ground, an upside-down food bowl, or any other object of that size that can be stabilized on the ground. With the client standing beside the dog, a treat can be used to turn the dog's head away from the direction in which it will turn as the client takes short steps sideways in the direction to which the dog will turn (Figure 10.14). In other words, if the dog is going to step to the right, the client should be on the left side of the dog, luring the dog's head to the left while stepping to the dog's right. The dog should circle three times around the perch in each direction. The perch can then be gradually elevated to elbow height, for example by using a footstool, an upside-down storage bin, or other stable objects.

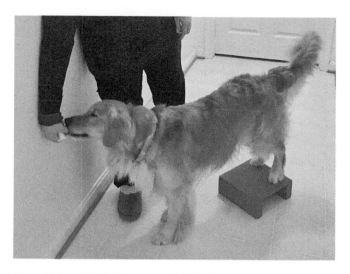

Figure 10.14   A dog working with its pelvic limbs on a perch. The dog should circle three times around the perch in each direction. The perch can be gradually elevated to elbow height, for example by using a foot stool, an upside-down storage bin, or other objects.

Case Study 10.1   Obedience dog with performance decline

Signalment: 5 y.o. MN Golden Retriever that competes in obedience (has Utility Dog title) and hunt tests (working on Master Hunter title).

History: The patient is a very stable, consistent obedience competitor. The client is in her 70s and has arthritis, so she trains and competes in obedience with the patient only indoors (usually on rubber mats on concrete) so that she can ambulate more easily. The patient has been slowing down on his approach to the jumps in obedience, using the wrong thoracic limb as lead when jumping and turning, and limping for a few steps when getting up from a rest, but otherwise

seems healthy. The client noticed that the patient's feet have developed bumps (Figure 10.15). The patient is fed high-quality grain-free dry dog foods and receives no supplements.

Clinical examination: The patient was lame on the left forelimb (grade 2 on a scale of 6) immediately after resting and more so (grade 4/6) after the joints of the left thoracic limb (including the toes) were held in flexion for a full minute before trotting. Swellings on the foot were firm and painful on hyperflexion or hyperextension of the affected joints. There was pain on palpation of the palmar sesamoid of the left 5th

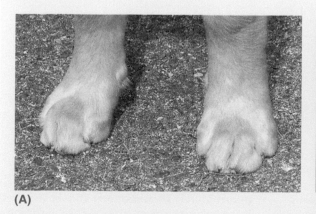

(A)

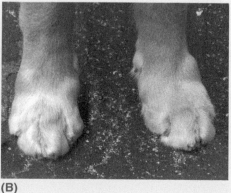

(B)

Figure 10.15   Patient's front feet at 18 months of age (**A**) and at 5 years of age (**B**). Source: Photos by William Huffman.

(*Continued*)

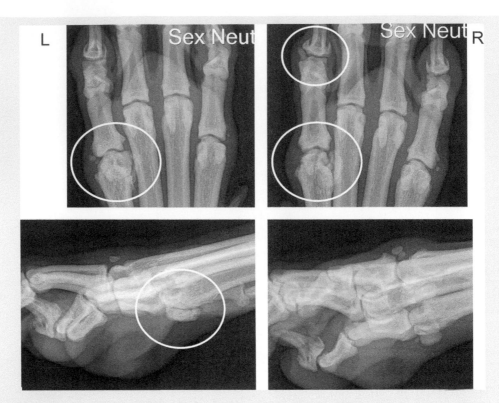

Figure 10.16   VD, lateral and oblique radiographs showing arthritic changes in the metacarpophalangeal joints of P2 and P5 on both front feet and the distal interphalangeal joint of P2 of the right front foot and degenerative changes of the palmar sesamoid of P2 of the left front foot.

metacarpophalangeal joint. VD, lateral, and oblique radiographs showed arthritic changes in the metacarpophalangeal joints of P2 and P5 on both front feet, the distal interphalangeal joint of P2 of the right front foot, and degenerative changes of the palmar sesamoid of P2 of the left front foot (Figure 10.16).

Recommendations

- Three weeks rest, with two 10-minute on-leash walks per day to maintain condition but no training or competition. Gradually increased exercise thereafter.
- Rehabilitation consisting of focused high-energy sound wave (shock wave) therapy, laser, joint mobilizations, and at-home passive range of motion.
- Heat and massage treatments daily with 30 minutes rest afterward.

- Rx: NSAIDs for 10 days then as needed before and after periods of intense training and competition, supplementation with joint-protective nutraceuticals for remainder of life.
- Train and compete only at venues with appropriate footing. Train at full jump height only 30% of the time. Remainder of the time train at 50% to full jump heights.

Outcome: The patient showed no evidence of lameness after the first week of therapy. By 4 weeks after diagnosis, the swellings in the feet had reduced in size by about 50% and the patient was much more active. The client elected to train and compete with the dog only minimally because of her own lack of mobility, and the dog remained comfortable for the rest of his life (he lived to age 14 years).

Core strengthening exercises

Beg/sit pretty. While sitting on a firm, nonslip surface, food is used to lure the dog onto its haunches with the thoracic limbs in the air (Figure 10.17A). Once the dog can stay in

this position for 15 seconds, rhythmic then nonrhythmic perturbations can be applied by moving the treat from side to side or by pushing on the back, shoulders, or chest to place the dog off-balance (Figure 10.17B).

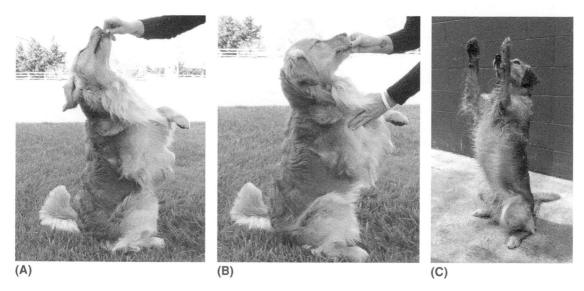

(A)   **(B)**   **(C)**

Figure 10.17   Dogs demonstrating the beg. With the dog nibbling on a treat, the client moves the food up and back until it is in a position over the base of the dog's tail (**A**). The food is then moved in all directions to off-balance the dog. To increase the difficulty, the client can gently push on the dog's shoulders, chest, and back to off-balance the dog, causing the dog to work the core muscles harder to maintain itself in the beg position (**B**). The dog can raise one or both feet to increase difficulty—note the strength and stability in this dog's core (**C**).

In addition, if the dog already knows how to wave or do high-nines, these exercises can be added to the beg exercise to off-balance the dog (Figure 10.17C). The exercise is then made more difficult by sequentially having the dog perform the exercise on a soft, level surface (bed, couch, air mattress), then on hills (facing the dog up, down, or sideways in each direction), and finally on an egg-shaped physioball with the client moving the ball rhythmically, then nonrhythmically.

Most dogs require several months to develop enough strength to proceed through all stages. This exercise is very difficult, but clients should be encouraged to keep working on it, since attempting and failing means that the muscles are working to overload, which is necessary to build strength. The dog should be worked to failure on this exercise with a training session never having more than three attempts. The client should not progress to the next surface until the dog can complete three 15-second begs with perturbations.

Clients with chondrodystrophic dogs such as Dachshunds or Corgis frequently are told not to let their dogs beg because of a belief that there is increased risk of spinal injury. In addition, some canine sports medicine/rehabilitation professionals worry that this exercise

puts the dog in an unnatural position, placing more stress on the facet joints. Evidence by Butterman and colleagues (1992) on the stressors placed on the facet joints while dogs are sitting up on their haunches indicates that the loads described here are not excessive; in fact, they are substantially less than occur when a dog is ascending or descending stairs. Athletic dogs do place themselves in a vertical position frequently when taking off or landing from jumps, when landing from contact obstacles in agility, especially when using a 2-on, 2-off contact performance, and when jumping over ditches and other obstacles when retrieving, and so forth. In these circumstances the dog's spinal column is not only vertical but has the added pressures of concussion.

The exercise described here carefully and in a nonconcussive manner strengthens the very muscles that will help athletic dogs deal with unexpected flexion and extension as well as concussion on the spine. With careful progression, this exercise significantly strengthens the core muscles, thus helping protect against the hyperflexion and hyperextension of the vertebrae that is thought to contribute to disc degeneration, spondylosis, and intervertebral disc disease (IVDD). Having said that, one caution for this exercise is that it should not be undertaken by dogs with acute back pain or chronic back pain of unknown origin.

Diagonal leg lifts. From a standing position, one of the dog's thoracic limbs should be lifted into an elbow-flexed position with the client holding the dog at the distal radius and ulna so that the carpus is not in flexion. At the same time the client should lift the diagonally opposite pelvic limb into flexion under the body holding at the distal tibia (Figure 10.18). The client should be sure not to abduct the limbs. The dog should be held in this position for 30 seconds and then the legs placed gently on the ground and the other two limbs lifted. This should be repeated twice for each set of diagonally opposite limbs. It can help to place food on the ground in front of the dog so that the dog does not laterally flex the spine. If the dog starts to lean on the client's hand, they should briefly drop their hand while still holding the leg so that the dog recognizes that it cannot support itself that way. The exercise is made more difficult by rhythmically then nonrhythmically perturbing the patient by gently bumping the dog with the client's knee or elbow.

Once the dog can perform three sets of 30-second lifts of each pair of limbs with perturbations, the client can extend the thoracic limb cranially and/or the pelvic limb caudally to add additional challenge; balance perturbations can then be performed with the dog in this position.

This exercise can also be made more difficult by sequentially having the dog perform the exercise on a soft, level surface (bed, couch, air mattress), then on hills (facing the dog up, down, or sideways in each direction), and finally on an egg-shaped physioball, as described for the beg exercise. However, progressing from one surface to the next should not be performed until the patient can successfully complete this exercise on the surface with both rhythmic and nonrhythmic perturbations with the legs in extension for a set of three 30-second repetitions on each pair of legs.

One side leg lifts. This exercise is the same as the above exercise, except that the thoracic and pelvic limbs on the ipsilateral side of the dog's body are lifted.

Roll over. Most dogs will begin to roll over if they are lying down and a treat is placed near the top of the scapula, in a position that allows the dog to nibble on it (Figure 10.19). As the dog's nose reaches toward its shoulder, the food is moved toward the dog's spine slowly, always letting the dog keep nibbling. This results in the dog naturally rolling over. Dogs should be taught to roll three times in each direction. To increase the difficulty of this exercise, the dog can be taught to roll up an incline. This is another exercise that, like begging, requires

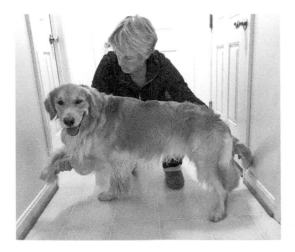

Figure 10.18 Diagonal leg lifts. Diagonally opposite thoracic and pelvic limbs are lifted into a flexed position and held there for 30 seconds. The exercise is then repeated for the other diagonally opposite pair of limbs.

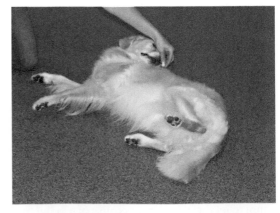

Figure 10.19 In the early stages of training a dog to roll over, food is held at the dog's shoulder to encourage the dog to roll over.

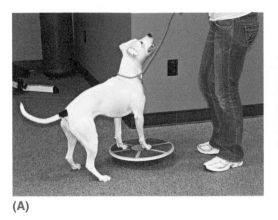
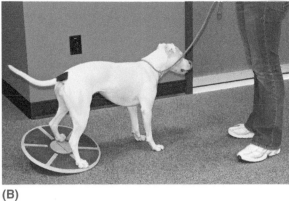

(A)   (B)

Figure 10.20   (**A, B**) Wobble boards can help build core strength. A single large board that fits the dog's entire body can be used or two smaller wobble boards, with the thoracic limbs on one and the pelvic limbs on the other.

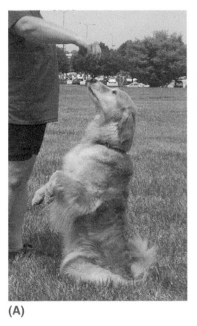
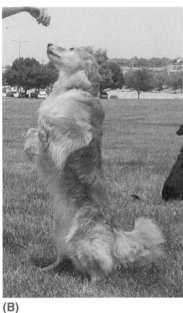
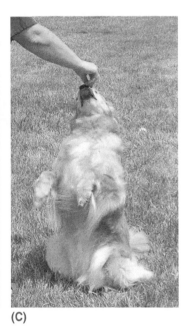

(A)   (B)   (C)

Figure 10.21   (**A**) The beg-stand-beg. Using food, the dog is lured from a beg into a stand (**B**), and back into the beg position without putting its front feet on the ground (**C**). Source: Photos by Sandra Murley.

significant strength to complete. Clients might need to try for several weeks before the dog is strong enough to roll over completely and certainly to roll up an incline.

Wobble board. Dogs can be encouraged to sit, stand, or lie down and to transition between those positions with their thoracic limbs, pelvic limbs, or all four limbs on a large wobble board. Once the dog is confident on the board, playing a game of tug increases the strength component considerably. In addition, two smaller wobble boards can be used, with the thoracic limbs on one and the pelvic limbs on the other (Figure 10.20).

Pelvic limb strengthening exercises

Beg-stand-beg. One of the best indoor exercises for strengthening the pelvic limbs is to have the dog first sit in the beg position then raise itself to a two-legged stand on the pelvic limbs, standing as still as possible for 15 seconds, and then lowering back down to the beg position without letting the thoracic limbs touch the ground (Figure 10.21). This

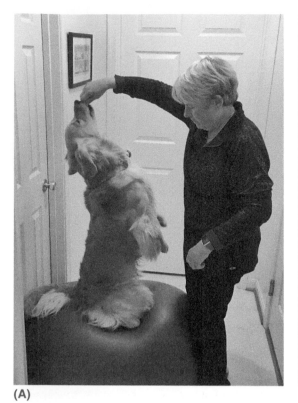
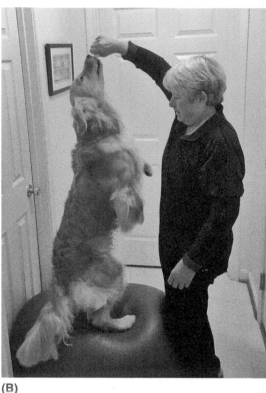

(A)   **(B)**

Figure 10.22   In the most advanced stage of the beg-stand-beg, a dog can do the exercise on a soft, egg-shaped physioball, transitioning from a sit (**A**) to a stand (**B**) and back.

exercise should not be attempted until all levels of the beg on all surfaces can be performed. As with the simple beg, this exercise is made significantly more difficult by having the dog perform it on progressively more difficult surfaces, moving from a solid surface to a soft surface, then hills, then on a physioball (Figure 10.22). The dog should be limited to raising itself three times from the beg position in any given session. This exercise should not be performed by dogs with acute injuries or undiagnosed pain of the pelvic limbs or spine.

Thoracic limbs on perch. The dog places its thoracic limbs on an elevated perch (Figure 10.23). This can be a box that is raised 3–4″ off the ground, an upside-down food bowl, or any other object of that size that can be stabilized on the ground. As with the same exercise with the dog's pelvic limbs on a perch, the client should turn the dog's head away from the direction to which it will step. The dog should circle three times around

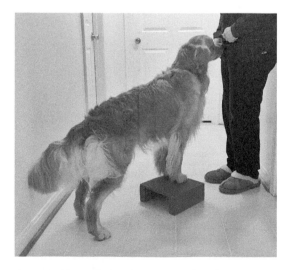

Figure 10.23   A dog working with its front feet on a perch. Once the dog can circle three times around the perch in each direction, the perch can be gradually elevated to elbow height.

the perch in each direction. The perch can then be gradually elevated to elbow height, for example by using a footstool, an upside-down storage bin, or other objects.

Pushing against a bungee cord. With the dog wearing a nonrestrictive harness (one that leaves the thoracic limbs free to extend fully forward) and standing on a nonslip surface, the client stands behind the dog and attaches a bungee cord to the harness. The dog is encouraged to lean forward to get a treat or its dinner (Figure 10.24). This works best if the food is placed in a bowl elevated to approximately the dog's elbow height. The dog uses its pelvic limbs to push against the bungee cord toward the food.

Outdoor strength exercises

Outdoor strengthening exercises such as those described below are tremendously beneficial for dogs psychologically and of course do build strength; however, unlike the indoor exercises, they generally cannot be targeted at specific muscle groups, they almost all involve concussion, and working to overload usually means exhausting the dog, which should be avoided due to the increased risk of injury. Nonetheless, the psychological benefits of these exercises make them a must for dogs.

Most of these exercises combine both strength and aerobic components.

Whole body strength exercises

Hiking. Hiking over varied terrain, especially over hilly terrain, is one of the best ways to strengthen all the muscles in a dog's body. Playing chase and dodge as a part of the hike also builds strength.

Jump chutes. Another way to build overall strength in agility and obedience dogs that already know how to jump is to have the dog jump over a series of jumps set up in a straight line (jump chutes) or in a large diameter circle. The height of the jumps and the distances between the jumps can be varied to increase the challenge.

Retrieving on land or water. Retrieving objects on land or in water over distances up to 50 yards (45 m) is another excellent outdoor strength exercise (Figure 10.25). The latter exercise can be made more difficult by having the dog run through cover of varying depths and densities and over/across obstacles such as creeks, low fences, or ditches.

Cavaletti poles. A very effective way to build overall strength outdoors is to have the dog trot over cavaletti ground poles placed parallel to each other approximately as far apart as the

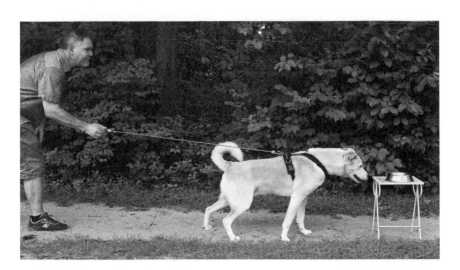

Figure 10.24 With the dog wearing a nonrestrictive harness (one that leaves the forelimbs free to extend forward) and a bungee attached, the dog is encouraged to lean forward to get a treat or its dinner. Source: Photo by Roseann Baars.

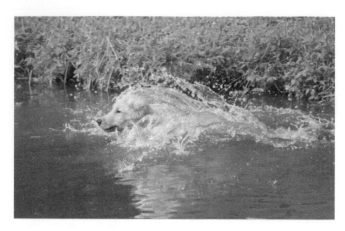

Figure 10.25   Retrieving over short distances in the water is an excellent exercise as the dog gains strength pushing in and out against the water.

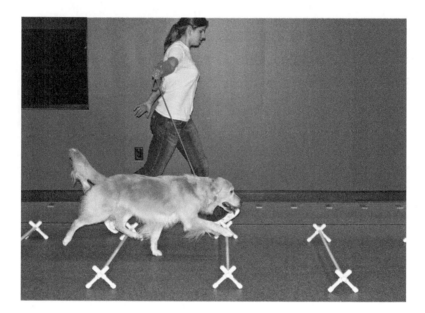

Figure 10.26   Trotting over cavaletti poles spaced about as far apart as the dog's height at the withers, then over gradually increasing distances, is an excellent overall strengthening exercise.

dog's height at the withers (Figure 10.26) (see Chapter 2). The distance between the poles is gradually increased 0.5–1″ at a time so that the dog must increase the force with which it pushes off with the thoracic and pelvic limbs and use the core musculature to suspend itself over the ever-increasing distance. To add an additional strength component, the height of the cavaletti can be increased to approximately the height of the dog's carpus.

Plyometrics. Plyometrics are exercises in which muscles exert maximum force in short inter-

vals of time, with the goal of increasing power (speed-strength). Bounding from side to side over a low jump is one way to accomplish this (Figure 10.27). Generally, only experienced trainers can get their dogs to land and take off immediately, spending minimal time on the ground.

Pelvic limb strength exercises

Running up hills. Having a dog retrieve an object while running up progressively

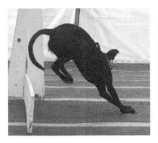
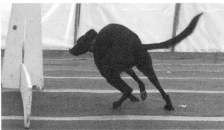
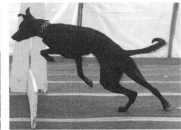

Figure 10.27   Plyometrics involves repeated exertion of maximal force in a short period of time. In this image the dog is landing from a jump then immediately taking off again. Source: Courtesy of Amanda Joudrey-LeBlanc.

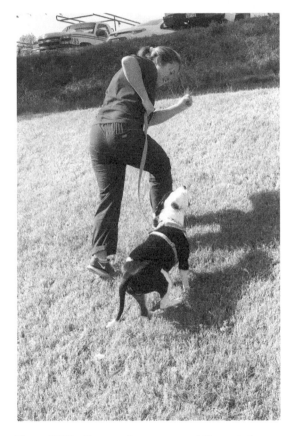

Figure 10.28   Dog running up a steep hill targets the pelvic limbs for strengthening. Having a dog retrieve an object while running up progressively steeper hills is another way to accomplish this. Source: Photo courtesy of Nicole Chun.

steeper hills (Figure 10.28) is an excellent way to target the pelvic limbs for strengthening. When the hills are very steep, it is a good idea to come down the hill more slowly to avoid concussion on the thoracic limbs.

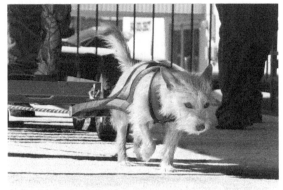

Figure 10.29   Weight-pulling predominantly strengthens the pelvic limbs. This game can be played by dogs of all sizes. Source: Photo by Debbie Maicach.

Pulling weights. The pelvic limbs can also be strengthened by having a dog pull weights or pull a sled over snow or a wheeled cart over the ground (Figure 10.29).

Timing of strength training

After a muscle is fatigued, its overworked fibers need time to rest and rebuild themselves before they can be productively stressed again. The failure to allow for adequate rest between strength-training sessions can lead to muscular injuries and diminished results (Zatsiorsky & Kraemer, 2006). One way to deal with this is to use split training. This involves fully exhausting individual muscle groups during a workout, then allowing several days for the muscle to fully recover. Muscles are worked roughly twice per week and allowed roughly 72 hours to recover (Zatsiorsky & Kraemer, 2006). Recovery of certain muscle groups is usually achieved on days while training other groups. For example, a client can train thoracic limb exercises on

Mondays and Thursdays, core muscles on Tuesdays and Fridays, and pelvic limb exercises on Wednesdays and Saturdays, taking a break on Sundays. In this way, all muscle groups are allowed the necessary recovery time.

Endurance (aerobic) training

Endurance training generally involves training the aerobic metabolic pathways for energy production, as well as cardiovascular and respiratory capacity. Endurance training modifies both the cardiovascular and musculoskeletal systems. Long-term endurance training induces many cardiovascular adaptations in the dog, including decreasing heart rate and increasing interventricular septal thickness and heart weight (Stepien et al., 1998). Skeletal muscle and the nervous system also adapt to exercise, with changes in the molecular structure of muscle fiber types (Seene et al., 2009) and the strengthening of connections between neurons with enhanced firing frequency and spinal reflexes and improvements in learning and memory (Folland & Williams, 2007; Morgan et al., 2015; Cassilhas et al., 2016). Additional goals of endurance training are to increase the lactate threshold in the muscles (the exercise intensity at which lactic acid starts to accumulate in the blood stream) and Vo_{2max} (maximal oxygen consumption—the point

during exercise at which oxygen consumption remains at a steady state despite an increase in workload) (Hiruntrakul et al., 2010). For more information on the physiology of exercise, see Chapter 3.

Endurance or aerobic exercise can be achieved by having a dog trot for at least 20 minutes continuously on land or swim continuously for at least 5 minutes. The most commonly employed endurance exercise is roadwork, in which the trotting dog is accompanied by the client, who can run alongside (Figure 10.30), use inline skates, a bike, a human- or electric-powered scooter, and so on. It is always best for the dog to be in the trot gait for these exercises, as this is the only gait that exercises both sides of the dog's body equally and requires each leg to function alone without assistance from the contralateral limb. If a dog is going to do roadwork at high frequency or duration, an effort should be made to have the dog work on a forgiving surface such as a grass or wood chip path, rather than on concrete or asphalt.

Dogs can be encouraged to swim around the edge of a pool by using treats that float on water (many dry dog biscuits do) or by having the dog on a leash with the client walking around the edge of the pool. Trained retrievers can be sent to retrieve a planted bumper at distances of 200 yards (180 m) or more (referred to as a blind retrieve). Dogs can also

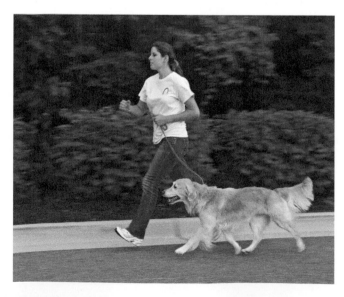

Figure 10.30   Dog performing endurance exercise (roadwork) accompanied by client.

be encouraged to follow a kayak or canoe by using verbal praise and treats.

Land treadmills can be used for endurance conditioning as long as the treadmill is at least 2.5 times the length of the dog's body from the manubrium to the ischiatic tuberosity (Figure 10.31). With most larger dogs this rules out the use of treadmills designed for humans. Because trotting on a treadmill does not exercise as many muscles as trotting over ground, and because having the legs pulled out from under the body is thought to affect the musculature differently from using the limbs to power across the ground (Van Caekenberghe *et al.*, 2013), treadmills should not constitute the main method for endurance conditioning in canine athletes that specialize in endurance events

such as mushing, field trials, and herding trials. They can, however, be an outstanding alternative during inclement weather and can provide variety in training. Other cautions for use of the treadmill include not having the treadmill face a wall or other solid surface, not harnessing a dog to a treadmill, and using treadmills only with dogs that enjoy the practice.

Underwater treadmills can add a significant amount of resistance to the training regimen of a canine athlete. As with land treadmills, the dog should predominantly be gaited at a trot, although bursts of faster speeds can be added for variety. This exercise provides a nice combination of both strength and endurance. See Chapter 9 for more information on the use of underwater treadmills.

Balance between strength and endurance training

Dogs should receive strength and endurance training in proportion to the amount of each type of activity the dog is required to perform in its sport(s) or job. Figure 10.32 shows a continuum between endurance and strength sports in dogs and the points on that continuum at which the most common canine performance events lie. Performance events that require mainly endurance include mushing, herding, and field trials. Performance events that have both endurance and strength components include upper level (masters) hunt tests and tracking. Performance events that

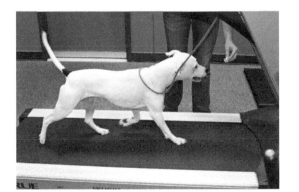

Figure 10.31   Dog exercising on a land treadmill. This treadmill is just large enough at 2.5 times the length of the dog's body. Notice that the dog is trotting.

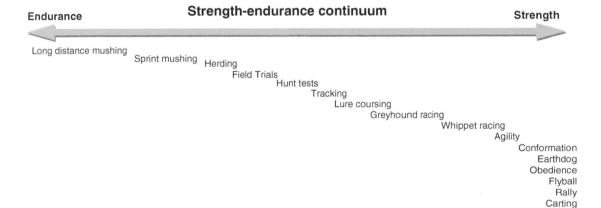

Figure 10.32   The strength-endurance continuum. Competitions that require mainly endurance are on the left side and those that require mainly strength are on the right.

require predominantly strength include flyball, obedience, agility, weight-pulling trials, and other activities that require only short (less than a minute) bursts of movement.

Most of the clients seen by rehabilitation professionals in a typical practice participate in sports that involve predominantly strength. Likewise, most working dogs perform activities that require strength rather than endurance. Nonetheless, dogs that compete only in strength-type activities such as obedience or flyball still benefit from some endurance training—a minimum of three 20-minute trots a week is a good starting point.

Note: Endurance should not be mistaken for stamina. Stamina is the ability to keep working at an activity (whether it involves strength or endurance activities) for long periods of time. Endurance implies increased oxidative capacity and muscular adaptations for performing long-term aerobic activities. For example, a person who can work out with weights for an hour might have exceptional stamina, but might not have the aerobic capacity to run for more than 40 seconds. From that point of view, all performance and working dogs should ideally have excellent stamina.

Certainly, there is significant overlap between strength and endurance training, and athletes benefit from experiencing both forms of exercise. For example, a study in human athletes showed that strength training can lead to enhanced long-term (>30 minutes) and short-term (<15 minutes) endurance capacity in both well-trained individuals and highly trained top-level endurance athletes, especially with the use of high-volume, heavy-resistance strength training protocols. The enhancement in endurance capacity appears to involve training-induced increases in the proportion of type IIA muscle fibers as well as gains in maximal muscle strength and rapid force characteristics (rate of force development), while likely also involving enhancements in neuromuscular function (Aagaard & Andersen, 2010).

Proprioception and balance

Proprioception is the ability to sense the spatial orientation of various parts of the body, including the head, legs, and feet, and to make movement adjustments accordingly. The proprioceptive

sense is thought to be provided by information from sensory neurons located in the inner ear (information on motion and orientation) and stretch receptors located in the muscles and the joint-supporting ligaments (for information on stance see Wodowski *et al.*, 2016).

There are specific nerve receptors for this form of perception called proprioceptors. Messages from these receptors are sent up the spinal cord and are read and interpreted by the brain, allowing the dog to make coordinated movements such as landing from a jump, climbing over debris, or grasping an object in the jaws. Just like all nerves, those that govern proprioception can be trained. In other words, connections between neurons in those pathways can be strengthened and their numbers of synapses increased. With practice, dogs can improve their proprioceptive abilities, making them less susceptible to injury and able to work on complex tasks for longer periods of time without tiring.

One of the best and most deceptively simple body awareness exercises is to have the dog step over the rungs of a ladder placed on the ground (Figure 10.33). It is best for the dog to move quite slowly, which gives it time to think about the placement of the feet. Once the dog can walk forward without touching the edges or the rungs, the dog can be moved forward then immediately backward. Likewise, these exercises can be performed on hills (with the dog moving in all four directions) to increase the difficulty. Another variation is to have the dog step sideways with only the front feet or only the rear feet stepping between the rungs. Search and rescue dogs can benefit from practicing stepping on (rather than between) the rungs of a ladder.

Other proprioceptive exercises include having a dog walk along a plank, step over PVC poles scattered randomly over the ground (Figure 10.34), and having dogs back up over various terrain such as sand, wood chips, and deep grass. The use of rocker boards and wobble boards to improve balance is discussed in Chapter 8.

Preparation and recovery (warm-ups and cool-downs)

Warming up prior to exercise improves performance (Fradkin *et al.*, 2010; Huang *et al.*, 2011),

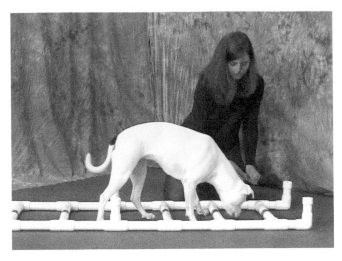

Figure 10.33   One of the best and most deceptively simple body awareness exercises is to have the client walk the dog over a ladder placed on the ground.

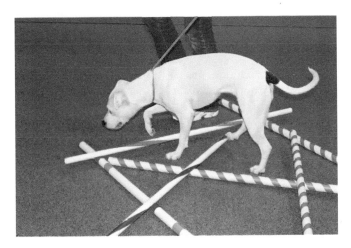

Figure 10.34   By stepping over randomly oriented poles on the ground, dogs can improve the awareness of foot placement (proprioception).

flexibility (Zakas *et al.*, 2006), and propriocep-tion (Magalhaes *et al.*, 2010). Appropriate warm-ups before sports are also thought to reduce the incidence and severity of injuries (Bien, 2011; Samukawa *et al.*, 2011), although it is also clear that not all warm-ups are helpful (Stojanovic & Ostojic, 2011). Warm-ups should include movements that recapitulate what the athlete will do when performing, so warm-ups should be different for dogs with different performance expectations or jobs (Amiri-Khorasani *et al.*, 2011). In a large meta-study of dynamic (in which the body is moved through the motions that will occur during the sport or job)

versus static (in which the limbs are passively moved into a stretched position) stretching in human athletes, it was concluded that static stretching should be avoided as the sole activity in a warm-up routine (Simic *et al.*, 2012). In another study, dynamic stretching was shown to be supe-rior to static stretching for improving athletic per-formance in sports that involved flexibility and jumping (Perrier *et al.*, 2011).

A good warm-up for dogs preparing to par-ticipate in events requiring jumping and active movements, such as agility, flyball, retrieving, and so on, might include the following: 2–3 min-utes of walking then trotting, some dodging

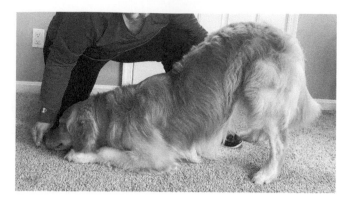

Figure 10.35   The play bow extends the spine dorsoventrally.

from side to side and/or tugging, then dynamic stretching using gradually more active movements such as wave, bow, spin, and beg that recapitulate the flexion and extension that the dog will use in the activity. These may also include practice jumps in the case of agility dogs. Once the dog is fully warmed up, which can be identified by seeing the dog lightly panting, the dog can be put through some motions that actively stretch the soft tissues of the vertebral column, including the play bow (Figure 10.35) to extend the spine and the hunch (Figure 10.36) to flex the spine; and lateral spinal stretches (Figure 10.37) to laterally flex the spine.

A good cool-down consists of gradually reduced exercise, such as some trotting followed by walking, then a brief whole-body rubdown, and potentially performing passive range of motion on joints that have been injured in the past.

Often, working dogs such as police dogs are not able to warm up before they engage in sudden activity. In this case, it is important to provide the dog with a cool-down period and watch carefully for signs of injury such as stiffness during the cool-down or when moving again after a rest period.

Skill training

Skill training consists of the specific training that is required to teach the dog to successfully compete in performance events. Clients will know more than the rehabilitation professional about the specifics of training their dogs. However, it is important to remind them that skill training

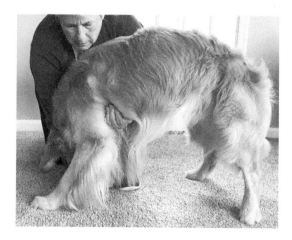

Figure 10.36   The hunch flexes the spine dorsoventrally.

should not be the only form of fitness training that their dogs receive. For dogs that are recovering from an injury or surgery, it is important to provide as detailed information as possible regarding how the client should retrain the dog for the specific requirements of the sporting event in which it will participate. For this reason, a detailed skills retraining program is essential.

Retraining the canine athlete

The primary goal of physical rehabilitation is to heal and then to strengthen the affected muscles while making sure to support the rest of the body through the healing and strengthening process to prevent re-injury or subsequent secondary or compensatory injury. Physical rehabilitation should start with a complete diagnosis: not only a veterinary diagnosis that addresses

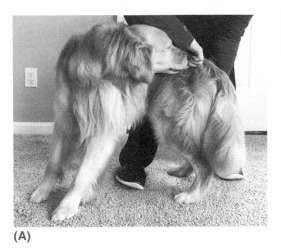
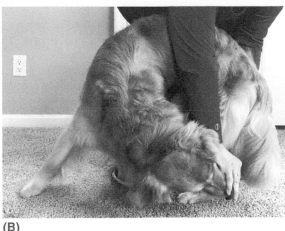

(A)   (B)

Figure 10.37   **(A, B)** Lateral flexion of the spine to both sides is accomplished by having the dog follow food along the lateral spine, pausing at the pelvis for 3 seconds, then moving the food down to the foot, pausing again for 3 seconds, then repeating in reverse.

the major problem, but also a list of secondary problems that might accompany the presenting problem or follow as a result of the presenting problem. Rehabilitation therapy might include any or all of manual therapy, physical modalities such as therapeutic ultrasound, transcutaneous electrical neuromuscular stimulation (TENS), laser, neuromuscular electrical stimulation (NMES), and/or magnetic field therapy as well as underwater treadmill, swimming, and therapeutic exercises. However, it should be a unified process that accounts for the dog's structure, fitness level, and future performance/working activities.

Once the dog has reached pet-level fitness, the canine athlete or working dog will need to begin to retrain in the activities that it must perform during its sport(s) or job. Sports retraining is the process of training the canine athlete to go from functional to competitive or just to full activity if the dog is not a competition sports or working dog. A human athlete might have a physical therapist to help in recovery after an injury or surgery, but will need the help of a sports medicine specialist to decide what exercises as well as how much and in what order they should be used to get back into condition for competition. Likewise, an agility dog that, for example, has had surgery for a fragmented medial coronoid process, will engage in a period of rehabilitation to strengthen the thoracic limb muscles and regain full flexion and extension of the elbow joint. At that point, a canine sports

medicine/rehabilitation professional can provide a detailed program of progressive at-home exercises and sport-specific training to help the dog regain its competitive physical condition and train the appropriate exercises in the appropriate order to continue the strengthening process and prevent re-injury.

A comprehensive retraining program starts with the four components that have already been discussed: strength, endurance, and proprioceptive exercises and a discussion of appropriate methods to warm up and cool down the dog. These provide the foundation for an all-around conditioning program for the dog going forward.

The skills retraining program should begin with the components of the dog's sport or work that are least stressful to the injured part of the body and best protect the dog from re-injury, then gradually progress to more complex physical requirements of the sport/job. For example, agility dogs that have had surgery for cranial cruciate ligament (CCL) insufficiency should start retraining in that sport using low jumps and straight-line sequences. Then they can gradually progress to tighter turns and higher jumps. Obstacles like the weave poles, which apply significant torque to the stifle joint, should be the last skills to retrain.

In addition, the client should be advised how to monitor the dog to determine whether the retraining program needs to be modified. This can happen with dogs that are so driven to work that they risk re-injury, because the dog is progressing more slowly than expected, or because other injuries surface that were masked by the more urgent injury. Depending on the injury, it takes weeks to months of retraining (three to four training sessions a week) to go from pet-level fitness to working dog fitness, although this is highly variable depending on the dog's injury, pre-injury fitness level, its age, size, the compliance and training experience of the client, and other factors.

It is essential that a canine sports medicine/rehabilitation professional who is developing a sports retraining program be knowledgeable about:

- Exercise physiology and nutrition for the canine athlete.
- Developmental conditions that affect a dog's performance, such as hip or elbow dysplasia, osteochondrosis, etc.
- Injuries that can occur in the canine athlete, such as CCL insufficiency, iliopsoas strain, medial shoulder instability, etc.
- Various surgical techniques that are used for repair of orthopedic injuries, such as the comparative risks and benefits of tibial plateau leveling osteotomy (TPLO), tibial tuberosity advancement (TTA), and extracapsular techniques for repair of CCL insufficiency.
- Principles of canine rehabilitation for developmental conditions, injuries, and surgical repair in the canine athlete.
- Drugs that can affect a dog's performance.
- The sports in which dogs compete. It is particularly important that the sports medicine/rehabilitation professional who is developing a retraining program be actively observing or competing in canine sports. They also should be familiar with current training techniques since those can impact a dog's return to competition or the potential for later re-injury. In addition, the professional should be very familiar with the muscles that are used for different aspects of the various canine sports.

The length of the sports retraining period depends on many factors, including:

- The dog's age. Older dogs often take a little longer to regain their competition condition.
- The dog's level of fitness when first entering

rehabilitation. Canine athletes have an edge over the average pet dog because they usually are in better muscular condition when injured. This is a significant advantage in rehabilitation, one that generally shortens the sports retraining period.
- The nature of the injury/surgery/illness. For example, a dog that has just been diagnosed with Addison's disease might see a canine sports medicine/rehabilitation professional to get a plan for training and competing in agility that will help minimize stress while maximizing muscle strength and overall fitness. This dog will likely be able to compete within weeks of diagnosis. In contrast, a dog that has had surgery for medial shoulder instability will require very specific, progressive exercises to gradually increase weight bearing and loading of the shoulder joint in the context of the specific sport(s) in which the dog competes to protect the shoulder from re-injury. The sports retraining period for this dog might be 2–3 months or longer depending on the dog's progress.

When designing a sports retraining regimen, it is important to consider the following factors:

- The age of the dog.
- Whether it is spayed/neutered and, if so, at what age.
- The sports in which the dog competes and the particular levels (e.g., what titles does the dog have?) or the specific tasks that a working dog must undertake.
- The client's goals in each sport.
- The dog's structure, including angulation of the thoracic and pelvic limbs, length of body relative to height at the withers, amount of bone, and so on.
- The dog's current level of fitness (muscle size and tone).
- The kinds of strength and endurance exercises the client worked on with the dog when it was healthy.
- Previous injuries or illnesses the dog has experienced, including stresses on other parts of the body due to compensation for the current condition.
- The food, supplements, and medications that the dog is receiving.

The canine sports medicine/rehabilitation professional should examine the client's dog *whole-istically*. In addition to providing information on fitness exercises and sports-specific training, the rehabilitation professional should advise the client on the following if appropriate:

- The patient's diet and any changes that might be made to improve healing and promote muscle strength. For example, the sports medicine/rehabilitation professional may advise the client on levels and digestibility of proteins and fats in the patient's diet to help provide the building blocks for healing and energy for exercise.
- Nutritional or other supplements that might aid in healing or prevent additional injury. A client might need advice on whether the patient should be administered joint-protective nutraceuticals, for example, as well as which ones are best and what dose is appropriate for the patient.
- Ancillary therapy such as massage, heat/ice treatments, and so on, that should be provided to promote healing and prevent re-injury.
- The most stressful activities of common sports. For example, the components of dog agility that produce the most stress on an injured canine body are:
  - ○ Sudden stops, such as fast 2-on, 2-off contacts (where the dog is trained to land with the two front feet on the

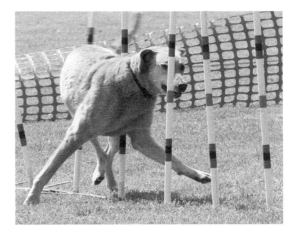

Figure 10.38 Dog showing the extreme lateral flexion that often occurs when dogs weave rapidly, particularly when landing on only one thoracic limb.

ground and the two rear feet on the obstacle), particularly on the A-frame, which meets the ground at a more acute angle than the other contact obstacles.
  - ○ Sharp turns such as serpentines, tight pinwheels, and 180- or 270-degree turns.
  - ○ Extreme lateral flexion of the spine, such as happens with dogs that do fast, one-footed weaves (Figure 10.38).

It is important to also be aware of the potential for obstacle-associated re-injury, such as falling off the dog walk or having one foot slip off the teeter or dog walk, even if the dog doesn't fall.

Case Study 10.2   Agility dog post shoulder rehabilitation retraining program

Signalment: 6 y.o. 35 lb intact male Border Collie.

History: The patient is one of the top five Border Collies in the country based on the AKC point system. He had a 3-month history of progressive left thoracic limb lameness and was diagnosed with moderate medial shoulder instability by arthroscopic examination. He underwent radiofrequency therapy followed by rehabilitation therapy three times per week for 2 months. Patient is now able to go up and down stairs, sit and stand quickly, and go for a 30-minute walk on leash that includes 10 minutes of trotting. The rehabilitation therapist feels that it is time for the patient to continue the rehabilitation program at home and to begin to retrain in preparation for agility competition.

Physical examination: The patient is in good physical condition and has not been allowed to gain weight during rehabilitation. Measurements of foreleg circumference 3 inches proximal to the olecranon process reveals equal circumference of both thoracic limbs. Abduction of the left thoracic limb with the patient in a standing position is approximately 22 degrees on the left and 30 degrees on the right. No pain or discomfort can be elicited.

Sports retraining plan

Strength exercises: Three stationary exercises are assigned for the whole body and each of the thoracic limbs, the core, and the pelvic limbs as follows:

Whole body:
- Rolling a peanut ball
- Sit-to-stand with elevated front
- Stand-down-stand without moving feet

(Continued)

Thoracic limbs:
- Wave
- High-nines
- Wheelbarrowing

Core:
- Beg
- Diagonal leg lifts
- One side leg lifts

Pelvic limbs:
- Beg-stand-beg
- Thoracic limbs on perch
- Pulling against a theraband

Endurance exercises: Begin with a 10-minute trot 3 days per week at a moderate speed. Increase to 15 minutes three times per week in 2 weeks, then 20 minutes three times per week at 4 weeks. Patient can swim 5 minutes every other day, swimming continuously rather than jumping in and out of the pool. Increase by a minute per week to 10 minutes maximum.

Proprioception exercises: Focus on retraining proprioception of the thoracic limbs. Exercises include walking forward, backward, and sideways with the thoracic limbs in the ladder.

Skill training: The patient will start agility training at 16 weeks after surgery, introducing the obstacles in the order shown in Table 10.2. In summary, this will involve, in order:

- Straight lines of widely spaced 8-inch jumps and tunnels ending at a low table.
- Wide circles of jumps, tunnels, tables, and the teeter.
- Large figure-eight-shaped sequences (inside diameter of loops = 20 ft) using the above obstacles. Increase jump height to 12 inches.

Table 10.2 Sample agility retraining program for a dog that jumps 24 inches*

Phase	Number of sessions per phase (one session per day)	Session duration	Number of obstacles per sequence	Obstacle types	Turns
I	5	• 10 minutes total • Minimum 30 s break (dog is sitting, standing still or lying down) between repetitions of the sequences	• Sequences of up to four obstacles only • One-jump collection work at 8″	• 8″ jumps, tunnels, 8″ tables • If using box method for contacts, start box work on the ground	Straight lines and wide curves, but no sharp turns (other than the ones used for the one-jump exercises)
II	8	• 12 minutes total • Minimum 30 s break between repetitions of the sequences	• Sequences of up to eight obstacles • One-jump work at 12″	• 12″ jumps, tunnels, 12″ tables, tire, teeter • Practice 2o2o contacts on travel board, start to elevate it up to 12″ • Continue box work for contacts low A-frame (4 ft)	• Up to 90-degree turns. Start with just one per training session and increase the number you do throughout this phase
III	10	• 15 minutes total • 30 s break between repetitions of the sequences	• Sequences of up to 12 obstacles • One-jump work at 16″	• 16″ jumps, tunnels, 16″ tables, tire, teeter, dog walk (2o2o) • Higher (5 ft) A-frame • Box on the A-frame • Channel weaves up to shoulder width, or: • Up to four poles if using 2 × 2 weave pole method (no more than four pole sets per training session)	• Up to 180-degree turns. Start with just one per training session and increase the number you do throughout this phase • No tight turns around jump stanchions

Table 10.2   (*Continued*)

Phase	Number of sessions per phase (one session per day)	Session duration	Number of obstacles per sequence	Obstacle types	Turns
IV	12	15 minutes total	• Sequences of up to 16 obstacles • One-jump work at 20″	• 20″ jumps, tunnels, 16″ tables, tire, teeter, dog walk (2o2o) • Full-height A-frame • Start removing the lower part of the box on the A-frame • Start to bend body in channel weave poles, or: • Six poles if using 2×2 method (no more than six pole sets per training session)	• Add sharper turns including tight turns around jump stanchions • Introduce just a few tight turns and gradually increase
V	12	20 minutes total	• Sequences of up to 20 obstacles	• 24″ jumps, tunnels, 16″ and 24″ tables, tire, teeter, dog walk (2o2o) • Full-height A-frame • Remove the rest of the box from A-frame • Start to bend body in channel weave poles, or: • 12 poles if using 2×2 method (no more than six pole sets per training session)	• Full variety of types of turns seen in a typical master/excellent course • Introduce just a few tight turns and gradually increase the number to a maximum of three in each sequence

*This is just a sample. Every retraining program should be individually designed for each dog, giving consideration to the dog's age, breed, structure, injury, the dog's response to treatment and rehabilitation, and the client's goals for the dog. 2o2o, 2-on, 2-off.

• Sequences with 90-degree turns on the flat, but not immediately after landing from an obstacle. Increase jump height to 16 inches. Add the dog walk and 2-on, 2-off contacts only if the patient does them gently. If the patient stops abruptly in a 2-on, 2-off position at the bottom of the A-frame and/or dog walk, switch to using a quick release or running contacts if possible.
• Add the A-frame if the patient has 2-on, 2-off contacts. Increase the jump height to 20 inches.
• Add weave poles last as they create the most torque on the shoulder.

Additional notes: The patient's shoulder should be iced for 10 minutes after exercise, whether skill training, competing, or fitness training. At-home heat and massage treatments followed by passive range of motion exercises should be performed daily, but not within 2 hours of exercise and icing. The patient should be given appropriate levels of protein (for tissue repair), fat (for energy and to provide a balance of omega-3 and omega-6 fatty acids for their anti-inflammatory activity), and should have the appropriate calcium:phosphorus balance (see Chapter 4). Patient should be taking high-quality joint-protective nutraceuticals, probiotics, omega-3 fatty acid supplements, and balanced antioxidants. Discuss the potential use of chiropractic adjustments and acupuncture with the client. Discuss ways to monitor the patient's progress including time to fatigue, muscle size and tone, and evidence of early subclinical lameness.

Case Study 10.2 is an example that provides the reader with basic principles. The specific exercises and their progression should be individualized for each dog depending on the many factors listed earlier.

Overtraining

Canine athletes can be overtrained, just as human athletes can. In human athletes, overtraining leads paradoxically to reduced fitness, poorer athletic performance, an increased chance of injuries, reduced resistance to infection, and depression (Purvis *et al.*, 2010; Winsley & Matos, 2011). Overtraining syndrome also occurs in sport horses, resulting in sustained loss of performance despite a heavy training program (Rivero *et al.*, 2008). The same problems can occur in dogs that are overtrained.

Three important variables of strength training are intensity, duration, and frequency. *Intensity* refers to the amount of work required to achieve the activity and can be both physical and psychological. *Duration* refers to the length of time over which the exercise occurs. *Frequency* refers to how many training sessions are performed in a given time period.

These variables are important because they are all interrelated, as the muscle has only so much strength and endurance and takes time to recover after significant use. Increasing one of these components by any significant amount might necessitate decrease of the other two. For example, increasing the height at which a dog jumps should be accompanied by a reduction of the number of reps, and might require more recovery time and therefore fewer workouts per week. Trying to push too much intensity, duration, and frequency at the same time will result in overtraining, and can eventually lead to injury and other health issues such as chronic soreness and general lethargy, illness, or even acute trauma such as avulsion fractures (MacKinnon, 2000). A high-medium-low formula can be used to avoid overtraining, with intensity, duration, or frequency being high, one of the others being medium, and the other being low (Coutts *et al.*, 2007).

To help prevent overtraining clients should be encouraged to:

(1) Vary the duration, frequency, and intensity of training throughout the week.
(2) Give the dog 1 day off from training every week.
(3) Give the dog a minimum of 1 month (30 consecutive days) off from training and competition every year. The dog should undertake no skill training during this time and only mild to moderate strength and endurance training. This last suggestion can be difficult for some clients to comply with.

Deconditioning

Canine athletes frequently take substantial breaks from competition, and it is of interest to know what effects those breaks might have on conditioning and a dog's strength and aerobic capacity. There are few studies of detraining in dogs, but studies in horses and humans can provide us with clues as to the potential effects of detraining in dogs. In one study, eight Canaan dogs were exercised on a treadmill until they achieved a level of fitness that allowed them to run 8.7 km/h at a 10° incline for 1 hour without their temperature elevating above 40 °C or their heart rate above 250 bpm. They then were put on a program of complete cage rest. Within 3–5 weeks, there was a significant loss in their fitness (ability to perform the above exercise) (Sneddon *et al.*, 1989).

In another study, yearling Thoroughbred horses were trained for 6 months, and then placed on pasture for 8 hours a day and stall rest at night for 10 weeks. The exercise that they obtained on pasture was sufficient to maintain the gains in Vo_{2max}, cardiac output, and stroke volume that were established during training (Mukai *et al.*, 2006).

In a study of the effects of detraining in humans, men and women underwent strength training for 9 weeks, then experienced detraining for 31 weeks. The detraining period consisted of cessation of the strength training protocol, while continuing daily activities of living. The strength gains established during the training period diminished only minimally during the first 12 weeks of detraining, but declined more between 12 and 31 weeks of detraining (Lemmer et al., 2000). Another study performed in young soccer players found that long-term detraining (>4 weeks) decreased oxygen uptake, Vo_{2max}, and aerobic and anaerobic running speeds (Melchiorri et al., 2014).

Similarly, a study performed in elite taekwondo athletes found 8-week detraining suppressed physiological stress but rapidly resulted in declines in athletic performance and health metabolic profiles, including reduced aerobic capacity, increased body fat, muscle loss, insulin resistance development, and elevated systemic inflammatory status. The inflammation state was positively associated with insulin resistance development, fat mass, central fat accumulation, and the decline in Vo_{2max} (Liao et al., 2016).

However, another study performed in elite women pole-vaulters found that after 28 days of inactivity, the rate of force development (RFD) and the ability to accelerate over very short distances (5 m) while sprinting improved after training cessation. Acceleration over longer distances (5–45 m) was impaired, while unloaded and loaded vertical jump tests suffered trivial to small changes. Further, this study concluded that detraining periods of approximately 1 month or even longer may be implemented in elite pole-vaulters without significantly impairing performance (Loturco et al., 2017). Together, these studies suggest that continued exercise, even of a relatively gentle nature, is essential to maintain levels of fitness that will shorten the length of time for recovery from an injury and return to competition sports.

Age-appropriate conditioning and sports training

Young, growing dogs undergo significant physical changes, especially during the first 12–18 months of life before the physes have closed. This means they have different capabilities for, and adaptations to, exercise. For this reason, training programs for young canine athletes should not be just scaled-down versions of adult

training programs. There are marked differences in coordination, strength, and stamina between puppies and adults. Puppies have lower anaerobic capabilities, are less metabolically efficient, and have less efficient thermoregulatory mechanisms (Bright, 2001).

For long-term health in canine athletes and working dogs, it is important to avoid intense and particularly concussive training until the physes are closed. The physes of different bones close at different ages (Table 10.3). The larger the breed, the later the physes close. In addition, it is well established that the physes of dogs that are spayed or neutered prior to puberty experience delayed closure (Salmeri et al., 1991). The best way to know whether the physes of a gonadectomized dog are closed is to perform a lateral radiograph of the stifle as the tibial tuberosity is the last physis in the body to close.

The difference in texture between the calcified bone and the uncalcified physes makes the physes susceptible to injury. The physis is the weakest area of the growing skeleton, weaker than the nearby ligaments and tendons that connect bones to other bones and muscles (Shire & Shultz, 2001). In a growing dog, a serious injury to a joint is more likely to damage a growth plate than the ligaments that stabilize the joint. An injury that would cause a sprain in an adult dog can injure the physis in a young

Table 10.3   Ages at which the physes close

Physis	Closure age (months)
Thoracic limb	
Tuber scapulae	4–7
Proximal humeral epiphysis	9–15.5
Humerus: lateral and medial condyles	6.25
Proximal radial epiphysis	4.5–11
Distal radial epiphysis	4.5–17
Pelvic limb	
Femoral head	4.3–18
Femoral distal epiphysis	4.5
Tibial condyles	4.75–13.75
Tibial tuberosity	4.75–14.5
Tibial distal epiphysis	4.5–16.5

Source: Adapted from Newton and Nunamaker, 1985.

dog. If a physis is injured, it can prematurely close, resulting in a shortening or malformation of the leg. This can limit or abrogate the dog's ability to have a performance or working career (Harasen, 2003).

While physeal injuries can be caused by an acute event, such as a fall or a blow to a limb, chronic injuries to the physes also can occur from overuse of young growing bones. Canine sports medicine/rehabilitation professionals have observed that agility dogs that are taught to weave or jump at a young age and are trained repetitively while young have an increased risk of chronic injuries, particularly to the spine, later in life. Agility dogs, particularly those of larger, more heavy-set breeds such as Golden Retrievers, that present with career-ending lumbosacral disease frequently have a history of being eager, fast weavers that were overtrained as young dogs. This condition appears to be much less common in dogs that begin intensive agility training when physically mature. Overuse or repetitive trauma injuries represent approximately 50% of all pediatric sport-related injuries (Valovich McLeod *et al.*, 2011). There is a significant need for research to increase our understanding of the effects of physically taxing sports on canine athletes.

Research on the effects of resistance training on young human athletes suggests that moderate strength training can be beneficial in children (Fedewa & Ahn, 2011; Gunter *et al.*, 2012). Coaches who place young athletes on strength-training programs must ensure that the athletes are properly taught the appropriate skills, are provided with a well-controlled, progressive program, and are not subjected to repetitive stresses.

For endurance training such as long-distance running, the story may be a bit different. Running depends on aerobic power—the ability to transport oxygen from the air to produce energy in the muscle cells. Endurance training can increase aerobic power in adults by up to 30%. But in children, the maximum increase, even with very hard training, is only about 10% (Borms, 1986; Zauner *et al.*, 1989). The cardiovascular system of a preadolescent youngster is simply not mature enough to adapt well to the physiological stress of long-distance running.

Furthermore, while long-distance running does not seem to harm the cardiopulmonary systems of children, overuse or repetitive trauma injuries represent a large percentage of all pediatric sports-related injuries (Valovich McLeod *et al.*, 2011). Again, maturity is an issue. Up to about age 16, the growing cartilage in the long leg bones and surrounding the joints is relatively soft. Continuous foot-to-road pounding can easily injure the cartilage during miles of training (Loud *et al.*, 2005). In addition, a child's leg bones can grow very rapidly, particularly during puberty. When this happens, the muscles and tendons that span the joints stretch, rather than grow. As a result, the tissue can get very tight, like taut elastic bands, increasing the risk of injuries.

There are psychological considerations as well. For many children, intense training can lead to problems like anxiety and chronic fatigue (Winsley & Matos, 2011). Such problems can easily take the fun out of the activity and could foster an unhealthy attitude toward sport, exercise, and physical fitness in general.

Bones grow and function the same, whether they make up the skeleton of a child or a dog. We can learn a great deal from studies that have been performed in human athletes because people can clearly identify where and how much they hurt and can verbalize their emotions about training. Hopefully, more studies in dogs will be performed in the future.

Guidelines for the types of exercise to which puppies and growing dogs can be exposed are provided in Table 10.4. These guidelines err on the side of caution, preventing young dogs from experiencing extremes of physical activity because of the problems that can develop in young adult and middle-aged dogs that are trained and exercised excessively prior to the closure of growth plates. Some dogs are driven to exercise even at young ages and will push themselves beyond the limits of safety. Be sure to set boundaries for your clients' dogs with the goal of increasing their longevity in performance.

Table 10.4 Age-appropriate conditioning and sports training

Age	Activities				Comments
	Strength	Endurance	Proprioception	Skills	
Under 6 months	• Short walks or hikes • Gentle tugging • Chasing an object dragged on the ground • Supervised play with appropriate-sized dogs • Short swimming periods	None	• Ladder work • Perch work • Spinning to the R and L • Play on a variety of surfaces • Wobble boards • Back up	• Skill training, such as sit, down, stand, stay, and touch • Early jump training with jumps no higher than carpus height • No agility weave pole training	Young puppies should not be exercised with the specific intent of increasing strength or endurance. Much of their exercise should be self-directed play
6 months to growth plate closure	All of the above, plus strength training exercises, beginning with moderate exercise and gradually increasing the frequency, duration, and intensity	None	All of the above, plus: • Ladder work on soft surfaces, hills • Side-stepping over ladder	• Jump training using gradually increasing jump heights from carpus to elbow height. Jump exercises that teach how to judge distance, collect and extend strides, how to use lead legs, etc. • No agility weave pole training that causes the spine to flex laterally	High impact and endurance training should be delayed until the physes have fully closed
After growth plate closure (approximately 14 months for intact dogs, 20 months for dogs that are prepubertally gonadectomized)	Planned strength training 4 to 6 days a week including all of the above, plus: • Beg and beg/stand/beg • Jump grids	• Begin aerobic exercise with three 20-minute jogs a week and gradually increase the frequency and duration of endurance training • Swimming • Gradually longer distances/times	All of the above	• Increase jumps to competition height • Begin agility weave pole training and build gradually • Begin repetitive flyball box work and build gradually	By this age, dogs are fully grown, although they still have relatively immature muscles, ligaments, and tendons, so the duration, frequency and intensity of exercise should be increased gradually

References

Aagaard, P. & Andersen, J. L. 2010. Effects of strength training on endurance capacity in top-level endurance athletes. *Scand J Med Sci Sports*, 20 (Suppl. 2), 39–47.

Acevedo, L. M. & Rivera, J. L. 2006. New insights into skeletal muscle types in the dog with particular focus towards hybrid myosin phenotypes. *Cell Tissue Res* 323(2), 283–303.

Amiri-Khorasani, M., Abu Osman, N. A., & Yusof, A. 2011. Acute effect of static and dynamic stretching on hip dynamic range of motion during instep kicking in professional soccer players. *J Strength Cond Res*, 25, 1647–1652.

Bach, J. F., Rozanski, E. A., Bedenice, D., Chan, D. L., Freeman, L. M., Lofgren, J. L., *et al.* 2007. Association of expiratory airway dysfunction with marked obesity in healthy adult dogs. *Am J Vet Res*, 68, 670–675.

Bauer, N. B., Er, E., & Moritz, A. 2012. Effect of submaximal aerobic exercise on platelet function, platelet activation, and secondary and tertiary hemostasis in dogs. *Am J Vet Res*, 73, 125–133.

Bien, D. P. 2011. Rationale and implementation of anterior cruciate ligament injury prevention warm-up programs in female athletes. *J Strength Cond Res*, 25, 271–285.

Borms, J. 1986. The child and exercise: an overview. *J Sports Sci*, 4, 3–20.

Braund, K. G., Hoff, E. J., & Richardson K. E. 1978. Histochemical identification of fiber types in canine skeletal muscle. *Am J Vet Res*, 39(4), 561–565.

Bright, J. M. 2001. The cardiovascular system. In: Hoskins, J. D. (ed.), *Veterinary Pediatrics: Dogs and Cats from Birth to Six Months*, 3rd edn. Philadelphia: W.B. Saunders, pp. 103–134.

Budsberg, S. C. & Bartges, J. W. 2006 Nutrition and osteoarthritis in dogs: does it help? *Vet Clin North Am Small Anim Pract*, 36(6),1307–1323, vii.

Buttermann, G. R., Schendel, M. J., Kahmann, R. D., Lewis, J. L., & Bradford, D. S. 1992. In vivo facet joint loading of the canine lumbar spine. *Spine*, 17, 81–92.

Cassilhas, R. C., Tufik, S., & de Mello, M. T. 2016. Physical exercise, neuroplasticity, spatial learning and memory. *Cell Mol Life Sci*, 73(5), 975–983.

Coutts, A., Reaburn, P., Piva, T. J., & Murphy, A. 2007. Changes in selected biochemical, muscular strength, power, and endurance measures during deliberate overreaching and tapering in rugby league players. *Int J Sports Med*, 28, 116–124.

Cowey, S. & Hardy, R. W. 2006. The metabolic syndrome: A high-risk state for cancer? *Am J Pathol*, 169, 1505–1522.

Davison, L. J., Holder, A., Catchpole, B. & O'Callaghan, C. A. 2017. The canine POMC gene, obesity in Labrador Retrievers and susceptibility to diabetes mellitus. *J Vet Intern Med*, 31, 343–348.

Fedewa, A. L. & Ahn, S. 2011. The effects of physical activity and physical fitness on children's achievement and cognitive outcomes: a meta-analysis. *Res Q Exerc Sport*, 82, 521–535.

Fisher, J. P., Carlson, L. & Steele, J. 2016. The effects of muscle action, repetition duration, and loading strategies of a whole-body, progressive resistance training programme on muscular performance and body composition in trained males and females. *Appl Physiol Nutr Metab*, 41, 1064–1070.

Folland, J. P. & Williams, A. G. 2007. The adaptations to strength training: morphological and neurological contributions to increased strength. *Sports Med*, 37, 145–168.

Fradkin, A. J., Zazryn, T. R., & Smoliga, J. M. 2010. Effects of warming-up on physical performance: a systematic review with meta-analysis. *J Strength Cond Res*, 24, 140–148.

German, A. J. 2006. The growing problem of obesity in dogs and cats. *J Nutr*, 136(7 Suppl.), 1940S–1946S.

Gosselin, J., Wren, J. A. & Sunderland, S. J. 2007. Canine obesity: an overview. *J Vet Pharmacol Ther*, 30(Suppl. 1), 1–10.

Gunter, K. B., Almstedt, H. C., & Janz, K. F. 2012. Physical activity in childhood may be the key to optimizing lifespan skeletal health. *Exerc Sport Sci Rev*, 40, 13–21.

Gupta, R. C., Canerdy, T. D., Lindley, J., Konemann, M., Minniear, J., Carroll, B. A., *et al.* 2012. Comparative therapeutic efficacy and safety of type-II collagen (UC-II), glucosamine and chondroitin in arthritic dogs: pain evaluation by ground force plate. *J Anim Physiol Anim Nutr (Berl)*, 96(5), 770–777.

Harasen, G. 2003. Common long bone fractures in small animal practice — part 1. *Can Vet J*, 44, 333–334.

Harridge, S. D. 2007. Plasticity of human skeletal muscle: gene expression to *in vivo* function. *Exp Physiol*, 92, 783–797.

Hawke, T. J. & Garry, D. J. 2001. Myogenic satellite cells: physiology to molecular biology. *J Appl Physiol*, 91, 534–551.

Hiruntrakul, A., Nanagara, R., Emasithi, A., & Borer, K. T. 2010. Effect of once a week endurance exercise on fitness status in sedentary subjects. *J Med Assoc Thai*, 93, 1070–1074.

Huang, J. S., Pietrosimone, B. G., Ingersoll, C. D., Weltman, A. L., & Saliba, S. A. 2011. Sling exercise and traditional warm-up have similar effects on the velocity and accuracy of throwing. *J Strength Cond Res*, 25, 1673–1679.

Knuttgen, H. G. 2003. What is exercise? A primer for practitioners. *Phys Sportsmed*, 31, 31–49.

Kumar, S., Pattanaik, A. K., Sharma, S., Jadhav, S. E., Dutta, N., & Kumar, A. 2017. Probiotic potential of a lactobacillus bacterium of canine faecal-origin and its impact on select gut health indices and immune response of dogs. *Probiotics Antimicrob Proteins*, Feb 10. doi: 10.1007/s12602-017-9256-z. [Epub ahead of print]

Kunst, C. M., Pease, A. P., Nelson, N. C., Habing, G., & Ballegeer, E. A. 2014. Computed tomographic identification of dysplasia and progression of osteoarthritis in dog elbows previously assigned OFA grades 0 and 1. *Vet Radiol Ultrasound*, 55, 511–520.

Latorre, R., Gil, F., Vázquez, J. M., Moreno, F., Mascarello, F. & Ramirez, G. 1993. Morphological and histochemical characteristics of muscle fibre types in the flexor carpi radialis of the dog. *J Anat*, 182 (Pt 3), 313–320.

Lemmer, J. T., Hurlbut, D. E., Martel, G. F., Tracy, B. L., Ivey, F. M., Metter, E. J., *et al.* 2000. Age and gender responses to strength training and detraining. *Med Sci Sports Exerc*, 32, 1505–1512.

Liao, Y. H., Sung, Y. C., Chou, C. C., & Chen, C. Y. 2016. Eight-week training cessation suppresses physiological stress but rapidly impairs health metabolic profiles and aerobic capacity in elite Taekwondo athletes. *PLoS ONE*, 11(7), e0160167.

Loturco, I., Pereira, L. A., Kobal, R., Martins, H., Kitamura, K., Cal Abad, C. C. & Nakamura, F. Y. 2017. Effects of detraining on neuromuscular performance in a selected group of elite women pole-vaulters: a case study. *J Sports Med Phys Fitness*, 57(4), 490–495.

Loud, K. J., Gordon, C. M., Micheli, L. J., & Field, A. E. 2005. Correlates of stress fractures among preadolescent and adolescent girls. *Pediatrics*, 115, e399–e406.

Louis, E., Raue, U., Yang, Y., Jemiolo, B., & Trappe, S. 2007. Time course of proteolytic, cytokine, and myo-statin gene expression after acute exercise in human skeletal muscle. *J Appl Physiol*, 103, 1744–1751.

MacDougall, J. D., Gibala, M. J., Tarnopolsky, M. A., MacDonald, J. R., Interisano, S. A., & Yarasheski, K. E. 1995. The time course for elevated muscle protein synthesis following heavy resistance exercise. *Can J Appl Physiol*, 20, 480–486.

MacKinnon, L. T. 2000. Special feature for the Olympics: effects of exercise on the immune system: overtraining effects on immunity and performance in athletes. *Immunol Cell Biol*, 78, 502–509.

Magalhaes, T., Ribeiro, F., Pinheiro, A., & Oliveira, J. 2010. Warming-up before sporting activity improves knee position sense. *Phys Ther Sport*, 11, 86–90.

Maitland, M. E. 2012. Purposeful exercise, including bicycle transportation, improves health. *Clin J Sport Med*, 22, 292–293.

Marsella, R., Santoro, D., & Ahrens, K. 2012. Early exposure to probiotics in a canine model of atopic dermatitis has long-term clinical and immunological effects. *Vet Immunol Immunopathol*, 146(2), 185–189.

Martí-Angulo, S., García-López, N., & Díaz-Ramos, A. 2014. Efficacy of an oral hyaluronate and collagen supplement as a preventive treatment of elbow dysplasia. *J Vet Sci*, 15(4), 569–574.

Martin, L. J., Siliart, B., Dumon, H. J., & Nguyen, P. G. 2006. Hormonal disturbances associated with obesity in dogs. *J Anim Physiol Anim Nutr (Berl)*, 90, 355–360.

Mason, O. J. & Holt, R. 2012. Mental health and physical activity interventions: a review of the qualitative literature. *J Ment Health*, 21, 274–284.

Maxwell, L. C., Barclay, J. K., Mohrman, D. E., & Faulkner, J. A. 1977. Physiological characteristics of skeletal muscles of dogs and cats. *Am J Physiol*, 233(1), C14–18.

Melchiorri, G., Ronconi, M., Triossi, T., Viero, V., de Sanctis, D., Tancredi, V., *et al.* 2014. Detraining in young soccer players. *J Sports Med Phys Fitness*, 54(1), 27–33.

Menor-Campos, D. J., Molleda-Carbonell, J. M., & Lopez-Rodriguez, R. 2011. Effects of exercise and human contact on animal welfare in a dog shelter. *Vet Rec*, 169, 388.

Miyabe, M., Gin, A., Onozawa, E., Daimon, M., Yamada, H., Oda, H., *et al.* 2015. Genetic variants of the unsaturated fatty acid receptor GPR120 relating to obesity in dogs. *J Vet Med Sci*, 77(10), 1201–1206.

Morgan, J. A., Corrigan, F., & Baune, B. T. 2015. Effects of physical exercise on central nervous system functions: a review of brain region specific adaptations. *J Mol Psychiatry*, 18, 3(1), 3.

Mukai, K., Ohmura, H., Hiraga, A., Eto, D., Takahashi, T., Asai, Y., & Jones, J. H. 2006. Effect of detraining on cardiorespiratory variables in young thoroughbred horses. *Equine Vet J Suppl*, 36, 210–213.

Newton, C. D., & Nunamaker, D. M. (eds) 1985. *Textbook of Small Animal Orthopaedics*. Philadelphia: JB Lippincott. Available at: http://cal.vet.upenn.edu/projects/saortho/appendix_c/appc.htm [accessed 16 December 2017].

Perrier, E. T., Pavol, M. J., & Hoffman, M. A. 2011. The acute effects of a warm-up including static or dynamic stretching on countermovement jump height, reaction time, and flexibility. *J Strength Cond Res*, 25, 1925–1931.

Phillips, S. M., Tipton, K. D., Aarsland, A., Wolf, S.E., & Wolfe, R. R. 1997. Mixed muscle protein synthesis and breakdown after resistance exercise in humans. *Am J Physiol*, 273, E99–107.

Purvis, D., Gonsalves, S., & Deuster, P. A. 2010. Physiological and psychological fatigue in extreme conditions: overtraining and elite athletes. *PM R*, 2, 442–450.

Raichlen, D. A., Foster, A. D., Gerdeman, G. L., Seillier, A., & Giuffrida, A. 2012. Wired to run: exercise-induced endocannabinoid signaling in humans and cursorial mammals with implications for the 'runner's high'. *J Exp Biol*, 215, 1331–1336.

Rivero, J. L., van Breda, E., Rogers, C. W., Lindner, A., & van Oldruitenborgh-Oosterbaan, M. M. 2008. Unexplained underperformance syndrome in sport horses: classification, potential causes and recognition. *Equine Vet J*, 40, 611–618.

Salmeri, K. R., Bloomberg, M. S., Scruggs, S. L., & Shille, V. 1991. Gonadectomy in immature dogs: effects on skeletal, physical, and behavioral development. *J Am Vet Med Assoc*, 198, 1193–1203.

Samukawa, M., Hattori, M., Sugama, N., & Takeda, N. 2011. The effects of dynamic stretching on plantar flexor muscle-tendon tissue properties. *Man Ther*, 16, 618–622.

Seene, T., Kaasik, P., & Umnova, M. 2009. Structural rearrangements in contractile apparatus and resulting skeletal muscle remodelling: effect of exercise training. *J Sports Med Phys Fitness*, 49, 410–423.

Shire, P. K. & Shultz, K. S. 2001. The skeletal system in veterinary pediatrics. In: Hoskins, J. D. (ed.), *Veterinary Pediatrics: Dogs and Cats from Birth to Six Months*, 3rd edn. Philadelphia: W.B. Saunders, pp. 402–423.

Simic, L., Sarabon, N., & Markovic, G. 2012. Does pre-exercise static stretching inhibit maximal muscular performance? A meta-analytical review. *Scand J Med Sci Sports*, 23(2), 131–148.

Sneddon, J. C., Minnaar, P. P., Grosskopf, J. F., & Groeneveld, H. T. 1989. Physiological and blood biochemical responses to submaximal treadmill exercise in Canaan dogs before, during and after training. *J S Afr Vet Assoc*, 60, 87–91.

Stepien, R. L., Hinchcliff, K. W., Constable, P. D., & Olson, J. 1998. Effect of endurance training on cardiac morphology in Alaskan sled dogs. *J Appl Physiol*, 85, 1368–1375.

Stojanovic, M. D. & Ostojic, S. M. 2011. Stretching and injury prevention in football: current perspectives. *Res Sports Med*, 19, 73–91.

Valovich McLeod, T. C., Decoster, L. C., Loud, K. J., Micheli, L. J., Parker, J. T., Sandrey, M. A., & White, C. 2011. National Athletic Trainers' Association position statement: prevention of pediatric overuse injuries. *J Athl Train*, 46, 206–220.

van Caekenberghe, I., Segers, V., Willems, P., Gosseye, T., Aerts, P., & de Clercq, D. 2013. Mechanics of overground accelerated running vs. running on an accelerated treadmill. *Gait Posture*, 38(1), 125–131.

Vina, J., Sanchis-Gomar, F., Martinez-Bello, V., & Gomez-Cabrera, M. 2012. Exercise acts as a drug; the pharmacological benefits of exercise. *Br J Pharmacol*, 167, 1–12.

Warren, B. S., Wakshlag, J. J., Maley, M., Farrell, T. J., Struble, A. M., Panasevich, M. R., & Wells, M. T. 2011. Use of pedometers to measure the relationship of dog walking to body condition score in obese and non-obese dogs. *Br J Nutr*, 106(Suppl. 1), S85–S89.

Winsley, R. & Matos, N. 2011. Overtraining and elite young athletes. *Med Sport Sci*, 56, 97–105.

Wodowski, A. J., Swigler, C. W., Liu, H., Nord, K. M., Toy, P. C., & Mihalko, W. M. 2016. Proprioception and knee arthroplasty: a literature review. *Orthop Clin North Am*, 47(2), 301–309.

Xu, J., Bourgeois, H., Vandermeulen, E., Vlaeminck, B., Meyer, E., Demeyere, K., & Hesta, M. 2015. Secreted phospholipase A2 inhibitor modulates fatty acid composition and reduces obesity-induced inflammation in Beagle dogs. *Vet J*, 204(2), 214–9.

Zakas, A., Doganis, G., Zakas, N., & Vergou, A. 2006. Acute effects of active warm-up and stretching on the flexibility of elderly women. *J Sports Med Phys Fitness*, 46, 617–622.

Zatsiorsky, V. M. & Kraemer, W. J. 2006. *Science and Practice of Strength Training*, 2nd edn. Champaign, IL: Human Kinetics Publishers.

Zauner, C. W., Maksud, M. G., & Melichna, J. 1989. Physiological considerations in training young athletes. *Sports Med*, 8, 15–31.

Zou, C. & Shao, J. 2008. Role of adipocytokines in obesity-associated insulin resistance. *J Nutr Biochem*, 19, 277–286.

11 Veterinary Orthotics and Prosthetics

Patrice M. Mich, DVM, MS, DABVP, DACVAA, DACVSMR, CCRT, and Martin Kaufmann, C-Ped, BSBA

Summary

The use of veterinary orthotic and prosthetic (V-OP) devices is a rapidly emerging, therapeutic strategy. Just as veterinary medicine has evolved to include advanced dentistry, joint replacements, chemotherapy, and stereotactic radiation, it is in turn evolving toward the application of advanced biomechanics and technology for the treatment of limb loss and loss of limb function. Knowledge of the components of normal quadruped gait guides treatment of pathomechanical deficiencies. Quadrupeds who suffer loss of limb function or a loss of limb are biomechanically distinct from bipeds with similar loss. An orthosis is any medical device attached to the body to support, align, position, prevent or correct deformity, assist weak muscles, or improve function (Deshales, 2002). These devices provide protected motion within a controlled range, prevent or reduce severity of injury, prevent or relieve contracture, allow lax ligaments and joint capsules to shorten and approach normal distensibilty, and provide functional stability for an unstable limb segment. Prosthetic limbs provide the opportunity to return quadripedal motion by replacing a limb segment.

Use of V-OP devices requires the proper application of biomechanical concepts not previously considered in veterinary medicine; these include three-point correction and force coupling. Further, design of these devices requires a thorough understanding of quadripedal locomotion and veterinary patients previously not considered in the human orthotics and prosthetics (H-OP) industry. Thus V-OP requires a unified effort between veterinary professionals and device fabricators. Proper case management includes thorough examination for clarification of the movement disorder, complete diagnosis including primary and secondary deficiencies, veterinary prescription, device fabrication, device fitting and adjustment, client education, and veterinary follow-up for continued care. With this approach, veterinary patients, in particular the canine ones, are good candidates for these devices.

Canine Sports Medicine and Rehabilitation, Second Edition. Edited by Chris Zink and Janet B. Van Dyke.
© 2018 John Wiley & Sons, Inc. Published 2018 by John Wiley & Sons, Inc.

Historical perspective and the advent of veterinary orthotics and prosthetics (V-OP)

The use of orthotics and prosthetics to assist humans in ambulation and functional independence was first recorded in 2700 BC (Seymour, 2002). In the past century, veterinary medicine has advanced in technology and sophistication coincident with the increasing value and importance of companion animals. State-of-the-art veterinary health care now includes a new industry called veterinary orthotics and prosthetics (V-OP). This industry has been emerging for the past decade. The acronym distinguishes it from the human specialty, referred to as H-OP.

The techniques and materials used in H-OP have been used in the establishment of V-OP. These include mechanical hinges, composite high-temperature plastics, carbon fiber, custom prosthetic feet/hands and dynamic motion-assist mechanics. Additional design, manufacturing methods, and componentry are required to account for quadruped ambulation and the significantly greater magnitude of force generated by veterinary patients relative to human patients. With a clear understanding of the intricacies of quadrupedal and tripedal biomechanics, the proper application of V-OP aids in ambulation, recovery from injury, and functional independence.

Specific advances in the manufacturing and design process have improved V-OP solutions over the past decade. The 20th century saw a dramatic increase in the ability to manufacture human orthoses and prostheses more efficiently (Klasson, 1985). Specifically, the advent of computer-aided design (CAD) systems provided the orthotic and prosthetic industry with tools to bring subjective design creativity to an objective application of biomechanics (Fairley, 2013).

State of V-OP practice: empiricism versus science

The use of V-OP devices is a rapidly emerging, therapeutic strategy. The goal of this chapter is to introduce basic concepts for the novice practitioner. First a bit about terminology: colloquial language refers to these devices as *orthotics* or *prosthetics*. Perhaps we put too fine a point on it, but the appropriate nouns are *orthosis* and *prosthesis* with the plural of each *orthoses* and *prostheses*. The former are adjectives as in *orthotic device* and *prosthetic limb*. Further, an orthosis is defined as any medical device attached to the body to support, align, position, immobilize, prevent or correct deformity, assist weak muscles, or improve function (Deshales, 2002). A prosthesis, by contrast, is an artificial device used to replace or augment a missing or impaired part of the body. This may include heart valves, ligaments or dental implants, among others. For this reason, we use the term prosthetic limb for clarity. By definition, a prosthesis may concurrently act as an orthosis, while the converse cannot be said. A term for the former is *prosthosis*.

Traditionally, veterinarians have been quite adept at fashioning orthopedic assistive devices from any number of on-hand materials such as PVC pipes, aluminum rods, thermoplastics, and fiberglass/plaster casting. Just as veterinary medicine has evolved to include advanced dentistry, joint replacements, chemotherapy, and stereotactic radiation, it is in turn evolving toward the application of advanced biomechanics and technology for the treatment of limb loss and loss of limb function. The potential advantages afforded by biomechanically appropriate, custom orthoses and prostheses over homemade, improvised devices include: (1) improved management of primary pain generators associated with functional impairments; (2) improvement in the accuracy/appropriateness of biomechanical therapeutics, which may allow for greater activity and a significant decrease in secondary and iatrogenic pain; (3) return to active lifestyle, resulting in decreased obesity and associated comorbidities; (4) improvement in quality of life and functional independence; and (5) the availability of treatment options where none existed before (Marcellin-Little *et al.*, 2015). All of these can prevent a premature decision to euthanize.

An internet search in January 2017 found as many as 18 companies offering custom and off-the-shelf devices for veterinary patients. A search of internet chat groups and blogs found the most commonly discussed devices were for canine cranial cruciate injury. Coincident to this increased interest in devices, technology is changing with the use of CAD,

3-D modeling, and 3-D printing simplifying product development. Unfortunately, innovation is outpacing science. A search of the scientific literature, also in January of 2017, revealed 16 V-OP papers, six of which were related to equine patients (shoeing practices), three were small animal review articles (Adamson *et al.*, 2005; Mich, 2014; Marcellin-Little *et al.*, 2015), five were canine case reports or case series (Levine & Fitch, 2003; Case, 2013; Hardie & Lewallen, 2013; Tomlinson *et al.*, 2014; Carr, 2016), one survey (Hart *et al.*, 2016), and one computer simulation of stifle orthosis for canine cranial cruciate ligament (CCL) insufficiency (Bertocci *et al.*, 2017). Interestingly, the earliest report was the use of an orthotic treatment for tibiotarsal deformity in an elephant (Siegel, 1973). A study of client satisfaction with one type of CCL orthosis as compared with tibial plateau leveling osteotomy indicated high client satisfaction for both interventions (Hart *et al.*, 2016). There is anecdotal evidence for the use of these devices, but there is a clear deficit in terms of evidence-based documentation of efficacy and a need for more publications to advance the field.

The literature on prosthetic limbs has focused on osteointegration as a means of supplanting the socket-based prosthesis for human patients (Drygas *et al.*, 2008; Fitzpatrick *et al.*, 2011; Devasconcellos *et al.*, 2012). From the standpoint of basic science, there is an upsurge in the evaluation of canine limb dysfunction/loss pathomechanics; this may drive future controlled clinical trials as we begin to understand the quality of life implications of such injuries. The old maxim that "dogs do great on three legs" is being scrutinized and may prove a gross overstatement (Kirpensteijn *et al.*, 1999; Abdelhadi *et al.*, 2013; Hogy *et al.*, 2013; Jarvis *et al.*, 2013; Fuchs *et al.*, 2014; Goldner *et al.*, 2015). To date, all published studies are short term; long-term studies are needed to thoroughly examine the impact of these deficiencies.

Much of what is known and applied in the practice of V-OP is gleaned from centuries of work in the human field. Despite the paucity of studies specifically related to V-OP, by integrating H-OP experience with good science already documenting the pathomechanics of limb dysfunction and loss in the canine, there seems to be adequate basis for pursuing V-OP even as we wait for science to catch up.

Applied biomechanics and control systems

Equations and terminology

$F = MA$: force (F) is the product of mass (M) and acceleration (A).

$Mo = FD$: moment (Mo*) is the product of force and the perpendicular distance (D) from ground reaction force vector to the pivot point (joint).

Moment (Mo*): the tendency of a force to rotate an object about an axis. This force can arise outside the body (e.g., gravity, splint, orthosis) or can be created by the body (e.g., muscles, tendons, ligaments, joint capsules) (Figure 11.1).

Ground reaction force (GRF): the equal and opposite force to the total body force (TBF) exerted by the ground during any phase of weight bearing.

Lever arm: the perpendicular distance from the axis of rotation to the line of action of the force (e.g., the pes is the distal lever arm for the tarsus, while the manus is the distal lever arm for the carpus).

Torque: a measure of the turning force on an object.

Total body force (TBF): sum of the gravitational (vertical) force and inertial (horizontal) forces acting upon the body's center of mass. The TBF vector terminates through the middle of the anatomic structure in contact with the ground (e.g., the metacarpal or metatarsal pad in stance). For practical purposes the thoracic limb TBF vector originates in the mid-pectoral girdle, while the pelvic limb TBF vector originates at the sacroiliac joint. These locations shift with movement.

Veterinary orthotic and prosthetic devices create external moments for the body when the body is unable to create an adequate internal moment to resist forces acting upon a joint.

---

* Though moment is generally listed as "M", we have used Mo here to differentiate it from mass.

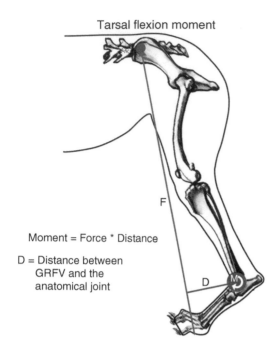

Figure 11.1 The relative position of the tarsus joint to the ground reaction force vector (GRFV) is responsible for the production of the tarsal flexion moment.

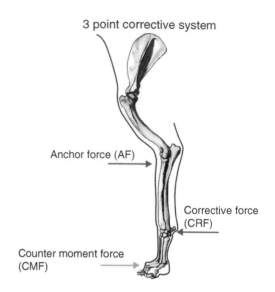

Figure 11.2 Coaptation is required to produce a three-point corrective system to create an external moment capable of resisting an unstable internal moment.

Common internal moment deficiencies include carpal hyperextension, tarsal valgus from shearing injury, and Achilles mechanism injury. Here the Achilles mechanism (internal moment) is unable to resist tarsal flexion created by the flexion moment acting against the tarsus (Figure 11.1). By employing mechanical control systems to the body, these devices stabilize joints either statically (no range of motion) or dynamically (range of motion possible). There are three general types of control systems: (1) three-point corrective system (3PCS); (2) modified three-point corrective system (M3PCS); and (3) force coupling (FC). While each control system is used for specific conditions, each system facilitates a common mechanical goal of creating an external moment to support or stabilize an affected anatomical joint or limb segment.

Three-point corrective systems

An orthosis applies a 3PCS (Figure 11.2), the most commonly used system, to stop, resist, or guide rotation of two limb segments about the shared point of rotation (joint). This system con-

sists of a corrective force (CRF) that is opposed by the proximal counter force and the distal counter force. The CRF is applied in direct opposition to the level and direction of joint instability. The purpose of the CRF is to resist the direction of instability presented by the deficient limb segment or joint. For example, traumatic palmar fibrocartilage injury results in carpal hyperextension in weight bearing. The instability is in the sagittal plane directed caudally at the carpus; the CRF for this injury would be at the same level directed cranially.

The counter forces are presented on the opposite side of the limb from the CRF location. The proximal counter force is known as the anchor force (AF) and the distal counter force is known as the counter moment force (CMF). These counter forces are positioned as far proximally and distally as functionally possible from the affected joint center to maximize the lever arm.

The sum of the two counter forces is equal to the magnitude of force acting at the corrective force location: $CRF = AF + CMF$. The equation $T = LF$ describes the relationship of lever arm to torque where T equals torque, L equals lever arm length, and F equals force. Increasing the length of lever arm by applying the counter force far away from the corrective force reduces the magnitude of force at each counter force location. Subsequently, the corrective force will also be reduced. Likewise, if the counter force locations are applied closer to the corrective force location (shorter lever arm), the magnitude of force at the corrective force location will be increased (Figure 11.3).

An increase in lever arm length creates a mechanical advantage and a reduction of force required. Reduced force is important because all forces are applied to the mechanical structure (skeleton) through the soft tissues, which are vulnerable to shear and pressure injury. In our example the ideal AF would be the proximal cranial antebrachium and the ideal CMF would be the distal manus (Figure 11.2).

Modified three-point corrective system

The M3PCS is similar to the 3PCS with a modification of the corrective force location. Rather than presenting a single point of corrective force to the affected joint, the M3PCS splits the corrective force location into a proximal and a distal component. This technique avoids bony prominences or anatomic joints that restrict desired contact with the limb. Furthermore, the addition of a second corrective force location distributes the total magnitude of force acting on the limb over a larger surface area. Increasing surface area decreases point pressure and soft tissue trauma.

In our example of carpal hyperextension, the accessory carpal bone interferes with direct access to the carpus. To apply a cranially directed corrective force to the carpus, the CRF would be applied directly against the accessory carpal bone. Pressing directly against the small surface area of a bone with tendon attachments is not desirable due to the increased risk of pressure sores and patient discomfort. The corrective force location is split into two points of contact just proximal and just distal to the accessory carpal bone (Figure 11.4).

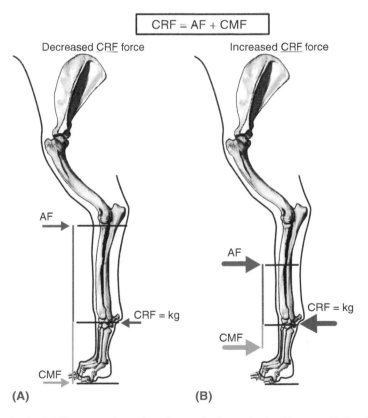

$$CRF = AF + CMF$$

Decreased CRF force   Increased CRF force

AF

AF

CRF = kg

CRF = kg

CMF

CMF

(A)   **(B)**

Figure 11.3 The length of a rigid lever arm determines the required magnitude of force applied to the lever arm to create the desired moment at the pivot point. Longer rigid lever arms (**A**) lead to smaller CRF, and shorter rigid lever arms to greater CRF (**B**). AF, anchor force; CMF, counter moment force; CRF, corrective force.

Modified 3 point corrective system

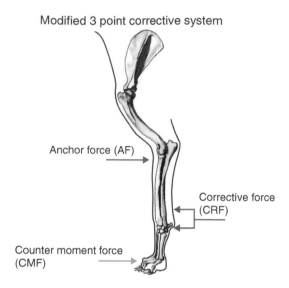

Anchor force (AF)

Corrective force
(CRF)

Counter moment force
(CMF)

Figure 11.4   When the desired corrective force (CRF) location is obscured by a bony structure, the CRF can be split into proximal and distal components placed superior and inferior to the bony structure.

Force coupling control system

Force coupling allows both orthoses and prostheses to guide and control motion about and within a joint (or motion segment) without limiting the range of motion desired at the joint.

Orthosis force coupling

In orthopedic force coupling, two bones are linked together with a shared joint axis. An example is the femur and crus united by the stifle. The stifle joint allows osteokinematic motion (flexion and extension) as well as arthrokinematic motion (movement within the joint such as rolling, spinning, and sliding translation over the joint surface).

A force coupling is defined as two lever arms joined at a pivot point with two forces applied at either end of each lever arm causing the lever arms to rotate about an imaginary axis in the center of each lever arm (Figure 11.5A). Thus, there are two force couples, one for each lever arm. To obtain balance in this system, each force couple is of

equal magnitude and they are linked about a mechanical hinge between the two lever arms. In this scenario, the action of the couples about the hinge is completely dictated by the physical limitations of the hinge.

An orthosis force coupling control system allows osteokinematic motion to persist (flexion and extension rotation) while controlling arthokinematics at the joint level. The effect is to create osteokinematic rotation without translational displacement where translation means roll, spin, and slide over the joint surface. An example of displacement within a joint is the arthrokinematic instability resulting from CCL insufficiency. The tibia is translated cranially and internally (cranial drawer and internal rotation).

The use of an orthosis to control CCL insufficiency instability is the most common application of orthosis force coupling. This orthosis typically consists of two shell segments that communicate with the femur and crural bones, respectively, and are joined together with a mechanical hinge aligned with the anatomic hinge (stifle joint).

For the cranial cruciate stifle orthosis to effect control it must create a force couple that resists cranial tibial thrust and internal tibial rotation, preserves normal arthokinematics, enables normal osteokinematics, and ensures device suspension. Importantly, a 3PCS is not able to control arthokinematics and preserve the normal osteokinematics of a cranial cruciate-deficient stifle joint.

Figure 11.5B illustrates the combined four points of contact, two on the femur encouraging a cranially directed distal femur rotational force at the stifle, and two points of contact acting on the tibia encouraging a caudally directed force at the stifle. Because a static point of contact is unable to harness the power of force coupling, the system requires a dynamic force to counteract cranial tibial thrust. Dynamic stabilization motion is created through muscle contraction, creating expansion during both eccentric and concentric contraction. The contraction of muscles in the pelvic limb during stance phase of the gait creates a caudally directed force that is communicated through the orthosis straps and shell to the proximal cranial aspect of the tibia.

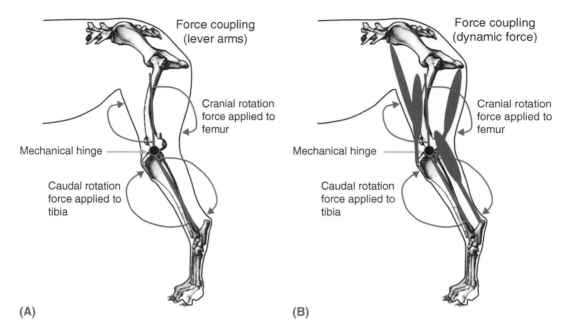

Figure 11.5   **(A)** A force couple is defined as two lever arms joined at a pivot point (mechanical hinge) with two forces applied at either end of each lever arm. These forces cause each lever arm to rotate about an imaginary axis in the center of each lever arm. A force couple control system allows coaptation to resist joint translation (arthokinematics) while enabling sagittal plane range of motion to persist (osteokinematics). **(B)** A force couple control system requires muscle contraction to create expansion force, producing dynamic force and enabling arthokinematic control while allowing osteokinematic motion.

Prosthesis force coupling

A prosthesis communicates with a patient's residual limb (residuum) through shell and strap contact to the body. During all phases of gait, the patient is either using the residuum to create prosthesis motion or to control prosthesis motion. In prosthesis force coupling, the connection between the residuum and the prosthesis can be thought of as a *joint*. At their intersection, the residuum and prosthesis are subject to forces applied by virtue of the GRF vector and the TBF vector, which shift in direction and magnitude with stance and gaiting. In all these events, the patient will present two points of contact (proximally and distally) to the prosthesis by utilizing their residual limb as a lever arm (Figure 11.6A). The points of contact will be presented in the same manner as the individual orthosis force coupling segment where the rotation about the lever arm is around an imaginary central axis and the lever arm can rotate in either direction (Figure 11.6B, C).

Prosthesis force coupling case example: subtotal amputation via an antebrachiocarpal disarticulation

The patient's distal residual limb segment includes the radius and ulna. The prosthesis provides socket communication with the residuum and extends distally to the ground recreating lost limb length. During swing phase, the patient will advance the prosthesis cranially with shoulder extension and elbow flexion for ground clearance. As the patient flexes the elbow joint, the residuum will contact the prosthesis along the distal cranial and proximal caudal aspect of the residuum creating a swing-phase force couple within the socket (Figure 11.7). During stance phase, the patient will create elbow extension resisting both (1) elbow flexion created from the GRF vector and the resulting flexion moment; and (2) the socket tendency to rotate caudally. The patient will communicate a force couple along the distal caudal and proximal cranial aspect of the residuum (Figure 11.8).

Prosthesis force coupling

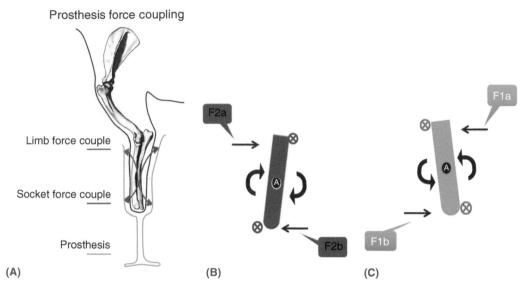

Limb force couple

Socket force couple

Prosthesis

(A)   **(B)**   **(C)**

Figure 11.6   (**A**) A prosthetic force couple requires the residuum to rotate in opposition to the rotational motion of the prosthetic socket. Through residuum counter rotation, the patient is able to control the movement of the prosthetic socket while creating purposeful stance-phase balance and propulsion while enabling the prosthetic socket to gain swing-phase clearance to the ground. (**B**) Diagram of the isolated force couple noted in (**A**), demonstrating contact points in swing phase (further illustrated in Figure 11.7). Refer to (**A**) for stance phase of gait where forces are neutral. (**C**) Diagram of the isolated force couple noted in (**A**), demonstrating contact points in the terminal or propulsive phase of gait (further illustrated in Figure 11.7).

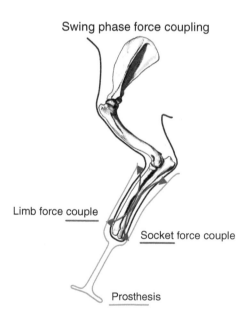

Swing phase force coupling

Limb force couple

Socket force couple

Prosthesis

Figure 11.7   The residuum communicates with the socket in two predicable locations during swing phase. The distal cranial aspect of the residuum produces the dominant force creating the force couple.

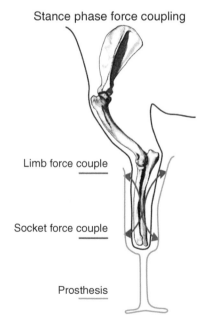

Stance phase force coupling

Limb force couple

Socket force couple

Prosthesis

Figure 11.8   The residuum communicates with the socket in two predicable locations during stance phase. The distal caudal aspect of the residuum produces the dominant force creating the force couple.

Case Study 11.1 Supination of front foot post digital amputation

Signalment: 13-y.o. FS German Shorthaired Pointer.

History: Patient injured left thoracic limb (LTL) manus on a hunting trip in 2008 at the age of 6 years. Over 3 years she developed pain and splaying of the second and third digits, which was managed medically. The second digit was amputated via metacarpophalangeal (MCP) disarticulation when medical management failed. Patient remained consistently lame postoperatively and within 6 months of the surgery the foot collapsed (digital arch) and the patient was no longer able to hunt. A surgical revision was performed with no improvement. Client noticed the right thoracic limb (RTL) foot collapsing (supination and digital collapse) as well, but not as severely. Presented for options to return to hunting, improve comfort, and protect the right thoracic foot from further injury.

Home environment: Single dog home, hardwood and carpeted floors, dog door, and two steps out to large yard.

Job: Hunting with client (waterfowl and pheasants).

Evaluation: General health: Unremarkable for age and breed. BCS 5/9.
   Conformation: WNL for breed with following exceptions: markedly splayed supinated digits 3-5 LTL; mildly splayed digits 2-5 with minor decrease in digital arch RTL; mild carpal valgus LTL. Mildly toed-out stance bilateral thoracic limbs typical of breed. In stance, LTL positioned relatively mediad (adducted) from shoulder, shifting total body force vector to lateral aspect of foot.
   Gait: Ambulatory × 4. Grade 2/5 LTL lameness.

Clinical evaluation: Orthopedic: Appendicular exam WNL with exception of noted splaying and supination; mild thickening of MCP joints 2 and 5 bilaterally except for absence of LTL 2nd digit (disarticulation at the MCP joint; no thickening or pain associated with the carpus).
   Neurological: WNL.
   Myofascial: Increased tone and myofascial sensitivity of the epaxial muscles of the neck and trunk as well as antigravity muscles of RTL (biceps brachii, supraspinatus, triceps group, digital flexors). Reduced flexibility of left pectoral muscles, latisimus dorsi, and brachiocephalicus.
   Biomechanical: Carpal goniometery in degrees:

Diagnostics: Radiographs of left manus including neutral lateral, stressed lateral (carpus), anteroposterior. Fragmented sesamoids RTL 2 and 5, LTL 5. Degenerative changes at these joints. No abnormalities associated with carpus. No evidence of sagittal plane pathology; increased extension of right carpus compensatory (weight shifting to RTL) with no soft tissue swelling noted radiographically.

Diagnosis: (1) Superficial and deep digital flexor failure with digital supination subsequent to amputation of left second digit by MCP disarticulation. (2) Bilateral MCP osteoarthritis secondary to chronic trauma of active lifestyle. (3) Mild superficial and deep digital flexor stretching/strain RTL due to compensatory overloading. (4) Right carpus not affected with hyperextension despite differences in midstance carpal angles (right +38° and left +28°). Difference due to overloading the RTL by compensating for the LTL.

V-OP goals:

(1)   Provide comfortable foot bed for LTL.
(2)   Limit splaying of digits of LTL.
(3)   Provide propulsion assist in absence of meaningful palmar-flexion function on LTL foot.
(4)   Improve LTL weight bearing to limit strain on RTL.

Case management: Rx: (1) Double-articulating carpus foot orthosis with custom insole for foot segment. The carpus component is only for suspension of the foot segment. (2) Rehabilitation for gait re-education, transitions, and long-term management of compensatory soft tissue issues.
   Mechanical principle: Propulsion assist (class 2 lever).
   Wearing schedule: Gradual break in over several weeks. To be used as sport/support orthosis for heavy activity (walks, play, hunting), but can be used all day and off at night if needed.

Case follow-up: Patient is comfortable in orthosis and wears it daily. Returned to hunting both seasons since device was fitted. At this time, client reports that her age, rather than her thoracic limbs, limits her hunting. At 18-month recheck, no progression in RTL pathology and LTL remains stable.

<Left stance (4 leg/3 leg)	Right stance (4 leg/3 leg)	Left PROM flex/ext	Right PROM flex/ext	Left walk*	Right walk*
+16/+20 +7 valgus	+15/+15 +5 valgus	40/+25	55/+25	25/28/24	33/38/28

*Initial contact/midstance/terminal stance (propulsion).

(Continued)

Take home points: (1) Digital amputation is not always a benign procedure. Secondary complications can be severe and lifestyle altering. (2) Although pathology may affect only the digits, an orthosis may require a proximal component for suspension; device design should minimally alter ROM and function of the proximal segments (e.g., low durometer hinges). (3) Thorough evaluation of all limbs is important to prevent over- and underdiagnosing concomitant pathology.

Computer-aided design and manufacturing

Biomechanically appropriate design is needed to apply these mechanical control systems. The field of orthotics and prosthetics has its roots in the artisan craftsman, such as black-smiths, woodworkers, and leather trades. Computer-aided drawing and 3-D designing is bringing the level of accuracy out of an art form into the realm of mechanical precision. With the advances in CAD software and modern manufacturing techniques, V-OP device fabrication has taken a significant step forward in integrating the aforementioned mechanical principles. The advantages of CAD in H-OP and now V-OP fabrication include design repeatability, consistent and intentional biomechanical force application, and speed in manufacturing. Sophisticated manufacturing technologies include handheld 3-D scanners that capture limb topography for digital sculpting, multiaxis carver machines to rapidly and accurately produce complex orthosis and prosthesis-positive models, and complete systems integration utilizing medical-grade 3-D printing (Fairley, 2013).

Is there a place for 3-D printing?

Fabrication of a hard-shell device can be accomplished by vacuum molding or 3-D printing. Traditionally H-OP and V-OP devices have been manufactured using the former. As a rapidly developing technology, 3-D printing brings innovation and interest for its potential use in V-OP. Importantly, a thorough understanding of quadrupedal biomechanics and the V-OP manufacturing process is required before delving into 3-D printing of V-OP devices. The goal of V-OP is to create a comfortable, well-fitting, biomechanically appropriate, and functional therapeutic device. Strict adherence to the principle that an animal patient must be evaluated and diagnosed is necessary for success. It is the view of the authors that these devices should be prescribed by a veterinarian as a durable medical device specifically indicated to treat a diagnosed pathology. A universal tenet of veterinary practice acts is that diagnosis and treatment of animal patients is the exclusive purview of licensed veterinarians. A V-OP solution has the potential to create therapeutic outcomes for a patient, but it has the potential to cause harm as well. Therefore, the application of such devices should be managed by a referring veterinarian, and ideally one who has gained a level of knowledge and experience in V-OP.

The manufacturing of a V-OP solution requires an understanding of anatomy, kinematics, kinetics, and biomechanics. At its core, the only role vacuum molding and 3-D printing serves is the actual manufacturing of a part or object. The design software and shape creation is separate from molding or printing of the device. Simply being able to manufacture a device is not enough to meet therapeutic goals. A close relationship between the prescribing veterinarian and a knowledgeable manufacturer provides the ideal framework for successful V-OP application regardless of the actual method of fabrication.

Materials

The material selected to fabricate a V-OP solution must meet or exceed the mechanical properties of the currently preferred materials polypropylene and laminated carbon fiber. Polypropylene is extruded in sheets creating a strength and molecular alignment superior to 3-D printing raw materials (Wong & Hernandez, 2012; Wu *et al.*, 2015). Carbon fiber lamination exceeds all other materials for the ability to create complex shapes with the greatest strength-to-weight characteristics (Tatar *et al.*, 2014; Jagannatha & Harish, 2015). At the time of this publication, 3-D printed materials are unable to match these characteristics.

Three-dimensional printers have their own version of sculpting software that could be adapted to the V-OP design. 3-D printing provides an opportunity to fabricate computer-aided V-OP designs without the technical skills required for manufacturing components with either plastics or carbon fiber. Because 3-D printing is readily available and relatively simple, individuals with little or no knowledge of V-OP, biomechanics, anatomy, or veterinary pathology can attempt to fabricate devices. 3-D printing and its novelty does not include the actual cost of manufacturing a V-OP device. If a 3-D printer were used in production for orthotics and prosthetics, the cost of those components would be astronomically expensive for clients, and, at the time of this publication, CAD along with fabrication from polypropylene or laminated carbon fiber is preferred. The authors are concerned about the fabrication and use of such devices without veterinary examination, diagnosis, and prescription. It is possible to inadvertently harm an animal patient or delay appropriate treatment.

Biomechanics and pathomechanics: the interrelationship between rehabilitation and V-OP

The application of mechanical devices is not a panacea and not without challenges. Return to functional independence requires re-education of the body as a whole, including muscles, nerves, and the mind. Early pioneers of H-OP did not anticipate the need for such rehabilitation. However, in modern practice it is clear a mechanical device must be coupled with rehabilitation to maximize its use and the patient's success. The aim of rehabilitation is to restore and preserve maximum independence of action and functionality (Geertzen *et al.*, 2001) (Figure 11.9).With respect to veterinary patients, an additional aim is to prolong active and comfortable life to prevent premature euthanasia.

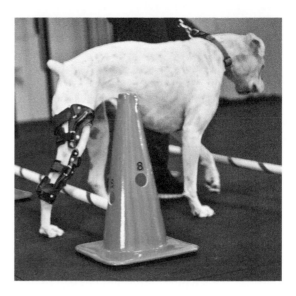

Figure 11.9 Boxer undergoing rehabilitation for cranial cruciate ligament insufficiency using a stifle orthosis.

Rehabilitation is a medical specialty concerned with the prevention, diagnosis, treatment, and management, by physical means, of disabling diseases, disorders, and injuries typically of a musculoskeletal, cardiovascular, neuromuscular, or neurological nature. Biomechanics encompasses anatomy, kinesiology, neurophysiology, mechanics, physics, and mathematics (Bedotto, 2006). Pathomechanics deals with the abnormal effect of static and dynamic forces on the body as a result of neurological, muscular, and skeletal disorders. It provides understanding of the underlying cause of gait deviation and the implication of forces acting on the injured body during movement: ground reaction force, inertia, and gravity. The specialty of orthotics and prosthetics addresses pathomechanics through the use of corrective forces including alignment of body position, muscular control, and external mechanical systems (Bedotto, 2006).

The application of an orthosis or prosthesis adds additional challenge to rehabilitative manipulation of movement. The comprehensive treatment of a pathomechanical injury requiring use of a device involves marrying the mechanics of the device with the mechanics of the body; the device must become part of the biomechanical system. The rehabilitation therapist plays an integral part in uniting the mechanics of body (muscle and nerve activation, and integration patterns) and device into the complex biomechanics of locomotion. In this paradigm, the therapist provides physical treatment and the prosthetist/orthotist provides the device or mechanical support. The physician (or veterinarian) orchestrates the larger therapeutic plan based on specific diagnosis and sequential evaluation. This united effort in human practice successfully aids the patient in regaining ambulation in a safe, efficient, and functional manner (Bechtol, 1967); the same goal can be met in our veterinary patients.

Modern technology is advancing the sophistication of V-OP devices. What is lacking is device-specific rehabilitation to enable our veterinary patients to fully realize device potential on par with human patients. The canine rehabilitation therapist must have a basic understanding of the purpose, mechanics, and limitations of the device. They must recognize complications in a timely manner to prevent injury and limit time out of the device. Likewise, the attending veterinarian (if the rehabilitation therapist is not the attending veterinarian) must understand short- and long-term rehabilitation goals, the biomechanics of therapeutic exercises, and the limitations of rehabilitation. The V-OP fabricator must understand the diagnosis and therapeutic goals so that device manufacture and adjustment are timely and appropriate. Ultimately, shared information and diverse expertise leads to intervention, device modifications/adjustments, and rehabilitation strategies that maximize patient comfort, endurance, and overall function (Pomeranz et al., 2006).

Implications of limb loss or dysfunction

Knowledge of the components of normal quadruped gait guides treatment of pathomechanical deficiencies. Quadrupeds who suffer loss of limb function or loss of a limb are biomechanically distinct from bipeds with similar loss. Asymmetrical loading of the remaining limbs and functional deficiencies such as loss of plantar and palmar flexor power in propulsion have not been quantified for veterinary patients. Conversely, kinetic and kinematic compensations in human amputees have been extensively studied. Amputation causes disruption of the human musculoskeletal system, resulting in asymmetrical biomechanics (Nolan et al., 2003;

Versluys et al., 2009; Nolan & Lees, 2000; Kent & Franklyn-Miller, 2011; Schoeman et al., 2011). The mechanical alterations of amputation or injury have implications for mobility and for the long-term health of joints, muscles, and spine. Both human and veterinary populations develop compensations for functional deficiencies, to maintain balance and locomotion (DeCamp, 1997; Kirpensteijn et al., 2000; Landman et al., 2004; Bockstahler et al., 2009; Prinsen et al., 2011; Abdelhadi et al., 2013; Hogy et al., 2013; Jarvis et al., 2013; Fuchs et al., 2014; Goldner et al., 2015). However, such compensatory movements are not necessarily efficient and frequently lead to short- and long-term complications.

The biomechanical implications of limb dysfunction or limb absence include intact limb breakdown and the development of pathology associated with myofascial tissue, joints (Fujisawa, 1999), and spine (Landman et al., 2004) by virtue of altered gait and structural support. In veterinary patients, these pathological changes lead to chronic pain, poor quality of life, and premature euthanasia. With these significant consequences in mind, alternative approaches such as subtotal or elective-level amputation, coupled with application of prostheses, become more appealing. Human medical practice provides perspective; preservation of normal proximal limb segments is paramount and amputation higher than is absolutely necessary is untenable—an example is the Syme's amputation technique for the human foot (Shurr & Cook, 1990).

Thoracic limb deficiency compensatory changes

Kinetic studies of canine gait have been available for decades both for normal (Budsberg et al., 1987, 1993, 1999; Riggs et al., 1993; McLaughlin & Roush, 1995; Lee et al., 1999; Bockstahler et al., 2009; Torres et al., 2013) and abnormal (DeCamp, 1997; Evans et al., 2003; Bockstahler et al., 2009) motion due to impairment. In the late 21st century three reports were published describing client satisfaction with amputation (Withrow & Hirsch, 1979; Carberry & Harvey 1987; Kirpensteijn et al., 1999). In 1999, Kirpensteijn et al. reported dog client satisfaction post amputation of a limb, where 42 of 44 dogs adapted satisfactorily to tripedal locomotion. However, 50% of respondents in this survey stated that they had serious objections to amputation, but it was concluded that these objections appeared to have been based more on emotional grounds than on rational judgment of facts. In these reports, any concerns expressed by the clients were attributed to comparison of the effects of similar surgery in humans and were seemingly attributed to unfounded client anthropomorphism. In 2015, Dickerson *et al.* published a retrospective telephone survey of client-perceived recovery from limb amputation, which was overall good over the time studied. Their findings correlate with others, indicating that dogs rapidly adjust to tripedal gaiting (Dickerson *et al.*, 2015).

Despite these studies, questions remain and over the past two decades tripedal gaiting studies have emerged, with several recent studies including kinematic evaluation (Kirpensteijn *et al.*, 2000; Hogy *et al.*, 2013; Jarvis *et al.*, 2013; Fuchs *et al.*, 2014; Goldner *et al.*, 2015). Interestingly, using force plate analysis, Kirpensteijn *et al.* objectively investigated tripedal canine ambulation, finding that control dogs carried 59.8% and 39.2% on the thoracic and pelvic limbs, respectively, whereas thoracic limb amputees carry 46.9% of their body mass on the remaining thoracic limb and 53.1% on the pelvic limbs. This study supported earlier work that showed that the thoracic limbs of quadrupeds are most important in braking forces, whereas the pelvic limbs primarily generate propulsion (Budsberg *et al.*, 1987; McLaughlin & Roush, 1995; Lee *et al.*, 1999). In contrast to the earlier study on client satisfaction, the Kirpensteijn *et al.* (2000) force plate study concluded that amputation of a limb causes significant changes in the gait of walking dogs. Kinetic differences were found to exist for both pelvic and thoracic limb amputees when compared with quadrupeds, but were greater in dogs undergoing thoracic limb amputation; these findings warrant thorough evaluation. A significant conclusion was that changes in gait caused by the amputation of a limb may lead to an increased incidence of orthopedic disease of the remaining limbs.

Thirteen years later, Jarvis *et al.* (2013) and Abdelhadi *et al.* (2013) reported similar changes in mass distribution in two different populations. Although the Abdelhadi *et al.* (2013) study simulated thoracic limb lameness (not amputation) and emphasized that comparisons should be drawn with caution, their conclusions may be relevant. They concluded that the long-term effects of load distribution and shift of the center of mass should be evaluated to establish prospects for patients with chronic lameness (or missing limbs). Jarvis *et al.* (2013) found that in dogs with a thoracic limb amputation, the vertebral column, carpus, and ipsilateral hip and stifle joints showed significant biomechanical changes compared with normal quadrupedal dogs. They concluded that altered motion of the vertebral column may have a long-term impact for an amputee because of increased demands on muscular control and trunk strength. Further, they noted that gait alterations and compensatory strategies may place thoracic amputees at increased risk for musculoskeletal injury in one of more of the remaining limbs.

The Jarvis study noted that a higher load was applied over a longer duration in stance phase of the gait for the remaining limbs. Cartilage degradation is presumed to progress faster with supraphysiological loading during cyclical movement, such as walking (Fujisawa *et al.*, 1999). This study also showed that the remaining limb had increased overall carpal joint range of motion, in particular hyperextension during stance phase. This change was attributed to increased distribution of body weight to this limb. Interestingly, the joint kinematics of the remaining elbow and shoulder remained relatively unchanged; therefore, the carpus of the thoracic limb amputee undergoes a significant increase in stress and strain, which is exacerbated by increased gait velocity. Lastly, this study showed that the ipsilateral pelvic limb of the thoracic limb amputee takes on a dual role of propulsion and braking and thus may be more susceptible to acute and chronic injury.

This important, objective work is in stark contrast to subjective assessment of patient outcomes. Although amputation is undoubtedly necessary in some cases, it may be appropriate to rethink our long-held paradigms. Consideration must be given to the data suggesting thoracic limb amputation is not benign (Figure 11.10).

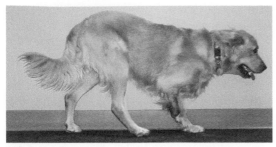

(A)

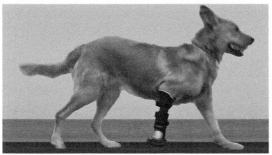

(B)

Figure 11.10 **(A)** The pathomechanical consequences of thoracic limb loss can be mitigated with the use of a properly fitted prosthesis. **(B)** A below-carpus prosthesis for amelia of the right thoracic limb distal to the radius and ulna. (B derived from video.)

Pelvic limb amputation compensatory changes

What about the pelvic limb? Kirpensteijn *et al.* (2000) found that after pelvic limb amputation the remaining pelvic limb carries 26% of total body weight, while the thoracic limbs each carry 37%. This implies that regardless of whether a pelvic or thoracic limb is amputated, the thoracic limbs carry an increased load (~17% for a thoracic limb amputation and 7% increase for each pelvic limb amputation) and that pelvic limb amputation may have less severe overload consequences than thoracic limb amputation. Further, one might intuitively suspect, based on this weight distribution disparity, that larger breed dogs would have more difficulty adapting to amputation than smaller breeds, although the 1999 Kirpensteijn *et al.* study did not support this. Conversely, Dickerson *et al.* (2015) found that client-assigned quality of life scores had significant negative correlations with preoperative body

condition score and body weight. More work is needed to expand on these findings, in particular additional kinematic data for long-term outcomes. However, until such studies are performed, it may be prudent to manage all prospective amputees with an eye toward prevention of overload regardless of limb, breed, weight, or body type.

Recent studies have examined the kinematic consequences of pelvic limb amputation. Although increased weight distribution is relatively small for the remaining pelvic limb, rotation forces about the transverse and sagittal axes of the trunk are altered. Pelvic limb amputation removes the normal contralateral limb support for the thoracic limb. In this regard, the limbs and the vertebral column (including their myofascial support structures) must compensate. Data support involvement of the spine; pelvic limb amputees laterally bend the vertebral column to place the remaining pelvic limb closer to the ipsilateral thoracic limb. Hogy *et al.* (2013) refer to this as a "unique laterally deviated gait when the pelvic limb is in propulsion." In this case, in contrast with the quadruped, the long axis of the thoracolumbar vertebrae is not parallel to forward motion.

Further findings salient to vertebral column motion included the cyclical movement of the head upward during propulsion of the contralateral thoracic limb. This was presumed to assist in elevation of the center of mass. The head was subsequently moved downward at the termination of contralateral thoracic limb swing phase and in to stance phase. Thus, there is increased cervical spine range of motion when compared with a quadruped. The remaining pelvic limb acts as a compliant strut, and is shifted cranially and medially to maintain stability and aid in propulsion. This causes increased flexion and rotation of the lumbosacral spine. The long-term implications of these spinal compensations are not known, and further studies are needed.

Hogy *et al.* (2013) also found that increased range of motion is present in the remaining tarsus. It was presumed that this is a compensatory mechanism to maximize efficient propulsion due to elastic recoil of the calcaneal tendon and associated musculature. This was confirmed by Goldner *et al.* in 2015. This additional stretch/loading of the calcaneal tendon and digital flexors may result in chronic strain of these soft tissues, in addition to the effect of supraphysiological loading of the tarsal joint structures themselves.

Fuchs *et al.* (2014) studied a simulated model of pelvic limb amputation in Beagles. They found that amputation led to an alteration in the forces exerted by the remaining pelvic limb and the ipsilateral forelimb. Changes in external forces lead to alterations in internal forces and moments acting on the joints, which may then lead to orthopedic problems. This supports the conclusions of Hogy *et al.* (2013) where the contralateral thoracic limb and the remaining pelvic limb were found to withstand greater forces and therefore greater wear on the joints and soft tissues. Both studies advocated for close monitoring of the intact support limbs, especially the diagonal pair. It was concluded that compensatory gaiting strategies may lead to increased wear on joints and soft tissues.

In 2015, Goldner *et al.* evaluated joint angular excursions, concentrating on the swing phase of gait. They found substantial kinematic changes in all three remaining limbs and in the axial skeleton. Their findings contradict Hogy *et al.* (2013) and Jarvis *et al.* (2013) in that they found compensatory mechanisms to require changes in all joint excursions and not just in the tarsus and carpus. Further, they found that changes were not limited to the weight-bearing (stance) phases, but that impacts were found in all aspects of the locomotor cycle. This study took the Hogy *et al.* (2013) study findings on pelvic inclination and lateralizing long axis torque a step further, noting that such compensation modifies trunk musculature not only in terms of moments, but also in neuromuscular recruitment patterns. They concluded that tripedal locomotion requires an overall concerted kinematic adjustment of the appendicular and axial musculoskeletal systems. This study recommended comprehensive and whole-body preventative, therapeutic, and rehabilitative care of canine amputees.

The studies reported here, both for thoracic and pelvic limb amputees, are helpful, however there are as yet no longitudinal studies documenting the potential for damage to soft tissues and joints in the amputee. Anecdotally, one author (PMM) routinely treats appendicular and axial myofascial pain syndromes, carpal hyperextension, carpal valgus and varus instability, superficial and deep digital flexor tendon failure, and osteoarthritis in pelvic and thoracic limb amputees. Further

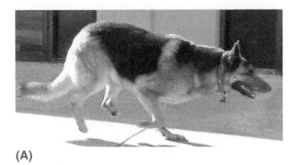

(A)

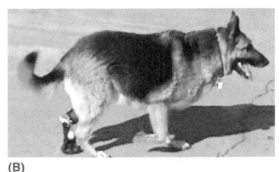

(B)

Figure 11.11   (A) The pathomechanical consequences of pelvic limb loss can be mitigated with the use of a properly fitted prosthesis. (B) Below-tarsus prosthesis for traumatic tarsometatarsal amputation. (Images derived from videos.)

studies are needed to quantify the incidence of such sequelae as well as to determine risk factors for breakdown and tissue damage, which may relate to conformation, breed, level of amputation, previous injury, and so on (Figure 11.11).

Orthotic devices

Splinting and bracing are described as passive immobilization to rest a limb segment in a fixed position (Heijnen *et al.*, 1997). The term coaptation refers to approximation and involves transmitting compressive (vertical) and bending (horizontal) forces through the engineered coaptation with specific mechanical purpose (Oakley, 1999). The resulting corrective forces are transmitted through skin to the bony structures beneath. Customized external coaptation can be used to provide limb segment stability before surgical repair and help prevent wounds or surgical failures caused by splinting, wet bandages, splint material fatigue/breakdown, and lack of patient tolerance of a splint. As a general rule, molded external coaptation devices (custom) are more efficient stabilizers of bones and joints than are premade devices (Piermattei *et al.*, 2006) due to patient-specific design and applied biomechanics. In closely approximating the patient's individual topography, custom devices disperse corrective forces over a larger surface area resulting in fewer soft tissue problems and better tolerance (Piermattei *et al.*, 2006).

An orthosis is any medical device attached to the body to support, align, position, prevent or correct deformity, assist weak muscles, or improve function (Deshales, 2002). These dynamic devices provide protected motion within a controlled range, prevent or reduce severity of injury, prevent or relieve contracture, allow lax ligaments and joint capsules to shorten and approach normal distensibilty, and provide functional stability for an unstable limb segment (American Academy of Orthopaedic Surgeons, 1987; Prokop, 2006) (Figure 11.12).

Surgical management of many orthopedic conditions in veterinary practice remains the standard of care and the preferred therapeutic choice. At the same time and for a variety reasons including financial, personal preference, advanced patient age, perceived increased anesthetic risk, comorbidities, or circumstances requiring a delay of surgery, a number of patients are not surgical candidates. Until recently, veterinarians had no viable option for these patients. V-OP provides choices using customized, articulated (as needed), external coaptation in the pre- or postoperative periods, as well as in lieu of surgical intervention (Box 11.1). Rehabilitation for these nonsurgical

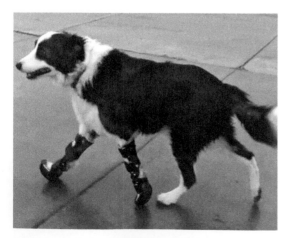

Figure 11.12   Bilateral, double-articulating, carpus/foot orthoses stabilize biplanar carpal instability (hyperextension of the radiocarpal joint and valgus due to medial collateral ligament injury). With proper rehabilitation, a normal trot can be achieved.

Box 11.1   Orthopedic conditions amenable to veterinary orthotic devices

Common problems amenable to thoracic limb orthoses

- Elbow: instability and osteoarthritis
- Carpus: hyperextension
- Carpus: bi- or triplanar instability
- Carpus: collateral ligament injury
- Carpus: arthrodesis postsurgical support
- Carpus: arthrodesis failure
- Carpus: prophylactic support for contralateral limb amputation
- Foot injuries including tendon laceration and digit amputation (e.g., adactyly, ectrodactyly, severe syndactyly, hypodactyly, or other limb reduction defects)
- Peripheral neuropathy
- Brachial plexus distal neuropathy

Common problems amenable to pelvic limb orthoses

- Stifle: cranial cruciate ligament rupture
- Stifle: patellar luxation (grades 1 and 2)
- Stifle: collateral ligament injury
- Tarsus: hyperextension
- Tarsus: collateral ligament injury
- Tarsus: failed Achilles tendon repair
- Tarsus: Achilles tendon rupture or avulsion postoperative support
- Tarsus: Achilles tendon sprain nonsurgical without complete disruption or avulsion
- Tarsus: Achilles tendon chronic plantigrade stance
- Tarsus: sciatic neuropathy (tarsal collapse)
- Foot injuries including tendon laceration and digit amputation
- Foot deformities (e.g., adactyly, ectrodactyly, severe syndactyly, hypodactyly, or other limb reduction defects)
- Degenerative myelopathy
- Peripheral neuropathy: sciatic nerve trauma (e.g., pelvic fracture, surgical collateral injury)
- Intervertebral disc disease, spinal canal stenosis, cervical spinal instability
- Fibrocartilagenous embolus

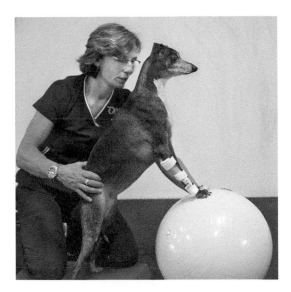

Figure 11.13 Use of the physioball to encourage stretch, balance, and proper weight bearing in a dog with moderate carpometacarpal hyperextension.

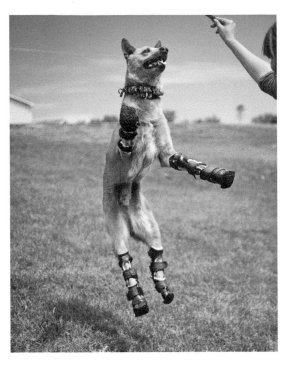

Figure 11.14 Dogs acclimate well to prosthetics as seen in this quad-prosthetic patient whose limbs were severely damaged by frostbite-induced vasculitis and necrosis at 6 weeks of age.

patients is as critical to successful outcomes as it is for surgical patients (Figures 11.9 and 11.13).With regard to patient selection, the majority of dogs will tolerate and acclimate to a properly designed, fitted, and adjusted orthosis. Chewing at a device is typically due to a behavioral propensity to chew objects or an ill-fitting device resulting in discomfort. Most dogs adapt to an orthosis as readily as they adapt to harnesses and collars.

Prosthetic devices

In general, it is advantageous to re-establish a normal quadruped structure whenever possible. Fortunately, veterinary patients are amenable to prosthetic limbs and adapt readily, especially when coupled with prosthetic-specific rehabilitation (Figure 11.14).Congenital defects, disease (e.g., neoplasia), and traumatic injuries can be successfully managed with custom prostheses (Box 11.2).For distal limb pathologies such as neoplasia, degloving injury, necrosis, or nonunion fractures, careful surgical planning provides the opportunity to preserve the functional proximal limb segments. Subtotal amputation is preferable therapy to traditional total limb amputation in many cases.

Box 11.2 Specific conditions amenable to veterinary prosthetic devices

Thoracic limb prosthetics

- Surgical subtotal amputation:
  - Midshaft radius ulna amputation (50% antebrachium required)
  - Radiocarpal disarticulation
  - Intercarpal disarticulation
  - Carpometacarpal disarticulation
  - Midshaft metacarpal amputation
  - Digital amputation
- Congenital dysmelias (e.g., congenital restriction (amniotic) band, amelia, meromelia)
- Traumatic limb amputation

Pelvic limb prosthetics

- Surgical subtotal amputation:
  - Tarsocrural disarticulation
  - Intertarsal disarticulation
  - Tarsometatarsal disarticulation
  - Metatarsal amputation
  - Digital amputation
- Congenital dysmelias (e.g., congenital restriction (amniotic) band, amelia, meromelia)
- Traumatic limb amputation

Case Study 11.2 Subtotal amputation and below carpus prosthesis

Signalment: 2-y.o. MC Yorkshire Terrier.

History: Patient suffered a catastrophic injury to right front foot after being bitten by another dog. Digits 2, 4, and 5 were amputated initially. Remained unwilling to use right thoracic limb (RTL); remaining digit painful on palpation.

Home environment: Multiple toy breed dogs in family, hardwood and carpeted floors, stairs, and outdoor yard.

Job: Companion dog.

Evaluation: General health: WNL for age and breed. BCS 4.5/9.

Conformation: WNL for breed and age. Weight shifted to left thoracic limb (LTL) and pelvic limbs. LTL shifted mediad (adducted) from glenohumeral joint.

Gait: Ambulatory × 3. Grade 5/5 RTL lameness.

Clinical evaluation: Orthopedic: Excellent ROM of remaining joints of RTL; normal ROM of remaining limbs.

Neurological: Unremarkable.

Myofascial: Muscles of cervical, thoracic, and lumbar epaxial; left lateral shoulder stabilizers (supraspinatus, infraspinatus, deltoideus); and pectoral muscles sensitive to palpation with restriction secondary to compensatory gait. Iliopsoas flexibility decreased due to cranial shifting of pelvic limbs.

Biomechanical: ROM of all appendicular joints WNL.

V-OP goals:

(1) Weight bearing on RTL by providing extension to the ground and mechanical foot to accommodate limb length discrepancy, provide propulsion assist, and align shoulders in frontal plane.
(2) Allow as much PROM and AROM as possible for RTL proximal joints.

Case management: Subtotal amputation of right foot performed via carpo-metacarpal disarticulation, preserving accessory carpal bone and pad. Suture line placed caudally. Perioperative pain management included regional nerve block (brachial plexus), NSAIDs, NMDA receptor antagonist, and gabapentin. Two weeks postsurgery, a fiberglass impression of RTL was obtained and prosthesis was prescribed.

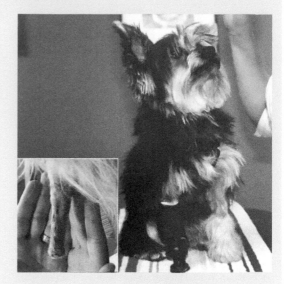

Figure 11.15 Thoracic limb below-carpus prosthesis with weight shift onto the prosthetic limb during a rehabilitation session. The inset shows the postoperative subtotal amputation at the level of the carpometacarpal joints.

Rx: (1) Below carpus prosthesis (Figure 11.15). (2) Rehabilitation for gait re-education; acclimation to activities of daily living including transitions, balance, and proprioception; recovery from myofascial sensitivity; and a long-term tripedal health maintenance plan.

Mechanical principle considerations: Device suspension; faux foot construction to facilitate braking and propulsion; and control of transverse plane motion of the residual limb within the device. No instabilities to control.

Wearing schedule: Gradual breaking in over 2–4 weeks with goal of day use only with breaks as needed during the day. Activity tolerated in device to be determined with tissue acclimation to device.

Case follow-up: Patient returned to full activity. Ambulatory × 4. Myofascial pain reduced significantly and managed with home massage therapy and conditioning exercises. Conformation improved with pelvic limbs repositioned beneath pelvis and weight bearing more evenly dispersed over all four limbs. Twice-yearly evaluations and device refurbishment as needed. At 3-year recheck patient continues to do well.

Take home point: Small patient size is not a factor in determining the necessity for a prosthesis or for the capability to fabricate a prosthesis.

The case for prosthetic limbs

Given the potential consequences of limb loss and the recent availability of prosthetic limbs for dogs, it seems prudent to offer this option for those patients and clients amenable to this approach. The biomechanics of the quadruped make design of prosthetic limbs an interesting challenge. The end goal is to provide a limb that allows as close to normal quadrupedal ambulation as possible. Angulation differences between the thoracic and pelvic limb, the mechanical role of different limbs in ambulation, breed differences, as well as level of subtotal amputation must all be considered.

The key for any prosthesis is suspension and retention of the device on the residual limb. Dogs create tremendous forces on their limbs during trotting, running, playing, and other daily activities. Device retention can be a challenge in the canine patient and proper design is critical to success. Currently there are two types of prosthetic limbs available: exoprostheses (socket-based) and endo-exoprostheses (e.g., Percutaneous Fixation To the Skeleton, PerFiTS™; Figure 11.16).

Exoprostheses provide a socket within which the residual limb rests; an extension provides contact to the ground via some form of foot component (Figures 11.10, 11.11, and 11.14). Importantly, in a properly designed exoprothesis, the total body force exerted through the limb and prosthesis is not borne on the distal end of the residual limb. This improves comfort and provides some protection for the residuum through the distribution of forces through a larger surface area. The advantage of exoprosthetic limbs over endoprostheses is their relatively low cost, simplicity of application, and adaptability to many levels of limb loss from foot to mid antebrachium or crus. Another advantage is the lack of a surgical implant, which could loosen or fail.

Endoprostheses employ a skeletally integrated implant to which a prosthesis is attached (Figure 11.16). There are two important advantages to this approach. First, there is no mechanical delay in gaiting; the forces applied to the prosthesis by virtue of gaiting are directly transmitted to the skeleton without a delay due to transmission first through fur, skin and muscle.

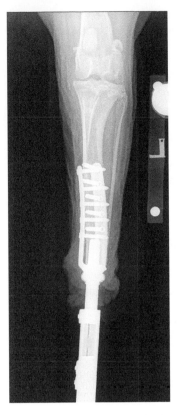

Figure 11.16 This PerFITS™ limb is an example of an endoprosthesis that employs a skeletally integrated implant to which a prosthesis is attached. Source: Image courtesy of Professor Noel Fitzpatrick.

An additional advantage is the potential for fewer soft tissue irritations because there is no socket. Although confounding, skin trauma is not an intractable sequelae of socket prosthesis in humans and animals. This is important because not all patients are amenable to interosseous techniques due to cost, injury level, or currently limited availability. In time these disadvantages may be overcome.

Rehabilitation is critical for the prosthesis patient during the adaptation period, whether using an exoprosthesis or an endo-exoprosthesis. For either patient there is no direct, anatomic contact to the ground, therefore control of the limb (GRF and TBF) is reversed. Control of the limb via the prosthesis comes from the top down (proximal intact limb) rather than ground up (prosthetic foot in the absence of a normal foot) and results in delayed feedback. Through gait patterning and proprioceptive retraining, along with strengthening, the prosthesis patient relearns proprioception, balance, gaiting at different speeds, and ambulation over varied terrain. Sensations transmitted through the device to the skeleton retrain the nervous system; this is called integration, and is critical to the best outcomes.

Given the consequences of limb loss in the short and long term it seems appropriate to *contemplate before we amputate* an entire limb when only the distal segment is beyond salvage. Example indications for a prosthesis include neoplasia, trauma, ectrodactyly, and partial agenesis. Preservation of at least 50% of the radius/ulna or tibia/fibula allows application of a socket-based prosthetic limb or intraosseous transcutaneous amputation prosthesis (ITAP) in dogs, cats, and other species. Subtotal amputation is possible at nearly every level of distal joint as well as distal trans-tibial and trans-radial levels. The basic tenet is to preserve as much limb as possible while providing a tension-free closure of the remaining tissues. The ideal level of amputation for each injury, the best techniques, and the advantages/disadvantages of each level are still being defined.

Considerations for patient and client selection

Most dogs adapt well to the use of a prosthetic limb. Although temperment is important, the use of a prosthetic limb typically does not require an extraordinarily tolerant animal. The ability to sit quietly while the limb is checked and for prosthetic limb donning and doffing is usually a simple matter of training. Just like human beings with prosthetic limbs, orientating to the prosthetic limb, learning to walk properly with the limb, as well as learning to navigate the environment are all accelerated with the help of a certified rehabilitation therapist.

Once fitted and properly adjusted, use of a prosthetic limb is relatively easy; at the same time, commitment to lifelong care of the residuum and the prosthetic limb is imperative. Like any animal with a chronic health issue, disabled animals require daily attention and maintenance. Marcellin-Little *et al.* (2015) noted that client-related contraindications of prosthesis use include a potential lack of interest, motivation, supervision, or financial ability. Some important issues to consider are:

(1) Client tolerance for financial commitment. At the time of writing, typical initial costs associated with this treatment plan are comparable with costs associated with common orthopedic surgeries. Lifetime expenses to consider include:
  (a) Anesthesia, surgery, and postoperative care if subtotal amputation or revision surgery is required.
  (b) Consultation appointment with V-OP provider (licensed veterinarian) to include assessment, treatment plan, device prescription, limb impression, or scan.
  (c) Device: some patients may require more than one device in their lifetime (e.g., puppies).
  (d) Fitting, follow-up, and adjustment appointments with V-OP provider (varies by case).
  (e) Professional rehabilitation.
  (f) Annual to biannual fit and function appointments.
  (g) Maintenance and repair.
(2) Client tolerance for time commitment:
  (a) The residual limb must be checked daily for skin irritation or breakdown.
  (b) A wearing schedule is established for each patient based on individual tolerances. This schedule should be meticulously followed and the device should never be left on for more than 12 hours without a significant break (consecutive hours tolerated in the device will vary among individuals); overnight wear is not appropriate.
  (c) Suitable activity while wearing the prosthetic limb is established over time; most dogs are able to resume a considerably more active lifestyle than a tripedal dog.
  (d) The prosthetic limb must be kept clean and in good working order at all times. The prosthetic patient needs regular health care including at least twice-annual check-ups specific to the device itself.
  (e) Rehabilitation and V-OP follow-up appointments are required.

A prosthetic limb is not for every dog or every client. Frequently, the limiting factors are related to client resources. Fortunately, with the establishment of expectations prior to moving forward with a prosthesis, many clients find the time and financial commitment manageable when considering the chronic health issues and costs associated with full limb amputation.

V-OP evaluation, objectives, and goal setting

It is important to establish a logical and thorough approach to V-OP patient evaluation. It is essential to dedicate extended time for the initial visit. This preliminary evaluation combines aspects of general physical, neurological, and orthopedic examinations as well as musculoskeletal and biomechanical evaluation (Box 11.3). The comprehensive assessment of each patient will likely result in a multipartite diagnosis; this is because the interrelated function of the whole body is considered rather than simply focusing on the chief complaint. The ultimate objective will be to provide an accurate diagnosis, appropriate prescription, and treatment plan to meet client and clinician expectations and goals.

Box 11.3 V-OP evaluation summary

- Observation outside
- Observation of free movement in exam room
- History: includes activity level (before and since the injury, structured and unstructured), home environment (flooring, stairs, yard, dog door, etc.), lifestyle (other animals, children, primary caregiver in the home)
- Client goal(s)
- Media acquisition (conformation, stance, gaiting) to include all four sides of the dog
- Examination:
  - General health examination
  - Neurological examination
  - Orthopedic examination
  - Myofascial examination (including specific flexibility)
  - Passive range of motion goniometry
- Diagnostic testing as needed (e.g., screening blood analysis and urinalysis, radiology, ultrasound, CT, MRI, SOD1 DNA testing)
- Comprehensive analysis resulting in diagnosis and prioritized rehabilitation problem list
- Prescription for V-OP device if appropriate

Components of the V-OP evaluation

Observation

Observation is essential and includes assessment of behavior in stance and ambulation. The ideal V-OP examination room is large with nonslip flooring and without an examination table. The patient should be allowed to explore the room freely while the history is taken. This provides time for acclimation and movement observation. The patient can also be examined while walking in an open area outside prior to entering the exam room. Props such as stairs, low hills or inclines are handy for challenged gaiting and mimicking the activities of daily living.

History and client goals

In addition to a thorough medical history including onset of injury, recent diagnostics performed, medications, supplements, and response to other therapies, the V-OP history should include information about past and present activity level, sport, or job, daily structured and nonstructured exercise, home and play environment (flooring, bedding, yard, stairs), and lifestyle (children, other pets, primary caregiver). These specific questions are important in determining the appropriateness of a prescribed V-OP device, its design, treatment plan, and implementation. For example, a home environment with hardwood floors versus carpeted floors may necessitate a different tread system; or a home in which the patient may freely roam at night may alter the wearing schedule of a device.

Next, client goals must be established. For example, is the intent to return a patient to world-class competition or is the intent an alternative to surgery because surgery, although recommended, is not possible? Of particular value is understanding why a client is seeking a V-OP therapeutic option. Common rationales for orthosis include: (1) no surgical alternative; (2) advanced age of the patient; (3) comorbidities; (4) poor anesthetic risk; or (5) financial constraints. It is important to establish client aims to select the appropriate therapy and to set realistic expectations. For example, in the case of a stifle orthosis for cranial cruciate insufficiency with meniscal damage, if financial constraints are the primary rationale for seeking a V-OP solution, the total expense of an orthosis, partial medial meniscectomy, and rehabilitation may not be within budget or it may not be less costly than surgical stabilization, partial medial meniscectomy, and rehabilitation.

Media acquisition for conformation, stance, and gaiting

Video is used for gait and active range of motion (AROM) analysis. Video capture is best performed in a long hallway (e.g. 30×5 feet) with a nonslip surface, or in an outdoor walkway. Obtaining video prior to examination can be beneficial as many patients tire significantly by the end of the comprehensive V-OP examination. Use of an electronic device (tablet or smart phone) with a gait analysis app permits slow motion viewing, still shots, and goniometry. At the time of this writing, commonly used apps include Coach's Eye™, Dartfish™, and Hudl™.

Media should be obtained from the level of the patient to reveal true motion without the distortion of perspective. Standard media obtained for each patient include combined transverse and frontal plane views (patient standing or moving toward and away from the camera) and sagittal plane views (patient standing or moving to the left and then to the right). Each view should incorporate the whole patient to further analyze the patient's top line, all limbs in relation to one another, and the trunk. Importantly, the dog should be moving at an even and steady pace, not pulling or lagging behind, and not leaning in either direction. Limiting any distractions in the area is helpful, as is keeping a loose, but controlled, leash.

The V-OP practitioner should evaluate each video for conformation, gait abnormalities, pathology, and measurement data (goniometry/osteokinematics). Good-quality media are necessary to make a proper diagnosis, prescription, and treatment plan; therefore, taking the time to capture good images is worthwhile. Additionally, this media is important for comparison as the treatment progresses.

While not all images are required for each patient, common video clips include four-leg and three-leg challenge stance and gaiting at walk and trot. For the former, the patient is positioned in a square stance with body weight evenly distributed over all limbs and the head facing directly forward. Video acquisition from all sides is ideal. Three-leg challenge stance, which simulates AROM loading, is acquired by lifting each limb sequentially. This is an isometric method of assessing internal moments used by the patient to resist external moments.

The second method of assessing internal moments is by gaiting at the walk and trot. Since the act of gaiting loads each limb differently, and with more force than stance (Kirpensteijn et al., 2000; Abdelhadi et al., 2013; Fischer et al., 2013; Hogy et al., 2013; Jarvis et al., 2013; Fuchs et al., 2014), these images can reveal the severity of instability or weakness as well as more subtle changes not seen in stance. Using a gait analysis app, goniometry and limb alignment can be assessed. By observing gait phases, information can be noted on (1) sagittal, frontal, and transverse plane conformation; and (2) ambulation abnormalities such as circumduction, varus, valgus, base-narrow or -wide, toed-in or turned-out feet, or cow-hocks.

Lastly, while assessing conformation and gaiting it is critical to assess the line of progression (LOP) for each limb. LOP describes the orientation of the proximal limb and the distal limb in stance and ambulation in the forward plane. LOP reveals alterations in the frontal and transverse planes. For many dogs the normal LOP for the thoracic and pelvic limbs is from the second or third digit due to a natural tendency for mild external rotation (toeing out). The Border Collie is an excellent example. If a V-OP device is prescribed attempting to create an LOP corresponding to the third or fourth digit (the cranial-most aspect of the foot), a forced internal rotation would be incurred predisposing to gaiting impairment and possible wounds from the device. Rather, with natural LOP in mind, the foot shell component should accommodate external rotation while the ground contact (sole of the device) realigns LOP in the forward plane.

Examination

The V-OP examination includes a general health assessment noting the presence of comorbidities that may supersede or impact the current issue. Neurological evaluation may be cursory or complete depending upon presenting complaint, signalment, and patient condition. Evaluation of cranial nerves, spinal reflexes, conscious proprioception, and postural reactions reveals additional information that aids in decision making, prescription, therapeutic plan, expectations, and prognosis, regardless of whether the presenting complaint is primarily neurological. For example, a Doberman Pinscher that presented for Achilles tendinopathy with concomitant evidence of cervical myelopathy may or may not be a candidate for an orthosis or may require specific design and rehabilitation prescription adjustments.

A thorough orthopedic examination is important to document primary and secondary orthopedic issues. For example, patients presented for an acute on chronic carpal hyperextension injury may exhibit contralateral carpal hyperextension. This may be secondary to temporary overloading with decreased weight bearing on the acutely affected limb. These cases resolve with treatment of the affected limb and weight-bearing equilibration over the paired thoracic limbs. Alternatively, contralateral carpal hyperextension may represent a second unstable joint requiring treatment. This can be distinguished by assessing the passive range of motion (PROM) relative to a video analysis of AROM, or by treating the first issue and re-evaluating the second within a few weeks. If the PROM is normal compared with the AROM, often the carpal hyperextension is dynamic and due to temporary overloading and/or weakness.

Special tests are included in the orthopedic examination. In the pelvic limb, these include tests for patellar stability because patellar luxation is not uncommon in skeletally immature pelvic limb amputees or in dogs with congenital pelvic limb deformity. Cranial drawer and tibial thrust are important general stifle tests easily performed. The Ortolani and Barden tests are performed to assess hip laxity. Lastly, the Achilles tension test is used to evaluate the integrity and flexibility of the Achilles complex. In the thoracic limb, particular attention is paid to the elbow and PROM testing should include supination and pronation of the antebrachium to test for elbow pain.

The next component of V-OP evaluation is myofascial examination. Muscle symmetry as well as lean muscle mass are assessed. Patterns of hypertrophy and atrophy can be important diagnostic clues. Deeper palpation and mobilization can reveal myofascial trigger points, muscle tension, and pain, as well as tendon or ligament laxity. These are important points for treatment planning and follow-up assessment.

The last portion of the evaluation is PROM goniometry. As a minimum, PROM should be measured for the major joints of the affected and contralateral limb. Additionally, any restrictions in flexibility (muscle or tendon), joint laxity (ligament, joint capsule, muscle atrophy, denervation), or alterations in the osteokinematics of the other limbs should be explored with goniometry.

Diagnostics, analysis, and diagnosis

Common diagnostic tests salient to the V-OP evaluation include radiography (survey and stressed views), MRI, CT, and ultrasonography. Not uncommonly, bilateral impairment is found, for example in CCL insufficiency, Achilles mechanism injury, and elbow dysplasia.

Critical analysis of videos using the analysis applications mentioned above is invaluable in diagnosing, assessing severity, prognosticating, and following treatment progression.

Laboratory work, including complete blood count, serum chemistry, urinalysis, and thyroid titer, can be helpful especially in the aged patient. Additionally, ancillary tests such as the SOD1 genetic test for degenerative myopathy may be beneficial when concomitant neurological signs are noted.

The purposes of this comprehensive V-OP evaluation are to ascertain all primary and secondary issues relevant to the presenting complaint, to determine the appropriateness of a V-OP device, and to align client and therapeutic goals with the proposed device. Observation, media analysis, diagnostic imaging, and laboratory results are vital in achieving these purposes. The clinician must determine if the proposed device will accommodate a nonresolvable issue (e.g., chronic Achilles tendinopathy with plantigrade stance in a 13-year-old dog) or whether the device will augment a treatment plan with intent to heal (e.g., acute Achilles tendinopathy in a 2-year-old field trial dog).

Prescription and treatment plan

The treatment plan includes device and rehabilitation prescription as well as a follow-up plan. The prescription format may vary from manufacturer to manufacturer. The key components are noted in Box 11.4.

The rehabilitation prescription should guide the canine rehabilitation professional. Setting specific goals and benchmarks should guide therapy. Common rehabilitation goals for the V-OP patient include: training the client and patient in proper donning and doffing, device acclimation, transitions, gait re-education, balance and proprioception adaptations, strength improvement, fitness/endurance, and return to/refinement of activities of daily living (e.g., stairs, dog door, car rides).

Follow-up evaluation

Follow-up is essential and client expectations must be aligned appropriately at the outset. Nearly all custom devices require adjustment in the first weeks of use. This is because customization can only be so accurate and is strongly dependent on accuracy in fiberglass impression. Additionally, as the patient acclimates, minor changes in fit due to muscle loss or development, material stretching, improved gaiting and limb alignment, and skin condition may require attention. Dogs with a thin hair coat or skin are especially vulnerable to irritation. The use of socks and friction-reducing powders can be helpful.

In the months after fitting the device, adjustments may be needed as the patient acclimates, heals, and progresses in the rehabilitation plan. Two excellent examples of this are dynamic Achilles orthoses and postop partial carpal arthrodesis orthoses. Both are designed to allow a gradual increase in range of motion of the affected joint as healing progresses. For patients whose devices are intended for lifelong use (e.g., CCL insufficiency, subtotal amputation, failed tarsal arthrodesis), follow-ups are typically provided every 6–12 months. The purposes are to (1) assess patient condition overall and status of the injury; and (2) assess the condition of the device to ensure it continues to meet fit and function needs. Replacement of worn components such as straps, pads, or tread is common. During these appointments it is important to assess the original injury and determine whether the device continues to meet therapeutic goals. In some cases, changes in patient condition or excessive wear of the device require a new device.

Box 11.4   V-OP prescription

- Signalment (breed, age, gender, weight, body condition score)
- Affected limb(s) including laterality
- Diagnosis including severity
- Style of device
  - e.g., simple one-joint orthosis: carpus, tarsus, stifle, elbow
  - e.g., combination orthosis: stifle–tarsus or elbow–carpus
  - e.g., simple prosthesis: above carpus, above tarsus
  - e.g., combination prosthesis: below carpus with elbow cuff and articulation, below metatarsals with crural cuff and articulation
  - e.g., prosthosis (combination of prosthesis and orthosis)
- Device components
  - e.g., articulation(s)
  - e.g., foot segment if needed, with or without heel
  - e.g., type of extension and foot for prosthesis
  - e.g., motion limiters
- Intended use
  - e.g., short term with intent to heal
  - e.g., post-surgical support (alternative to serial casting)
  - e.g., permanent solution with no intent to heal
- Intended wearing schedule
  - e.g., sport use only (support device)
  - e.g., all day use
  - e.g., 24/7 use

Finding a V-OP fabricating partner

H-OP and V-OP scope of practice

As the veterinarian develops a V-OP practice it is important to thoroughly understand how H-OP devices are prescribed and the training required to appropriately direct fabrication. As of 2017, no certification specific to V-OP exists. No veterinary practice acts in the United States specifically address the use of these devices. Veterinary practice acts also do not specify prescription characteristics or discuss the characteristics of the doctor–patient–client relationship for the use of V-OP devices. Likewise, there are no standards or regulations for V-OP fabricators.

At the same time, H-OP as an industry or profession does not limit the scope of practice to human patients. As such, H-OP fabricators and practitioners can and do provide devices to non-human patients with no additional training in quadruped mechanics and pathomechanics. This is concerning because such individuals may not have knowledge of veterinary patient behavior, anatomy, and pathology. The H-OP fabricator might fabricate a number of veterinary devices or fabricate a one-off as a favor to a veterinarian or client, or perhaps as an interesting project. However, the science and technology of veterinary biomechanics and V-OP have passed the stage of novelty and human interest. The potential risk to veterinary patients cannot be understated. These risks range from delay of appropriate therapy to iatrogenic injury, which can exceed the original injury in terms of severity and consequence. Clients risk the financial burden of a potentially inappropriate or harmful device.

Training, licensure, and certification

H-OP training and certification programs have been established chiefly by the American Board of Certification (ABC) and the Board of Certification (BOC) founded in 1948 and 1984, respectively (www.abcop.org/WhoWeAre/Pages/History.aspx; www.bocusa.org/about-boc). These certifying bodies are endorsed by the American Academy of Orthotists and Prosthetists (AAOP), which was founded in 1970 (www.oandp.org). The education standards endorsed by the AAOP are embodied within the *Standards and Guidelines for an Accredited Educational Program for the Orthotic and Prosthetic Practitioner*, developed by the National Commission on Orthotic and Prosthetic Education (NCOPE) (http://www.

ncope.org/view/?file=NCOPE_Policy). These standards were recognized by the American Medical Association's Council on Medical Education in 1993, and by the Commission on Accreditation of Allied Health Education Programs (CAAHEP). For experiential requirements, the AAOP endorses the completion of an NCOPE-accredited residency program prior to certification (http://www.oandp.org/page/licposition). For those individuals who undergo formal training, a 12–18-month residency is required (http://www.ncope.org/view/?file=2015_residency_standards; all websites in this paragraph accessed October 2017).

Surprisingly, ABC and BOC are voluntary certification programs, and licensure is required in only 15 states in the United States as of this writing. According to their website, the ABC believes that the provision of orthotic and prosthetic care should be vested in practitioners who have fulfilled requirements for ABC certification and that state licensure should embody equivalent requirements (www.abcop.org/State-Licensure/Pages/ABC-State-Licensure-Policy.aspx; accessed October 2017). The limited requirement for licensure in the United States implies that not all H-OP fabricators are adequately trained, certified, and licensed, and by extension the same can be said for V-OP fabricators. Fortunately, these certifications are considered a minimum among established H-OP practices.

For those who are licensed, there are several levels of training, certification, and codes of ethics limiting scope of practice including pedorthist (i.e., foot orthotic fabricator), orthotist and prosthetist (O and P) technician, fitter, and assistant. The ABC, BOC, and AAOP actively support the establishment of training and certifying standards for each of these levels and for all states. The AAOP endorses state licensure of orthotists and prosthetists as the preferred method of establishing patient protection mechanisms through legislated state standards (http:www.oandp.org/page/licposition; accessed October 2017). Until such a time as veterinary O and P fabrication and practice requirements are established, it is appropriate to assume the requirement of ABC certification in orthotics and prosthetics specifically as a minimum for fabricators of veterinary devices.

Prescription requirement

According to the BOC model licensure act for human practice, "A licensed orthotist, prosthetist, pedorthist or orthotic fitter may provide care or services only if the care or services are provided pursuant to an order from a licensed physician or licensed podiatrist" (www.bocusa.org/files/BOC_Model_Licensure_Act.pdf; accessed October 2017). Again, this is based on a model licensure act and is not required in all states. Unfortunately, at this time the same cannot be said for non-human patients or fabricators of devices for nonhuman patients. This means that clients can order V-OP devices without the guidance of a veterinarian, without a prescription, and without veterinary follow-up care. Devices are frequently ordered from online entities. Working with animal patients is not the same as working with human patients because of the vastly different biomechanics and pathomechanics of the quadruped. Just as cats are not small dogs, Chihuahuas are not small Greyhounds, and quadrupeds are absolutely not small people on all fours. Veterinary species are tremendously diverse and challenging for many reasons, not the least of which is that these patients are not verbally self-reporting and advocating. Therefore, a fabricator should be appropriately H-OP certified and have a great deal of veterinary patient experience before providing a device for any companion animal. Because of this, it is incumbent on the attending veterinarian to educate and advise their clients and to perform due diligence in selecting a fabricator. Although currently not regulated, prudent practice dictates that V-OP devices are prescribed by a veterinarian with a valid doctor-patient-client relationship and, further, that ongoing care be managed by a veterinarian.

Key questions to ask when selecting a reputable fabricator

The following are listed beginning with strongest recommendation:

(1) What is the certification type/scope of practice of the fabricator?
(2) What is the fabricator's veterinary caseload? Do they work with animals exclusively or work with animals as a side business? With what species has the fabricator worked?
(3) Does the fabricator require a prescription from a veterinarian with a valid doctor-patient-client relationship for *all* cases? This is a matter of professional ethics; in the opinion of the authors, if a prescription is required for a human patient, veterinary patients should receive the same standard of care.
(4) What level of support and customer service is available from the fabricator? This is particularly important for the novice V-OP veterinarian.
(5) Does the fabricator have a close working relationship with a collaborating veterinarian other than the prescribing veterinarian who can provide consultation and guidance with regard to animal health, locomotion, behavior, wound management, and rehabilitation?
(6) Does the collaborating veterinarian have advanced training in sports medicine, rehabilitation, and V-OP? There are several interest groups and specialty boards providing certification and continuing education for veterinarians. These include, but are not limited to, the Veterinary Orthopedic Society (VOS), American College of Veterinary Sports Medicine and Rehabilitation (ACVSMR), the American Association of Rehabilitation Veterinarians (AARV), the Canine Rehabilitation Institute (CRI), and NorthEast Seminars. Association with such organizations is ideal for any veterinarian providing frequent consultation to a V-OP fabricator.

Summary

V-OP is a novel and potentially significant addition to the practice of canine sports medicine and rehabilitation. It is not a panacea and is not for every client or patient. Thorough evaluation is required as a prelude to specific diagnosis and V-OP prescription.

Much work is needed to provide a scientific basis for the anecdotal advantages of V-OP devices. Current basic research supports moving forward, but clinical studies are lacking. Until such a time as a body of highest quality literature can be amassed, it is incumbent on veterinarians to communicate with their clients about these options and guide them in seeking knowledgeable V-OP providers (veterinarians) and responsible fabricators. State practice acts should be amended and enforced to address the prescription and use of V-OP devices. Training and certification programs should be developed to educate those veterinarians interested in providing these solutions, and fabricators should be held to the same standards required in H-OP, even as H-OP requirements and licensure are becoming more stringent.

References

Abdelhadi, J., Wefstaedt, P., Galindo-zamora, V., Anders, A., Nolte, I. & Schilling, N. 2013. Load redistribution in walking and trotting Beagles with induced forelimb lameness. *Am J Vet Res*, 74(1), 34–39.

Adamson, C., Kaufmann, M., Levine, D., Millis, D. L. & Marcellin-little, D. J. 2005. Assistive devices, orthotics, and prosthetics. *Vet Clin North Am Small Anim Pract*, 35, 1441–1451, ix.

American Academy of Orthopaedic Surgeons. 1987. *The Use of Knee Braces*. Position Statement 1124. Rosemont, IL: AAOS.

Bechtol, C. O. 1967. The fitting of a lower-extremity prosthesis in the immediately postamputation period: a new challenge in rehabilitation. *Arch Phys Med Rehabil*, 48, 145–146.

Bedotto, R. A. 2006. Biomechanical assessment and treatment in lower extremity prosthetics and orthotics: a clinical perspective. *Phys Med Rehabil Clin N Am*, 17, 203–243.

Bertocci, G. E., Brown, N. P. & Mich, P. M. 2017. Biomechanics of an orthosis-managed cranial cruciate ligament-deficient canine stifle joint predicted by use of a computer model. *Am J Vet Res*, 78(1), 27–35.

Bockstahler, B. A., VOBORNIK, A., Müller, M. & Peham, C. 2009. Compensatory load redistribution in naturally occurring osteoarthritis of the elbow joint and induced weight-bearing lameness of the forelimbs compared with clinically sound dogs. *Vet J*, 180(2), 202–212.

Budsberg, S. C., Verstraete, M. C. & Soutas-little, R. W. 1987. Force plate analysis of the walking gait in healthy dogs. *Am J Vet Res*, 48(6), 915–918.

Budsberg, S. C., Jevens, D. J., Brown, J., Foutz, T. L., Decamp, C. E. & Reece, L. 1993. Evaluation of limb symmetry indices, using ground reaction forces in healthy dogs. *Am J Vet Res*, 54(10), 1569–1574.

Budsberg, S. C., Johnston, S. A., Schwarz, P. D., Decamp, C. E. & Claxton, R. 1999. Efficacy of etodolac for the treatment of osteoarthritis of the hip joints in dogs. *J Am Vet Med Assoc*, 214(2), 206–210.

Carberry, C. & Harvey, H. 1987. Owner satisfaction with limb amputation in dogs and cats. *J Am Vet Med Assoc*, 23, 227–232.

Carr, B. J. 2016. The use of canine stifle orthotics for cranial cruciate ligament insufficiency. *Veterinary Evidence*, 1(1).

Case, J. B. (2013). Gastrocnemius tendon strain in a dog treated with autologous mesenchymal stem cells and a custom orthosis. *Vet Surg J*, 42(4), 355–360.

Decamp, C. E. 1997. Kinetic and kinematic gait analysis and the assessment of lameness in the dog. *Vet Clin North Am Small Anim Pract*, 27(4), 825–840.

Deshales, L. D. 2002. Upper extremity orthoses. In: trombly, C. A. & radomski, M. V. (eds), *Occupational Therapy for Physical Dysfunction*, 5th edn. Baltimore, MD: Lippincott, Williams & Wilkins, pp. 313–349.

Devasconcellos, P., Balla, V. K., Bose, S., Fugazzi, R., Dernell, W. S. & Bandyopadhyay, A. 2012. Patient specific implants for amputation prostheses: design, manufacture and analysis. *Vet Comp Orthop Traumatol*, 25(4), 286–296.

Dickerson, V. M., Coleman, K. D., Ogawa, M., Saba, C.F., Cornell, K.K., Radlinsky, M.G. & Schmiedt, C.W. 2015. Outcomes of dogs undergoing limb amputation, owner satisfaction with limb amputation procedures, and owner perceptions regarding postsurgical adaptation: 64 cases (2005–2012). *J Am Vet Med Assoc*, 247, 786–792.

Drygas, K. A., Taylor, R., Sidebotham, C. G., Hugate, R. R. & McAlexander, H. 2008. Transcutaneous tibial implants: a surgical procedure for restoring ambulation after amputation of the distal aspect of the tibia in a dog. *Vet Surg*, 37, 322–327.

Evans, R., Gordon, W. & Conzemius, M. 2003. Effect of velocity on ground reaction forces in dogs with lameness attributable to tearing of the cranial cruciate ligament. *Am J Vet Res*, 64(12), 1479–1481.

Fairley, M. 2013. Cad/Cam's expanding potential. *The O&P Edge*. http://www.oandp.com/articles/2013-05_03.asp (accessed October 2017).

Fischer, S., Anders, A., Nolte, I. & Schilling, N. 2013. Compensatory load redistribution in walking and trotting dogs with hind limb lameness. *Vet J*, 197(3), 746–752.

Fitzpatrick, N., Smith, T. J., Pendegrass, C. J., Yeadon, R., Ring, M., Goodship, A.E. & Blunn, G.W. 2011. Intraosseous transcutaneous amputation prosthesis (ITAP) for limb salvage in 4 dogs. *Vet Surg*, 40(8), 909–25.

Fuchs, A., Goldner, B., Nolte, I. & Schilling, N. 2014. Ground reaction force adaptations to tripedal locomotion in dogs. *Vet J*, 201, 307–315.

Fujisawa, T., Hattori, T., Takahashi, K., Kuboki, T., Yamashita, A. & Takigawa, M. 1999. Cyclic mechanical stress induces extracellular matrix degradation in cultured chondrocytes via gene expression of matrix metalloproteinases and inter-leukin-1. *J Biochem*, 125(5), 966–975.

Geertzen, J. H., Martina, J. D. & Rietman, H. S. 2001. Lower limb amputation. Part 2: Rehabilitation: a 10 year literature review. *Prosthet Orthot Int*, 25, 14–20.

Goldner, B., Fuchs, A., Nolte, I. & Schilling, N. 2015. Kinematic adaptations to tripedal locomotion in dogs. *Vet J*, 204(2), 192–200.

Hardie, R. J. & Lewallen, J. T. 2013. Use of a custom orthotic boot for management of distal extremity and pad wounds in three dogs. *Vet Surg J*, 42(6), 678–682.

Hart, J. L., May, K. D., Kieves, N. R., Mich, P. M., Goh, C. S., Palmer, R. H. & Duerr, F.M. 2016. Comparison of owner satisfaction between stifle joint orthoses and tibial plateau leveling osteotomy for the management of cranial cruciate ligament disease in dogs. *J Am Vet Med Assoc*, 249(4), 391–398.

Heijnen, L., Roosendaal, G. & Heim, M. 1997. Orthotics and rehabilitation for chronic hemophilic synovitis of the ankle. An overview. *Clin Orthop Relat Res*, 343, 68–73.

Hogy, S. M., Worley, D. R., Jarvis, J. C., Hill, A. E., Reiser, R. F. & Haussler, K. K. 2013. Kinematic and kinetic analysis of dogs during trotting after amputation of a pelvic limb. *J Am Vet Med Assoc*, 74, 1164–1171.

Jagannatha, T. D., & Harish, G. (2015). Influence of carbon and glass fiber reinforcements on flexural strength of epoxy matrix polymer hybrid composites. *Int J Eng Res Applic*, 5(4), 109–112.

Jarvis, S. L., Worley, D. R., Hogy, S. M., Hill, A. E., Haussler, K. K. & Reiser, R. F. 2013. Kinematic and kinetic analysis of dogs during trotting after amputation of a thoracic limb. *Am J Vet Res*, 74, 1155–1163.

Kent, J. & Franklyn-miller, A. 2011. Biomechanical models in the study of lower limb amputee kinematics: a review. *Prosthet Orthot Int*, 35, 124–139.

Kirpensteijn, J., VAN DEN Bos, R. & Endenburg, N. 1999. Adaptation of dogs to the amputation of a limb and their owners' satisfaction with the procedure. *Vet Res*, 144, 115–118.

Kirpensteijn, J., VAN DEN Bos, R., VAN DEN Brom, W. E. & Hazewinkel, H. A. 2000. Ground reaction force analysis of large breed dogs when walking after the amputation of a limb. *Vet Rec*, 146(6), 155–159.

Klasson, B. 1985. Computer aided design, computer aided manufacture and other computer aids in prosthetics and orthotics. *Digital Resource Foundation for the Orthotics & Prosthetics Community*, 9, 3–11.

http://www.oandplibrary.org/poi/1985_01_003. asp (accessed October 2017).

Landman, M. A., DE Blaauw, J. A., VAN Weeren, P. R. & Hofland, L. J. 2004. Field study of the prevalence of lameness in horses with back problems. *Vet Rec*, 155, 165–168.

Lee, D. V., Bertram, J. E. & Todhunter, R. J. 1999. Acceleration and balance in trotting dogs. *J Exp Biol*, 202(24), 3565–3573.

Levine, J. M. & Fitch, R. B. (2003). Use of an ankle–foot orthosis in a dog with traumatic sciatic neuropathy. *J Small Anim Pract*, 44, 236–238.

Marcellin-little, D. J., Drum, M. G., Levine, D. & McDonald, S. S. 2015. Orthoses and exoprostheses for companion animals. *Vet Clin North Am Small Anim Pract*, 45(1), 167–183.

McLaughlin, R., Jr. & Roush, J. K. 1995. Effects of increasing velocity on braking and propulsion times during force plate gait analysis in grey-hounds. *Am J Vet Res*, 56(2), 159–161.

Mich, P. M. 2014. The emerging role of veterinary orthotics and prosthetics (V-OP) in small animal rehabilitation and pain management. *Top Companion Anim Med*, 29(1), 10–19.

Nolan, L. & Lees, A. 2000. The functional demands on the intact limb during walking for active trans-femoral and trans-tibial amputees. *Prosthet Orthot Int*, 24, 117–125.

Nolan, L., Wit, A., Dudzinski, K., Lees, A., Lake, M. & Wychowanski, M. 2003. Adjustments in gait symmetry with walking speed in trans-femoral and trans-tibial amputees. *Gait Posture*, 17, 142–151.

Oakley, R. E. 1999. External coaptation. *Vet Clin North Am Small Anim Pract*, 29, 1083–1095.

Piermattei, D., Flo, G. & Decamp, C. 2006. Fractures: classification, diagnosis, and treatment. In: Piermattei, D., Flo, G., Decamp, C. & Brinker, W. (eds), *Handbook of Small Animal Orthopedics and Fracture Repair*, 4th edn. St. Louis, MO: Saunder-Elsevier, pp. 25–159.

Pomeranz, B., Adler, U., Shenoy, N., Macaluso, C. & Parikh, S. 2006. Prosthetics and orthotics for the older adult with a physical disability. *Clin Geriatr Med*, 22, 377–394; ix.

Prinsen, E. C., Nederhand, M. J. & Rietman, J. S. 2011. Adaptation strategies of the lower extremities of patients with a transtibial or transfemoral amputation during level walking: a systematic review. *Arch Phys Med Rehabil*, 92, 1311–1325.

Prokop, L. L. 2006. Upper extremity orthotics in performing artists. *Phys Med Rehabil Clin N Am*, 17, 843–852.

Riggs, C. M., Decamp, C. E., Soutas-little, R. W., Braden, T. D. & Richter, M. A. 1993. Effects of subject velocity on force plate-measured ground reaction forces in healthy greyhounds at the trot. *Am J Vet Res*, 54(9), 1523–1526.

Schoeman, M., Diss, C. E. & Strike, S. C. 2012. Kinetic and kinematic compensations in amputee vertical jumping. *J Appl Biomech*, 28(4), 438–447.

Seymour, R. 2002. *Introduction to Prosthetics and Orthotics*. Philadelphia, PA: Lippincott, Williams & Wilkins, pp. 3–35.

Shurr, G. & Cook, T. 1990. Below knee amputations and prosthetics. In: *Prosthetics and Orthotics*. Norwalk, CT: Appleton and Lange, pp. 53–82.

Siegel, I. M. 1973. Orthotic treatment of tibiotarsal deformity in an elephant. *J Am Vet Med Assoc*, 163(6), 544–545.

Tatar, Y., Ramazanoglu, N., Camliguney, A. F., Saygi, E. K. & Cotuk, H. B. 2014. The effectiveness of shin guards used by football players. *J Sports Sci Med*, 13(1), 120–127.

Tomlinson, J. E. & Manfredi, J. M. (2014). Evaluation of application of a carpal brace as a treatment for carpal ligament instability in dogs: 14 cases (2008–2011). *J Amn Vety Med Assoc*, 244(4), 438–443.

Torres, B. T., Moëns, N. M., Al-nadaf, S., Reynolds, L. R., Fu, Y. C. & Budsberg, S. C. 2013. Comparison of overground and treadmill-based gaits of dogs. *Am J Vet Res*, 74(4), 535–541.

Versluys, R., Lenaerts, G., VAN Damme, M., Jonkers, I., Desomer, A., Vanderborght, B., *et al.* 2009. Successful preliminary walking experiments on a transtibial amputee fitted with a powered prosthesis. *Prosthet Orthot Int*, 33(4), 368–377.

Withrow, S. J. & Hirsch, V. M. 1979. Owner response to amputation of a pet's leg. *Vet Med Small Anim Clin*, 74(3), 332, 334.

Wong, K. V. & Hernandez, A. 2012. A review of additive manufacturing. *ISRN Mech Eng*, 2012, article ID 208760.

Wu, W., Geng, P., Li, G., Zhao, D., Zhang, H. & Zhao, J. 2015. Influence of layer thickness and raster angle on the mechanical properties of 3D-printed PEEK and a comparative mechanical study between PEEK and ABS. *Materials*, 8(9), 5834–5846.

12 Disorders of the Canine Thoracic Limb: Diagnosis and Treatment

Sherman O. Canapp, Jr, DVM, MS, DACVS, DACVSMR, CCRT, David Dycus, DVM, MS, DACVS, CCRP, and Kristin Kirkby Shaw, DVM, MS, PhD, DACVS, DACVSMR, CCRT

Summary

While thoracic limb lameness in the dog is very common, it can be extremely challenging and frustrating at times to determine the exact cause. An injury as simple as a digit sprain can throw off the entire musculoskeletal system, leading to secondary compensatory issues further up the limb and also affecting the rest of the body. When there are pathological changes in the shoulder and elbow at the same time, it can be very confusing as to which is the primary cause of pain and lameness.

In canine sports medicine practice it is no longer acceptable to state that the patient has a "shoulder condition" as its cause of lameness. We need to know not only the exact structure in the shoulder that is injured, but the specific area of that structure involved (i.e., muscle; muscle–tendon interface; tendon; or tendon insertion) as the treatments for each may vary. Advancements in diagnostic musculoskeletal ultrasound allow these challenging soft tissue injuries to be assessed down to the fiber pattern, and allow assessment of the patient's response to treatment over time. Another exciting development in canine sports medicine as it relates to thoracic limb conditions is the growing evidence for the use of biological therapies.

This chapter focuses primarily on the most common shoulder conditions in sporting, working, and companion dogs (supraspinatus tendinopathy, medial shoulder syndrome, biceps tendinopathy, and osteochondrosis dissecans).

Elbow dysplasia is a common cause of thoracic limb lameness in dogs. Early diagnosis and treatment is critical to slowing the progression of osteoarthritis. Unlike joint replacement for the hip, there has yet to be an established successful total elbow replacement technology for the dog, and the other advanced aggressive surgical techniques have shown less than favorable results long term. Therefore, a multimodal approach including arthroscopic treatments, rehabilitation therapy, medical management, weight management, joint supplements, and intra-articular injections including biological therapies (platelet-rich plasma and stem cell therapy) should be considered.

Canine Sports Medicine and Rehabilitation, Second Edition. Edited by Chris Zink and Janet B. Van Dyke.
© 2018 John Wiley & Sons, Inc. Published 2018 by John Wiley & Sons, Inc.

While not as common as injuries to the shoulder or elbow, injuries to the manus (carpus, metacarpal bones, phalanges, and sesamoid bones) can be just as frustrating and challenging to treat. Such injuries include hyperextension of the carpus, ligamentous sprains, fractures, or luxations.

Shoulder disorders

It is estimated that over 4.5 million people visit the doctor every year for shoulder pain associated with rotator cuff injuries (Oh *et al.*, 2007). Rotator cuff tears affect more than 40% of the population over the age of 50 with an economic cost of over US$3 billion annually (Tempelhof *et al.*, 1999; Mather *et al.*, 2013). Given that such a large percentage of the human population has shoulder conditions, it comes as no surprise that a substantial percentage of thoracic limb lameness in dogs involves the shoulder. Shoulder conditions are the most common causes of lameness in working, sporting, and performing dogs (Cullen *et al.*, 2013).

Although shoulder injury appears to be extremely common in both human and canine athletes, a report has shown that the structural and biomechanical characteristics of the joints of quadruped animals are quite different from those of humans (Sager *et al.*, 2009). With the coordinated action of over 25 muscles required for shoulder motion, the ensuing movement is complex, with the limb undergoing flexion, extension, rotation, abduction, and adduction (Marcellin-Little *et al.*, 2007). The potential for muscle and tendon injuries causing performance issues and lameness is significant when all muscular contributions to the joint are con-

sidered (Figure 12.1). One author's (SC) case database reveals the most common muscle and tendon sports-related injuries in the canine shoulder include subscapularis tendinopathy (a component of medial shoulder syndrome), supraspinatus tendinopathy, biceps tendinopathy, and infraspinatus myopathy.

Supraspinatus tendinopathy

Several degenerative disorders of the human and canine supraspinatus tendon have been identified, including rotator cuff tears, calcifying tendonitis or tendinosis (microtears), and tendinosis as a result of overuse (Fransson *et al.*, 2005). Tendinopathy has been adopted as a generic descriptive term for the clinical conditions in and around tendons arising from overuse (Sharma & Maffulli, 2005).

Degeneration of the supraspinatus tendon is thought to be a factor in the development of rotator cuff tears in humans (Danova & Muir, 2003). Overuse is likely an important factor in this disorder and has been supported in animal models. In these models of repetitive activity, the mechanical properties of supraspinatus tendons deteriorated as noted by a decreased modulus of elasticity and decreased

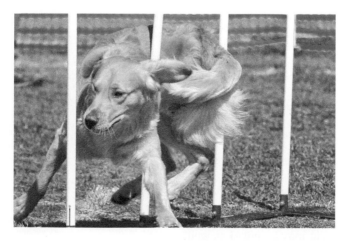

Figure 12.1   Golden Retriever performing the weave poles and demonstrating significant shoulder abduction, biomechanically stressing the medial compartment.

maximum stress to failure in the tendon (Carpenter *et al.*, 1998; Soslowsky *et al.*, 2000). Supraspinatus tendinopathies can be difficult to treat and often require lengthy management (Carpenter *et al.*, 1998; Soslowsky *et al.*, 2000).

Affected tendons contain discontinuous, disorganized fibers, and typically no acute inflammation is detected, explaining the often-noted lack of response to NSAIDs. Affected tendons that contain such fiber patterns, as noted on musculoskeletal diagnostic ultrasound, are seen as hypoechoic foci or *core lesions* (Schramme *et al.*, 2010). This term is now used for similar canine tendon lesions seen on diagnostic musculoskeletal ultrasound. A rapidly growing nodule develops within the supraspinatus tendon in chronic cases, compressing the biceps tendon and causing pain (Lafuente *et al.*, 2009).

Cause

It appears that repeated strain injury is an underlying cause of supraspinatus tendinopathy (ST). In performance dogs, repeated strain can result from hitting the ground or agility contacts on an outstretched thoracic limb, quick turns, and repetitive eccentric contractions as well as concentric contractions with the muscle in a lengthened state. Slipping, overstretching, and overuse of the muscle can also contribute.

Thus, dogs that perform agility are overrepresented in ST cases. In a recent retrospective study of dogs affected by ST, agility dogs made up 58% of the overall performance canine population (Canapp *et al.*, 2016a). Initiation of ST may in part be due to inflammation, but inflammation has not been seen to exacerbate the disease and was found to be absent when evaluating histology and tendon fibers (Canapp *et al.*, 2016a). Additionally, that study indicated that commonly occurring concurrent thoracic limb pathological changes have the potential to predispose dogs to ST. This suggests that ST can occur as a secondary condition.

Diagnosis

Patients with supraspinatus tendinopathies present with varying degrees of lameness, from a shortened stride length to a significant weight-bearing lameness. The lameness worsens with activity and is resistant to treatment. Atrophy of the supraspinatus muscle may be noted as well as pain on direct palpation over the tendon with flexion of the shoulder. ST presents unilaterally

more frequently than bilaterally (62% to 38%, respectively) (Canapp *et al.*, 2016a). No sex predisposition is apparent. A retrospective study found that dogs diagnosed with ST frequently had concurrent elbow (55%) and/or shoulder (62%) pathological changes (Canapp *et al.*, 2016a).

Mineralization within the tendon or bony remodeling at the point of insertion on the greater tubercle or along the region of the scapular notch to supraglenoid tubercle, may be noted radiographically in chronic cases (Figure 12.2). Although MRI is an excellent diagnostic modality for acute and chronic cases, musculoskeletal ultrasound can be a rapid, inexpensive means of diagnosis in the hands of experienced operators (Figure 12.3). Musculoskeletal ultrasound allows for a definitive diagnosis as well as serial evaluations to assess response to treatment. Musculoskeletal ultrasound features of ST cases are reported to include nonhomogenous echogenicity, (93% of cases), enlarged tendons (76%), and irregular fiber patterns (74%) (Canapp *et al.*, 2016a). Less common features include bone irregularity, bicipital tenosynovitis, and mineralization of the supraspinatus tendon, recorded in 19%, 16%, and 15% of cases, respectively. Identification of the core lesion was possible in 24% of cases.

Arthroscopic exploration can be performed to evaluate the shoulder and elbow for concurrent conditions. Although the supraspinatus tendon is extracapsular and cannot be directly evaluated via arthroscopy, a supraspinatus bulge causing biceps tendon contact/compression and a biceps tendon kissing lesion are commonly found

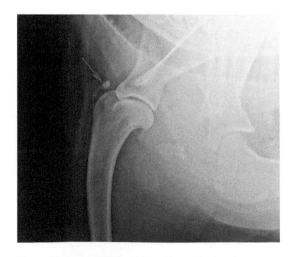

Figure 12.2   Lateral shoulder radiograph showing mineralization within the supraspinatus tendon (arrow).

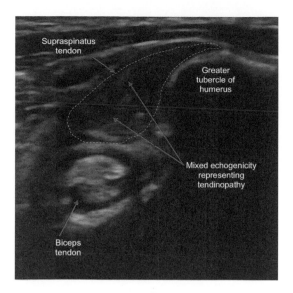

Figure 12.3   Ultrasound image demonstrating supraspinatus tendinopathy.

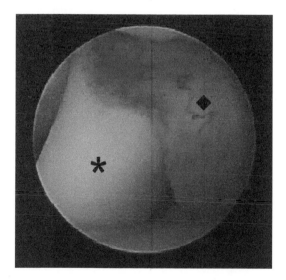

Figure 12.4   Arthroscopic view of a compressed biceps tendon (asterisk) secondary to a supraspinatus bulge (diamond).

(Figure 12.4). A study found that arthroscopy of the shoulder revealed a supraspinatus bulge in 82% of cases, which led to bicep impingement in 39% of affected dogs (Canapp *et al.*, 2016a). Other abnormalities commonly revealed by shoulder arthroscopy include subscapularis lesions (62%), medial glenohumeral ligament lesions (45%), labral tear (33%), cartilage defects (22%), and bone eburnation/osteophytosis (11%). Medial shoulder syndrome (MSS) was found in 62% of the dogs evaluated. Pathological changes in the

biceps were noted in 38% of cases, primarily bicipital tenosynovitis (29%). Elbow arthroscopy revealed 55% of elbows to have elbow lesions such as fragmented medial coronoid process (35%), medial coronoid disease (5%), and/or end stage medial compartment disease (15%).

Treatment

Acute cases can be treated with conservative medical management consisting of NSAIDs, controlled activity, and rehabilitation therapy (manual therapy, modalities, range of motion (ROM) with progression to stretching and strengthening exercises). However, these cases rarely present in the acute phase. Treatment for subacute and chronic cases is dictated by the findings of advanced diagnostics (ultrasound or MRI). A recent report revealed that 75% of subacute and chronic cases did not respond to conservative medical management, and 45.5% did not respond to rehabilitation (Canapp *et al.*, 2016b).

An inflammatory response is needed to jump-start the healing process. Reinitiating the inflammatory process increases circulation to the tendon. For this reason, NSAIDs and intra-articular corticosteroids are contraindicated. Rehabilitation therapies include soft tissue massage, heat, ultrasound therapy, and pain-free ROM/stretching. Shock wave therapy may also be considered (Danova & Muir, 2003). Further details are provided in Chapter 13.

Surgical intervention may be considered for dogs that do not respond to rehabilitation therapy. Surgically excising or debulking the supraspinatus nodule has been reported as a treatment option (Lafuente *et al.*, 2009). Surgical treatment should include arthroscopic exploration to evaluate and treat concurrent MSS if indicated. Unfortunately, whether surgical or conservative treatment is elected, it is common for dogs to have persistent or recurrent thoracic limb lameness.

When ST is moderate to severe, or when rehabilitation and conservative medical management has failed, biological therapies may be able to produce results. Good results using ultrasound-guided injections of combination platelet-rich plasma (PRP) and mesenchymal stem cells (MSC), such as cultured adipose-derived progenitor cells (ADPC) or bone marrow aspirate concentration (BMAC), into core lesions have been reported (Canapp, 2011). MSCs are capable of aiding tissue regeneration, initiating chemotaxis of progenitor cells, supplying growth factors, contributing to extracellular matrix formation, promoting angiogenesis, and providing anti-inflammatory and antifibrotic effects.

In a study of 55 dogs treated with ADPC/PRP, all had improved fiber patterns at 90 days post treatment, 82% showed a reduction in supraspinatus size, and 88% were sound with no significant difference in thoracic limb total pressure index (TPI).[1] Four months after treatment, 96% of the performance and sporting dogs were able to return to occupation (Canapp *et al.*, 2016b).

While there has been a positive response from the use of cultured adipose-derived stem cells, there have been many challenges clinically that made users look for alternative means of stem cell processing. These challenges included high morbidity associated with fat collection, 2-week turnaround time, shipping issues (such as contaminated, lost, or damaged cells in transit), as well as increasing laboratory costs. Due to the low morbidity of BMAC collection, quick in-house processing, lower costs, and success of BMAC/PRP in humans, some have elected to institute this mode of treatment.

Osteochondritis dissecans of the shoulder

Osteochondritis dissecans (OCD) of the humeral head occurs when the ossification process within the joint produces an excessive amount of cartilage. The excessive cartilage formation stems from failed transformation of cartilage to bone during endochondral ossification. As the cartilage accumulates, it becomes easily fissured by normal activity. These fissures lead to detachment of the cartilage from the humeral head, which creates a cartilage flap. OCD is generally considered to be hereditary and commonly occurs bilaterally in young dogs ranging from 5 to 12 months of age. OCD disproportionately affects large-breed male dogs (Rochat, 2012). Lameness generally presents gradually and becomes worse after exercise.

Cause

Shoulder OCD etiology is still being established, but two likely causes have been observed. The first is the rapid growth that occurs during adolescence. Early development is significantly influenced by hormones,

---

Case Study 12.1   Traumatic fragmented medial coronoid process

Signalment: 3-y.o. M/I Malinois (Police K9).

History: Presented with 2-month history of intermittent left thoracic limb lameness. Previous diagnosis: suspect mild shoulder soft tissue injury.

Examination: Gait: Mild weight-bearing lameness in left thoracic limb at walk.
    Posture: Stands slightly off-loading left thoracic limb.
    Palpation: Normal ROM all joints. Mild discomfort with full extension and abduction of left shoulder and on direct palpation over left medial coronoid process.
    Forelimb circumference: Left, 33 cm; right, 34 cm.
    Radiographic findings: shoulders and elbows WNL, no significant bone remodeling.

Arthroscopy: Left elbow: Fissure through tip of medial coronoid, nondisplaced subchondral fragment; mild humeroulnar incongruency; cartilage change distal medial humeral condyle WNL.
    Left shoulder: Mild inflammation of bicipital tendon sheath and cranial joint capsule; medial glenohumeral ligament and subscapularis tendon intact, no gross evidence of pathology.

Diagnosis: Traumatic fragmented medial coronoid process and mild bicipital tenosynovitis.

Treatment: Arthroscopic elbow debridement and curettage. Rechecks every 4 weeks postoperatively. Enrolled in rehabilitation program.
    4 weeks: Mild elbow joint effusion, generalized mild atrophy of left thoracic limb, ROM of left elbow and shoulder WNL, no pain or discomfort on palpation.
    8 weeks: Decreased joint effusion, improved muscle mass in left thoracic limb, ROM of left elbow and shoulder WNL, no pain or discomfort on palpation.
    12 weeks: Decreased joint effusion; increased muscle mass; left elbow and shoulder ROM WNL. No discomfort on direct palpation; no lameness noted. Gradual return to full duty.

Case follow-up: Active duty 4+ years postsurgery.

---

[1] Please refer to Chapter 2 for a comprehensive explanation of TPI and evaluating objective gait analysis.

nutrition, and genetics. Overnutrition, such as an excess of calcium, has been found to disrupt endochondral ossification and may be the cause for shoulder OCD (Hazewinkel *et al.*, 1985; Dammrich, 1991). The second factor that contributes significantly to shoulder OCD is trauma to the joint. Repetitive and concussive impacts commonly experienced by performance and working dogs likely increase the prevalence of shoulder OCD in that population.

Diagnosis

Slight to moderate lameness is common initially and many clients will not immediately notice the change in gait. When clients do start to notice lameness, it is not unusual for them to report it only as a unilateral lameness in the leg with the most severe symptoms. Lameness is reportedly worse after exercise, and stiffness is commonly reported after rest. Dogs will exhibit a shortened stride length at both a walk and a trot, and occasionally some will completely offload the painful limb. Palpation typically reveals pain along the caudal humeral head and during shoulder extension and flexion. A click can sometimes be noted during hyperextension of the shoulder and is likely associated with the coexistence of degenerative joint changes. Muscle atrophy is generally noted in long-term or severe cases. Additionally, it has been noted that the pain and lameness experienced is often predictive of the size and location of the OCD lesions. Dogs with a unilateral OCD lesion located caudocentrally on the humeral head showed a persistent lameness that did not occur when the lesion was located caudomedially (Olivieri *et al.*, 2007).

Radiographs can help to reveal OCD lesions that may appear as a surface cavity and cause the surface of the subchondral bone to seem flattened and/or abnormal in shape (Figure 12.5). Rarely, OCD lesions are not revealed by radiographs. In these cases, needle scope or musculoskeletal ultrasound is recommended to rule out OCD, especially for young dogs with shoulder pain and lameness that is indicative of shoulder OCD. Musculoskeletal ultrasound, although not a strong modality for diagnosing shoulder OCD, may reveal irregularities around the humeral head.

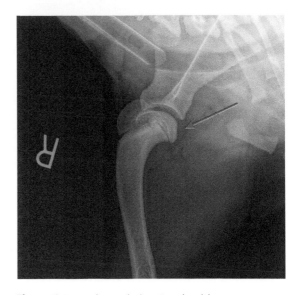

Figure 12.5   Radiograph showing shoulder osteochondritis dissecans lesion (arrow).

Treatment

Medical management consisting of NSAIDs and restricted activity may benefit a small number of dogs who present with mild OCD lesions, but most cases will require surgical treatment. Arthroscopy of the joint allows for removal of the osteochondral flap, debridement, and stimulation of fibrocartilage formation. Fibrocartilage formation within the lesion can be encouraged through abrasion arthroplasty, microfracture, or forage. Frequently, the flap fragments or breaks free entirely, which may cause secondary conditions such as bicipital tenosynovitis. On rare occasions, the flap is unable to be located and is reabsorbed (Olivieri *et al.*, 2007). Arthroscopy is minimally invasive, allows for extensive exploration of the joint, and allows for simultaneous bilateral treatment. Arthrotomy is not preferred as it may require a second surgical procedure should the flap not be found caudally. In severe cases with large lesions and/or severe joint inflammation, consideration may be given to biological therapies to improve healing and decrease inflammation (Mokbel *et al.*, 2011).

One author (SC) recommends follow-up to arthroscopic treatment consisting of eight biweekly intramuscular injections of polysulfated glycosaminoglycans (PSGAGs), lifelong oral joint protective agents, and weekly rehabilitation therapy to include manual therapy, physical modalities, and hydrotherapy. NSAIDs and pain medications can be prescribed postoperatively.

When treated surgically, shoulder OCD generally has an outstanding prognosis. Chronic long-term cases and dogs that have significant osteoarthritis may benefit from intra-articular injections of hyaluronic acid, PRP, or stem cell therapy.

Infraspinatus myopathy

Infraspinatus myopathy is normally seen in large-breed dogs, particularly working dogs that do hunting or herding and other very active dogs (Pettit, 1980). Although it remains an uncommon occurrence, contracture of the infraspinatus muscle is one of the two most frequently reported contractures in dogs, along with quadriceps contracture (Fossum, 2002; Harasen, 2005). The classic presentation of the contracture is unilateral, but there have been bilateral cases reported (Leighton, 1977; Slatter, 1985; Dillon *et al.*, 1989). Most present with an acute onset of shoulder lameness with work or exercise (Leighton, 1977; Slatter, 1985; Carberry & Gilmore, 1986; Dillon *et al.*, 1989; Denny, 1993; Siems *et al.*, 1998; Fossum, 2002).

Cause

Repetitive microtrauma, blunt trauma, and osteofascial compartment syndrome have been reported to cause infraspinatus contracture (Pettit *et al.*, 1978; Matava *et al.*, 1994). Early treatment is focused on surgical decompression by fasciotomy; however, if contraction has already occurred, tenectomy or myectomy may be necessary (Carmichael & Marshall, 2012; Rochat, 2012).

The hypothesis that an acute traumatic event with an incomplete rupture of the infraspinatus muscle may lead to fibrosis and contracture is supported by the histological findings of degeneration and atrophy of skeletal muscle with fibrous tissue replacement (Carmichael & Marshall, 2012; Rochat, 2012).

Diagnosis

The patient may present with a painful, non-weight-bearing shoulder lameness. The shoulder may be swollen. The initial pain and lameness usually resolve with rest and/or supportive treatment over a period of 1–4 weeks; however, signs of contracture may appear within several days to weeks after the initial trauma (Carberry & Gilmore, 1986). The initial injury to the infraspinatus muscle is not commonly recognized.

Affected patients typically present with no signs of systemic illness. With a mature contracture, adhesion of the tendon of insertion of the infraspinatus muscle to the adjacent joint capsule occurs. Patients have a weight-bearing lameness with circumduction of the affected thoracic limb and a characteristic flip-like action of the foot when placing the foot (Slatter, 1985; Carberry & Gilmore, 1986; Dillon *et al.*, 1989; Denny, 1993; Siems *et al.*, 1998). The affected thoracic limb is held with the shoulder in abduction and the elbow in adduction against the thoracic wall (Siems *et al.*, 1998). The distal thoracic limb and carpus are externally rotated and held in abduction (Slatter, 1985; Carberry & Gilmore, 1986). The patient typically is not painful on palpation and manipulation of the limb (Carberry & Gilmore, 1986; Siems *et al.*, 1998). The remaining shoulder muscles, primarily the supraspinatus and deltoid muscles, display disuse atrophy or may be contracted (Carberry & Gilmore, 1986; Dillon *et al.*, 1989; Denny, 1993; Fossum, 2002). A significantly decreased range of motion will be noted in the shoulder (Carberry & Gilmore, 1986). When the patient is placed in lateral recumbency with the affected limb up, a true infraspinatus contracture will cause the distal thoracic limb to remain in an abducted and externally rotated position off the floor and away from the body (Carmichael & Marshall, 2012; Rochat, 2012) (Figure 12.6).

Siems and colleagues (1998) reported a series of ultrasonographic findings of simultaneous bilaterally traumatized infraspinatus muscles in one dog. One muscle resolved without any complications, while the other progressed to contracture (Siems *et al.*, 1998). The ultrasonographic description of a contracted infraspinatus muscle is that of increased echogenicity when compared with the normal muscle (Slatter, 1985; Denny, 1993). MRI may be useful for diagnosing the condition in both the acute and chronic phases.

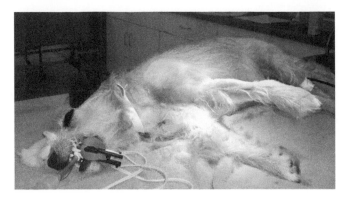

Figure 12.6   Dog with severe contracture of the infraspinatus tendon.

Treatment

In acute and subacute infraspinatus tendinopathies, rehabilitation including therapeutic ultrasound and stretching may help prevent contracture by maintaining the length and flexibility of the affected tissues.

Surgical release is required in mature contractures. Tenotomy of the tendon of insertion with release of capsular adhesions is most commonly performed. Complete transection of the infraspinatus tendon with partial tenectomy is required to restore motion in the affected limb and most often proves curative, with an immediate release of contracture and return to function of the shoulder joint (Slatter, 1985; Carberry & Gilmore, 1986; O'Neill & Innes, 2004). This treatment carries an excellent prognosis (Carberry & Gilmore, 1986; Slatter, 1985). Adhesions of the infraspinatus tendon to the joint capsule are commonly found and once dissected away seldom cause further issues (Carberry & Gilmore, 1986; Pettit *et al.*, 1978). Rehabilitation therapy is started prior to suture removal to prevent the formation of further adhesions (Carberry & Gilmore, 1986).

Biceps tendinopathy

Biceps tendinopathy (BT) was once thought to be the most common shoulder condition seen in performance dogs. However, through the use of advanced diagnostics and improved palpation techniques, the biceps tendon is often found to be a secondary finding (i.e., impingement and

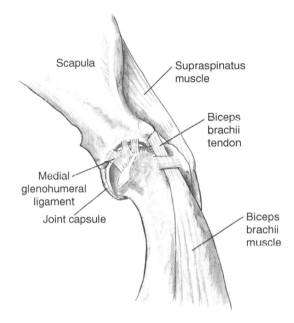

Figure 12.7   Anatomy of the canine shoulder. Source: Illustration by Marcia Schlehr.

compression from a supraspinatus tendon nodule or referred elbow pain at the point of insertion).

When BT is the primary diagnosis, it most often involves the biceps brachii muscle and its tendon where it crosses the shoulder joint (Figure 12.7). The actions of the biceps are elbow flexion, shoulder extension, and stabilization of the shoulder during standing and the weight-bearing phase of locomotion (Evans, 1993).

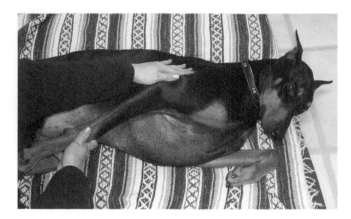

Figure 12.8   Example of a passive biceps stretch (shoulder flexion with elbow extension).

Cause

The cause of injury in performance dogs appears to be repeated strain injury, including two-on/two-off contacts in agility, landing vertically on the thoracic limbs following a misjudged jump, overstretching the muscle, quick turns, and repetitive contractions of the muscle with the shoulder flexed and/or elbow extended. The tendon can be injured via strain from overloading, leading to degeneration or disruption (Wernham *et al.*, 2008). Disruption can occur from a single, less-than-maximum load that injures some fibers without complete failure of the tendon. Because the blood supply to the tendon is poor, healing time is protracted (Sharma & Maffulli, 2005). Degeneration of the tendon may be initiated by repetitive strain (Sharma & Maffulli, 2005). Continuous reinjury of the biceps tendon may sufficiently weaken it such that the surrounding tendons become inflamed and/or develop microtears, ultimately leading to shoulder joint instability (Gilley *et al.*, 2002).

Diagnosis

Complaints of difficulty with quick turns and reluctance to jump are common in performance dogs with BT. Agility dogs present with complaints regarding performing two-on/two-off contacts and knocking bars with their thoracic limbs.

Patients often have a shortened stride and a weight-bearing lameness that can range from subtle to severe. The lameness worsens with

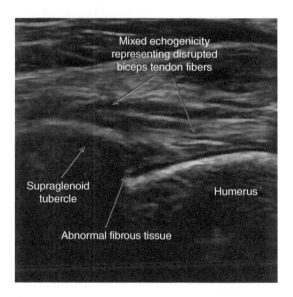

Figure 12.9   Ultrasound image demonstrating disrupted hypoechoic biceps tendon fibers.

activity. Direct palpation over the biceps tendon may elicit a pain response. Pain and spasm may be noted when performing the biceps stretch (flexing the shoulder with the elbow in extension) (Gilley *et al.*, 2002) (Figure 12.8). A bony avulsion may be detected radiographically. Chronic cases may reveal mineralization of the tendon or sclerosis within the bicipital grove (Gilley *et al.*, 2002). MRI and ultrasound may be used to identify acute and chronic cases (Gilley *et al.*, 2002; Wernham *et al.*, 2008) (Figure 12.9). Shoulder arthroscopy is an excellent diagnostic modality as well as therapeutic tool, if indicated (Wernham *et al.*, 2008) (Figure 12.10).

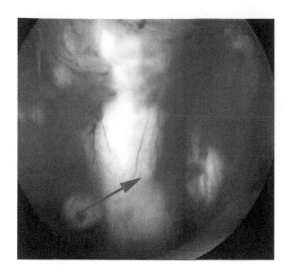

Figure 12.10 Arthroscopic image of severe bicipital tenosynovitis (arrow).

Treatment

Conservative medical management and rehabilitation therapy are recommended for acute cases. Conservative medical management should include controlled activity, NSAIDs, and cryotherapy. Intra-articular injections including hyaluronic acid, cortisone, PRP, or stem cell therapy may also be considered (Cookson & Kent, 1979; Gilley *et al.*, 2002; Marcellin-Little *et al.*, 2007; Wernham *et al.*, 2008). If a core lesion is noted, ultrasound-guided biological therapies (PRP, stem cell therapy, or combination therapy) may be considered.

Surgical treatment is recommended for biceps avulsions or tears and for cases that are nonresponsive to medical management and rehabilitation therapy. Surgical treatment includes arthroscopic reattachment for bony avulsions or an arthroscopic release for severe tendinopathies or tears.

Medial shoulder syndrome

A common cause of thoracic limb gait-related issues and lameness in performance, working, and active dogs is MSS. This condition is similar to rotator cuff injuries in humans, including ligament disruption, tendinopathy, labral and capsular tears, or disruption. Such shoulders are not unstable, instead they show evidence of sprain and strain injury leading to discomfort and dysfunction. Subscapularis tendinopathy is the most common component of MSS.

The human thrower's shoulder must be lax enough to allow extremes of motion but secure enough to provide stabilization of the shoulder (Arrington & Miller, 1995; Slatter, 1985). The same is true for the canine athlete that performs many extremes of range of motion and requires appropriate stabilization. Signs of MSS can range from performance-related problems such as refusing tight turns to a weight-bearing lameness. MSS involves multiple components of the shoulder joint and requires a thorough evaluation to confirm. It is important to identify and treat this condition early to obtain the best long-term results, and to prevent further sprain and strain injury, which can lead to shoulder instability and progression of osteoarthritis.

Cause

Medial shoulder syndrome is believed to be related to chronic strain and sprain due to repetitive activity or overuse rather than trauma. Repetitive agility dog activities such as jump–turn combinations and weave poles are performed regularly during practice and at trials. These maneuvers place the shoulder near its end range of abduction (Figure 12.11) and stress the soft tissue of the medial shoulder complex. Mishaps on agility equipment or simply slipping on wet surfaces can also contribute to the trauma inflicted on the shoulder. The cumulative effects of the microtrauma occurring to the shoulder structures can lead to performance issues, discomfort, and lameness. Overuse of the shoulder support structures can lead to degeneration of the tissues, reducing tensile strength and predisposing them to fraying, disruption, and eventually complete breakdown (Maganaris *et al.*, 2004; Marcellin-Little *et al.*, 2007). When instability, subluxation, or luxation occurs, a diagnosis of medial shoulder instability is made.

Diagnosis

Presenting history will vary from avoiding tight turns during performance to intermittent thoracic limb lameness that worsens with exercise and heavy activity. In some cases, a severe

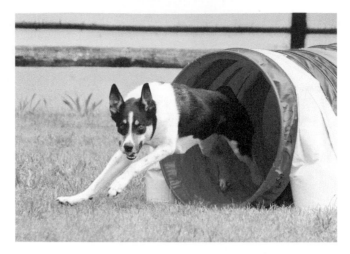

Figure 12.11 Agility maneuvers such as repeated jump–turn combinations and performing the weave poles at fast speeds place stress on the soft tissues of the medial shoulder. Source: Photo by Rich Knecht Photography.

weight-bearing lameness may be noted. A history of a lack of response to rest and NSAIDs is also common.

Patients present with a unilateral lameness ranging from a mildly shortened stride in the affected thoracic limb at a walk or trot to a significant weight-bearing lameness (Marcellin-Little *et al.*, 2007). In chronic cases, atrophy may be noted with thoracic limb circumference decreased in the affected limb as compared with the contralateral limb (Figure 12.12). Decreased extension in the shoulder is common. Shoulder muscle spasm and discomfort on abduction are consistent findings. To appropriately engage the components of the craniomedial shoulder, the elbow and shoulder must be placed in full extension with concurrent abduction of the thoracic limb. The scapula at the level of the acromion process must be stabilized with the evaluator's hand to achieve a passive stretch of the craniomedial shoulder components. In severe cases, a slight thud or subluxation may be felt when abducting the shoulder. If a concurrent supraspinatus tendinopathy is present, pain may be noted when placing the shoulder into flexion (direct stretch of the supraspinatus) or on direct palpation of its tendon and/or point of insertion.

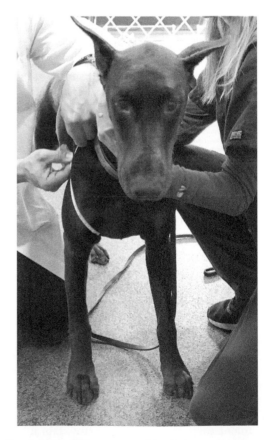

Figure 12.12 Measurement of forelimb muscle mass using a Gulick girthometer.

The shoulder abduction test (Cook *et al.*, 2005a), although originally described with patients under sedation in lateral recumbency, may be performed with similarly consistent results on awake and standing patients. A goniometer is held with its stable arm parallel to the spine of the scapula, the center of rotation over the shoulder joint, and its free arm extending over the axis of the humerus in contact with the skin. With the elbow and shoulder held in extension, the thoracic limb is abducted to its physiological limit and the measurement obtained as shown in Figure 12.13. The same technique is applied to the contralateral shoulder for comparison. Using this palpation technique, it has been reported that a normal mean shoulder abduction angle is approximately 30 degrees (Cook *et al.*, 2005a). Although this report revealed that dogs with medial shoulder instability had abduction angles significantly larger than 30 degrees, a

more recent study showed an inconsistent correlation between abduction angles and medial compartment pathological changes identified arthroscopically (Cook *et al.*, 2005a; Devitt *et al.*, 2007). Patients with MSS rarely show evidence of instability but rather show signs of dysfunction and pain associated with craniomedial pathological changes including varying degrees of subscapular tendinopathy, medial glenohumeral ligament disruption, craniomedial capsular lesions, and labral tears. The contralateral shoulder usually does not show signs of dysfunction, pain, or spasm on abduction.

A complete work-up includes history, signalment, gait analysis, orthopedic and neurological examinations, abduction angle tests, hematology, biochemical profile, urinalysis, arthrocentesis, and imaging modalities. Diagnostic musculoskeletal ultrasound can identify pathological changes in the medial compartment such as

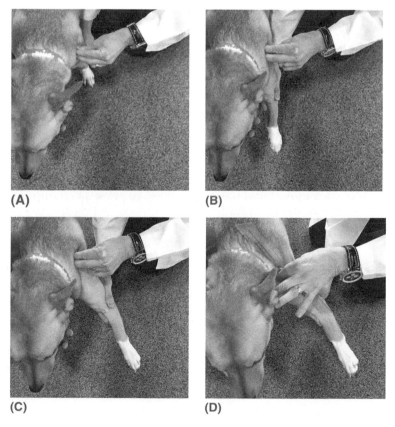

(A)   **(B)**

(C)   **(D)**

Figure 12.13 Orthopedic examination for medial shoulder instability. (**A**) Isolation of the glenohumeral joint with the examiner's fingers on the acromial process. (**B**) With the joint isolated, the glenohumeral joint is then extended. (**C**) Abduction of the glenohumeral joint is then performed, while stabilizing the scapula against the body wall. (**D**) Goniometry is used to determine the abduction angle.

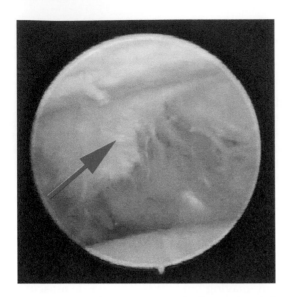

Figure 12.14   Arthroscopic image of a disrupted medial glenohumeral ligament (arrow) and subscapularis tendon.

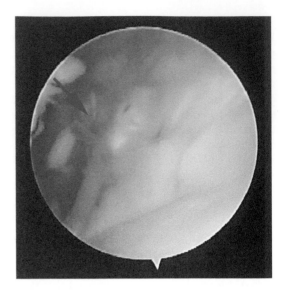

Figure 12.15   Arthroscopic image demonstrating mild to moderate disruption/fraying, hypertrophy, and neovascularization of the subscapularis tendon (arrow) (mild medial shoulder syndrome).

joint capsule thickening, effusion, subscapularis tendon, and medial glenohumeral ligament pathological changes. Based on the results of the orthopedic evaluation and musculoskeletal ultrasound findings, an arthroscopy may be considered. Arthroscopy allows for direct observation of the major intra-articular structures with magnification, dynamic evaluation of tissues during shoulder ROM tests, and palpation of intra-articular tissues using arthroscopic instrumentation. Arthroscopic exploration with evaluation of intra-articular structures provides a definitive diagnosis of MSS, as shown in Figure 12.14 (Devitt *et al.*, 2007; Sager *et al.*, 2009).

Treatment

Based on the results of the orthopedic examination, abduction angle tests, and arthroscopic scoring, patients are placed into one of three treatment categories: mild, moderate, or severe.

Mild MSS

Mild pathological changes include inflammation without fraying, disruption, or laxity of the medial glenohumeral ligament and subscapularis tendon and joint capsule (Figure 12.15). Patients with mild MSS are placed in a shoulder support system or *hobbles* and prescribed rehabilitation therapy (Marcellin-Little *et al.*, 2007).

Moderate MSS

Most MSS cases seen by one author (SC) in performance, working, and active dogs are moderate. Arthroscopic findings include subscapularis tendinopathy (disruption, fraying, core lesion), medial glenohumeral ligament lesions (fraying or disruption; Figure 12.16), craniomedial joint capsule focal synovial proliferation and/or disruption, and labral lesions (fraying, disruption, tears). In some cases where there is a concurrent supraspinatus tendinopathy (62% of cases; Canapp *et al.*, 2016a), a bulge of the supraspinatus tendon with impingement on the biceps tendon may be found. Arthroscopic treatment will vary depending on the tissues involved and the severity of disease. Treatment may include radiofrequency-induced thermal capsulorrhaphy (RITC). This technique has altered significantly in recent years due to the detrimental effects that can occur with aggressive application (Cook *et al.*, 2005b). A single-pass striping technique, developed based on current applications in humans, is currently used instead of the previous multipass paintbrush technique

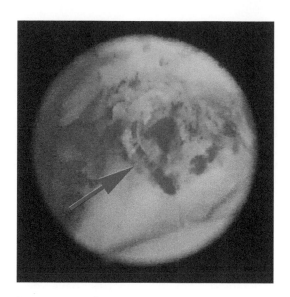

Figure 12.16 Arthroscopic image of moderate disruption of the subscapularis tendon (arrow) (moderate medial shoulder syndrome).

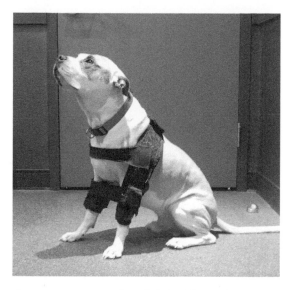

Figure 12.17 Dog with medial shoulder syndrome in a forelimb hobble system.

(Abrams, 2001). The radiofrequency energy delivered during treatment causes DNA wind-up and collagen contracture, which shrinks and tightens the tissues on contact. Second-look arthroscopy has revealed increased vascularity, tissue tightening, and a more normal fiber pattern in the treated tissues. Optimal shrinkage without necrosis of the tissue occurs between 65 and 75 °C (Abrams, 2001).

For the initial 2 weeks following treatment, the mechanical stiffness of the tissue is significantly decreased. The mechanical properties return to near normal by 6–12 weeks postop, after the tissues have undergone active cellular repair from the surrounding uninjured tissue (Miniaci & Codsi, 2006). Dogs are placed in a shoulder support system/hobbles (Figure 12.17) for 3 months while carrying out a rehabilitation therapy program. To prevent recurrence, a shoulder-strengthening program and a preventative maintenance program are used.

During the initial phases of the postoperative period, treatment to the shoulder is minimal. Following radiofrequency treatment, the tissues must be allowed to heal. Modalities or medications that are anti-inflammatory are not recommended since the inflammatory process is required as part of the healing process.

Biological therapies (PRP and stem cell combination therapy) may be used with arthroscopic treatment, based on severity. Other reported treatment options include suture imbrications or stabilization using a specialized fiber band and buttons technique (Abrams, 2001; O'Neill & Innes, 2004; Cook *et al.*, 2005b; Marcellin Little *et al.*, 2007; Sager *et al.*, 2009).

Severe MSS and medial shoulder instability

Severe MSS, which is much less common, is often associated with trauma. Patients typically have signs of craniomedial compartment laxity with shoulder abduction angles greater than 65 degrees. Complete tears of the medial glenohumeral ligament and severe disruption of the subscapularis tendon, joint capsule, and labrum may be noted on arthroscopic evaluation. In these cases, reconstruction of the medial compartment by direct tissue reapposition using synthetic capsulorrhaphy, bone/soft tissue anchors, and/or TightRope® stabilization (Arthrex Inc.) is indicated (Figure 12.18). Postoperative management consists of a spica splint for 2 weeks followed by the application of a shoulder support system for 2–3 months. Biological therapies (PRP and stem cell therapy) may be considered to augment the surgical repair in severe cases. Rehabilitation therapy is required for 4–6 months.

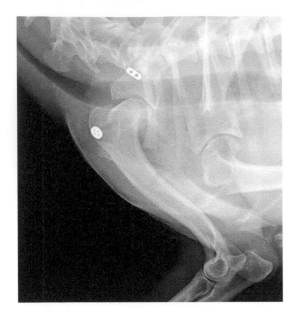

Figure 12.18   Postoperative radiograph of a shoulder reconstruction using a prosthetic ligament and anchor system (severe medial shoulder instability).

Additional shoulder disorders

Shoulder conditions that occur less commonly but that should be considered during the work-up include infraspinatus tendinopathy, teres major strains, shoulder dysplasia, glenoid fractures, osteoarthritis, frozen shoulder (Carr *et al.*, 2016), osteosarcoma, and synovial cell sarcoma. Conditions that may cause referred shoulder pain and resemble shoulder conditions include caudal cervical disease and brachial plexus masses.

Elbow disorders

Elbow dysplasia

Elbow dysplasia is a common cause of thoracic limb lameness in companion dogs. The term dysplasia simply means an abnormality in development (Blood & Studdert, 1999). Elbow dysplasia encompasses three distinct syndromes that result from abnormal growth and development: ununited anconeal process (UAP), fragmented medial coronoid process (FCP), and osteochondrosis (Wind & Packard, 1986; Schulz & Krotscheck, 2003; Trostel *et al.*, 2003b). The pathogenesis responsible for these

growth disturbances is not completely understood, but is thought to be due to asynchronous growth of the radius and ulna with genetic and nutritional origins (Wind & Packard, 1986; Schulz & Krotscheck, 2003; Trostel *et al.*, 2003b). Other developmental conditions of the elbow that are not classically included in the definition of elbow dysplasia include incomplete ossification of the humeral condyle (IOHC) and ununited medial epicondyle (UME) (Marcellin-Little *et al.*, 1994; de Bakker *et al.*, 2011).

Ununited anconeal process

Pathophysiology

The pathophysiology of UAP is incompletely understood. Several theories have been proposed, including nutritional deficiency, trochlear notch dysplasia, trauma, osteochondrosis, metabolic deficiencies, and hormonal effects (Corley *et al.*, 1968; Krotscheck *et al.*, 2000; Schulz & Krotscheck, 2003; Trostel *et al.*, 2003b). Evidence suggests that incongruous growth of the radius and ulna, such that the radius is relatively longer than the ulna, results in abnormal pressure on the ossification center of the anconeal process, leading to failure of the anconeal process to fuse to the proximal ulna (Wind & Packard, 1986; Schulz & Krotscheck, 2003). The anconeal process normally fuses with the ulna by 20 weeks of age (Corley *et al.*, 1968).

A genetic basis for UAP has been postulated and German Shepherd Dogs are overrepresented, with an incidence of 18–30% reported (Wind & Packard, 1986). Other large, giant, and chondrodystrophic breeds can be commonly affected as well (small-breed dogs do not have a separate center of ossification at the anconeal process) (Wind & Packard, 1986; Trostel *et al.*, 2003b). Male dogs may be predisposed, and the condition is bilateral in up to 30% of dogs (Wind & Packard, 1986; Trostel *et al.*, 2003b). Other developmental conditions of the elbow do not commonly occur in conjunction with UAP; although one study found that 16% of dogs with UAP also had FCP (Meyer-Lindenberg *et al.*, 2006).

Diagnosis

Diagnosis of UAP cannot be made until a dog is older than 20 weeks (Corley *et al.*, 1968). Most

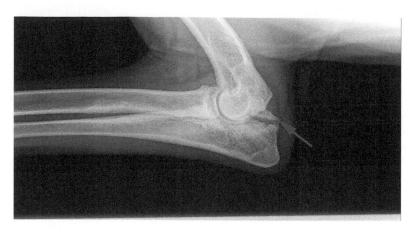

Figure 12.19   Radiographic image of an ununited anconeal process (arrow).

dogs present for progressive and intermittent thoracic limb lameness at 5-12 months of age (Wind and Packard, 1986; Trostel et al., 2003b). Physical exam findings include moderate to severe weight-bearing lameness (typically unilateral), pain and crepitus on palpation and PROM assessment of the elbow, and palpable effusion, sometimes marked, of the lateral aspect of the humeroulnar joint (Wind and Packard, 1986; Trostel et al., 2003b).

Flexed lateral radiographs reveal the UAP (Cook & Cook, 2009a) (Figure 12.19). A full series of elbow radiographs of both limbs should be obtained. Advanced imaging is not necessary to diagnose UAP; however, CT and arthroscopy may be performed to evaluate for concurrent conditions as radiographs have been shown to miss the concurrent diagnosis of FCP in 50% of dogs with UAP (Meyer-Lindenberg et al., 2006).

Treatment

Several surgical treatment options have been recommended for UAP (Krotscheck et al., 2000; Pettitt et al., 2009). Osteotomy of the proximal ulna is intended to relieve the excessive pressure of the humeral condyle on the anconeus. Performed alone, it has been shown to result in radiographic union of the anconeal process in 12-100% of dogs (Pettitt et al., 2009). Lag screw fixation of the anconeal process has also been recommended, alone and in combination with proximal ulnar osteotomy (Krotscheck et al., 2000; Pettitt et al., 2009). Recent studies suggest

that the best outcome is achieved with combined lag screw fixation and proximal ulnar osteotomy (Pettitt et al., 2009). If the diagnosis of UAP is made after maturity and adequate compression of the processes cannot be achieved, excision of the anconeal process is advised, if clinically warranted, and can result in excellent long-term function (Roy et al., 1994).

Postoperative care and rehabilitation is similar to that in the treatment of all elbow conditions and is discussed elsewhere in this book.

Fragmented coronoid process

Pathophysiology

Fragmentation of the medial coronoid process of the ulna is the most commonly diagnosed developmental disorder of the elbow (Trostel et al., 2003a; Temwichitr et al., 2010). There is substantial evidence to show a genetic component to the disorder, with particular over-representation in Labrador Retrievers, Bernese Mountain Dogs, and Rottweilers (Trostel et al., 2003a, 2003b; Temwichitr et al., 2010). The incidence of FCP in Labradors is 18–50% (Temwichitr et al., 2010). The exact mode of inheritance has not been determined but there is a strong familial association. A sex predilection has been reported with a male to female ratio of between 2:1 and 3:1 (Trostel et al., 2003a). FCP occurs bilaterally in 50–90% of dogs and concurrent osteochondrosis has been reported in up to 60% of cases (Trostel et al., 2003a).

The pathogenesis of FCP is not completely understood (Danielson et al., 2006). Several theories have been investigated including defective osteochondral ossification, abnormalities of the trabecular bone of the coronoid process, and biomechanical influences including radioulnar incongruity (Trostel *et al.*, 2003a; Danielson *et al.*, 2006; Temwichitr *et al.*, 2010). A wide spectrum of FCP can be seen ranging from large, discrete osteochondral fragments to small cartilage fissures that are only appreciated with advanced imaging or histopathology (Danielson *et al.*, 2006; Fitzpatrick & Yeadon, 2009). Regardless of the underlying etiology, FCP inevitably results in the development and progression of osteoarthritis, particularly within the medial compartment or humeroulnar articulation of the elbow (Clements *et al.*, 2006; Fitzpatrick & Yeadon, 2009).

Diagnosis

Dogs commonly present at 4–12 months of age, although some may not show clinical signs until later in life after degenerative joint disease becomes severe (Trostel *et al.*, 2003a; Fitzpatrick & Yeadon, 2009). Juvenile dogs with FCP typically have an insidious onset of mild to severe weight-bearing lameness that is aggravated by activity. Often, they will shift weight to the unaffected or less severely affected limb, with the affected limb held with the elbow adducted and foot abducted or externally rotated. This is commonly confused with a valgus limb deformity (Trostel *et al.*, 2003a). There may be muscle atrophy, and some patients may have the appearance of overdeveloped hindquarters due to increased weight bearing through the pelvic limbs. Joint effusion is rarely appreciated with FCP or osteochondrosis. Pain can be elicited with supination of the antebrachium with the elbow in flexion or extension (Trostel *et al.*, 2003a; Fitzpatrick & Yeadon, 2009). Deep palpation over the biceps brachii insertion near the medial coronoid commonly results in a pain response (Fitzpatrick & Yeadon, 2009). As degenerative changes of the joint develop, fibrous thickening of the medial compartment, crepitus, and loss of range of motion can be appreciated. These clinical findings are identical to those seen with osteochondrosis, and clinical exam alone is unlikely to differentiate the two (Trostel *et al.*, 2003a; Fitzpatrick & Yeadon, 2009).

A series of elbow radiographs is recommended initially. However, discrete visualization of a fragmented coronoid process is not possible (Moores *et al.*, 2008; Cook & Cook, 2009a; Punke *et al.*, 2009). Rather, secondary signs such as sclerosis of the subchondral bone at the semilunar notch and enthesiophyte formation on the dorsal anconeal process are seen (Danielson *et al.*, 2006; Cook & Cook, 2009a). Studies have shown radiographs to be highly insensitive to diagnosing FCP and, therefore, advanced imaging should be recommended (Danielson *et al.*, 2006; Moores *et al.*, 2008; Cook & Cook, 2009a; Punke *et al.*, 2009).

CT is very effective for diagnosing and characterizing FCP (as well as osteochondrosis) but is not capable of evaluating the articular cartilage (Moores *et al.*, 2008; Cook & Cook, 2009a). Arthroscopy is recommended alone or in combination with CT to assess the integrity of the articular cartilage as well as radioulnar congruity (Moores *et al.*, 2008; Punke *et al.*, 2009). MRI can be used to evaluate the elbow and is more sensitive than CT for evaluating the surrounding soft tissues, subchondral and medullary bone, cartilage, and bone–cartilage interface (Cook & Cook, 2009a; Baeumlin *et al.*, 2010).

Treatment

In one author's (SC) opinion, arthroscopic treatment should be considered as soon as the condition is diagnosed. If there are questions regarding a definitive diagnosis, arthroscopy would allow for confirmation of the condition while at the same time providing treatment. Depending on the severity of disease, arthroscopic treatments typically include fragment removal (taking the "pebble out of the shoe"; Figure 12.20); subtotal coronoidectomy (removing unhealthy coronoid tissue); abrasion arthroplasty (stimulating the subchondral bed for the formation of fibrocartilage); resurfacing (shaving down areas that are in conflict or abnormally communicating); and microfracture or micropicking (to open channels into the subchondral bone to assist in fibrocartilage formation). Even older patients in which osteoarthritic progression is noted can benefit from arthroscopic treatment before they enter into a formal rehabilitation program. With the advancement of arthroscopic instrumentation,

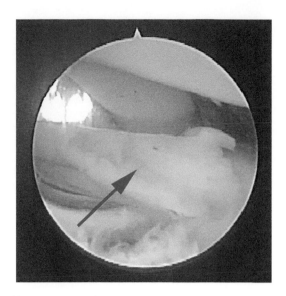

Figure 12.20 Arthroscopic image of a traumatic fragmented medial coronoid process (arrow), showing removal of the fragment with a grasper.

dogs of any size (even as small as 5 lbs (2.25 kg)) are candidates for treatment.

At the completion of the arthroscopic procedure and while still under anesthesia, an intra-articular injection of hyaluronic acid as a synovial fluid replacement or postsurgical lavage is recommended. This allows for restoration of the joint to a more normal physiological state (Mathies, 2006; Hempfling, 2007). Biological therapies (PRP and stem cell therapy) could also be considered as a post-arthroscopic treatment to decrease inflammation and aid in tissue healing (Guercio *et al.*, 2012; Zhu *et al.*, 2013; Beitzel *et al.*, 2015; Kilincoglu *et al.*, 2015).

When significant (>4 mm) radioulnar incongruity is detected arthroscopically, an ulnar osteotomy may be performed to facilitate the development of congruency (Fitzpatrick & Yeadon, 2009). Some surgeons have advocated for performing a subtotal coronoidectomy (SCO) (Fitzpatrick & Yeadon, 2009). The biceps ulnar release procedure (BURP), in which the insertion of the biceps brachii on the medial ulna is transected, has been suggested as a method of decreasing excessive rotational stress on the medial coronoid process (Fitzpatrick & Yeadon, 2009). Long-term results of SCO and BURP are not yet available.

Despite surgical intervention, patients with FCP will develop degenerative joint disease/osteoarthritis of the medial compartment of the elbow (Fitzpatrick & Yeadon, 2009; Fitzpatrick *et al.*, 2009c; Burton *et al.*, 2011). Surgical techniques continue to be investigated as means of long-term treatment of medial compartment diseases. Sliding humeral osteotomy involves a transverse osteotomy of the humeral diaphysis with the distal humerus translated medially and stabilized with a plate. The aim of this procedure is to transfer biomechanical load from the medial to lateral compartment. Preliminary clinical results show promising short-term outcomes (Fitzpatrick *et al.*, 2009c).

Total elbow joint replacement has been investigated for many years. There has been difficulty in designing the optimal implant system, and significant morbidity has been reported in initial studies (Conzemius, 2009). One study showed that good long-term outcomes are possible with a nonconstrained total elbow replacement (Conzemius, 2009). Clinical outcomes associated with initial use of partial joint replacement (Canine Unicompartmental Elbow, CUE®) is in clinical trials and long-term results have been reported (Cook *et al.*, 2015).

Traumatic fragmented medial coronoid process

Traumatic fragmented medial coronoid process (TFCP) appears to occur commonly in performance, working, and active dogs with no limitations of age, size, or breed.

Cause

There is no definitive etiology for TFCP, although three theories exist. The first suggests that increased repetitive load arises from the force generated by contraction of the biceps/brachialis muscle complex. This force rotates the medial coronoid into the radius. It is theorized that, as a result of this repetitive loading, microcracks develop, disturbing the mechanical properties of the bone (fatigue microdamage). If proper healing does not take place, fatigue fractures of the subchondral trabecular bone eventually occur (Danielson *et al.*, 2006). Further, loss of osteocytes, indicated by decreased osteocyte density, has been strongly linked with the presence of microdamage after fatigue loading, and may play an important role in the pathogenesis of TFCP (Verborgt *et al.*, 2000). A second theory speculates that these dogs are predisposed due to underlying elbow dysplasia, in particular incongruency. Elbow incongruity such as radioulnar step defects, humeroulnar incongruency/conflict, and varus deformity of the humerus causes abnormal contact patterns in the elbow, specifically at the coronoid–trochlear articulation, which is theorized to increase the load on the medial coronoid process (Punke *et al.*, 2009). The third theory proposes that microfractures of the bone below the cartilage (subchondral fractures) result from abnormal repetitive loading, such as landing from jumps, or hitting contacts or flyball boxes (Boettcher *et al.*, 2009). Recent research may elicit some clarification on these competing theories.

One study excluded dogs that showed any radiographic or arthroscopic evidence of FCP due to elbow dysplasia or other intra-articular pathological changes. Dogs under 2 years of age were also excluded because elbow dysplasia related to medial compartment disease, osteochondrosis, or osteochondritis dissecans may not present until 18 months of age. Clinical records of dogs that experienced acute unilateral non-weight-bearing lameness associated with a traumatic and concussive event were reviewed. Arthroscopy of these dogs revealed a single, large, displaced or nondisplaced fragment with no other lesions or elbow pathological changes present (Figure 12.21). This research suggests that while TFCP can accompany elbow disease and dysplasia as a secondary condition, TFCP itself can present in dogs with no genetic predisposition and should be deemed a clinically distinct disease unrelated to elbow dysplasia (Tan *et al.*, 2016). Secondary osteoarthritis will progress if left untreated. Damage to the cartilage such as softening, fibrillation, fissuring, erosions, and additional subchondral bone microcracks and fragmentation may occur. Over time, frictional abrasion (kissing lesions) may occur as a result of free fragments disrupting opposing surfaces, including the medial aspect of the humeral condyle and radial head.

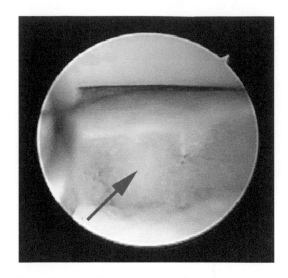

Figure 12.21 Arthroscopic image of a traumatic fragmented medial coronoid process (arrow).

Diagnosis

Patients with TFCP present with a history of subtle intermittent lameness to significant acute unilateral lameness. Bilateral presentation is uncommon. The lameness is exacerbated with increased activity and exercise. Onset is insidious, although, on occasion, acute onset following a jump-down may be reported. Severity of the lameness may be progressive. Affected dogs gait in a manner consistent with elbow pain. A lack of response to rest and NSAIDs is common.

Discomfort is elicited on direct palpation of the medial compartment of the elbow joint, specifically the medial coronoid process. Patients are reluctant to allow full elbow flexion, and discomfort is noted on hyperflexion. In chronic cases, full flexion may not be obtained. Crepitus is rare. Carpal flexion with external rotation while extending the elbow may exacerbate the pain response. Joint effusion distal to the lateral or medial epicondyle of the humerus may be detected.

Misdiagnosis as biceps tendinopathy is common, based on the pain response to shoulder extension or the biceps stretch test. This pain response may be due to the simultaneous hyperextension of the elbow when the shoulder is placed in extension. Elbow extension causing tension in the biceps/brachialis muscle complex may exert pressure on the medial coronoid and inflamed joint capsule, creating a pain response. A similar response is noted during the biceps stretch test in which the shoulder is flexed and the elbow is extended. Direct palpation of the proximal biceps tendon as well as other shoulder assessment tests are necessary to rule out shoulder conditions.

Radiographs are often unrewarding (Cook & Cook, 2009a). In chronic cases, radiographs may reveal secondary evidence of bony remodeling and, in particular, sclerosis of the ulnar notch is a highly sensitive indicator of suspected fragmented medial coronoid process (Danielson *et al.*, 2006).

Advanced diagnostic imaging modalities such as CT, MRI, nuclear scintigraphy, and arthroscopy may confirm the diagnosis (Cook & Cook, 2009a; Cook & Cook, 2009b). Arthroscopic evaluation offers the advantage of magnified direct observation of the major intra-articular structures, dynamic evaluation of the tissues during ROM, and palpation of intra-articular tissues using arthroscopic instrumentation to make a definitive diagnosis as well as allowing for treatment with one anesthetic event (Fitzpatrick *et al.*, 2009a). In a small percentage of cases, advanced imaging may indicate fragmentation of the medial coronoid process not found on arthroscopic observation. In these cases, the fissures are believed to be beneath the cartilage surface of the coronoid process (Fitzpatrick *et al.*, 2009a).

Treatment

Arthroscopy may include a combination of techniques such as fragment removal, debridement of injured tissues, abrasion arthroplasty, forage, microfracture, and subtotal coronoid ostectomy as dictated by progression and severity (Fitzpatrick *et al.*, 2009a). Arthroscopic treatment is believed to cause less soft tissue trauma, reduce surgery time, decrease the risk of infection, and speed recovery time as compared with traditional arthrotomy (Hoelzler *et al.*, 2004). Following the arthroscopy, at the time of closure, intra-articular injection of hyaluronic acid as a postsurgical lavage and synovial fluid replacement is recommended. This is intended to restore the joint to a more normal physiological condition. Injection of PRP could also be considered in place of hyaluronic acid to further help with inflammation and joint restoration.

Postoperative bandaging is not suggested as PROM and early return to function are recommended. NSAIDs are prescribed for 14 days to decrease inflammation and discomfort. Twice-weekly intramuscular injections of PSGAGs are prescribed for 4 weeks. Oral joint protective agents such as glucosamine, chondroitin sulfate, and avocado/soybean unsaponifiables are recommended as a daily supplement for life. Prospects of returning to normal activity and competition are improved with early detection and treatment. Treatment for progression of elbow osteoarthritis will be covered later in this chapter.

Case Study 12.2   Biological therapy for supraspinatus tendinopathy with concurrent injuries

Signalment: 9-y.o. F/S Labrador Retriever. Agility dog.

History: Presented with intermittent right thoracic limb lameness. Nonresponsive to rest, NSAIDs, rehabilitation therapy, and activity restriction.

Examination: Gait: Shortened stride in right thoracic limb at walk and trot.

Palpation: Bilateral discomfort in shoulder extension/ flexion. Discomfort and spasm during right shoulder abduction and increased abduction angle. Mild discomfort of bilateral supraspinatus during passive stretch. Mild sensitivity over right medial coronoid process.

Radiographs: Right elbow: sclerosis within ulnar notch; fragmented medial coronoid. Left shoulder: mineralization of supraspinatus tendon. Right shoulder and left elbow WNL.

Diagnostic ultrasound: Left shoulder: generalized, hypoechoic, mottled fiber pattern of the supraspinatus with a large distinct hyperechoic focus at the point of insertion on the greater tubercle. Enlargement of the supraspinatus tendon. Mild biceps contact and impingement. Thin joint capsule. Fibrous tissue deep within joint. Infraspinatus tendon, teres minor, and biceps WNL. Right shoulder: generalized, hypoechoic, mottled fiber pattern and enlargement of supraspinatus tendon. Contact with biceps. Thickened joint capsule. Fibrous tissue deep within joint. Infraspinatus tendon, teres minor, and biceps WNL.

Arthroscopy: Right elbow: Single non-displaced fragment on medial coronoid process. Grade 5 cartilage lesions on humeral condyle and radial head.

(Continued)

Left shoulder: Significant inflammation and tenosynovitis of biceps tendon. Severe supraspinatus bulge. Severe inflammation, fraying, and disruption along subscapularis tendon, medial glenohumeral ligament, medial labrum, and caudal glenoid labrum. Moderate inflammation and disruption of synovium. Mild craniomedial laxity. Caudal glenoid slab fracture.

Right shoulder: Significant inflammation and tenosynovitis of biceps tendon. Severe supraspinatus bulge. Moderate inflammation, fraying, and disruption along subscapularis tendon, MGL, medial labrum, and caudal glenoid labrum. Mild to moderate inflammation and disruption of synovium. Mild craniomedial laxity.

Diagnosis: Bilateral supraspinatus tendinopathy (left > right), bilateral medial shoulder syndrome (left > right), left caudal glenoid slab fracture, severe medial compartment disease (right elbow).

Treatment: Bilateral radiofrequency treatment performed to medial joint capsule, subscapular tendon, medial glenohumeral ligament, and in the region of the supraspinatus bulge. Excision of right caudal glenoid slab fracture. Right elbow arthroscopic debridement and fragment excision. Ultrasound-guided injections of bone marrow-derived stem cell and platelet-rich plasma into both supraspinatus tendons, both shoulders, right elbow, and right biceps. Hobbles applied.

Enrolled in rehabilitation program 7 days following injections and application of hobbles. Diagnostic ultrasound and physical examination rechecks performed 6, 12, and 16 weeks postoperatively.

6 weeks: Diagnostic ultrasound shows improved homogenous fibers of bilateral supraspinatus tendinopathy. Decreased inflammation, biceps impingement, and fibrous tissue within shoulder joint. Joint capsule WNL. Biceps insertionopathy remains consistent with hobbles use. Palpation shows improved comfort on shoulder ROM. Moderate muscle atrophy due to hobbles usage and lack of strength training. Mild restriction in scapular thoracic region, elbow, and carpi. Mild effusion in right elbow.

12 weeks: Hobbles removal. Diagnostic ultrasound shows significantly decreased inflammation and significantly improved homogenous fibers of bilateral supraspinatus tendinopathy. Bilateral supraspinatus WNL. No biceps impingement. Decreased fibrous tissue within shoulder joint. Joint capsule WNL. Biceps insertionopathy remains, but consistent with use of hobbles. Palpation shows improved ROM in shoulder, elbow, and carpus.

16 weeks: Diagnostic ultrasound shows resolution of bilateral supraspinatus tendinopathies, no inflammation present, and decreased fibrous changes in both supraspinatus tendon insertions. Right biceps insertionopathy at the point of origin resolved and shows a significant improvement of fiber pattern. Palpation reveals shoulder and elbow ROM WNL. No discomfort noted.

Agility retraining initiated.

Case follow-up: 6-, 12-, and 18-month follow-up calls with no reports of lameness or performance-related issues.

Osteochondrosis/osteochondritis dissecans of the elbow

Pathophysiology

Osteochondrosis is defined as the failure of endochondral ossification resulting in a discrete lesion of thickened and degenerative cartilage (Trostel *et al.*, 2002). Mild forces on the abnormal cartilage can result in shearing of the cartilage flap from the underlying bone, referred to as osteochondritis dissecans (OCD). The flap of cartilage can remain attached to the defect or can become dislodged into the joint. Osteochondrosis/OCD can occur in the shoulder, stifle, tarsus, and elbow. Within the elbow, the most common location for osteochondrosis to develop is the distal medial humeral condyle (Trostel *et al.*, 2002; Fitzpatrick *et al.*, 2009b).

The underlying cause of osteochondrosis has not been firmly established, but may be related to overnutrition, rapid growth, excess dietary calcium, ischemia, hormonal influences, or trauma. A genetic component is also likely. The condition is most commonly seen in large- and giant-breed male dogs such as Bernese Mountain Dogs and Labrador Retrievers. Bilateral disease occurs in 20–50% of dogs and osteochondrosis and FCP commonly occur within the same joint (Trostel *et al.*, 2002; Fitzpatrick *et al.*, 2009b, 2009c).

Diagnosis

The clinical history and physical exam findings of dogs with osteochondrosis/OCD is similar to that of FCP (Trostel *et al.*, 2002; Fitzpatrick & Yeadon, 2009). Four-view radiographs of the elbow are often sufficient to diagnose osteochondrosis, where the lesion is seen as a lucency of the distal medial humeral condyle (Cook & Cook, 2009a). Advanced imaging techniques such as CT, MRI, and arthroscopy are often used to evaluate dogs for concurrent FCP and to evaluate the articular cartilage (Cook & Cook, 2009a).

Treatment

Surgical removal of the osteochondrosis/OCD fragment is recommended (Trostel *et al.*, 2002; Fitzpatrick & Yeadon, 2009; Fitzpatrick *et al.*, 2009b). After fragment removal, curettage and osteostixis of the subchondral bone is performed to encourage ingrowth of fibrocartilage (Fitzpatrick & Yeadon, 2009). Long-term osteoarthritis is expected. Osteochondral autographs and allographs have been used to replace the osteochondrosis defect with hyaline cartilage (Fitzpatrick *et al.*, 2009b). Fitzpatrick *et al.* (2009b) showed promising short-term results using the osteochondral autograph transfer system. Sliding humeral osteotomy, total elbow joint replacement, and CUE® may also be used in the long-term management of medial compartment disease secondary to osteochondrosis/OCD (Fitzpatrick & Yeadon, 2009; Cook, 2012b).

Long-term management of elbow dysplasia and osteoarthritis

Nonsurgical or complementary therapy for the long-term management of patients with elbow dysplasia and osteoarthritis involves a multimodal approach including weight management, activity modification, chondroprotectants, pain management, omega-3 fatty acids, therapeutic modalities (such as laser therapy, shock wave therapy, pulsed electromagnetic field therapy), therapeutic exercises, acupuncture, manual therapy, and intra-articular injections (biological therapies, hyaluronic acid, cortisone, etc.) (Canapp *et al.*, 2009).

Intra-articular injections of biologics should be considered as a treatment option for elbow dysplasia. Biological therapies for managing significant osteoarthritis may be done in conjunction, in lieu of, or after arthroscopic treatment. Products such as hyaluronic acid, PRP, and stem cell therapies have been reported to be used successfully for osteoarthritis in humans, horses, and dogs (Guercio *et al.*, 2012; Vilar *et al.*, 2013; Zhu *et al.*, 2013; Beitzel *et al.*, 2015; Kilincoglu *et al.*, 2015; Meheux *et al.*, 2016). Patients with persistent postop intra-articular

symptoms (e.g., effusion, discomfort, or lameness) and those who are intolerant or nonresponsive to NSAIDs may also benefit from intra-articular therapy (Figure 12.22).

Ununited medial epicondyle

An ununited medial epicondyle is not considered to be a component of elbow dysplasia but is a developmental condition of the canine elbow. The etiology of UME is thought to be either failed fusion of the ossification center of the medial humeral condyle or osseous metaplasia of the flexor tendon origins (Paster *et al.*, 2009). The condition occurs in Labradors, with a prevalence of 15% (Paster *et al.*, 2009). German Shepherds and English Setters are also frequently affected. UME is generally unilateral; however, histological studies suggest that the underlying pathological changes affect both elbows (Paster *et al.*, 2009). Patients present with a history of lameness and pain localized to the elbow, however, UME may be an incidental finding. Craniocaudal radiographs demonstrate the lesion although the condition may not be evident until dogs reach middle age (Paster *et al.*, 2009). Surgical resection of the ossified bodies has been recommended; however, little evidence exists regarding long-term results of surgical intervention. Importantly, it has been shown that UME is not associated with the development of radiographic signs of osteoarthritis (Paster *et al.*, 2009). Rather, it is an extra-articular condition and carries a better prognosis than other disorders of the elbow.

Incomplete ossification of the humeral condyle

Incomplete ossification of the humeral condyle is a developmental condition that primarily affects Spaniel breeds, with a reported polygenic recessive mode of inheritance (de Bakker *et al.*, 2011; Hattersley *et al.*, 2011). Labrador Retrievers and Rottweilers are also overrepresented. The underlying pathophysiology is a failure of the two ossification centers of the humeral condyle to fuse (de Bakker *et al.*, 2011; Hattersley *et al.*, 2011). Normally, complete fusion should occur by 70 ± 14 days of age

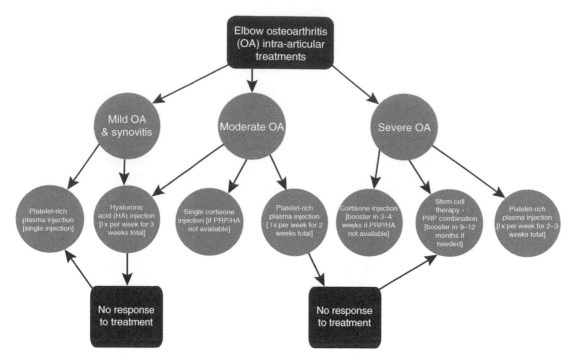

Figure 12.22   Elbow osteoarthritis intra-articular treatment algorithm.

(de Bakker *et al.*, 2011; Hattersley *et al.*, 2011). IOHC occurs bilaterally in approximately 90% of dogs and male dogs are most commonly affected (de Bakker *et al.*, 2011; Hattersley *et al.*, 2011). Concurrent FCP has been reported in 25–56% of Spaniels with IOHC (de Bakker *et al.*, 2011). IOHC can be diagnosed on plain radiographs using a 15-degree craniomedial/caudolateral view; however, CT has been shown to be more sensitive and specific (Farrell *et al.*, 2011). The condition is most commonly diagnosed when a patient presents for a lateral humeral condylar fracture following minimal trauma, although a history of lameness prior to fracture is not uncommon (Hattersley *et al.*, 2011).

It is reasonable to recommend prophylactic screening of predisposed breeds after 6 months of age, particularly those that will be participating in sporting events. If IOHC is diagnosed prior to humeral condylar fracture, a lag screw can be placed across the condyles to help prevent future fracture, although this procedure may be associated with significant morbidity (Hattersley *et al.*, 2011). Furthermore, it is important that these animals are removed from the breeding pool and care be taken to avoid high-impact activities.

Radius curvus

Proper development and alignment of the thoracic limb and elbow require that the radius and ulna grow at a synchronous rate. The distal physis of the radius is responsible for 60–70% of the bone's overall length, whereas the distal ulnar physis is responsible for 85% of the ulna's length (Carrig, 1975). The conical shape of the distal ulnar physis makes it susceptible to type V Salter–Harris fractures following minimal trauma (Fox, 1984). Hypertrophic osteodystrophy and a retained cartilaginous core can also lead to premature closure of this physis (Fox, 1984). When distal ulnar growth is arrested during the critical period of growth (<8 months of age), valgus limb deformity or radius curvus occurs (Carrig, 1975; Fox, 1984) (Figure 12.23).

The primary mechanism for the resulting deformity is the constrained or bow-string effect of the ulna on the radius as it continues to grow. This leads to cranial and medial bowing of the radius, hyperextension and subluxation of the carpus, and external rotation of the foot (Fox, 1984). The most clinically significant effect of this deformity is the development of elbow

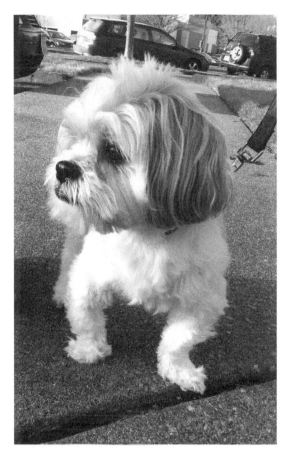

Figure 12.23   Shih Tzu with radius curvus.

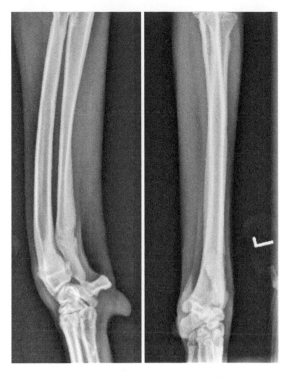

Figure 12.24   Radiographs of a dog with radius curvus.

incongruity, and, in extreme cases, luxation of the proximal ulna (Boudrieau, 2003).

Diagnosis of radius curvus is based on physical examination and radiographs (Figure 12.24). Characterization and quantification of the deformity can be made by comparing radiographs or CT images of the affected and nonaffected limbs (Crosse & Worth, 2010).

The decision to intervene surgically depends on the patient's functional mobility and degree of elbow incongruity, which will lead to osteoarthritis despite surgery (Boudrieau, 2003; Crosse & Worth, 2010). The surgical technique depends on the age of the patient at the time of growth arrest and surgeon preference (Boudrieau, 2003). When closure of the distal ulnar physis is diagnosed prior to significant radial deformity, and substantial growth of the limb remains, a distal ulnar ostectomy can be performed to remove the tethering effect of the ulna (Boudrieau, 2003). After radial deformity has occurred, a dynamic or static corrective ostectomy/osteotomy of the radius can be performed along with ulnar ostectomy (Boudrieau, 2003). If considerable length discrepancy exists between the limbs, distraction osteogenesis can be performed along with correction of the deformity.

Carpal, metacarpal, and digit injuries

Injuries of the manus (carpus, metacarpal bones, phalanges, and sesamoid bones) are less common than those of the shoulder or elbow in performance dogs; however, they can be just as challenging to diagnose and treat. The anatomy of the manus is complex with fibrous, ligamentous, and tendinous components that not only act as shock absorbers for the thoracic limb during weight bearing but also help to maintain appropriate flexion and extension of the limb throughout the gait cycle. Many of the mechanisms of injury to the manus and the best treatment options are poorly understood. Furthermore, the scientific literature is based largely on observational studies and *in vitro* biomechanical studies.

Carpal injuries

Cause

The most common cause of carpal injury appears to be acute hyperextension (Figure 12.25) that results from excessive loading of the limb due to traumatic events from falls, including jumping down from heights or with a twisting motion at the limb (Kapatkin *et al.*, 2012). Fractures along with luxations/subluxations often will occur concurrently with ligamentous injuries. The fractures tend to be intra-articular in nature and as such fit the criteria for anatomic reconstruction and internal rigid fixation. Acute injuries tend to result in a significant to non-weight-bearing lameness.

Chronic repetitive sprains and strains to the supportive structures of the joint occur over time. These stressors do not usually cause an acute significant lameness but rather an inconsistent to low-grade consistent lameness. The mechanical properties of the carpal ligaments have been evaluated. The accessoro-metacarpal ligaments have the highest elastic modulus, which likely contributes to preventing hyperextension. The intra-articular palmar radiocarpal and palmar ulnocarpal ligaments have the second highest elastic modulus and are responsible for restricting cranial and caudal instability. The lowest elastic modulus is found in the medial and lateral collateral ligaments, which support valgus and varus deviation. Failure was documented in all of these ligaments and revealed that 58% fail at the mid-ligament, 23% are a result of avulsion, and close to 19% fail at the bone–ligament interface (Shetye *et al.*, 2009).

Injuries

Carpal injuries can be broadly classified into sprains, strains, luxations, fractures, or a combination of these injuries. Many variations of carpal injury can occur including: (1) hyperextension (Figure 12.26A) with disruption of the palmar ligaments with or without disruption of the joint capsule; (2) hyperflexion (Figure 12.26B) with rotation of the dorsal ligaments and collateral ligaments with or without disruption of the joint capsule; and (3) medial or lateral collateral ligament injuries or degeneration of the carpal ligaments as a result of disease processes (immune-mediated disease, metabolic disease, etc.). Flexor carpi ulnaris (FCU) injuries can range from strains to core lesions or complete disruption and avulsion.

A sprain is an injury to a ligament that can occur in the mid-portion of the ligament or at its attachment to the bone. Historically, sprains can be classified into three grades of severity. Grade 1 sprains are mild and are described as an overstretching of the ligament without disruption or loss of function of the ligament. Grade 2 sprains are moderate in severity and are described as a partial tear of the ligament. The general continuity of the ligament is intact although the strength of the ligament is significantly reduced. Grade 3 sprains are severe and result from complete disruption or tearing of the ligament, resulting in instability of the joint. Since ligaments have a poor blood supply and require the formation and organization of collagen for their repair, ligament healing times can be quite lengthy (Dirks & Warden, 2011). Studies show that ligaments regain between 50% and 70% of their original strength after 1 year (Bishop & Bray, 1993; Frank, 1996; Frank *et al.*, 1999). If a gap forms or is present at the junction of the ligament ends during healing, permanent ligament elongation and subsequent instability may result even if an intact ligament reforms (Hildebrand & Frank, 1998).

Carpal hyperextension injuries occur due to damage to the flexor retinaculum and palmar

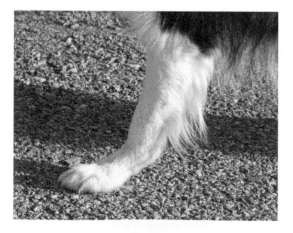

Figure 12.25   Dog with carpal hyperextension.

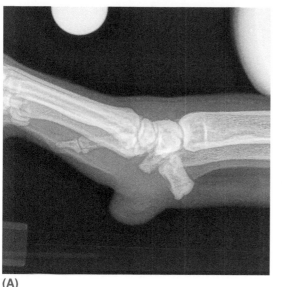
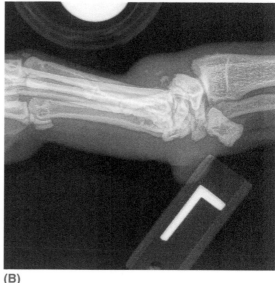

(A)   (B)

Figure 12.26   (A) Stress radiograph of a left carpal hyperextension injury. (B) Radiograph of a carpal subluxation with damage to the dorsal carpal ligaments.

fibrocartilage that results in loss of palmar support and secondary hyperextension. Commonly, carpal hyperextension injuries result from trauma due to falls, stepping in a hole, or from a twisting motion at the limb. One author (DD) has noted unilateral and bilateral carpal hyperextension injuries as a result of chronic overloading of the carpi due to pelvic limb impairment such as chronic cranial cruciate ligament injuries. The degree of damage (grade 1, 2, or 3) will dictate the appropriate treatment; however, conservative management of grade 3 carpal hyperextension injuries is rarely successful and surgical fixation is recommended (pancarpal or partial carpal arthrodesis).

Luxations and subluxations can involve the disruption of multiple ligaments (Figure 12.26B) as well as the joint capsule, and most will require surgical intervention consisting of either a pancarpal or partial carpal arthrodesis (Kapatkin *et al.*, 2012). The level of luxation in dogs in one report has been shown to be 31% at the antebrachiocarpal joint, 22% at the middle carpal joint, and 47% at the carpometacarpal joint (Parker *et al.*, 1981), while in another report the authors suggest the distribution to be 10% antebrachiocarpal, 50% middle carpal, and 40% carpometacarpal (Piermattei *et al.*, 2006).

Common fractures associated with carpal injuries in sporting and agility dogs include the attachment sites for the collateral ligaments (avulsion fractures) and compression or shear fractures. Fractures of these sites result in joint instability when stressed on palpation or during weight bearing. Fractures of the carpal bones can also occur and can be difficult to diagnose on standard radiographs. Radial carpal bone fractures have been shown to occur in active dogs that have not sustained significant trauma, and male dogs tend to have a predilection. Boxers, English Springer Spaniels, Setters, and Pointers may be at an increased risk and the theory for this is due to incomplete fusion of the centers of ossification in the radial carpal bone of these breeds (Li *et al.*, 2000; Tomlin *et al.*, 2001; Gnudi *et al.*, 2003). Traumatic radial carpal bone fractures are commonly associated with the right carpus of racing Greyhounds (Johnson & Piras, 2005). Right accessory carpal bone fractures are also commonly diagnosed in racing Greyhounds, likely due to the accessory carpal bone acting as a fulcrum for the palmar carpal ligaments and the flexor tendons thus preventing hyperextension. Accessory carpal bone fractures have been broken down into five types based on the location (Johnson, 1987; Johnson *et al.*, 1989; Johnson & Piras, 2005).

Currently, there are no data on the incidence, treatment, or outcome after fracture of the ulnar or carpal bones. Diagnosis can be difficult due to small fragmentation of the bones.

Medial and lateral collateral ligament sprains can occur due to acute trauma, repetitive trauma with breakdown over time, or conformational abnormalities leading to chronic strain of the ligaments. Much as with carpal hyperextension injuries, the degree of damage (grade 1, 2, or 3) will dictate the appropriate course of treatment. FCU strains may be the result of acute tendinitis, implying an inflammatory condition from acute traumatic tendon fiber tearing, or the result of chronic tendinosis, leading to a tendinopathy. Most chronic FCU tendinopathies are the result of overuse and a dysfunctional repair response. In these conditions, breakdown of the collagen matrix is involved and there is no inflammation within the tendon (Dirks & Warden, 2011). High-level or prolonged periods of tensile stress due to repetitive, intense activities can lead to collagen breakdown. Because of the lack of inflammatory activity in these conditions, most patients are unresponsive to rest and NSAIDs. Although it seems counterintuitive, initiating an inflammatory response is necessary to activate the healing process.

Diagnosis

Diagnosing carpal injures can be challenging, especially for mild sprain and strain conditions. The diagnosis is based on a comprehensive orthopedic evaluation and various imaging techniques. Lameness can range from a chronic, intermittent, low-grade lameness to an acute, non-weight-bearing lameness. It is important to evaluate patients at both the walk and the trot if they are weight bearing on the limb. Attention should be given to the carpus during the stance phase of the gait to evaluate for evidence of carpal hyperextension (Figure 12.25). Palpation may reveal soft tissue swelling, discomfort, crepitus, decreased range of motion, or instability when stressed (flexion, extension, varus or valgus). In cases of a mild (grade 1–2) strain of the ligamentous structures, instability may not be present. As part of a complete orthopedic evaluation palpation of the contralateral limb should be used as a reference in determining abnormal motion.

Imaging choices and techniques will vary depending on the injury. Radiographic changes are often nonspecific and may reveal soft tissue swelling within the region of injury. In chronic cases of medial or lateral collateral strains, enthesiophyte formation may be noted (Langley-Hobbs et al., 2007). For possible ligamentous instability or luxation/subluxation, stress radiographs can be beneficial and may reveal evidence of medial or lateral joint space widening, carpal hyperextension (Figure 12.26A), or dorsal subluxation (Figure 12.26B). Attention should be paid to the carpal bones for any evidence of fractures or fragmentation. Unfortunately, carpal bone fractures can be difficult to diagnose on standard radiographic views. Additional views such as oblique or skyline may help in diagnosing a carpal fracture. The authors recommend always taking radiographs of the contralateral nonaffected carpal joint for comparison. In cases of suspected carpal fractures or other osseous pathological changes, a CT scan can be performed (Gnudi et al., 2003). In cases of ligamentous or other soft tissue injury an MRI or ultrasound are often required for a definitive diagnosis. For soft tissue lesions such as an FCU strain, medial or lateral collateral ligament injury, or other ligamentous injuries the authors (SC and DD) prefer to begin with diagnostic musculoskeletal ultrasound. Ultrasound allows for minimally invasive direct visualization of the supporting structures and evaluation of the architecture of the tissues for objective grading of the injury such as a grade 1, 2, or 3 strain (Figure 12.27). Furthermore, ultrasound allows for easy follow-up in response to treatment. For cases where ultrasound is nondiagnostic or more information needs to be obtained an MRI may be recommended (Figure 12.28).

Treatment

Treatment options for carpal injuries will vary based on which tissue is damaged. For example, with carpal bone fractures, if there is enough bony purchase for an implant, then lag screw or Kirschner wire fixation can be attempted after absolute anatomic reconstruction since these fractures are intra-articular (Kapatkin et al., 2012). If the fragment is small, it

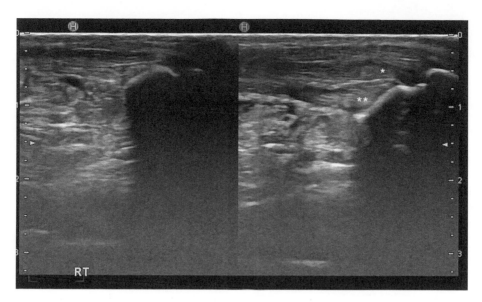

Figure 12.27   Ultrasound images of a normal and grade 2 flexor carpi ulnaris (FCU) strain. The image on the left is the normal FCU while the image on the right reveals damage to both the humeral and ulnar components of the FCU where it attaches to the accessory carpal bone. One asterisk reveals thickening of the humeral component of the FCU where it attaches to the accessory carpal bone, and two asterisks reveal thickening of the ulnar component with fiber disruption of the ulnar component of the FCU. Source: Image courtesy of Dr. Deb Canapp.

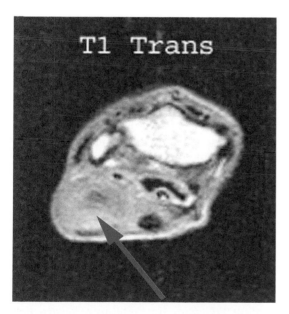

Figure 12.28   MRI of a flexor carpi ulnaris (FCU) tendinopathy. The arrow shows disruption of the FCU tendon.

is often excised (Kapatkin *et al.*, 2012). Following fracture of a carpal bone, osteoarthritis is expected even after anatomic repair (Forward

et al., 2008). Many of the repair methods for carpal bone fractures are not rigid enough for full weight bearing immediately postoperatively. For this reason, a bivalve cast or palmar splint is typically recommended for 6–8 weeks.

For ligamentous injuries (FCU, medial, lateral, dorsal, or palmar injuries) the treatment will vary based on the degree of damage; however, for treatment to be successful, a definitive diagnosis is essential. Mild to moderate ligament sprains (grade 1 and 2) are amenable to external support from coaptation with palmar splints, specialized support wraps (Figure 12.29) or orthoses (Figure 12.30) for 6–8 weeks along with formal rehabilitation therapy. Exercise restriction as well as medical management consisting of NSAIDs and analgesics is also recommended. External support allows for immobilization of the joint, preventing further injury to the affected ligament and facilitating healing. Specialized support wraps and custom orthotics are designed and manufactured for the patient to ensure accurate and comfortable fit. For more severe cases, a functional hinged orthosis may be used, allowing for controlled range of motion (Figure 12.30). In cases of grade 2+ injuries where there is partial fiber

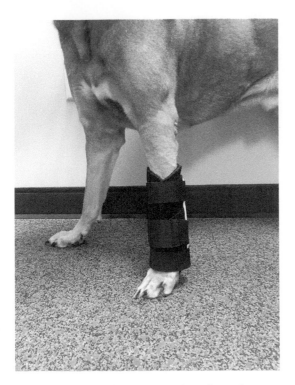

Figure 12.29   Carpal support wrap for a dog with a grade I flexor carpi ulnaris tendinopathy.

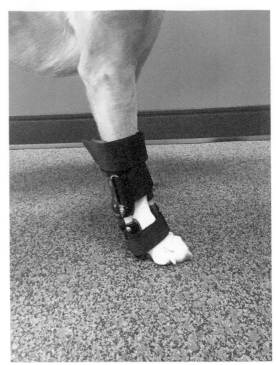

Figure 12.30   Custom carpal orthosis for a dog with a grade 2 carpal hyperextension injury following biological therapy.

disruption, or in chronic cases where there is evidence of core lesions and reorientation of the fiber pattern to suggest fibrous tissue, biological therapies may be used. The authors prefer to use a combination of mesenchymal stem cells (either bone marrow or adipose tissue) combined with PRP. The stem cells and PRP combination is injected directly into the lesion using ultrasound guidance. A more in-depth discussion on biological therapies can be found elsewhere in this textbook (see Chapter 16). Following treatment with biological therapies, the carpus is immobilized in a custom, hinged, controlled ROM orthosis for 12–16 weeks. Initially, the orthosis is locked-out to prevent any range of motion, then every 4–6 weeks there is gradual dynamization of the orthosis to allow the ligament to heal. Formal rehabilitation therapy is begun 2 weeks following biological therapies and continued until the patient can return to normal function. Recheck ultrasound is recommended at 4, 8, and 12 weeks

post biological therapies to evaluate tissue healing.

Severe sprains (grade 3 or those unresponsive to conservative management) or luxations resulting in instability usually require surgical intervention. Surgical correction can be augmented with biological therapies. If the ligament cannot be primarily repaired, a prosthetic ligament can be used via placement of bone tunnels or bone screws at the origin and insertion of the collateral ligaments. The long-term outcome with these techniques is not known (Kapatkin *et al.*, 2012), but one author (DD) has had good success with prosthetic ligamentous fixation. Following ligamentous reconstruction or prosthetic ligament repair, external coaptation with a lateral or palmar splint is recommended for 6–8 weeks to protect the fixation and allow healing and fibrous tissue development. Severe ruptures or avulsions of the FCU require surgical treatment consisting of tenorrhaphy or reattachment with or without

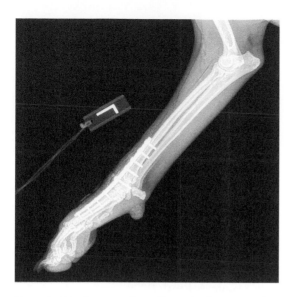

Figure 12.31 Postoperative radiograph of a pancarpal arthrodesis for a severe radiocarpal luxation. Figure 12.26(A) shows the preoperative image.

biological therapies, followed by a custom orthosis and rehabilitative therapy. In cases such as carpal hyperextension or irreparable fractures, carpal fusion (arthrodesis) may be needed. Depending on the area of injury either a partial carpal arthrodesis or a pancarpal arthrodesis (Figure 12.31) may be needed. Pathological changes involving the middle carpal or carpometacarpal joint, or disruption of the palmar ligaments, can be stabilized with a partial carpal arthrodesis. This allows for stabilization of the joint while maintaining the motion of the radiocarpal joint. When there is instability of the radiocarpal joint, pancarpal arthrodesis is usually indicated. The procedure of arthrodesis can be performed by long-term stabilization with an external skeletal fixator, plate and screws or internal pins and wire. One author (DD) prefers to perform a minimally invasive pancarpal arthrodesis with a pancarpal arthrodesis plate and fluoroscopic-guided assistance. Because this approach causes less tissue trauma to the patient resulting in less morbidity and quicker return to weight bearing. This is completed by making three small incisions: one incision at the carpus to allow removal of the articular cartilage and placement of a bone graft (Figure 12.32), and then two stab incisions for placement of the plate (Figure 12.33). There

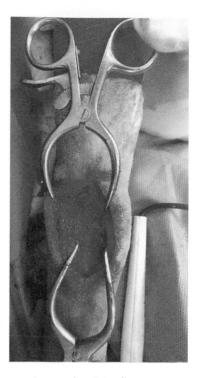

Figure 12.32 Image of a minimally invasive pancarpal arthrodesis. The first small incision over the carpus has been made, the articular cartilage has been removed and a bone graft has been packed into the carpus to promote fusion.

is debate regarding postoperative external coaptation with splinting following carpal arthrodesis; however, most surgeons still prefer to immobilize the fixation for at least 4–8 weeks following repair to prevent cycling of the implants and premature breakdown. Radiographs should be performed, initially every 4 weeks, until 16 weeks after arthrodesis, and then every 8 weeks until fusion is noted. Typically, fusion times range from 20 to 24 weeks postoperatively; however, patients are slowly returned to normal function beginning 16 weeks postoperatively. It is currently unknown if implant removal is needed following fusion in working dogs or canine athletes. In one author's (DD) opinion the implants can remain unless problems occur such as implant breakdown, pain if the carpus hits objects while working or performing, or evidence of postoperative infection.

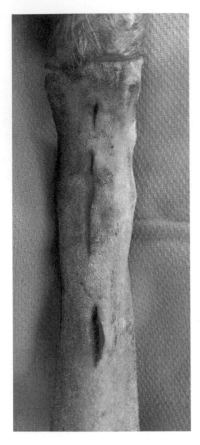

Figure 12.33   Immediate postoperative image following a minimally invasive pancarpal arthrodesis using the pancarpal arthrodesis plate. Note the three small incisions used for the procedure.

Metacarpal and sesamoid injuries

Cause

The most common injuries are metacarpal fractures. Currently, there are few studies evaluating metacarpal fractures, and of those available most are retrospective in nature (Muir & Norris, 1997; Kapatkin *et al.*, 2000). It appears that the cause of metacarpal fractures is usually trauma. Metacarpal fractures are more common than metatarsal fractures and most fractures occur in the middle or distal regions of the bones (Muir & Norris, 1997). In racing Greyhounds a specific distribution of metacarpal fractures has been described likely due to stress and possibly fatigue leading to fissures and ultimately a fracture (Bellenger *et al.*, 1981).

Metacarpal fractures in racing Greyhounds usually occur at metacarpal V on the left and metacarpal II on the right.

Sesamoid disease consists of fractures and fragmentation. There is conflicting evidence in the literature on whether these conditions are different or the same (Kapatkin et al., 2012). Racing Greyhounds and Rottweilers are the two most common breeds to have a clinical lameness associated with sesamoid disease, while in many other breeds it may be an incidental finding (Cake & Read, 1995). Theories for sesamoid disease include trauma, congenital disorders of ossification, osteoarthritis from abnormal forces, and osteonecrosis from vascular compromise. Sesamoids II and VII have fewer vascular foramina than the other sesamoids (Cake & Read, 1995).

Diagnosis

Dogs with metacarpal fractures may exhibit varying degrees of lameness from non-weight bearing in the acute phases to intermittent lameness with chronic fractures. Swelling may be noted with pain and crepitus upon palpation in acute cases. In chronic cases a callus or firm fibrous tissue may be palpated at the fracture site. Given the lack of soft tissue coverage, wounds should be carefully evaluated. Radiographs are the mainstay in diagnosing metacarpal fractures (Figure 12.34). Attention should be paid to the number of metacarpals fractured and the degree of displacement.

Patients with sesamoid disease can have variable degrees of lameness, pain, swelling, and effusion. With chronic disease, there may be thickening with a reduction in joint flexion. It is very important to rule out other orthopedic disease conditions in the thoracic limb before assuming the lameness is due to sesamoid disease. Radiographs are needed to document evidence of sesamoid disease (Figure 12.35); however, the diagnosis can sometimes be challenging on standard orthogonal radiographic projections. Oblique views are typically needed to identify the fracture or fragmentation. Findings include two or more fragments with sharp or smooth borders, osteophytosis, or dorsal displacement, and in

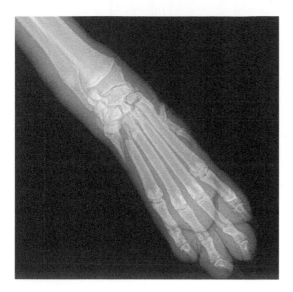

Figure 12.34 Radiograph of a dog with a proximal diaphyseal long oblique fracture of metacarpal V. The patient also sustained fractures of carpal bone II and digit I, and a carpometacarpal luxation at metacarpals II–IV. Source: Image courtesy of Dr. Justin Harper.

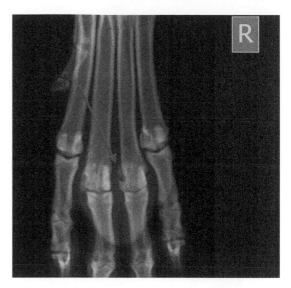

Figure 12.35 Radiograph of a 1-year-old Dalmatian with evidence of a sesamoid fracture (arrow). If needed, oblique views can be obtained to further identify sesamoid fracture(s)/fragmentation. Source: Image courtesy of Dr. Aldo Vezzoni.

chronic cases soft tissue calcification (Cake & Read, 1995).

Treatment

Specific treatment options for metacarpal fractures are based more on clinical intuition than on concrete data because of the paucity in the scientific literature. Current guidelines have been adopted from human literature on metatarsal fractures. Surgical management is recommended if two or more metacarpal fractures are present in the same manus, if the fractures involve both of the primary weight-bearing bones (metacarpals III and IV), if the fractures are articular, if the fracture fragments are displaced more than 50%, if the fracture involves the base of metacarpal II or V, and/or if the patient is a large breed, athletic, working, or show dog (Wernham & Roush 2010). Conservative treatment consists of a splint and bandage using a modified Robert Jones bandage. Attempts to improve alignment and apposition of the fractures should be made prior to external coaptation. Radiographs should be taken every 4 weeks until clinical union; if there is evidence of delayed union, malunion, or nonunion, then surgical fixation may need to be performed.

Surgical fixation of metacarpal fractures is largely similar to any other bony fixation. For avulsion fractures of the base of metacarpals II and V, lag screw fixation with an antirotational pin or a tension band fixation can be used. It is important to surgically stabilize these fractures as they serve as an insertion site of collateral ligaments and failure to repair can result in varus or valgus malunions. Diaphyseal fractures can be stabilized with intramedullary Kirschner wires or plate fixation (Figure 12.36). One author (DD) prefers to use 1.1 mm plates or 1.5 mm locking plates for metacarpal fractures.

To date there is only one study comparing long-term outcome for the treatment of sesamoid disease (Mathews *et al.*, 2001). The most commonly affected breed in that study was the Rottweiler, followed by the Labrador Retriever and Australian Cattle Dog. A better clinical outcome with significantly fewer degenerative changes was found in those patients that were treated conservatively versus surgically (Mathews *et al.*, 2001). Conservative management consists of exercise restriction for 6–8 weeks along with analgesics as needed. A splint or bandage could be applied but the efficacy of external coaptation is unknown. Surgery is limited to removal of the fragment or the entire sesamoid.

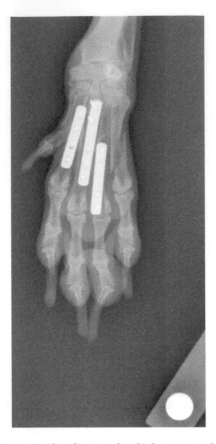

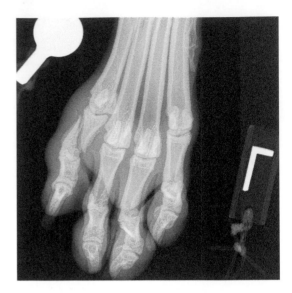

Figure 12.37   Radiograph of a Doberman Pinscher with a long oblique fracture of thoracic limb digit V P2. Note the soft tissue swelling surrounding the fracture.

Figure 12.36   Plate fixation of multiple metacarpal fractures involving both primary weight-bearing bones (metacarpals III and IV). This patient was stabilized with surgery using a 1.1 mm plating system. Source: Image courtesy of Dr. Simon Roe.

The approach and removal disturbs the joint capsule, cruciate ligaments, and intersesamoidean ligaments, as well as the medial and lateral ligaments, resulting in instability of the joint (Mathews *et al.*, 2001). In nonresponsive cases, one author (DD) has used fluoroscope-guided steroid or biological therapies injections with good success.

Digit injuries

Cause

Digit injuries include fractures, luxations, and ligamentous injuries. The true incidence of these injures as well as the outcome is unknown (Kapatkin *et al.*, 2012). It is suspected that many digit injuries are a result of trauma; however, ligamentous injuries can be due to excessive

work over time. Digit fractures can occur during a sharp turn when the toes are in an otherwise fixed position, stepping in a hole, and knocking the digits on hard surfaces (rocks, tree stumps, etc.) during training or competition. Ligamentous injuries can occur during fast sharp turns on uneven or slippery terrain. The toes are often splayed out to gain as much traction as possible. In these situations, the toe can experience significant torque at an unnatural angle resulting in damage to the collateral ligaments.

Diagnosis

Patients with digit injuries will commonly have a severe weight-bearing to non-weight-bearing lameness. With acute injuries, significant swelling may be noted with pain and crepitus on manipulation of the digit. With chronic ligamentous injuries, there may be swelling at the site of injury as well as pain on manipulation. It is important to pay close attention to the webbing of the digits for any evidence of penetrating trauma or evidence of an open fracture especially on the palmar surface. Radiographs are the mainstay for determining the presence of digit fractures (Figure 12.37), luxations, and degree of soft tissue swelling. If a fracture or

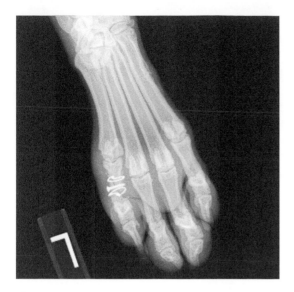

Figure 12.38   Postoperative radiograph of the same patient from Figure 12.37. The fracture was stabilized with a 1.0 mm lag screw and two cerclage wires.

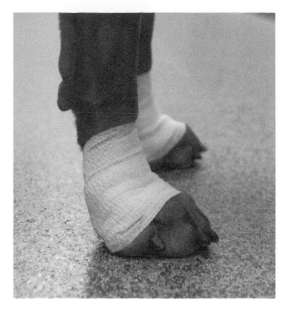

Figure 12.39   Image of a digital wrap to prevent additional damage and allow healing following a grade 2 digital collateral ligament injury. Note that the wrap is placed on both front feet although the injury was localized to the right thoracic limb. Source: Image courtesy of Dr. Deb Canapp.

luxation is not seen, a penetrating foreign body or ligamentous injury should be considered. Diagnostic musculoskeletal ultrasound can be used to determine the presence and severity (grade 1–3) of a ligamentous injury.

Treatment

Treatment of digit fractures is commonly conservative, using a splint and bandage for 6–8 weeks. For external coaptation alone to be successful, the fracture must be stabilized a joint above and a joint below the fracture. It can be challenging to fully immobilize digit fractures, resulting in micro-motion, which may delay healing. Radiographs should be taken every 4 weeks to ensure appropriate healing. Fractures that fail to heal with conservative management, as well as those in large patients, in those with multiple digit fractures, or in canine athletes and working dogs may benefit from surgical fixation (Figure 12.38). Following surgical fixation, external coaptation with a splint is recommended to protect the repair. In patients with failed conservative or surgical treatment or for fractures of digit P3, digit amputation can be considered.

Ligamentous injuries to the digits are common in working and sporting dogs. The diagnosis can be suspected if other orthopedic conditions have been ruled out. The authors prefer to confirm the diagnosis with diagnostic musculoskeletal ultrasound. Treatment of ligamentous injuries is typically conservative in nature with rest, analgesics, and external coaptation with a splint. Unfortunately, ligamentous injuries tend to heal poorly and require a significant amount of time to form appropriate fibrous tissue (approximately 2–4 months). To mitigate the morbidity associated with external coaptation and splints, a novel digital wrap can be used (Figure 12.39). The wrap consists of two to three layers of an elastic, nonstick wrap such as Vet-Wrap®. It is placed with enough tension to restrict lateral toe movement, but not so tight as to cause abrasions or swelling. In most cases the wrap is placed on both feet so that the dog does not focus on the injured limb and chew at the bandage (an E-collar may be needed in some patients). In cases where healing is not progressing as expected or the tissues fail to heal, ultrasound-guided or fluoroscope-guided injections of biological therapies or steroids can be used to aid in providing comfort and facilitate tissue healing.

References

Abrams, J. S. 2001. Thermal capsulorrhaphy for instability of the shoulder: concerns and applications of the heat probe. *Instr Course Lect*, 50, 29–36.

Arrington, E. D. & Miller, M. D. 1995. Skeletal muscle injuries. *Orthop Clin North Am*, 26, 411–422.

Baeumlin, Y., DE Rycke, L., VAN Caelenberg, A., VAN Bree, H. & Gielen, I. 2010. Magnetic resonance imaging of the canine elbow: an anatomic study. *Vet Surg*, 39, 566–573.

Beitzel, K., Allen, D., Apostolakos, J., Russell, R. P., McCarthy, M. B., Gallo, G. J., *et al.* 2015. US definitions, current use, and FDA stance on use of platelet-rich plasma in sports medicine. *J Knee Sur*, 28(1), 29–34.

Bellenger, C. R., Johnson, K. A., Davis, P. E. & Ilkiw, J. E. 1981. Fixation of metacarpal and metatarsal fractures in greyhounds. *Aust Vet J*, 57, 205–211.

Bishop, P. B. & Bray, R. C. 1993. Abnormal joint mechanics and the proteoglycan composition of normal and healing rabbit medial collateral ligament. *J Manipulative Physiol Ther*, 16(5), 300–305.

BLOOD, D. C. & Studdert, V. P. 1999. *Saunders Comprehensive Veterinary Dictionary*, 2nd edn. London: W. B. Saunders, p. 368.

Boettcher, P., Werner, H., Ludewig, E., Grevel, V. & Oechtering, G. 2009. Visual estimation of radioulnar incongruence in dogs using three-dimensional image rendering: an in vitro study based on computed tomographic imaging. *Vet Surg*, 38, 161–168.

Boudrieau, R. 2003. Fractures of the radius and ulna In: Slatter, D. (ed.), *Textbook of Small Animal Surgery*. 3rd edn. Philadelphia, PA: Saunders, 1965–1972.

Burton, N. J., Owen, M. R., KIRK, L. S., Toscano, M. J. & Colborne, G. R. 2011. Conservative versus arthroscopic management for medial coronoid process disease in dogs: a prospective gait evaluation. *Vet Surg*, 40, 972–980.

Cake, M. A & Read, R. A. 1995. Canine and human sesamoid disease. *Vet Comp Orthop Traumatol*, 8, 70–75.

Canapp, S. Supraspinatus tendinopathy: regenerative medicine for supraspinatus tendinopathy, update on canine orthopedic devices. In: *Veterinary Arthrology Advancement Association (VA3) Annual Symposium*, August 18–20, 2011, Bonita Springs, FL.

Canapp, S., Acciani, D., Hulse, D., Schulz, K. & Canapp, D. 2009. Rehabilitation therapy for elbow disorders in dogs. *Vet Surg*, 38, 301–307.

Canapp, S., Canapp, D., Carr, B., Cox, C. & Barrett, J. 2016a. Supraspinatus tendinopathy in 327 dogs: a retrospective study. *Veterinary Evidence*, 1(3).

Canapp, S., Canapp, D., Ibrahim, V., Carr, B., Cox, C. & Barrett, J. 2016b. The use of adipose derived progenitor cells and platelet rich plasma combination for the treatment of supraspinatus tendinopathy in 55 dogs: a retrospective study. *Front Vet Sci*, 3, 61.

Carberry, C. A. & Gilmore, D. R. 1986. Infraspinatus muscle contracture associated with trauma in a dog. *J Am Vet Med Assoc*, 188, 533–534.

Carmichael, S. & Marshall, W. 2012. Muscle and tendon disorders. In: Tobias, K. M., Johnston, S. A. (eds), *Veterinary Surgery: Small Animal*. St. Louis, MO: Elsevier, p. 1129.

Carpenter, J. E., Flanagan, C. L., Thomopoulos, S., Yian, E. H. & Soslowsky, L. J. 1998. The effects of overuse combined with intrinsic or extrinsic alterations in an animal model of rotator cuff tendinosis. *Am J Sports Med*, 26, 801–807.

Carr, B. J., Canapp, S. O., Canapp, D. A., Gamble, L.-J. & Dycus, D. L. 2016. Adhesive capsulitis in eight dogs: diagnosis and management. *Front Vet Sci*, 3, 55.

Carrig, C. 1975. The effects of asynchronous growth of the radius and ulna on the canine elbow joint following experimental retardation of longitudinal growth of the ulna. *J Am Anim Hosp Assoc*, 11, 560.

Clements, D. N., Carter, S. D., Innes, J. F. & Ollier, W. E. 2006. Genetic basis of secondary osteoarthritis in dogs with joint dysplasia. *Am J Vet Res*, 67, 909–918.

Conzemius, M. 2009. Nonconstrained elbow replacement in dogs. *Vet Surg*, 38, 279–284.

Cook, C. R. & Cook, J. L. 2009a. Diagnostic imaging of canine elbow dysplasia: a review. *Vet Surg*, 38, 144–153.

Cook, J. 2012b. Sports medicine for the canine elbow: what really helps? In: *Proceedings, 28th Annual International Canine Sports Medicine Symposium*, Orlando, FL.

Cook, J. L. & Cook, C. R. 2009b. Bilateral shoulder and elbow arthroscopy in dogs with thoracic limb lameness: diagnostic findings and treatment outcomes. *Vet Surg*, 38, 224–232.

Cook, J. L., Renfro, D. C., Tomlinson, J. L. & Sorensen, J. E. 2005a. Measurement of angles of abduction for diagnosis of shoulder instability in dogs using goniometry and digital image analysis. *Vet Surg*, 34, 463–468.

Cook, J. L., Tomlinson, J. L., Fox, D. B., Kenter, K. & Cook, C. R. 2005b. Treatment of dogs diagnosed with medial shoulder instability using radiofrequency-induced thermal capsulorrhaphy. *Vet Surg*, 34, 469–75.

Cook, J. L., Shulz, K. S., Karnes, J. G., Franklin, S. P., Canapp, S. O., Lotsikas, P. J., *et al.* 2015. Clinical outcomes associated with the initial use of the Canine Unicompartmental Elbow (CUE) Arthroplasty System®. *Can Vet J*, 56, 971–977.

Cookson, J. C. & Kent, B. E. 1979. Orthopedic manual therapy—an overview. Part I: the extremities. *Phys Ther*, 59, 136–146.

Corley, E. A., Sutherland, T. M. & Carlson, W. D. 1968. Genetic aspects of canine elbow dysplasia. *J Am Vet Med Assoc*, 153, 543–547.

Crosse, K. R. & Worth, A. J. 2010. Computer-assisted surgical correction of an antebrachial deformity in a dog. *Vet Comp Orthop Traumatol*, 23, 354–361.

Cullen, K. L., Dickey, J. P., Bent, L. R., Thomason, J. J. & Moens, N. M. 2013. Survey-based analysis of risk factors for injury among dogs participating in agility training and competition events. *J Am Vet Med Assoc*, 243(7), 1019–1024.

Dammrich, K. 1991. Relationship between nutrition and bone growth in large and giant dogs. *J Nutr*, 121, S114–S121.

Danielson, K. C., Fitzpatrick, N., Muir, P. & Manley, P. A. 2006. Histomorphometry of fragmented medial coronoid process in dogs: a comparison of affected and normal coronoid processes. *Vet Surg*, 35, 501–509.

Danova, N. A. & Muir, P. 2003. Extracorporeal shock wave therapy for supraspinatus calcifying tendinopathy in two dogs. *Vet Rec*, 152, 208–209.

de Bakker, E., Samoy, Y., Gielen, I. & VAN Ryssen, B. 2011. Medial humeral epicondylar lesions in the canine elbow. A review of the literature. *Vet Comp Orthop Traumatol*, 24, 9–17.

Denny, H. R. 1993. *A Guide to Canine and Feline Orthopaedic Surgery*, 3rd edn. Boston, MA: Blackwell Scientific Publications, 199–200, 334–336.

Devitt, C. M., Neely, M. R. & Vanvechten, B. J. 2007. Relationship of physical examination test of shoulder instability to arthroscopic findings in dogs. *Vet Surg*, 36, 661–668.

Dillon, E. A., Anderson, L. J. & Jones, B. R. 1989. Infraspinatus muscle contracture in a working dog. *N Z Vet J*, 37, 32–34.

Dirks, R. C. & Warden, S. J. 2011. Models for the study of tendinopathy. *J Musculoskelet Neuronal Interact*, 11(2), 141–149.

Evans, H. E. 1993. *Miller's Anatomy of the Dog*, 3rd edn. Philadelphia, PA: W. B. Saunders.

Farrell, M., Trevail, T., Marshall, W., Yeadon, R. & Carmichael, S. 2011. Computed tomographic documentation of the natural progression of humeral intracondylar fissure in a cocker spaniel. *Vet Surg*, 40, 966–971.

Fitzpatrick, N. & Yeadon, R. 2009. Working algorithm for treatment decision making for developmental disease of the medial compartment of the elbow in dogs. *Vet Surg*, 38, 285–300.

Fitzpatrick, N., Smith, T. J., Evans, R. B., O'riordan, J. & Yeadon, R. 2009a. Subtotal coronoid ostectomy for treatment of medial coronoid disease in 263 dogs. *Vet Surg*, 38, 233–245.

Fitzpatrick, N., Yeadon, R. & Smith, T. J. 2009b. Early clinical experience with osteochondral autograft transfer for treatment of osteochondritis dissecans of the medial humeral condyle in dogs. *Vet Surg*, 38, 246–260.

Fitzpatrick, N., Yeadon, R., Smith, T. & Schulz, K. 2009c. Techniques of application and initial clinical experience with sliding humeral osteotomy for treatment of medial compartment disease of the canine elbow. *Vet Surg*, 38, 261–278.

Fossum, T. 2002. *Small Animal Surgery*, 2nd edn. St. Louis, MO: Mosby, pp. 1164–1167.

Forward, D. P., Davis, T. R. & Sithole, J. S. 2008. Do young patients with malunited fractures of the distal radius inevitably develop symptomatic post-traumatic osteoarthritis? *J Bone Joint Surg Br*, 90, 629–637.

Fox, S. 1984. Premature closure of distal radial and ulnar physes in the dog 1. Pathogenesis and diagnosis. *Compend Contin Educ Vet*, 6, 128–139.

Frank, C. B. 1996. Ligament healing: current knowledge and clinical applications. *J Am Acad Orthop Surg*, 4(1), 74–83.

Frank, C. B., Hart, D. A. & Shrive, N. G. 1999. Molecular biology and biomechanics of normal and healing ligaments—a review. *Osteoarthritis Cartilage*, 7(1), 130–140.

Fransson, B. A., Gavin, P. R. & Lahmers, K. K. 2005. Supraspinatus tendinosis associated with biceps brachii tendon displacement in a dog. *J Am Vet Med Assoc*, 227, 1416, 1429–1433.

Gilley, R. S., Wallace, L. J. & Hayden, D. W. 2002. Clinical and pathologic analyses of bicipital tenosynovitis in dogs. *Am J Vet Res*, 63, 402–407.

Guercio, A., Di Marco, P., Casella, S., Cannella, V., Russotto, L., Purpari, G., *et al.* 2012. Production of canine mesenchymal stem cells from adipose tissue and their application in dogs with chronic osteoarthritis of the humeroradial joints. *Cell Biol Int*, 36(2), 189–194.

Gnudi, G., Mortellaro, C. M. & Bertoni, G. 2003. Radial carpal bone fracture in 13 dogs. *Vet Comp Orthop Traumatol*, 16, 178–183.

Harasen, G. 2005. Infraspinatus muscle contracture. *Can Vet J*, 46, 751–2.

Hattersley, R., McKee, M., O'Neill, T., Clarke, S., Butterworth, S., Maddox, T., *et al.* 2011. Postoperative complications after surgical management of incomplete ossification of the humeral condyle in dogs. *Vet Surg*, 40, 728–733.

Hazewinkel, H. A. W., Goedegebuure, S. A., Poulos, P. W. & Wolvekamp, W. T. C. 1985. Influences of chronic calcium excess on the skeletal development of growing Great Danes. *J Am Anim Hosp Assoc*, 21, 377–391.

Hempfling, H. 2007. Intra-articular hyaluronic acid after knee arthroscopy: a two-year study. *Knee Surg Sports Traumatol Arthrosc*, 15, 537–546.

Hildebrand, K. A. & Frank, C. B. 1998. Scar formation and ligament healing. *Can J Surg*, 41(6), 425–429.

Hoelzler, M. G., Millis, D. L., Francis, D. A. & Weigel, J. P. 2004. Results of arthroscopic versus open arthrotomy for surgical management of cranial cruciate ligament deficiency in dogs. *Vet Surg*, 33, 146–153.

Johnson, K. A. 1987. Accessory carpal bone fractures in the racing Greyhound: classification and pathology. *Vet Surg*, 16, 60–64.

Johnson, K. A. & Piras, A. 2005. Fractures of the carpus. In: Johnson, A. L., Houlton, J. E. F. & Vannini, R. (eds), *AO Principles of Fracture Management in the Dog and Cat*. Davos, Switzerland: AO Publishing, pp. 341–348.

Johnson, K. A., Dee, J. F. & Piermattei, D. L. 1989. Screw fixation of accessory carpal bone fractures in racing Greyhounds: 12 cases (1981–1986). *J Am Vet Med Assoc*, 194, 1618–1625.

Kapatkin, A. S., Howe-Smith, R. & Shofer, F. 2000. Conservative versus surgical treatment of metacarpal and metatarsal fractures in dogs. *Vet Comp Orthop Traumatol*, 13, 123–127.

Kapatkin, A. S., Garcia-Nolen, T. & Hayash, I. K. 2012. Carpus, metacarpus, and digits. In: Tobias, K. & Johnston, S. (eds), *Veterinary Surgery Small Animal*, 1st edn. St. Louis, MO: Saunders-Elsevier, pp. 785–800.

Kilincoglu, V., Yeter, A., Servet, E., Kangal, M. & Yildrim, M. 2015. Short term results comparison of intraarticular platelet-rich plasma (PRP) and hyaluronic acid (HA) applications in early stage of knee osteoarthritis. *Int J Clin Exp Med*, 8(10), 18807–18812.

Krotscheck, U., Hulse, D., Bahr, A. & Jerram, R. 2000. Ununited anconeal process: lag-screw fixation with proximal ulnar osteotomy. *Vet Comp Orthop Traumatol*, 13, 212–216.

Lafuente, M. P., Fransson, B. A., Lincoln, J. D., Martinez, S. A., Gavin, P. R., Lahmers, K. K. & Gay, J. M. 2009. Surgical treatment of mineralized and nonmineralized supraspinatus tendinopathy in twenty-four dogs. *Vet Surg*, 38, 380–387.

Langley-Hobbs, S. J., Hamilton, M. H. & Pratt, J. N. 2007. Radiographic and clinical features of carpal varus associated with chronic sprain of the lateral collateral ligament complex in 10 dogs. *Vet Comp Orthop Traumatol*, 20, 324–330.

Leighton, R. L. 1977. Tenotomy for infraspinatus muscle contracture. *Mod Vet Pract*, 58, 134–135.

Li, A., Bennett, D., Gibbs, C., Carmichael, S., Gibson, N., Owen, M., *et al.* 2000. Radial carpal bone fractures in 15 dogs. *J Small Anim Pract*, 41, 74–79.

Maganaris, C. N., Narici, M. V., Almekinders, L. C. & Maffulli, N. 2004. Biomechanics and pathophysiology of overuse tendon injuries: ideas on insertional tendinopathy. *Sports Med*, 34, 1005–1017.

Marcellin-Little, D. J., Deyoung, D. J., Ferris, K. K. & Berry, C. M. 1994. Incomplete ossification of the humeral condyle in spaniels. *Vet Surg*, 23, 475–487.

Marcellin-Little, D. J., Levine, D. & Canapp, S. O., Jr. 2007. The canine shoulder: selected disorders and their management with physical therapy. *Clin Tech Small Anim Pract*, 22, 171–182.

Matava, M. J., Whitesides, T. E., Jr., Seiler, J. G., 3rd, Hewan-Lowe, K. & Hutton, W. C. 1994. Determination of the compartment pressure threshold of muscle ischemia in a canine model. *J Trauma*, 37, 50–58.

Mather, R. C., Koenig, L., Acevedo, D., Dall, T. M., Gallo, P., Romeo, A., *et al.* 2013. The societal and economic value of rotator cuff repair. *J Bone Joint Surg Am*, 95(22), 1993–2000.

Mathews, K. G., Koblik, P. D. & Whitehair, J. G. 2001. Fragmented palmar metacarpophalangeal sesamoids in dogs: a long-term evaluation. *Vet Comp Orthop Traumatol*, 14, 7–14.

Mathies, B. 2006. Effects of Viscoseal, a synovial fluid substitute, on recovery after arthroscopic partial meniscectomy and joint lavage. *Knee Surg Sports Traumatol Arthrosc*, 14, 32–39.

Meyer-Lindenberg, A., Fehr, M. & Nolte, I. 2006. Co-existence of ununited anconeal process and fragmented medial coronoid process of the ulna in the dog. *J Small Anim Pract*, 47, 61–65.

Meheux, C. J., McCulloch, P. C., Lintner, D. M., Varner, K. E. & Harris, J. D. 2016. Efficacy of intra-articular platelet-rich plasma injections in knee osteoarthritis: a systematic review. *Arthroscopy*, 32(3), 495–505.

Miniaci, A. & Codsi, M. J. 2006. Thermal capsulorrhaphy for the treatment of shoulder instability. *Am J Sports Med*, 34, 1356–1363.

Mokbel, A., El-Tookhy, O., Shamaa, A., Sabry, D., Rashed, L. & Mostafa, A. 2011. Homing and efficacy of intra-articular injection of autologous mesenchymal stem cells in experimental chondral defects in dogs. *Clin Exp Rheumatol*, 29, 275–284.

Moores, A. P., Benigni, L. & Lamb, C. R. 2008. Computed tomography versus arthroscopy for detection of canine elbow dysplasia lesions. *Vet Surg*, 37, 390–398.

Muir, P. & Norris, J. L. 1997. Metacarpal and metatarsal fractures in dogs. *J Small Anim Pract*, 38, 344–348.

Oh, L. S., Wolf, B. R., Hall, M. P., Levy, B. A. & Marx, R. G. 2007. Indications for rotator cuff repair: a systematic review. *Clin Orthop Rel Res*, 455, 52–63.

Olivieri, M., Ciliberto, E., Hulse, D. A., Vezzoni, A., Ingravalle, F. & Peirone, B. 2007. Arthroscopic treatment of osteochondritis dissecans of the shoulder in 126 dogs. *Vet Comp Orthop Traumatol*, 1, 65–69.

O'Neill, T. & Innes, J. F. 2004. Treatment of shoulder instability caused by medial glenohumeral ligament rupture with thermal capsulorrhaphy. *J Small Anim Pract*, 45, 521–524.

Parker, R. B., Brown, S. G. & Wind, A. P. 1981. Pancarpal arthrodesis in the dog: a review of forty-five cases. *Vet Surg*, 10, 35.

Paster, E. R., Biery, D. N., Lawler, D. F., Evans, R. H., Kealy, R. D., Gregor, T. P., *et al.* 2009. Un-united medial epicondyle of the humerus: radiographic prevalence and association with elbow osteoarthritis in a cohort of Labrador Retrievers, *Vet Surg*, 38, 169–172.

Pettit, G. D. 1980. Infraspinatus muscle contracture in dogs. *Mod Vet Pract*, 61, 451–452.

Pettit, G. D., Chatburn, C. C., Hegreberg, G. A. & Meyers, K. M. 1978. Studies on the pathophysiology of infraspinatus muscle contracture in the dog. *Vet Surg*, 7, 8–11.

Pettitt, R. A., Tattersall, J., Gemmill, T., Butterworth, S. J., O'Neill, T. J., Langley-Hobbs, S. J.,*et al.* 2009. Effect of surgical technique on radiographic fusion of the anconeus in the treatment of ununited anconeal process. *J Small Anim Pract*, 50, 545–548.

Piermattei, D. L., Flo, G. L. & Decamp, C. E. 2006. *Brinker, Piermattei and Flo's Handbook of Small Animal Orthopedics and Fracture Repair, 14*, 4th edn. Philadelphia, PA: Saunders-Elsevier.

Punke, J. P., Hulse, D. A., Kerwin, S. C., Peycke, L. E. & Budsberg, S. C. 2009. Arthroscopic documentation of elbow cartilage pathology in dogs with clinical lameness without changes on standard radiographic projections. *Vet Surg*, 38, 209–212.

Rochat, M. C. 2012. The shoulder. In: Tobias, K. M. & Johnston, S. A. (eds), *Veterinary Surgery: Small Animal*. St. Louis, MO: Elsevier, pp. 694–696, 707.

Roy, R., Wallace, L. & Johnston, G. & 1994. A retrospective long term evaluation of ununited anconeal excision on the canine elbow. *Vet Comp Orthop Traumatol*, 7, 94–97.

Sager, M., Herten, M., Ruchay, S., Assheuer, J., Kramer, M. & Jager, M. 2009. The anatomy of the glenoid labrum: a comparison between human and dog. *Comp Med*, 59, 465–475.

Schramme, M., Kerekes, Z., Hunter, S. & Labens, R. 2010. MR imaging features of surgically induced core lesions in the equine superficial digital flexor tendon. *Vet Radiol Ultrasound*, 51, 280–287.

Schulz, K. & Krotscheck, U. 2003. Canine elbow dysplasia. *In*: Slatter, D. (ed.), *Textbook of Small Animal Surgery*, 3rd edn. Philadelphia, PA: W. B. Saunders, pp. 1927–1952.

Sharma, P. & Maffulli, N. 2005. Tendon injury and tendinopathy: healing and repair. *J Bone Joint Surg Am*, 87, 187–202.

Shetye, S. S., Malhotra, K., Ryan S. D. & Puttlitz, C. M. 2009. Determination of mechanical properties of canine carpal ligaments. *Am J Vet Res*, 70, 1026–1030.

Siems, J. J., Breur, G. J., Blevins, W. E. & Cornell, K. K. 1998. Use of two-dimensional real-time ultrasonography for diagnosing contracture and strain of the infraspinatus muscle in a dog. *J Am Vet Med Assoc*, 212, 77–80.

Slatter, D. 1985. *Textbook of Small Animal Surgery*, 2nd edn. Philadelphia, PA: W. B. Saunders.

Soslowsky, L. J., Thomopoulos, S., Tun, S., Flanagan, C. L., Keefer, C. C., Mastaw, J. & Carpenter, J. E. 2000. Overuse activity injures the supraspinatus tendon in an animal model: a histologic and biomechanical study. *J Shoulder Elbow Surg*, 9, 79–84.

Tan, D., Canapp, S. O., Leasure, C., Dycus, D. L. & O'Donnell, E. 2016. Traumatic fracture of the medial coronoid process in 24 dogs. *Vet Comp Orthop Traumatol*, 4, 325–329.

Tempelhof, S., Rupp, S. & Seil, R. 1999. Age-related prevalence of rotator cuff tears in asymptomatic shoulders. *J Shoulder Elbow Surg*, 8, 296–299.

Temwichitr, J., Leegwater, P. A. & Hazewinkel, H. A. 2010. Fragmented coronoid process in the dog: a heritable disease. *Vet J*, 185, 123–129.

Tomlin, J. L., Pead, M. J., Langley-Hobbs, S. J. & Muir, P. 2001. Radial carpal bone fracture in dogs. *J Am Anim Hosp Assoc*, 37, 173–178.

Trostel, C., McLaughlin, R. & Pool, R. 2002. Canine lameness cause by developmental orthopedic diseases: osteochondrosis. *Compend Contin Educ Vet*, 24, 836–854.

Trostel, C., McLaughlin, R. & Pool, R. 2003a. Canine lameness caused by developmental orthopedic diseases: fragmented medial coronoid process and ununited anconeal process. *Compend Contin Educ Vet*, 25, 112–120.

Trostel, C., McLaughlin, R. & Pool, R. 2003b. Canine elbow dysplasia: anatomy and pathogenesis. *Compend Contin Educ Vet*, 25, 754–762.

Verborgt, O., Gibson, G. J. & Schaffler, M. B. 2000. Loss of osteocyte integrity in association with microdamage and bone remodeling after fatigue in vivo. *J Bone Miner Res*, 15, 60–67.

Vilar, J. M., Morales, M., Santana, A., Spinella, G., Rubio, M., Cuervo, B. & Carrillo, J. M. 2013. Controlled, blinded force platform analysis of the effect of intraarticular injection of autologous adipose-derived mesenchymal stem cells associated to PRGF-Endoret in osteoarthritic dogs. *BMC Vet Res*, 9, 131.

Wernham, B. G. & Roush J. K. 2010. Metacarpal and metatarsal fractures in dogs. *Compend Contin Educ Vet*, 32, E1–7.

Wernham, B. G., Jerram, R. M. & Warman, C. G. 2008. Bicipital tenosynovitis in dogs. *Compend Contin Educ Vet*, 30, 537–552.

Wind, A. & Packard, M. 1986. Elbow incongruity and developmental elbow diseases in the dog: Part II. *J Am Anim Hosp Assoc*, 22, 725–730.

Zhu, Y., Yuan, M., Meng, H. Y., Wang, A.Y., Guo, Q.Y., Wang, Y. & Peng, J. 2013. Basic science and clinical application of platelet-rich plasma for cartilage defects and osteoarthritis: a review. *Osteoarthritis Cartilage*, 21(11), 1627–1637.

13

Evaluation and Rehabilitation Options for Orthopedic Disorders of the Canine Thoracic Limb

Sasha A. Foster, MSPT, CCRT

Summary

Rehabilitation evaluation of orthopedic conditions includes six components: capturing subjective data, obtaining objective findings, completing a problem list, developing an assessment, building a treatment plan, and re-evaluating for treatment efficacy. Capturing subjective data occurs with the client and includes the client's subjective perception of the patient's current condition, history of the present injury, the client's goals for their animal, and a thorough medical history from the referring veterinarian including diagnostics and medications. Objective data are then obtained during the hands-on portion of the evaluation and includes posture, function, strength, gait, palpation, passive range of motion, muscle flexibility, clearing the spine, joint play, and special tests. Findings from each of these areas are placed on a problem list. The problem list is critically analyzed by the therapist to develop a working hypothesis, an assessment, that explains all the findings on the problem list. The assessment may be an expansion of the primary orthopedic diagnosis, including the sequelae of the primary diagnosis, and it may also include underlying physical limitations that may not be associated with the primary orthopedic condition. To build the treatment plan, the problem list is prioritized starting with pain, then primary tissue type injured, followed by sequelae. The treatment plan is then executed and may include modalities, manual therapies, and therapeutic exercise, each of which follows physiologically based levels of frequency, intensity, and duration. Treatment efficacy is then re-evaluated within a session and over a course of treatment to ensure treatment effectiveness. Treatments may be modified within a treatment session or over the course of a treatment plan. When re-evaluation reveals the patient has reached the rehabilitation goals, they are discharged to a health maintenance program.

Canine Sports Medicine and Rehabilitation, Second Edition. Edited by Chris Zink and Janet B. Van Dyke.
© 2018 John Wiley & Sons, Inc. Published 2018 by John Wiley & Sons, Inc.

Overview of orthopedic rehabilitation

Current evidence in canine rehabilitation indicates that, when treated by a certified rehabilitation professional, rehabilitation is safe and may improve outcomes in postoperative tibial plateau leveling osteotomy (TPLO) (Romano & Cook, 2015). Historically, postsurgical outcomes of TPLO without rehabilitation indicate that dynamic and static weight bearing of the surgical limbs return to control limb levels, but that passive range of motion of the stifle, active range of motion of the stifle, and thrust force from the ground remain inferior to the control limb (Molsa et al., 2014). Another study supported these finding by indicating that thigh circumference and stifle range of motion do not return to control limb measurements 1–5 years after TPLO surgery (Moeller et al., 2010). The historical standard practice of crate rest after orthopedic surgery may need to be re-evaluated as a study has shown that crate rest-induced cartilage atrophy is not reversed (Kiviranta et al., 1994; Haapala et al. 1999). Because these studies indicate standard orthopedic care without rehabilitation may have lasting negative impacts on the patient, early intervention rehabilitation should be considered (Marsolais et al., 2002). Studies are currently showing that, after surgery for a cruciate-deficient stifle, early intervention may prevent muscle atrophy, build muscle mass and strength, and increase stifle flexion and extension range of motion (Monk et al., 2006).

Sequencing the orthopedic evaluation

For all rehabilitation, from acute postoperative care through return-to-sport conditioning, a thorough evaluation must be completed. Proper sequencing of the six components of the rehabilitation evaluation—capturing subjective data, obtaining objective findings, completing a problem list, developing an assessment, building a treatment plan, and re-evaluating to determine if the treatment plan is effective—assists the therapist with capturing detailed information while promoting a lasting therapeutic relationship with the client and patient.

At the initial meeting, the therapist greets the client in a warm and friendly manner taking breed-specific preferences for patient interaction into consideration. For all patients, initially avoiding direct eye contact and physical interaction helps the patient perceive the therapist as nonintrusive. The therapist then leads the client and patient into the therapy room, allowing the patient the freedom to become familiar with the new setting. As the patient explores the environment, the therapist interviews the client capturing subjective data and medical history. The objective evaluation, which may be done with or without the client present, begins with the hands-off elements of the exam including posture, function, strength, and gait. If the patient is provided with rewards in the form of food or toys during the initial phases of the evaluation they may be more agreeable to the manual portions of the exam which include muscle and bone palpation, passive range of motion, muscle flexibility, fascial mobility, clearing the spine, joint play, and special tests. Patient preference for body position (standing, sitting, or lying) and order of manual exam elements is respected and modified to meet a particular patient's behavioral needs. To avoid pain and fear responses early in the examination, the involved limb is typically evaluated last.

Findings from each of the objective exam areas are placed on a problem list and the therapist critically analyzes the list to develop an assessment. The assessment is a working hypothesis that explains all the findings on the problem list. It may be an expansion of the primary orthopedic diagnosis, including the sequelae of the primary diagnosis, and it may also include underlying physical limitations that may not be associated with the primary orthopedic condition.

The treatment plan is then developed based on the prioritized problem list. For each problem on the list, the primary tissue type and the chronicity of the injury is determined. Common injured tissue types for orthopedic treatments may include muscle, tendon, ligament, joint capsule, intra-articular structures (cartilage and meniscus), and bone. Chronicity of injury is defined in three phases of healing: (1) acute, recent onset with effusion and/or edema; (2) subacute, with tissue effusion/edema resolved but time to tissue healing not yet complete; and (3) chronic, with tissue primarily healed.

With the prioritized problem list in place, including tissue type injured and chronicity of injury for each problem, the treatment plan is then developed. Treatment interventions may include modalities, manual therapies, and therapeutic exercise—all of which should include intensity, frequency, and duration of treatment intervention.

Within a session and throughout a treatment plan, re-evaluation of treatment interventions should be completed allowing modifications to the plan of care for the most effective outcomes. A home exercise program should always be part of the treatment plan and it should include principle-based frequency, intensity, and duration for each exercise. When a follow-up evaluation reveals that the patient has reached the client's rehabilitation goals for their dog, the patient is discharged to a health maintenance program.

Specific guidelines for determining injury location and tissue type

Consideration of anatomy, osteokinematics, and arthrokinematics during each objective test will guide the therapist to a deeper understanding of the injury location and tissue type that will, in turn, promote more efficacious treatment plans. A thorough evaluation observes muscle origins and insertions and their impact on normal passive range of motion, or osteokinematic movement, including: scapular protraction (scapula moves away from the midline) and retraction (scapula moves toward the midline); glenohumeral flexion, extension, abduction, adduction, and internal and external rotation; elbow flexion and extension; carpal flexion, extension, supination, and pronation; and manus flexion and extension. Limitations in osteokinematic motion at a joint may indicate a limitation in joint play, or arthrokinematic motion. Normal arthrokinematic movement includes glenohumeral joint cranial, caudal, medial, lateral, internal, and external rotational glides; elbow (ulnar) glides toward flexion or extension; elbow (radius) cranial and caudal glides; carpal palmar and dorsal glides; and manus plantar and dorsal glides. Each of these arthrokinematics requires joint capsule stability, which is maintained via the inherent integ-

rity of the joint capsule and surrounding ligaments that provide additional resistance to external forces. Ligamentous stability in the thoracic limb includes the medial and lateral collateral ligaments of the glenohumeral joint that prevent excessive medial and lateral glides, respectively, of the humerus in the glenoid fossa; the medial and lateral collateral ligaments of the elbow, carpus, and digits that counteract varus and valgus forces through each of these joints; and the oblique ligament of the elbow that may counteract hyperextension forces. Keen observation of anatomy, osteokinematics, and arthrokinematics in each of the following tests will assist the therapist with the critical thinking skills to develop a precise problem list and the correct treatment plan.

Posture

The purpose of postural evaluation is to determine positional inequities that may lead the therapist to further evaluate particular areas of the body. Posture is observed with the patient in a natural static standing position. The therapist describes appendicular skeletal posture from the front, side, back, and top of the patient. The therapist first takes into consideration head position relative to back height and midline. Changes in neck position may change the posture of the entire body, predisposing the thoracic limbs, spine, and pelvic limbs to compensatory issues. For example, due to a number of multi-joint muscles including the brachiocephalicus and omotransversarius, primary or compensatory injuries of the thoracic limb can affect neck position, which in turn can affect active and passive range of motion which, over time, may limit cervical spine facet joint arthrokinematics. Position of the scapulae on the thorax should then be reviewed taking into consideration breed-specific angulation (visit www.akc.org for breed-specific angulation). Inequities in scapular position can indicate tightness, weakness, or injury to the muscles that connect the scapula to the thorax including the serratus ventralis cranial and caudal fibers, rhomboids, and cranial and caudal heads of the trapezius.

Postural evaluation of the peripheral limbs is then completed, taking care to note the standing angle of the glenohumeral, elbow, and

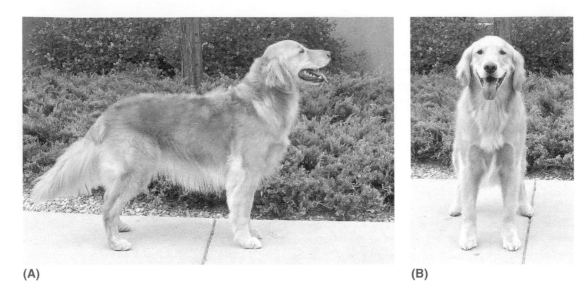

(A)   **(B)**

Figure 13.1   Postural assessment from the front and side of a young, injury-free dog. **(A)** Side view. **(B)** Front view. Note the position of the scapula on the thorax, the angulation of the thoracic limb joints, and the position of the head and top line in comparison with the geriatric patient shown in Figure 13.2.

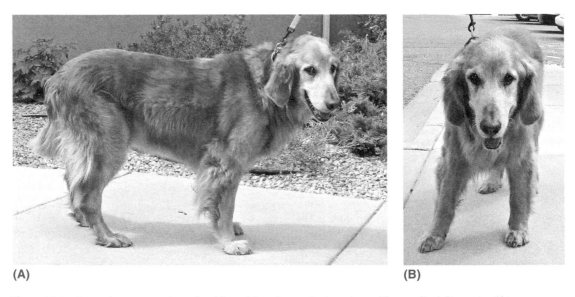

(A)   **(B)**

Figure 13.2   Postural assessment from the side and front in a geriatric patient with a medical diagnosis of hip osteoarthritis. **(A)** Side view. **(B)** Front view. Physical therapy postural assessment reveals scapulae dorsally positioned on the thorax, extension of the shoulder and elbow joints, and hyperextension of the carpal joints (likely using the passive tension of flexor carpi ulnaris), all of which help maintain a passive energy-efficient standing position. The head and top line positions indicate offloading of the pelvic limbs, increasing weight through the thoracic limbs, and offloading of the right thoracic limb.

carpal joints relative to the contralateral limb and relative to each other. Abnormal standing angles or inequities from side to side can indicate primary injuries. For example, compare Figure 13.1 of a young, injury-free dog to Figure 13.2 of a geriatric patient. The low head carriage of the geriatric dog may indicate a primary injury in the cervical spine, thoracic limbs, or pelvic limbs and the increased right thoracic limb abduction and external rotation indicates partial weight bearing of the right thoracic limb. These postural findings could lead a therapist to further examine the cervical spine and right thoracic limb in detail. See Chapter 15 for an evaluation of the pelvic limbs.

Function

The purpose of the functional assessment is to critically analyze functional transitions that may indicate primary or secondary physical limitations. Functional assessment should, at a minimum, include lateral recumbence-to-sit, sternal-to-sit, sit-to-stand (Figure 13.3), and stand-to-sit. Additionally, it may include movement on curbs, ramps, stairs, and into and out of the client's primary vehicle. Movement abnormalities during each of these functional activities can provide important information regarding injury location. For example, refusal to assume and maintain a sternal recumbent position may indicate decreased glenohumeral joint flexion, hypermobility of the glenohumeral joint, or hypomobility of the elbow joint. Further evaluation is indicated, including muscle and bone palpation, passive range of motion, muscle flexibility, fascial mobility, clearing the spine, joint play and special tests of passive range of motion (osteokinematics), flexibility, joint play (arthrokinematics), and palpation and special tests of the thoracic limbs.

Clinical findings will lead to a problem list that will then lead to an assessment and treatment plan. For example, if thoracic limb lameness increases when a dog is walking downstairs, the therapist would further evaluate the shoulder joint. During the course of the evaluation the therapist may find decreased shoulder joint flexion, decreased cranial glide joint play of the glenohumeral joint, and pain on palpation of the biceps tendon—leading the therapist to hypothesize that biceps brachii is the primary tissue type injured. In best practice, these clinical findings would then lead to further diagnostics prior to development of a treatment plan.

Strength

Skeletal muscle provides strength to maintain posture and move joints while absorbing external forces and distributing loads (Hill, 1950). The purpose of strength testing is to determine baseline force-producing capacity of a particular skeletal muscle group and to analyze, in the problem list, if more strength is required to meet the client's goals for the patient. Prior to strength testing, quality of muscle bulk must be observed to determine whether atrophy is present. If atrophy is noted, limb circumference is measured with a Gulick tape measure taking particular note of the area measured to allow for

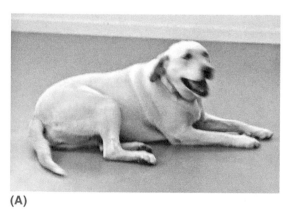

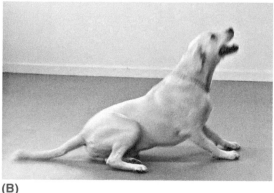

(A)   (B)

Figure 13.3 Functional assessment of the thoracic limb requires observation of the primary functional activities needed for daily living. Here a dog is attempting to stand by first **(A)** swinging the head in preparation for standing, and **(B)** struggling to extend the pelvic limbs and elevate the pelvis. As this geriatric patient with a medical diagnosis of hip osteoarthritis moves from sit to stand, the cranial placement of the feet and the extended position of the elbows indicate likely caudal shoulder muscle concentric contraction pulling the body to stand. This posturing decreases the need to actively flex the shoulder and elbow joints indicating possible arthrokinematic issues that need to be assessed in the evaluation. (Images derived from video.)

valid remeasurements, which are taken throughout the course of treatment to determine whether muscle bulk is returning within an expected time frame. Current evidence regarding validity and reliability of Gulick measurements is inconsistent. In one study, intra-rater reliability improved when the tester used the same device for repeat measurements (Baker *et al.*, 2010). Another study indicated that thigh circumference measurements with a Gulick may not produce a valid measurement (Bascunan *et al.*, 2016). Muscle strength must be tested separately as muscle circumference is not directly correlated with muscle torque (Stevens *et al.*, 2004). See Chapter 5 for a detailed description of Gulick measurements.

In human physical therapy, strength has been determined with a manual muscle test (MMT), a 1–5 rating scale requiring volitional open-chain muscle contraction through full joint range of motion (Perry *et al.*, 2004). In the canine patient, the traditional MMT cannot be used. To strength test the canine patient, closed-chain contractions must be observed in a functional standing position and the data captured in the canine manual muscle test (C-MMT) developed by this author. This test requires rigorous study

to determine validity and rater reliability. Three categories of strength are defined:

- <3/5 (poor): the muscle group is unable to provide the force required to maintain a static standing position;
- 3/5 (fair): the muscle group is able to provide the force required to maintain a static standing position;
- 3+/5 (good): the muscle group is able to provide more force than is required to maintain a static standing position.

For C-MMT strength testing, a stifle-height box or step is required. The strength test is initiated from the least strenuous testing position to the most strenuous testing position. To complete the test (Figure 13.4), the dog is positioned in a standing position and the limb opposite the testing limb is lifted into a non-weight-bearing position; the therapist observes the standing limb. If the limb is unable to maintain the position, as observed by increased dorsal glide of the scapula (weakness of serratus ventralis), increased shoulder flexion (weakness of biceps and supraspinatus), increased elbow flexion (weakness of triceps), increased carpal extension

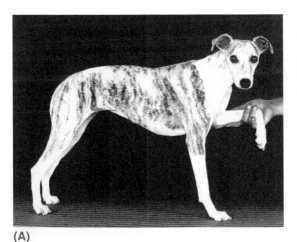
(A)

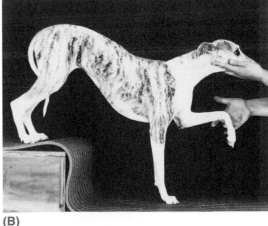
(B)

Figure 13.4 Canine manual muscle testing allows the therapist to determine baseline isometric strength in a functional standing position. (**A**) The patient is placed in a standing position and the contralateral limb is lifted into a non-weight-bearing position. The therapist observes changes in the position of the scapula on the thorax and changes in the joint angle as the contralateral limb is lifted. Inability to maintain scapular and joint angles indicates a strength score of <3/5. The ability to maintain the position requires further testing. (**B**) The patient is placed in a standing position with the pelvic limbs on a box increasing weight bearing through the thoracic limbs. The contralateral limb is lifted into a non-weight-bearing position. The therapist observes changes in the position of the scapula on the thorax and changes in the joint angle as the contralateral limb is lifted. Inability to maintain scapular position and joint angles indicates a strength score of 3/5. Ability to maintain the position indicates a strength score of 3+/5.

(weakness of carpal flexors), or any combination of these or other signs of weakness, the strength score is <3/5 (poor). The test is then completed on the contralateral limb. If the patient is able to maintain the position without compensation on either of the thoracic limbs, the strength score is at least 3/5 (fair). The limb must then be tested in a more strenuous position with the patient's pelvic limbs placed on the box, thus increasing the weight, and therefore the force the muscles must produce, into the thoracic limbs. With the pelvic limbs on the box, the thoracic limb test is repeated with the therapist observing whether the thoracic limb is able to maintain the standing position with the pelvic limbs on the box. If the patient is unable to maintain the position the strength score is 3/5 (fair). If the patient is able to maintain the position the strength score is 3+/5 (good). When completing the C-MMT, attention must be given to musculoskeletal issues that may interfere with the test such as facet joint dysfunction, which would prevent the patient from comfortably placing the pelvic limbs on the box.

More objective strength test scores may be obtained with surface electrode electromyography (EMG). Clinical limitations include time constraints, the need to shave each muscle group, and the paucity of research directly correlating canine EMG measures and muscle force production. Further studies are required to develop canine objective strength measures that are valid and reliable.

Gait

Gait evaluation is used to examine lameness and movement quality. Gross lameness and decreased weight bearing can commonly be seen subjectively. During gait analysis, movement quality includes measurements of the gait cycle phases such as swing phase and stance phase. Observational data from gait evaluation guides the therapist to in-depth evaluation of specific areas. For example, observation of a right thoracic limb decreased stance phase may lead the therapist to a detailed assessment of the right thoracic limb, cervical spine, and thoracolumbar spine. Historically, it was thought that subjective capture of low-grade lameness may improve with the use of slow motion cameras but recent evidence suggests slow motion capture compared with real-time video does not improve the accuracy or consistency of subjective gait analysis (Lane *et al.*, 2015). Currently, the gold standard for objective measurements of gait analysis is the force plate (Voss *et al.*, 2007) but novel devices such as inertial sensors may be able to provide alternative and more real world objective measures of gait and movement (Duerr *et al.*, 2016). See Chapter 2 for gait analysis.

Passive range of motion

Evaluation of passive range of motion (PROM) guides a therapist to a deeper understanding of a patient's osteokinematic baseline. PROM evaluation includes objective goniometric measurements and subjective descriptions of the *end-feel* (see Chapter 6). The objective goniometric measurement determines if the range of motion is normal, and, if not, the subjective end-feel determines which tissue is limiting the full range of motion. Research has shown that objective goniometric measurements are both valid and reliable when tested with a universal goniometer (Jaegger *et al.*, 2002). Studies comparing universal goniometers with electronic goniometers currently on the market also indicate the universal goniometer to be superior to the electronic goniometer in reliability (Thomas *et al.*, 2006).

Subjective descriptions of tissues that may limit range of motion include effusion (boggy end-feel), cartilage (crepitus), joint capsule (hard capsular end-feel), ligament (hard ligamentous end-feel), tendon (elastic end-feel), and meniscus (springy or click end-feel). For the highest quality goniometric objective measurement, the nonaffected side is measured first. Of tremendous importance during range of motion testing is ensuring all muscles surrounding the joint are on slack so a valid joint osteokinematic measurement can be obtained. In general, if testing flexion, placing the proximal and distal joints into a flexed position will place the multi-joint muscles on slack. If testing extension, placing the proximal and distal joints into an extended position will improve PROM testing. It is important to note that there are ranges of motion where one-joint muscles cannot be placed on slack and this may influence the quantity of goniometric motion and quality of end-feel; this is the case with glenohumeral joint flexion stretching the supraspinatus, and glenohumeral joint abduction stretching the subscapularis. With the multi-joint muscles on slack, the joint is gently moved into the testing range of motion and overpressure is applied to assess for pain, restriction, or hypermobility. Overpressure should not be applied to a joint that is hypermobile or has an empty (painful) end-feel. When end range is determined, the goniometer is placed over the joint with the stationary arm on the proximal bony landmark, the point of rotation over the joint, and the movable arm on the distal bony landmark (Figure 13.5). The goniometric measurement is recorded and the subjective end-feel is noted.

An increase or decrease in PROM from the nonaffected side to the affected side, and from one session to the next, leads a therapist to further assess the affected joint. For example, a limitation in goniometric elbow flexion with a hard capsular end-feel may lead the therapist to carefully assess joint play to determine if the articular surfaces, joint capsule, or both are causing the limitation. The treatment for hypomobile joints generally includes joint mobilization manual therapy. Once completed, the joint is remeasured to determine whether the treatment improved the joint range of motion. An absence of improvement in range of motion in a session and from one session to the next will lead a therapist to reassess the cause of the restriction and change their treatment plan accordingly. See Chapter 6 for detailed information on PROM measurements.

Flexibility

Objective evaluation of flexibility allows the therapist to determine baseline passive muscle extensibility. To test flexibility, the patient assumes a relaxed side lying position. Slowly, the therapist guides the limb into the stretched position, stabilizing the origin of the muscle and moving the insertion of the muscle in the direction opposite to the concentric action of the muscle. As the therapist passively lengthens the muscle, they evaluate the subjective quality and quantity of extensibility throughout the available range of motion. Careful consideration is given to multi-joint muscles, as they require precise hand placement to stabilize the origin or insertion of the

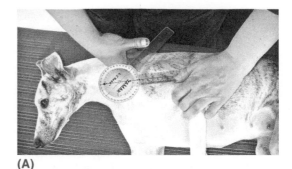

(A)

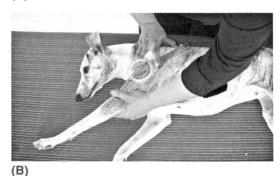

(B)

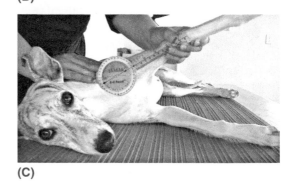

(C)

Figure 13.5   (**A**) When completing the goniometric measurement for flexion of the glenohumeral joint, the therapist must keep in mind that range of motion limitations may be due to joint capsule involvement, joint play restrictions, or, due to the origin and insertion of the supraspinatus, musculotendinous involvement. (**B**) When completing the goniometric measurement for glenohumeral joint extension, the therapist carefully stabilizes the scapula to ensure assessment of joint end-feel. Without stabilization, the scapula glides on the thorax creating a false-positive hypermobility measurement. (**C**) When completing the goniometric measurement for glenohumeral joint abduction, the therapist carefully stabilizes the scapula against the thorax to prevent a false-positive hypermobility measurement. The therapist also is careful to prevent unintentional external rotation of the joint, which may involve the subscapularis tendon.

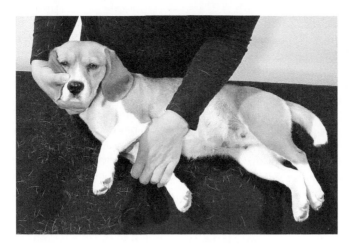

Figure 13.6 Passive stretch assessment of the brachiocephalicus requires stretching the distal insertion of the muscle with the elbow extended and the shoulder flexed. This position is then maintained or stabilized, allowing the therapist to assess the quality and amount of muscle extensibility as the cervical spine is guided into side bending and the atlanto-occipital joint is moved into flexion.

Table 13.1   Muscle open-chain concentric actions from an anatomically neutral position

Muscle	Muscle open-chain actions
Rhomboids	Scapular dorsal glide
Trapezius, cranial head	Scapular dorsocranial glide
Trapezius, caudal head	Scapular dorsocaudal glide
Omotransversarius	Scapular cranial glide + cervical spine side bending
Subscapularis	Glenohumeral adduction
Serratus ventralis, cranial fibers	Scapular ventrocranial glide
Serratus ventralis, caudal fibers	Scapular ventrocaudal glide
Supraspinatus	Glenohumeral extension
Infraspinatus	Glenohumeral abduction + external rotation
Biceps brachii	Glenohumeral extension + elbow flexion
Brachiocephalicus	Cervical spine side bending + glenohumeral extension
Deltoids	Glenohumeral flexion + abduction
Latissimus dorsi	Glenohumeral flexion + adduction + internal rotation
Superficial pectoral	Glenohumeral adduction
Deep pectoral	Glenohumeral flexion + adduction + internal rotation
Teres major	Glenohumeral flexion + adduction + internal rotation
Triceps	Elbow extension + shoulder flexion
Brachialis	Elbow flexion
Carpal and digital flexor muscle group	Carpal flexion + digit flexion
Carpal and digital extensor muscle group	Carpal extension + digit extension

muscle while manually moving multiple joints to place the muscle on stretch. For example, to stretch the brachiocephalicus, the therapist places the dog in lateral recumbency, stabilizes the insertion of the muscle by flexing the shoulder of the down limb, and, maintaining this position, stretches the muscle by placing the cervical spine in lateral flexion and atlanto-occipital joint flexion (Figure 13.6). Outcomes from flexibility testing—such as decreased flexibility and pain during the flexibility test—provide the therapist with information about specific muscle primary injuries as well as secondary compensatory issues. Thorough objective assessment of thoracic limb muscle flexibility includes testing all the muscles listed in Table 13.1.

Palpation

Palpation provides the therapist with a subjective evaluation of specific tissues including bone, muscle, fascia, and ligaments. By manually challenging the tissues, palpation assessment provides the therapist with information regarding the specific tissue type and location of edema, heat, pain, tone, and tightness. Palpation findings help specify the anatomic structure and chronicity of a primary or secondary orthopedic injury. For example, during the evaluation of the thoracic limb, palpation assessment of the latissimus dorsi requires pressing the fingertips into the muscle tissue along the ventral boarder of the muscle from origin to insertion and through the muscle belly from the proximal caudal border of the humerus into the thoracodorsal fascia (Figure 13.7). A positive response to palpation, including the subjective feeling of edema, heat, and tone as well as visible pain or muscle spasm, leads the therapist to further assess the scapulothoracic and glenohumeral joints and thoracolumbar areas. Thorough objective palpation includes all joints, muscles (Table 13.1), and bony landmarks of the thoracic limb.

Clear the spine

Clearing the spine is required before initiating joint play examination as it is unknown at this time if, in the canine model, mobilizing the facet joints of the spine has a negative impact on the disk or the nerve roots. The purpose of clearing the spine is to capture significant pain or neurological signs that would contraindicate joint play tests. Clearing the spine is initiated with the dog in standing; the conscious proprioception test is completed (see Chapter 17). If the patient displays delayed or absent conscious proprioception reactions, this is noted in the objective portion of the evaluation, and joint play tests are not completed. Next, active range of motion of the spine is completed. If during the course of active range of motion the patient demonstrates significant pain, this is noted in the evaluation, and joint play tests are not completed.

Joint play

The purpose of joint play assessments of the thoracic limb is to determine arthrokinematic quality and quantity and joint capsule integrity. By stabilizing one side of the joint and mobilizing the other, a therapist feels for abnormal joint surface qualities such as crepitus, a decreased quantity of bone-on-bone movement, and joint capsule hyper- or hypomobility that may be affecting osteokinematic range of motion. For example, decreased cranial glide of the humeral head in the glenoid fossa may be limiting shoulder joint flexion (Figure 13.8). The therapist must determine if this limitation

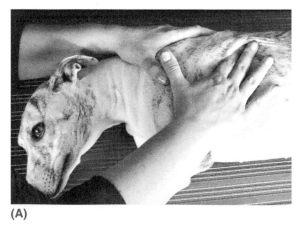

(A)

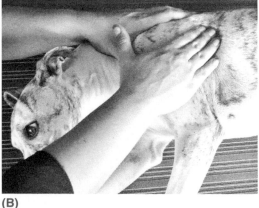

(B)

Figure 13.7   **(A)** Manual palpation of the latissimus dorsi muscle challenges the muscle tissues along the ventral border of the muscle from origin to insertion, feeling for tissue changes including edema, heat, tone, pain, and muscle spasm. **(B)** Manual palpation of the latissimus dorsi also challenges tissues in the central portion of the muscle belly, paying particular attention to areas of pain and tightness that may indicate trigger points.

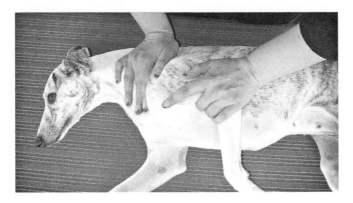

Figure 13.8   If, during the course of range of motion assessment, a restriction in glenohumeral joint flexion is noted, the therapist will assess joint glides. Assessment of the cranial glide requires stabilizing the scapula then gliding the head of the humerus cranially, the arthrokinematic movement associated with glenohumeral joint flexion. If a restriction is noted during joint play, the therapist carefully captures manual assessment data including joint surface quality and end-feel, the outcomes of which will guide the treatment plan.

is due to joint surface abnormalities, joint capsule restrictions, or musculotendinous restrictions of the biceps or supraspinatus. Determination of joint play requires extensive manual therapy training as subjective capture of joint movement quality and quantity is a learned skill and incorrect application of manual forces through a joint can be injurious. See Chapter 6 for further discussion of joint play techniques.

Special tests

Special tests for the thoracic limb consist primarily of ligament stress tests to determine baseline joint stability. They include the medial shoulder instability test, elbow varus and valgus stress tests, and carpal varus and valgus stress tests. All tests are completed in a closed-pack position with the ligaments positioned for highest tensile resistance.

Development of the rehabilitation assessment

At completion of evaluation, the problem list is developed by describing the location, tissue type, and chronicity of each clinical finding. Location is described as precisely as possible in specific anatomic terms so that a second therapist could immediately locate the injury. Tissue type is delineated in very clear terms

differentiating muscle belly, musculotendinous junction, tendon, ligament, joint capsule, cartilage, or bone. The chronicity of injury must be determined for each impairment location and is defined as acute, subacute, or chronic.

At completion of the problem list, the therapist critically analyzes the list and prioritizes the problems in descending order from the most painful tissues to primary tissues to compensatory tissues. The outcome of this critical analysis leads the therapist to write an assessment, the hypothesis that supports all of the problems on the list. For example, a primary diagnosis may be "left glenohumeral joint osteochondritis dissecans (OCD) lesion with surgical excision," and the rehabilitation problem list may be "left glenohumeral joint acute pain due to postoperative edema with compensatory pain in left biceps brachii at musculotendinous junction, left latissimus dorsi decreased flexibility, and palpation pain of bilateral paraspinals T6-L2." Analysis of the problem list will often reveal complex iterations of location, tissue type, and acuity, requiring the therapist to carefully consider treatment options for the most efficacious interventions.

Development of the treatment plan

Using the rehabilitation problem list as the template, a treatment plan is developed to meet the client's goals for the patient. Each treatment in the care plan includes intensity, frequency, and duration, and dosing parameters that are based on anatomic, physiological, and biomechanical principles. The therapist must consider the need to modify treatment parameters throughout the plan of care since the location, tissue type, and acuity of the injury has a profound impact on intensity, frequency, and duration of all types of treatment interventions.

Types of treatment interventions

Treatment interventions can be divided into three categories: modalities, manual techniques, and therapeutic exercise.

Modalities are the application of technologies that affect cellular physiology in well-defined ways to diminish pain, promote soft tissue healing, improve muscle extensibility, and facilitate muscle strengthening. See Chapter 7 for details.

Manual techniques are the application of hands-on treatments that mechanically and physiologically affect tissues to decrease pain, increase circulation, reduce swelling, increase soft tissue extensibility, and normalize joint mobility. Although modalities can generally be safely performed with minimal education, the application of manual treatments requires extensive training, as incorrect application of mechanical forces through soft tissue can be detrimental. See Chapter 6 for details.

Therapeutic exercise is the application of precise movements to recruit specific skeletal muscles in functional ways and includes balance, strength, and endurance exercises. Proper application of therapeutic exercise requires a thorough understanding of muscle origins and insertions, type of muscle contractions, muscle fiber type, motor recruitment, and motor timing. For example, the exercises demonstrated in Figure 13.9 are specific for the subscapularis and superficial pectoralis, two muscles that provide dynamic stability to the medial joint line of patients diagnosed with medial shoulder instability. See Chapter 8 for details. Application of exercises without consideration of muscle anatomy and physiology can, at minimum, prevent return of function, and, at worst, exacerbate an underlying condition.

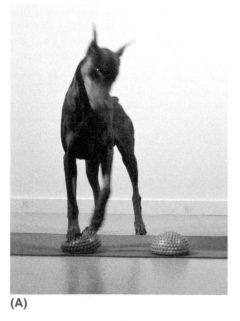 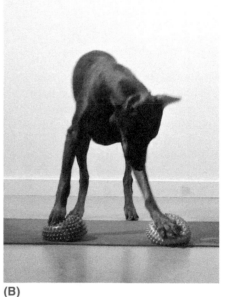

(A)   **(B)**

Figure 13.9   **(A, B)** Therapeutic exercise planning takes into consideration the origin and insertion of the muscle, the type of muscle contraction required, and the intensity, frequency, and duration of the exercise. This exercise demonstrates concentric superficial pectoral and subscapularis contraction of the ipsilateral limb and eccentric contraction of the same muscles of the contralateral limb. This exercise may be appropriate for the strengthening (chronic) phase of treatment for medial shoulder instability. (Images derived from video.)

Common injuries by tissue type

There are five types of tissues that may sustain injury and can be treated by the therapist: muscle/tendon, ligament, intra-articular structures (meniscus and cartilage), joint capsule, and bone. A comprehensive understanding of the physiological mechanisms of healing for each tissue must be incorporated into the treatment plan, allowing the therapist to determine whether the course of healing is following a normal physiological path or if reassessment and change in treatment plan are required (see Chapter 3 for more details). Table 13.2 provides an outline of treatments per tissue type, and Table 13.3 an outline of treatment guidelines.

Muscle injuries

Muscle is comprised of a contractile component—the muscle fibers—and an elastic component consisting of connective tissues and tendon. When the muscle voluntarily contracts, the connective tissues absorb and dissipate the energy of the contraction allowing for smooth and supple movement (Nordin & Frankel, 1989). When the muscle passively elongates, the elastic components elongate first followed by the musculotendinous junction (Wright *et al.*, 1982). Understanding these mechanical properties of muscle assists a therapist in determining if one or both of the muscle components is involved in the injury. Treatment is initiated on the correct muscular component(s) with the treatment plan including rehabilitation of the entire muscle and all compensatory issues related to the primary injury.

Three types of muscle injuries are commonly seen—surgical injuries, strain injuries (i.e., tendinitis), and chronic extensibility injuries (i.e., tendinosis). Surgical incisions may cause damage to the contractile component or the elastic component of the muscle. Determining which tissue is involved requires an anatomic understanding of the surgery. Acute treatment of surgical incisions includes modalities and soft tissue retrograde massage to decrease edema. Subacute treatment includes modalities to increase circulation and promote tissue healing followed by scar massage to correctly align collagen fibers. Chronic treatment requires returning the soft tissues to their previous strength while addressing compensatory issues related to the primary injury (Table 13.3).

External injuries to muscles in the form of loads exceeding the inherent force of the muscle causing strain injuries can affect the contractile or elastic components. Differentiating the components requires an assessment of active muscle contraction in descending order of muscle tension produced (Norkin & Levange, 1983), concentrically, isometrically, and eccentrically, with observation of joint position that may place the elastic components on stretch. For example, assessment of possible biceps injury may test a foot shake (concentric), single limb

Table 13.2 Common thoracic limb diagnoses per tissue type

Diagnosis	Primary injury tissue type
Biceps tendinopathy	Muscle, elastic, and/or contractile components
Carpal hyperextension	Ligament
	Muscle, elastic, and/or contractile components
Carpal bone subluxation	Ligament
Fragmented coronoid process (FCP)	Bone
	Cartilage
	Joint capsule
	Muscle, elastic, and/or contractile components
Infraspinatus contracture	Muscle, elastic, and/or contractile components
Medial shoulder syndrome	Ligament, grade I, II, or III
	Muscle, elastic, and/or contractile components
Osteochondrosis dessicans (OCD)	Cartilage
Supraspinatus tendinopathy	Muscle, elastic, and/or contractile components
Teres major strain	Muscle, elastic, and/or contractile components
Ununited anconeal process (UAP)	Bone
	Cartilage
	Joint capsule
	Muscle, elastic, and/or contractile components

Table 13.3   Primary tissues injuries and treatments by acuity

Type of tissue	Acuity	Common problem list	Possible treatments
Muscle contractile components	Acute	1. Pain due to inflammation 2. Decreased extensibility 3. Decreased strength	1. Modalities 2. Modalities and stretching 3. Pain-free isometric strengthening
	Subacute	1. Pain due to tissue injury 2. Decreased extensibility 3. Decreased strength	1. Modalities 2. Modalities and stretching 3. Pain-free concentric strengthening
	Chronic	1. Decreased extensibility 2. Decreased strength	1. Modalities and stretching 2. Eccentric strengthening
Muscle elastic components	Acute	1. Pain due to inflammation 2. Decreased extensibility	1. Modalities 2. Modalities, stretching, and manual therapy
	Subacute	1. Pain due to tissue injury 2. Decreased extensibility	1. Modalities 2. Modalities, stretching, and manual therapy
	Chronic	1. Decreased extensibility	1. Modalities, stretching, and manual therapy
Ligament, grades I and II	Acute	1. Pain due to inflammation 2. Joint instability	1. Modalities 2. Stabilization with bracing and pain-free isometric muscular stabilization
	Subacute	1. Pain due to inflammation 2. Joint instability	1. Modalities 2. Stabilization with bracing and pain-free concentric/eccentric muscular stabilization
	Chronic	1. Joint instability	1. Grade I – concentric/eccentric muscular stabilization 2. Grade II – bracing and concentric/eccentric muscular stabilization
Ligament, grade III	Acute	1. Pain due to inflammation 2. Joint instability	1. Modalities 2. Stabilization with bracing and isometric muscular stabilization
	Subacute	1. Pain due to inflammation 2. Joint instability	1. Modalities 2. Stabilization with bracing and muscular stabilization
	Chronic	1. Joint Instability	1. Stabilization with bracing and muscular stabilization
Joint capsule	Acute	1. Pain due to inflammation 2. Joint hypomobility[1]	1. Modalities and joint mobilizations 2. Joint mobilizations
	Subacute	1. Joint hypomobility	1. Modalities and joint mobilizations
	Chronic	1. Joint hypomobility	1. Modalities and joint mobilizations
Intra-articular cartilage	Acute	1. Pain due to inflammation 2. Joint hypomobility	1. Modalities and joint mobilizations 2. Joint mobilizations including compression
	Subacute	1. Joint hypomobility	1. Modalities and joint mobilizations
	Chronic	1. Joint hypomobility	1. Modalities and joint mobilizations
Peripheral nerves	Acute	1. Pain due to inflammation and nerve damage 2. Atrophy prevention	1. Modalities 2. Modalities including electrical stimulation
	Subacute	1. Pain due to nerve damage 2. Atrophy Prevention	1. Modalities 2. Modalities including electrical stimulation
	Chronic	1. Decreased connective tissue extensibility 2. Weakness	1. Modalities and stretching 2. Therapeutic exercise

[1] For joint hypermobility see "Ligament."

stance (isometric), and push-up (eccentric) to observe if increasing muscle tension increases pain. Close observation of pain response during this test is essential. Passive muscle extensibility is tested as it helps differentiate whether contractile or elastic components are painful. For example, beginning the biceps stretch with the gleno-humeral joint in neutral and very slowly stretch-ing the biceps allows the therapist to note quality of extensibility and onset of pain response. Further assessment with palpation is then needed to determine the precise location of injury.

Treatment of strain injuries must follow a pre-cise course of treatment to promote tissue healing and prevent muscle cells from adaptive shorten-ing, predisposing the patient to chronic tendino-sis injuries. Acute injuries require immediate resolution of edema with modalities and pain-free active contractions to prevent collagen mis-alignment and disuse atrophy. The subacute phase of healing requires pain-free increases in strength training intensity while preventing

re-exacerbation of the primary injury, which is best achieved with concentric contractions. The chronic phase of healing demands return of strength using eccentric contractions, which promote tis-sue extensibility while producing the highest loads through the muscle tissues (Verrall et al., 2011). Throughout the course of treatment, reas-sessment is required to determine whether tissues are following a normal course of healing. Patients that do not follow a normal course of healing are reassessed to determine the correct rehabilitation diagnosis and/or the treatment plan is modified to promote healing and to avoid re-exacerbation.

The underlying mechanism of chronic mus-cle extensibility injuries is adaptive cellular changes in both contractile and elastic fibers that histologically have little or no evidence of inflammation (Khan et al., 1999). Unlike tend-initis injuries, where the acute treatment regime goal is to decrease inflammation, treatment of chronic adaptive shortening requires instigating an inflammatory response to coax the tissues

---

Case Study 13.1 Acute-on-chronic biceps tendinopathy

Signalment: 10-y.o. F/S Labrador Retriever.

Diagnosis: Radiographic right glenohumeral joint OA.

Subjective findings: Acute onset of right thoracic limb (RTL) head-bobbing lameness 3/5, significantly worse upon waking, improves throughout the day, but worse after play and 30-minute walks. Five-year history of intermittent RTL lameness.

Objective findings: Posture: right scapula craniodorsal positioning on thorax.

Function: refusal to maintain sternal position, lameness increases down stairs.

Strength: <3/5 (poor) strength RTL isometric contraction.

Gait: RTL decreased stride length end of stance phase.

Palpation: heat and pain on medial glenohumeral joint line, discomfort on supraspinatus muscle belly, pain at origin of biceps brachii tendon, pain and spasm in latissimus dorsi and teres major.

Range of motion: glenohumeral joint flexion 70 degrees with empty end-feel, extension 150 degrees with hard capsular end-feel, abduction 40 degrees with hard capsular end-feel.

Flexibility: biceps decreased flexibility and pain, supraspinatus decreased flexibility, omotransversarius decreased flexibility.

Joint play: 2/6 cranial glide of humerus on glenoid fossa.

Assessment: From a rehabilitation perspective, the primary limiting factors to highest level of function include right biceps brachii pain and decreased flexibility with compensatory supraspinatus muscle overuse and shortening. Chronicity of injury leads therapist to suspect this is an acute-on-chronic biceps tendinopathy with adaptive shortening of the cranial joint capsule exacerbating the underlying gleno-humeral joint OA with compensatory overuse pain and tightness in the supraspinatus, latissimus dorsi, and teres major.

Plan of care:
Acute phase:

(1) Decrease edema: laser 4.0 J/cm² to target tis-sues including glenohumeral joint and biceps tendon.

(2) Decrease acute pain: TENS 5 Hz, 160 μs pulse width, 20 minutes, nerve roots of musculocu-taneous nerve (C6, C7, C8).

(3) Begin reversal of adaptive shortening of gleno-humeral joint capsule: grade I–IV cranial joint glides.

(4) Begin reversal of decreased extensibility of muscle tissue: soft tissue mobilization and stretching.

(5) Implement home exercise program: slow walking daily for 10 minutes followed by biceps and supraspinatus pain-free stretches held for 30 seconds (Table 13.3).

into a healing phase that allows the therapist to complete soft tissue work, including cross-friction massage and stretching, thus modifying adaptively shortened tissues. As the tissues remodel, gentle strengthening, motor timing (the sequencing of a type of muscle contraction), and motor control of exercises (the graded intensity of a muscle contraction) are initiated to return the muscle to pain-free functional contractions. Completion of the healing phase of treatment includes eccentric strengthening exercises to return the muscle to full strength (Verrall *et al.*, 2011) (Table 13.3).

Ligament and joint capsule injuries

Ligaments are comprised of nonextensible parallel collagenous fibers with minimal vascular supply. Their purpose is to stabilize joints, preventing excessive motion. When the external forces on a ligament exceed the physiological load, fiber failure occurs in the form of fiber disruption. Grade I ligament injuries are microtears that will present as pain without joint instability. Grade II tears produce severe pain and minor to moderate joint instability. Grade III tears are severely painful at onset with decreasing pain following the injury and gross joint instability (Nordin & Frankel, 1989). The joint instability of grade II and III tears allows for increased displacement of the joint surfaces causing further ligament fiber disruption, excessive pressure to the joint capsule, increased force on tendons, and abnormally high stresses on articular cartilage. In the canine model this has been shown to modify forces through the joint structures and cause deterioration of articular cartilage (Marshall & Olsson, 1971).

Multiple factors affect the biomechanical properties of ligaments including aging, pregnancy and the postpartum period, mobilization, and immobilization. These factors are considered as they impact the course of treatment and anticipated physiological outcomes. Aging causes a decrease in tensile strength of the ligament due to declining collagen content, placing older patients at higher risk for ligament injuries. Overall body condition and fitness should meet or exceed the physical activities of patients. This is particularly true in canine athletes and older patients that may be completing activities that exceed the abilities

of their muscles to protect the joints, placing the stabilizing ligaments at risk for injury. Pregnancy and the postpartum period see a release of relaxin, which increases the distensibility of ligaments (Goldsmith *et al.*, 1994). In the dog, mobilization and exercise has been shown to increase the tensile strength of ligaments (Montgomery, 1989) while, in the primate model, immobilization for 8 weeks was found to decrease the tensile strength of ligaments by up to 39%. The same study showed that a reconditioning program of 12 months was required to reach pre-immobilization tensile strength (Noyes, 1977). Biomechanical properties of the ligament and factors affecting ligament integrity are considered when creating a treatment plan, including fiber alignment for optimal force resistance and decreased vascularity. Treatment plans first consider the grade of ligament rupture. Conservative nonsurgical approach of ligament sprains greater than grade I require external stabilization of the joint with bracing such as a hobble-type support for the glenohumeral joint with medial shoulder instability. The course of treatment includes edema management with modalities and manual therapy in the acute phases followed by a graded return of strength in the muscles supporting the hypermobile joint, such as subscapularis and superficial pectoral strengthening for medial shoulder instability (Table 13.3).

Intra-articular injuries

Articular cartilage, by virtue of its viscoelastic characteristics, distributes loads through the joint and allows for smooth arthrokinematics. In canine subjects, exercise groups (running for 1 hour at 15% incline for 5 days per week for 15 weeks) showed an increase in stifle cartilage thickness compared with crated controls (Kiviranta *et al.*, 1988). Lubrication is diminished with injury to the articular cartilage, as stress and strain forces are not distributed evenly during loading. Canine studies have shown that immobilization-induced atrophy of cartilage does not improve after 50 weeks of activity resumption (Kiviranta *et al.*, 1994; Haapala *et al.*, 1999). Impairment of force distribution causes compensatory changes in osteokinematic movement. Therefore any impairment of articular cartilage can have a deleterious

Case Study 13.2   T8 facet joint and rib dysfunction

Signalment: 3-y.o. F/I Border Collie, training for national agility team. Began knocking bars in training 3 weeks ago. No qualifying runs three weekends in a row. Consistently completes a physical therapy conditioning program.

Diagnosis: Thoracic back pain. Thoracolumbar and coxofemoral radiographs negative.

Objective findings: Palpation: from T6 to wings of the ilium, muscle spasm in spinalis and longissimus; right iliocostalis lumborum muscle spasm and pain; thoracic muscle spasms during extension active range of motion; T8–T9 dorsoventral glide joint play restriction 2/6; right rib 8 and 9 dorsoventral glide restriction with discomfort; right latissimus dorsi and serratus ventralis decreased flexibility.

Assessment: Precipitous decline in jump quality of unknown etiology beginning 3 weeks ago. Possible T8–T9 facet joint hypomobility and rib dysfunction causing decreased thoracic active range of motion into extension and soft tissue restrictions which may be limiting jumping quality.

Plan of care:
Acute phase:

(1)   Normalize mobility of T8–T9 facet joint and ribs: grade III and IV mobilizations to normalize joint arthrokinematics.
(2)   Normalize flexibility of latissimus dorsi and serratus ventralis: laser 4 W, 8 J/cm² to muscles from origin to insertion followed by stretching, hold 30 seconds, repeat × 2
(3)   Spine mobility home exercise program (HEP): concentric spine extensors exercise to maintain facet and rib mobility, 20 repetitions, twice daily; eccentric latissimus dorsi exercises to

promote natural deceleration of glenohumeral joint extension required for jumping, 10 repetition, twice daily; stretch latissimus dorsi and serratus ventralis, one repetition, hold 30 seconds, twice daily.
(4)   Activity restriction: no agility training, in particular jumping, until follow-up appointment in 1 week.

Subacute phase: Reassess and modify plan of care as needed. If facet and rib mobility remain normalized, begin subacute treatment. If joint mobility is not normalized, treat with joint mobilizations again and reassess HEP.

(1)   Strength training HEP: continue concentric spine extension exercises adding rotation and side bending with spine extension, 20 repetitions, twice daily; eccentric latissimus dorsi exercises with spine in extended position to prepare for jump training, 20 repetitions, twice daily; stretch latissimus dorsi and serratus ventralis, one repetition, hold 30 seconds, twice daily.
(2)   Activity restriction: resume agility training, low jump height, until follow-up appointment in 1 week.

Chronic phase: Reassess and modify plan of care as needed. If joint mobility remains normalized begin chronic treatment.

(1)   Resume physical therapy-based conditioning program continuing eccentric latissimus dorsi exercises with spine extended.
(2)   Educate client to palpate for paraspinal pain, which may indicate a joint mobility issue and need for follow-up treatment.
(3)   Activity restriction: none, resume agility training without restriction.

effect on all aspects of function and movement. Treatment plans should consider the biomechanical properties of cartilage including the need for manual compression forces to normalize the inherent viscoelasticity of remaining healthy cartilage (Kiviranta *et al.*, 1987) and the limited capacity for regeneration of damaged cells. Treatment plans should also consider the spectrum of musculoskeletal compensatory changes related to arthrokinematic anomalies (Table 13.3).

Peripheral nerve injuries

Each component of peripheral nerves—nerve fibers, connective tissues, and vascular structures—has specific biomechanical properties that are considered when developing a treatment plan for peripheral nerve injury. Axons alone are very vulnerable to compression and stretching injuries (Rydevik & Nordborg, 1980). Three layers of connective tissues, the endoneurium, perineurium, and epineurium, provide resistance to compression and stretch. The thickness of connective tissue can increase or decrease along a single nerve (Topp & Boyd, 2012). For example, where a nerve passes over bone the connective tissues may be thicker, providing a measure of protection.

Treatment of peripheral nerve injuries takes into consideration the cause of the injury—compression, stretching, or vascular compromise. Compression injuries can cause numbness, pain, and muscle weakness (Sunderland, 1978). Stretching injuries can cause severe functional deficits as axons rupture before connective tissues can resist the stretch force (Lundborg & Rydevik, 1973). Such functional deficits can be seen in diagnoses such as brachial plexus avulsions. Vascular injuries are often due to insult to the highly vascular connective tissues resulting in interstitial pressure changes causing axon damage (Spencer *et al.*, 1975). The treatment of peripheral nerves addresses the cause of the injury and is chosen to best promote the body's natural healing process for the highest level of functional return. Acute treatment emphasizes edema control, pain management, and atrophy prevention. Subacute treatment uses modalities to promote nerve healing while beginning pain-free functional strengthening to prevent atrophy and promote nerve healing. Chronic-phase treatment emphasizes continued modalities for nerve healing as well as therapeutic exercises to return to the highest level of function. Care is taken to ensure pain management is provided throughout the course of treatment as healing nerves often temporarily increase nerve pain and sensory anomalies (Table 13.3).

Treatment efficacy and modifications

Throughout the treatment plan, reassessment of treatment efficacy is completed and treatment interventions modified as needed. Because each tissue follows a physiological process and timeframe for healing, these parameters are used as guidelines to determine treatment effectiveness. Healing that appears to be too rapid may be a transition from the subacute to chronic phase of healing, and not true physiological healing. Healing that takes longer than the natural timeframe may indicate incorrect rehabilitation diagnosis, inaccu-

rate application of modalities, misuse of manual techniques, or incorrect therapeutic exercise prescription. Complete tissue healing should occur within a normal physiological time frame and is followed by a home health maintenance program to maintain strength, balance, and endurance gained in the rehabilitation process.

Treatment efficacy is a response to thorough evaluation, development of the problem list, and implementation of the treatment plan. The rehabilitation process requires continual reassessment to determine whether progress is being made within a normal physiological timeframe. Because of the myriad internal and external factors affecting the healing process, including but not limited to response to medication, diet, comorbidities, home environment, activity restriction, or home exercise compliance, reassessment is required at each follow-up visit to clarify whether new limitations should be added to the problem list and to determine whether the current plan of care requires modification. After reassessment and treatment plan modifications, portions of treatments such as the application of modalities, therapeutic exercises, and stretching can be delegated to support staff. Because of the need for continual reassessment, protocols, as developed by the team of veterinary specialists including a physical therapist, should be used as treatment guidelines and not as treatment plans. Using a problem-based, critical thinking process throughout the rehabilitation plan of care will ensure the most efficacious outcomes.

Webliography

World Association for Laser Therapy (WALT). 2010. *Dosage Recommendations*. Dose table 780–860nm for low level laser therapy WALT 2010. https://waltza. co.za/wp-content/uploads/2012/08/Dose_ table_780-860nm_for_Low_Level_Laser_Therapy_ WALT-2010.pdf (accessed November 2017).

References

Baker, S. G., Roush, J. K., Unis, M. D. & Wodiske, T. 2011. Comparison of four commercial devices to measure limb circumference in dogs. *Vet Comp Orthop Traumatol*, 23(6), 406–410.

Bascunan, A. L., Kieves, N., Goh, C., Hart, J. & Regier, P. 2016. Evaluation of factors influencing thigh circumference measurement in dogs. *Vet Evidence*, 1(2), 1–12.

Duerr, F. M., Pauls, A., Kawcak, C., Haussler, K., Bertocci, G., Moorman, V. & King, M. 2016. Evaluation of inertial measurement units as a novel method for kinematic gait evaluation in dogs. *Vet Comp Orthop Traumatol*, 29(6), 475–483.

Goldsmith, L. T., Lust, G. & Steinetz, B. G. 1994. Transmission of relaxin from lactating bitches to their offspring via suckling. *Biol Reprod*, 50(2), 258–265.

Haapala, J., Arokoski, J. P., Hyttinen, M. M., Lammi, M., Tammi, M., Kovanen, V., Helminen, H. J. & Kiviranta, I. 1999. Remobilization does not fully restore immobilization induced articular cartilage atrophy. *Clin Orthop Relat Res*, 362, 218–229.

Hill, A. V. 1950. The series elastic component of muscle. *Proc R Soc Lond B Biol Sci*, 137, 273–280.

Jaegger, G., Marcellin-Little, D. J. & Levine, D. 2002. Reliability of goniometry in Labrador Retrievers. *Am J Vet Res*, 63(7), 979–986.

Khan, K. M., Cook, J. L., Bonar, F., Harcourt, P. & Astrom, M. 1999. Histopathology of common tendinopathies. Update and implications for clinical management. *Sports Med*, 27, 393–408.

Kiviranta, I., Jurvelin, J., Tammi, M., Saamanen, A. M. & Helminen, H. J. 1987. Weight bearing controls glycosaminoglycan concentration and articular cartilage thickness in the knee joints of young beagle dogs. *Arthritis Rheum*, 30, 801–809.

Kiviranta, I., Tammi, M., Jurvelin, J., Saamanen, A. M. & Helminen, H. J. 1988. Moderate running exercise augments glycosaminoglycans and thickness of articular cartilage in the knee joint of young beagle dogs. *J Orthop Res*, 6, 188–195.

Kiviranta, I., Tammi, M., Jurvelin, J., Arokoski, J., Saamanen, A. M. & Helminen, H. J. 1994. Articular cartilage thickness and glycosaminoglycan distribution in the young canine knee joint after remobilization of the immobilized limb. *J Orthop Res*, 12, 161–167.

Lane, D. M., Hill, S. A., Huntingford, J. L., Lafuente, P., Wall, R. & Jones, K.A. 2015. Effectiveness of slow motion video compared to real time video in improving the accuracy and consistency of subjective gait analysis in dogs. *Open Vet J*, 5(2), 158–165.

Lundborg, G. & Rydevik, B. 1973. Effects of stretching the tibial nerve of the rabbit. A preliminary study of the intraneural circulation and the barrier function of the perineurium. *J Bone Joint Surg Br*, 55, 390–401.

Marshall, J. L. & Olsson, S. E. 1971. Instability of the knee. A long-term experimental study in dogs. *J Bone Joint Surg Am*, 53, 1561–1570.

Marsolais, G. S., Dvorak, G. & Conzemius, M. 2002. Effects of postoperative rehabilitation on limb function after cranial cruciate ligament repair in dogs. *J Am Vet Med Assoc*, 220(9), 1325–1330.

Moeller, E. M., Allen, D. A., Wilson, E. R., Linberger J. A. & Lenenbauer, T. 2010. Long-term outcomes of thigh circumference, stifle range-of-motion, and lameness after unilateral tibial plateau levelling osteotomy. *Vet Comp Orthop Traumatol*, 23(1), 37–42.

Molsa, S. H., Hyytiainen, A. K., Hielm-Bjorkman, H. K. & Laitinen-Vapaavouri, O. M. 2014. Long-term functional outcome after surgical repair of cranial cruciate ligament disease in dogs. *BMC Vet Res*, 10, 266.

Monk, M. L., Preston, C. A. & Mcgoan, C. M. 2006. Effects of early intensive postoperative physiotherapy on limb function after tibial plateau leveling osteotomy in dogs with deficiency of the cranial cruciate ligament *Am J Vet Res*, 67, 529–536.

Montgomery, R. D. 1989. Healing of muscle, ligaments and tendons. *Semin Vet Med Surg Small Anim*, 4(4), 304–311.

Nordin, M. & Frankel, V. H. 1989. *Basic Biomechanics of the Musculoskeletal System*, 2nd edn. Philadelphia, PA: Lippincott Williams & Wilkins, pp. 65–66.

Norkin, C. & Levange, P. 1983. *Joint Structure and Function: A Comprehensive Analysis*. Philadelphia, PA: F. A. Davis Company.

Noyes, F. R. 1977. Functional properties of knee ligaments and alterations induced by immobilization: a correlative biomechanical and histological study in primates. *Clin Orthop Relat Res*, 123, 210–242.

Perry, J., Weiss, W. B., Burnfield, J. M. & Gronley, J. K. 2004. The supine hip extensor manual muscle test: a reliability and validity study. *Arch Phys Med Rehabil*, 85, 1345–1350.

Romano, L. S. & Cook, J. L. 2015. Safety and functional outcomes associated with short-term rehabilitation therapy in the post-operative management of tibial plateau leveling osteotomy. *Can Vet J*, 56(9), 942–946.

Rydevik, B. & Nordborg, C. 1980. Changes in nerve function and nerve fibre structure induced by acute, graded compression. *J Neurol Neurosurg Psychiatry*, 43, 1070–1082.

Spencer, P. S., Weinberg, H. J., Raine, C. S. & PRINEAS, J. W. 1975. The perineurial window—a new model of focal demyelination and remyelination. *Brain Res*, 96, 323–329.

Stevens, J. E., Walter, G. A., Okereke, E., Scarborough, M. T., Esterhai, J. L., George, S. Z., et al. 2004. Muscle adaptations with immobilization and rehabilitation after ankle fracture. *Med Sci Sports Exerc*, 36, 1695–1701.

Sunderland, S. 1978. *Nerve and Nerve Injuries*, 2nd edn. Edinburgh: Churchill Livingstone.

Thomas, T. M., Marcellin-Little, D. J., Roe, S. C., Laxcelles, B. D. & Brosey, B. P. 2006. Comparison of measurements obtained by use of an electrogoniometer and a universal plastic goniometer for the assessment of joint motion in dogs. *Am J Vet Res*, 67(12), 1974–1979.

Topp, K. S. & Boyd, B. S. 2012. Peripheral nerve: from the microscopic functional unit of the axon to the biomechanically loaded macroscopic structure. *J Hand Ther*, 25, 142–152.

Verrall, G., Schofield, S. & Brustad, T. 2011. Chronic Achilles tendinopathy treated with eccentric stretching program. *Foot Ankle Int*, 32, 843–849.

Voss, K. L., Imhof, J., Kaestner, S. & Montavon, P. M. 2007. Force plate gait analysis at the walk and trot in dogs with low-grade hindlimb lameness. *Vet Comp Orthop Traumatol*, 20(4), 299–304.

Wright, S., Neil, E. & Joels, M. 1982. Muscle and the nervous system. In: Keele, C. A. & Neil, E. (eds), *Samson Wright's Applied Physiology*, 13th edn. Oxford: Oxford University Press, pp. 248–259.

14 Disorders of the Pelvic Limb: Diagnosis and Treatment

Peter J. Lotsikas, DVM, DACVS-SA, DACVSMR, Faith M. Lotsikas, DVM, CCRT, David Hummel, DVM, DACVS-SA, Nina R. Kieves, DVM, DACVS-SA, DACVSMR, CCRT, Jonathan Dyce, MA, VetMB, MRCVS, DSAO, DACVS, and Patrick A. Ridge, BVSc, Cert VR, Cert SAS, MRCVS

Summary

Orthopedic conditions of the pelvic limb are some of the most frequently diagnosed causes of lameness in the dog. In the canine athlete as well as the active companion, acute stretch-induced muscle disorders are common occurrences, and are often under- or misdiagnosed. The pelvic limb muscle disorders section of this chapter reviews the anatomy, diagnosis, and treatment of muscle strains. The next section of the chapter addresses the primary arthropathies of the pelvic limb including hip dysplasia, hip luxation, and conditions of the stifle; and cranial cruciate disease, meniscal injury, and patellar luxation. For these conditions, both conservative and surgical management are discussed, as well as prognosis and appropriate recovery time for return to function. The chapter concludes with descriptions and treatment options for common tendon injuries of the pelvic limb including calcanean tendon injury and luxation of the superficial digital flexor tendon. While this chapter is intended to be an abbreviated explanation of various pelvic limb conditions, it provides the sports medicine-minded clinician the critical and pertinent information necessary to manage these common conditions and injuries.

Introduction

Orthopedic conditions of the pelvic limb are some of the most frequently diagnosed causes of lameness in the dog. Historically many causes of lameness have been attributed to joints and bones, rather than looking at the importance of individual soft tissue structures. As our understanding of rehabilitation therapy and sports medicine grows, new conditions are being identified, and conservative means of treatment rather than surgical options are being used.

Canine Sports Medicine and Rehabilitation, Second Edition. Edited by Chris Zink and Janet B. Van Dyke.
© 2018 John Wiley & Sons, Inc. Published 2018 by John Wiley & Sons, Inc.

This chapter offers an overview of some of the common pelvic limb conditions seen clinically; the first section discusses pelvic limb soft tissue injuries. A keen diagnostician will palpate all structures carefully to identify changes or discomfort in soft tissues that may have yet to be published as a specific condition. Applying knowledge of pertinent anatomy with function, physical examination findings, and appropriate diagnostic tools will provide an accurate and specific diagnosis, and proposal of treatment options.

Iliopsoas strain

Anatomy

The iliopsoas muscle represents the fusion of the psoas major and iliacus muscles (Figure 14.1). The psoas major muscle arises from the transverse processes of the lumbar vertebrae of the ventral lower spinal column at L2 and L3 and the bodies of L4 to L7. The iliacus muscle arises from the ventral surface of the ilium. The two muscles combine and have a common insertion on the lesser trochanter of the femur. The action of this muscle is hip flexion with external femoral rotation, and lumber flexion (Evans, 1993).

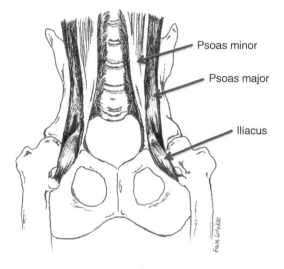

Psoas minor

Psoas major

Iliacus

Figure 14.1 Iliopsoas muscle anatomy. The iliopsoas muscle represents the fusion of the psoas major and iliacus muscles. Source: Illustration by Dr. Faith Lotsikas.

Pathophysiology

Iliopsoas muscle strains are believed to occur during eccentric contraction, when the muscle is contracting while lengthening (Breur & Blevins, 1997; Nielsen & Pluhar, 2005). The weakest area is the muscle–tendon junction, and strains most often occur at or near this junction. However, midbody and proximal psoas major injury may be noted as well. Iliopsoas strain may be a primary injury or secondary to an underlying orthopedic or neurological condition. Primary strains can occur as acute stretch-induced injuries or from chronic repetitive use. In performance dogs, there may be a long-standing cycle of microtearing, particularly if the strain is ongoing due to poor fitness, repetitive training, improper warm-ups, and/or fatigue compensation. Slipping into sudden abduction, jumping out of a vehicle or from give-way footing, and roughhousing with other dogs may be precipitating events in any type of dog.

Pes anserinus injury

Anatomy

The pes anserinus (Latin for "goose foot") is the conjoined tendon group of the sartorius, gracilis, semimembranosus, and semitendinosus muscles on the medial aspect of the proximal tibia. This web-like structure is unique in that the four muscles are innervated by three different nerves (femoral, obturator, and tibial, respectively). The four muscle groups also have very different functions (Evans, 1993). The cranial sartorius is a long muscle that spans from the ilium to the patella and cranial medial aspect of the tibia. Biomechanically, the sartorius primarily flexes the hip and the stifle, but the cranial belly also serves to extend the stifle. The gracilis is the only adductor to cross the stifle. The semimembranosus and semitendinosus extend the hip and tarsus and flex or extend the stifle (Evans, 1993).

Pathophysiology

Injury to this tendon group can cause lameness and pain on palpation of the proximal medial aspect of the stifle. Pain in this region may lead to an inaccurate suspicion of a cranial cruciate ligament (CCL) or medial collateral ligament injury. The authors also see this muscle group affected in canine athletes evaluated for performance issues that have been previously attributed to nonresponsive iliopsoas muscle strains.

The pes anserinus insertion site can serve as a source of discomfort following knee surgery, as tibial osteotomies (tibial plateau leveling osteotomy, tibial tuberosity advancement) require elevation and reattachment of this tendinous insertion.

Proximal sartorius strain

In performance dogs, proximal sartorius strains are appreciated as a primary condition or in conjunction with iliopsoas strains. In one author's (FL) experience the sartorius muscle is often the more painful culprit and more limiting factor for comfortable hip extension. The sartorius muscle, amongst other soft tissues, can also experience secondary strain due to compensation related to chronic lameness from other orthopedic or neurological conditions, or in the postoperative period. Within a sports medicine-heavy rehabilitation department, in which canine athletes are seen for maintenance therapies, the rehabilitation therapist may routinely find this region inflamed and in need of therapy despite the patient showing no overt lameness.

Diagnosis

Lameness associated with these muscle strains ranges from subtle intermittent offloading to significant even non-weight-bearing lameness, and is typically exacerbated by return to activity. A shortened stride and stiffness in the pelvis is a common presentation in fit dogs, whereas a more severe lameness may be noted in the companion or geriatric patient. Agility performance-related issues such as knocking bars with the pelvic limbs, avoidance of tight handling, and slowing within the weave poles are common complaints. In working dogs, the client may report reluctance to jump up for bite work or scaling heights, as well as fatigue appearing sooner than expected. With knowledge of soft tissue anatomy and understanding of

muscle function, specific muscle stretch tests can be used to help determine pain sources and appreciate reduced function. The clinician should palpate gently, being sensitive to muscle rigidity, prominence, and asymmetry, spasms or fine fasciculations, and stretch reluctance. If the patient is amenable to laying in lateral recumbency, muscle/tendon flexibility testing may be easier to appreciate as well as being more comfortable for the patient.

Iliopsoas

Tightening, discomfort, and spasm may be noted on direct palpation of the myotendinous unit (Figure 14.2), or when stretching the muscle by placing the hip in extension with abduction, or extension with internal rotation of the limb (Figure 14.3). Soft cupped hands can apply an upward, medially directed pressure to assess the body of the psoas. Most dogs will show discomfort when simply palpating the affected regions with superficial consistent pressure, thus heavy or deep pressure to induce a spasm is not recommended or necessary. The groin is a particularly sensitive region for normal dogs and one must be careful not to overread or create false reactivity. Lower spine discomfort and pelvic alignment should also be evaluated for their relationship to these muscle groups and potential correlation in treatments.

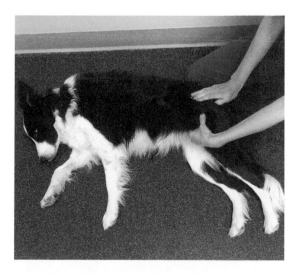

Figure 14.2 Tightness, discomfort, and spasm may be noted on direct palpation of the myotendinous unit of the iliopsoas.

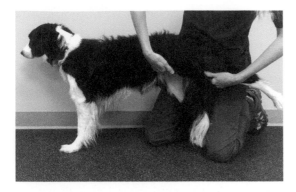

Figure 14.3 Tightness, discomfort, and spasm may be noted when stretching the iliopsoas muscle by placing the hip in extension with abduction, or extension with internal rotation of the limb.

Sartorius

Palpation in standing or lateral recumbency is achieved by cupping the hand across the cranial aspect of the femur and then tracing up the sartorius with the thumb placed laterally and remaining fingers placed medially. As the examiner approaches the proximal segment, near the iliac crest, a prominent and firm oval bulging is noted. Generally, the central portion of this prominence will be painful with pressure or stretch applied and the patient may shift or raise the leg. While placing the limb into hip extension, concurrent palpation of the sartorius may give the examiner the sense that the muscle is too taut to allow normal

---

Case Study 14.1   Chronic iliopsoas insertionopathy

Signalment: 7-y.o. MN Border Collie. Dual certified in Wilderness Air Scent (Live) and Human Remains Detection Land (Cadaver). Liam actively trains in a USAR environment to increase his agility and confidence for searching in various terrains (Figure 14.4).

Presenting complaint: Acute left pelvic limb lameness. Onset of lameness associated with a cadaver search. Pertinent medical history: right iliopsoas strain with quadriceps involvement 1 year and bilateral iliopsoas strains 4 years prior, each managed with rehabilitation.

Physical examination: Circumduction of both pelvic limbs during swing phase of gait. Able to sit square, but slightly off-weighting left pelvic limb while standing. Spasm and mild reaction elicited on palpation of left iliopsoas at midbody and insertion point on lesser trochanter. Mild muscle atrophy noted in both pelvic limbs and less paraspinal mass than expected in a working dog. Weakness appreciated in both pelvic limbs and core. Neck and shoulder tension noted but no orthopedic impairments noted. Tick-borne disease ruled out, normal cardiac status, no metabolic diseases.

Diagnostics: Radiographs: Radiographs of stifles, pelvis, and lumbar spine submitted for radiologist review. No significant abnormalities identified in lumbar spine. Coxofemoral joints WNL; femoral muscle mass symmetrical. Remodeling and fragmented appearance of left lesser trochanter. Stifle and tarsal joints appear symmetrical and WNL. Findings consistent with iliopsoas injury/enthesopathy. No other significant abnormalities appreciated (Figure 14.5).

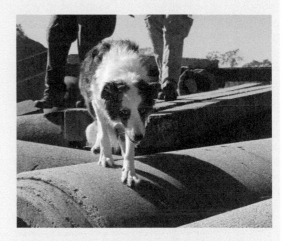

Figure 14.4   Patient working a rubble pile during training.

Musculoskeletal ultrasound: Mild focal swelling with decreased echogenicity and loss of echotexture noted at distal insertion of left iliopsoas. Remainder of insertion heterogonous with loss of echotexture and echogenic areas. Small indentation of lesser trochanter deep to a rounded bony body associated with insertion of the iliopsoas. Mildly uneven width of distal insertion of right iliopsoas with altered echogenicity and small echogenic foci (Figure 14.6).

Diagnosis: Acute exacerbation of bilateral chronic iliopsoas muscle injury with ongoing fibrotic replacement. Degree of echoarchitectural changes most pronounced on left iliopsoas.

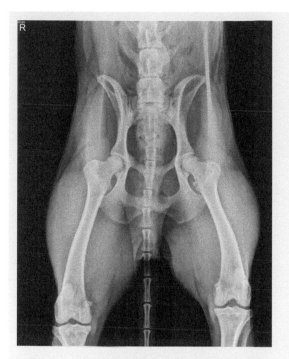

Figure 14.5 Ventrodorsal pelvis view. Note remodeling and fragmented appearance of left lesser trochanter.

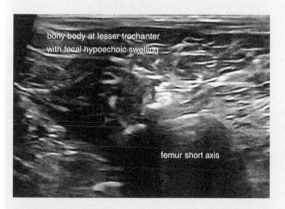

Figure 14.6 Ultrasonographic image of the iliopsoas insertion.

Treatment: Patient sedated and ultrasound-guided intralesional stem cell/autologous conditioned serum injected into both iliopsoas tendon insertions.

Postinjection rehabilitation therapy:

Week 1-2: Short-line leash walks for urination and defecation purposes no longer than 5 minutes each. Indoor and outdoor management to rest hip flexors by preventing jumping, playing, or excessive stair

use. Cryotherapy over the injection site q.i.d. for 4 days. Non-end-range passive stretching of the hip flexors as tolerated. Omega-3 fatty acids and Robaxin® prescribed. Diet reduced to reflect resting energy requirements.

Week 2-6: Weekly rehabilitation, starting week 2 for manual therapies, therapeutic ultrasound, and laser therapy. Client education: moist heat or warm-ups prior to massage and passive stretching performed b.i.d. Use tummy rubs to encourage active hip extension, and slowly add sartorius stretches. Passive stretching assigned: iliopsoas, sartorius, and hamstrings bilaterally, 5 reps of each for 15–30 seconds as tolerated. PROM of stifle, tarsus, and toes assessed daily. Passive stretching/ PROM thoracic limbs.

Initial therapeutic exercises minimized as early goals of therapy are pain reduction, healing, and regaining flexibility. Cookie stretches to hips, weight shifting on stable footing, play bows, and low front feet up performed o.d. to b.i.d. for first 4 weeks. Low repetitions, gradually increased. Calm indoor search games and seated thoracic limb tricks to offer distraction from boredom.

Flat terrain walks increased in 3–5-minute intervals weekly if no regression to circumduction or off-weighting. Discussed walking in controlled and deliberate manner without leash pulling, and advised monthly chiropractic.

Week 6-10: Bimonthly rehabilitation therapy results in no lameness or off-weighting. Patient demonstrates comfortable mobility despite expected loss of conditioning. Rehabilitation modalities remain unchanged. Goals switched to regaining strength while protecting healing tissues. Therapeutic exercise includes hill walking, figure-of-eights, and short-distance side hill walking. Limited jogging on long line after warm-up time. Patient taught to back consistently and straight for 10 steps, before progressing to doing this facing up and down slopes. One walk per day involves the additional hill work. Sit-to-stand work progresses to: hills or an indoor slope shifting weight to the rear, perch pivots in both directions, three-leg stands on stable footing progressing to wobble surface, walking cavalettis, and sit pretty.

Exercise routine mixes easier and harder categories, giving client flexibility to prevent boredom and provide rest periods. Bodywork reduced to once daily after exercise. Robaxin® D/C at 4 weeks. Dietary protein increased for increase in activity and muscle recovery.

(Continued)

Week 10-16: Rehabilitation therapy once monthly. Light cantering in a controlled environment for up to 5 minutes after 15 minutes of walking. Light tracking permitted on walks, including wooded terrains. Return to swimming/wading in water permitted for controlled periods once weekly, adjusting work to prevent fatigue.

Week 16: Patient remains sound with significant progress in fitness. Periodic recheck and rehabilitation therapy tune up is recommended at 3-month intervals. Client is taught proper warm-up/cool-down routines, and continues once weekly at-home bodywork to maintain suppleness and to monitor for early signs of strain recurrence.

Exercise now includes long-distance trotting, uphill sprints, increased water play, and swimming. Patient is transitioned to off-leash except in slippery conditions. Ongoing core work is encouraged while fine-tuning proprioception.

Case discussion: Due to the chronic history of iliopsoas strains, orthobiological intervention was chosen to augment rehabilitation therapy for this case. Manual therapies were very important as numerous muscle groups and the neck/spine had been compensating for some time. Endurance training remains an important part of the training regimen.

range of extension. To focally stretch test the sartorius, the stifle is first placed into flexion, then hip extension is slowly added. The sartorius stretch is not a large movement in the normal dog, however, when affected, a difference is appreciated in flexibility and comfort.

For muscle injuries, pelvic limb radiographs are generally unremarkable. Avulsion of the lesser trochanter may be noted in acute traumatic avulsions of the iliopsoas tendon, and mineralization within tendons sometimes can be seen in chronic cases.

Musculoskeletal ultrasonography is an excellent diagnostic modality to confirm the diagnosis, grade the severity of strain, and assist with prognosis. The skill of the diagnostician is paramount so as to not overinterpret ultrasonographic findings or dismiss a diagnosis because a grade I strain is ultrasonographically normal. Sequential imaging may assist the rehabilitation therapist make a decision regarding when to increase exercise, bearing in mind the importance of treating the patient rather than the image.

Treatment

Conservative medical management with rehabilitation therapy is recommended for acute and chronic muscle strains. At-home medical management includes short courses of NSAIDs, muscle relaxants, cryotherapy that transitions to moist heat, restricted activity to prevent ongoing damage, and controlled exercise to stimulate proper repair and body use. Administration

of NSAIDs beyond the first 24–48 hours has recently fallen out of favor in the human literature as there is increasing evidence that it may delay tissue healing and carries a risk of adverse reactions (Jones *et al.*, 2015).

In general, muscle relaxants are well tolerated and may facilitate easier passive and active stretching exercises. Pain management can promote limb use and thus reduce further contracture of the tissues that accompanies avoidance postures and guarding, particularly if the patient will not have the option of concurrent rehabilitation therapy.

Rehabilitation therapy is highly successful in the management of most strains, along with proper education and guidance of clients through the recovery process homework. Following recovery, as with any injury, proper conditioning and transition to sport as well as teaching injury prevention strategies may help prevent new or reoccurring strains. Rehabilitation involves use of physical modalities such as therapeutic ultrasound, phonophoresis, and laser therapy to aid tissue repair (see Chapter 7). Because these modalities also reduce pain and increase tissue extensibility, the rehabilitation therapist will often find the patient more receptive to manual therapies following their use. However, these modalities should be viewed as complements to skilled manual therapies and do not replace the importance of proper massage, the release of myofascial trigger points, and working with the patient to regain normal flexibility and range of motion through appropriate stretches and therapeutic exercises. Weekly to biweekly rehabilitation and reassessment allows adaptation of the therapeutic exercise plan and home care. Complementary therapies such as acupuncture and chiropractic are also often used to promote whole-patient wellness.

For muscle strains in which core lesions are noted, or those refractory to rehabilitation, ultrasound-guided injection with orthobiologics may be performed (see Chapter 16).

Surgical treatment by tenotomy may be warranted when there are irreversible changes to the myotendinous unit that are nonresponsive to medical management and rehabilitation therapy.

Gracilis and semitendinosus/semimembranosus myopathy

Myopathy of the gracilis, semitendinosus, or semimembranosus muscles may occur individually, or concurrently. There is usually no definitive episode reported by the client. There does appear to be some breed and age predilection, with highly active German Shepherd Dogs and Shepherd-related breeds between the ages of 3 and 7 years overrepresented (Vaughan, 1979; Lewis *et al.*, 1997; Steiss, 2002).

Anatomy

The gracilis, semitendinosus, and semimembranosus muscles form an extensive broad muscular sheet that is found superficially in the caudal portion of the medial thigh (Figure 14.7). The semitendinosus muscle arises from the ischiatic tuberosity and ends along the cranial border of the tibia. An aponeurosis also spreads out into the crural fascia and from its caudal border sends a well-developed reinforcing band to the calcanean tendon, which attaches to the tuber calcaneus. This muscle group is responsible for thigh adduction, hip extension, stifle flexion, and tarsal extension (Evans, 1993).

Pathophysiology

In most cases, the etiology of gracilis/semitendinosus myopathy is unknown. Numerous theories

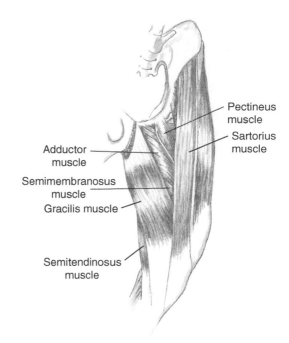

Figure 14.7   The gracilis, and lateral to that muscle, the semitendinosus and semimembranosus muscles, form an extensive broad muscular sheet that is found superficially in the caudal portion of the medial thigh. Source: Illustration by Marcia Schlehr.

exist, including acute trauma, chronic repetitive trauma, autoimmune disease, drug reaction, infection, neurogenic disorders, and vascular abnormalities (Taylor & Tangner, 2007). Ischemia secondary to indirect trauma may also lead to fibrosis and contracture (Taylor & Tangner, 2007). Histologically, muscle is replaced by dense, collagenous connective tissue.

A 2002 study involving canine athletes suggested that excessive activity can lead to muscle strains resulting in inflammation, edema, localized hemorrhage, and eventually fibrosis (Steiss, 2002). German Shepherd Dogs may be at greater risk of muscle strain during physical activity due to the increased angulation (flexion) at the stifle (Steiss, 2002).

Diagnosis

Presentation of gracilis, semitendinosus, or semimembranosus contracture is very unique and consistent in appearance. The diagnosis can be made with a thorough history, observation

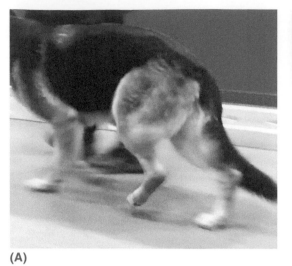
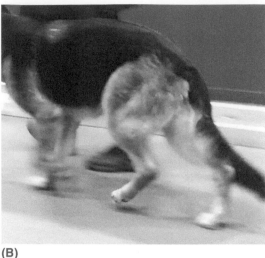

(A)   **(B)**

Figure 14.8   Dogs with gracilis myopathy have a characteristic pelvic limb gait abnormality. **(A)** Elastic medial rotation of the left rear foot and external rotation of the calcaneus. **(B)** 0.5 seconds later the foot has rotated laterally and the calcaneus medially. (Images obtained from video.)

of gait, and physical examination. Affected dogs have a pelvic limb gait abnormality character- ized by a shortened stride with lack of stifle extension and a rapid, elastic, medial rotation of the foot, internal rotation of the tarsus with external rotation of the calcaneus, and inter- nal rotation of the stifle during the mid to late swing phase of protraction (Figure 14.8).

A taut, firm band is palpable in the caudo- medial aspect of the thigh (this can be the gracilis or semitendinosus tendon). Pain and spasm may be noted when performing a stretch of the gracilis–semitendinosus muscle complex (hip flexion, stifle extension, and limb abduc- tion) (Figure 14.9). In many cases, the stifle physically cannot be fully extended during this stretch.

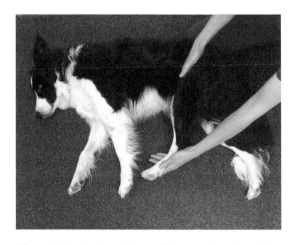

Figure 14.9   In dogs with gracilis myopathy, pain and spasm may be noted when performing a stretch of the gracilis–semitendinosus muscle complex (hip flexion, stifle extension, and limb abduction).

Treatment

For acute cases, conservative management and rehabilitation therapy consisting of NSAIDs, restricted controlled activity, cryotherapy switching to moist heat, and rehabilitation therapy is recommended. Dry needling has been found helpful in one author's (FL) opinion as an adjunctive therapy.

Unfortunately, it is rare for rehabilitation therapy to completely resolve the clinical signs associated with a gracilis/semitendinosus

myopathy, but improvement in quality of life and function is notable in our experience. With continued rehabilitation therapy and dedica- tion to a home maintenance program, working dogs with this condition can remain active and on duty. Teaching the client proper massage and stretching, as well as conditioning, warm- ups, and avoidance of repetitive strain activi- ties when possible is recommended as part of the ongoing rehabilitation effort.

Additional treatment options are limited for chronic or refractory cases. Eighteen dogs with gracilis or semitendinosus myopathy were treated with various methods (Lewis *et al.*, 1997). Eight received medical management either alone or prior to surgery. There was no apparent response. Fifteen dogs were treated with one or more surgical procedures. Lameness resolved following transection, partial excision, or complete resection of the affected muscle. However, it recurred 6 weeks to 5 months following surgery. Adjunctive medical treatment did not change the outcome. Myectomy of the entire gracilis muscle is no more successful as the gait abnormality may return within 3–5 months due to semitendinosus involvement (Lewis *et al.*, 1997).

Hip dysplasia

Pathophysiology

Hip dysplasia (HD) can be defined as abnormal development of the hip joint, resulting in coxofemoral laxity due to decreased coverage of the femoral head by the acetabulum and ineffective soft tissue stabilization of the joint (Demko & McLaughlin, 2005; Lopez, 2012). Abnormal kinematics result in joint capsule stretching, cartilage erosion, subchondral bone fracture, periarticular fibrosis, and new bone formation (Dassler, 2003). Disease progression results in degenerative and inflammatory changes characteristic of osteoarthritis (OA) (Dassler, 2003).

Hip dysplasia is the most common developmental orthopedic condition in dogs and is highly breed dependent (Witsberger *et al.*, 2008; Smith *et al.*, 2012). Despite attempts at eradication of the condition through selective breeding programs, the prevalence of HD remains very high within certain breeds (Coopman *et al.*, 2008; Witsberger *et al.*, 2008; Smith *et al.*, 2012). A review of over 1.2 million dogs between 1964 and 2003 reported the prevalence and risk factors for HD in over 50 breeds (Witsberger *et al.*, 2008). Newfoundlands, Rottweilers, German Shepherd Dogs, and retrievers are among the most commonly affected breeds, with prevalences up to 17% (Witsberger *et al.*, 2008). Smith and colleagues (2012) followed a colony of Labrador Retrievers over their life span and found that despite breeding for an expected HD incidence between 26% and 51%, in fact 98% of the dogs had evidence of HD at the time of death. These studies highlight the fact that HD is a complex condition with many factors involved in the development, progression, and recognition of the disease.

Hip dysplasia is a polygenic, heritable condition, in which the phenotypic expression can be influenced by reproductive status, age, body condition and conformation, diet, and other environmental factors (Spain *et al.*, 2004; Demko & McLaughlin, 2005; Witsberger *et al.*, 2008; Smith *et al.*, 2012). Castrated male dogs are significantly more likely to be affected by HD, and an association has been shown between gonadectomy at <5 months of age and the development of HD in both males and females (Spain *et al.*, 2004; Witsberger *et al.*, 2008).

Kealy, Smith and others found that the development and progression of HD was significantly delayed or decreased in dogs maintained at a lean body condition through caloric restriction compared to litter-matched pairs of a higher body condition score (Kealy *et al.*, 2002; Smith *et al.*, 2012). When all dogs in this study were pooled, a linear relationship was seen between age and prevalence of HD. A conclusion of this study was that selecting breeding dogs based on phenotype (young age, lean body condition) does not ensure elimination of the HD genotype (Smith *et al.*, 2012).

Diagnosis

Dogs with HD often show clinical signs following a bimodal curve: 4 months to 3–4 years and >7 years of age (Smith *et al.*, 2012; Witsberger *et al.*, 2008). Puppies and young dogs with HD present with a history of decreased activity or reluctance to jump or climb stairs, bunny-hopping gait, underdeveloped pelvic limbs with a narrow stance, and pain or vocalization with manipulation (Dassler, 2003; Demko & McLaughlin, 2005). Mature dogs with symptoms related to OA of the hips show varying degrees of lameness that is worse after rest and heavy exercise, reluctance to jump, pelvic limb atrophy, and behavior changes associated with pain (Demko & McLaughlin, 2005).

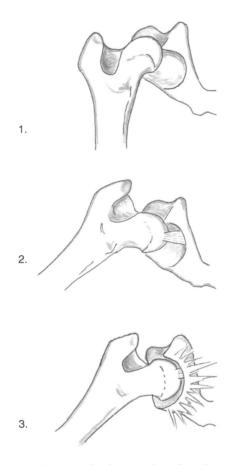

Figure 14.10 Passive hip laxity can be palpated in young dogs using the Ortolani maneuver. Source: Illustrations by Marcia Schlehr.

The diagnosis of HD is based on physical examination and radiographic findings (Demko & McLaughlin, 2005). Passive hip laxity can be palpated in young dogs using the Ortolani maneuver (Demko & McLaughlin, 2005; Gatineau *et al.*, 2012) (Figure 14.10). This test may be inaccurate in dogs younger than 4 months, as maximal laxity increases between the ages of 2 and 6 months (Smith *et al.*, 1998; Gatineau *et al.*, 2012).

The sensitivity and specificity of a positive Ortolani sign detected at 6 months for the development of hip OA at 2 years has been shown to be 100% and 50%, respectively (Gatineau *et al.*, 2012). In other words, all dogs with hip OA at 2 years had a positive Ortolani at 6 months, and half of the dogs with a positive Ortolani at 6 months showed radiographic signs of OA at 2 years. Furthermore, a negative

Ortolani sign at 6 months is significantly predictive of a lack of OA at 2 years (Gatineau *et al.*, 2012).

In mature dogs with HD, physical exam findings typically include uni- or bilateral weight-bearing pelvic limb lameness, pelvic limb muscle atrophy and gluteal weakness, prominence of the greater trochanter consistent with femoral head subluxation, decreased passive and active extension of the hip, and core muscle weakness (Bockstahler *et al.*, 2012; Demko & McLaughlin, 2005).

There are several radiographic views used to assess hip conformation and secondary OA (Powers *et al.*, 2010; Gatineau *et al.*, 2012; Verhoeven *et al.*, 2012). The standard ventrodorsal extended limb view is widely used (Figure 14.11), and is the view required by the Orthopedic Foundation for Animals (OFA) for breed screening.

There are several limitations to the ventrodorsal view and the OFA screening methodology. Positioning for this view underestimates the degree of joint laxity. Additionally, radiographs are given a subjective rating based on

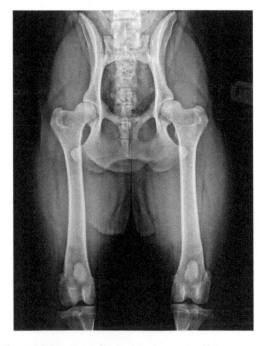

Figure 14.11 For radiographic diagnosis of hip dysplasia, the standard ventrodorsal extended limb view is widely used, and is the view required by the Orthopedic Foundation for Animals for breed screening.

assessment of joint conformation, laxity, and degenerative changes in dogs at least 2 years of age. Lastly, submission of radiographs to the OFA by breeders and veterinarians is optional; consequently, underestimation of the prevalence of HD is likely (Powers *et al.*, 2010; Gatineau *et al.*, 2012; Verhoeven *et al.*, 2012).

Other radiographic views have been developed to objectively diagnose HD earlier in the disease process (Powers *et al.*, 2010; Gatineau *et al.*, 2012; Verhoeven *et al.*, 2012). PennHIP® measures joint congruity by calculating the relative displacement of the femoral head from the acetabulum during coxofemoral distraction, thus accounting for passive joint laxity (Powers *et al.*, 2010). The calculated distraction index (DI) predicts the likelihood of developing OA compared with other dogs of the same breed (Runge *et al.*, 2010). PennHIP® has been validated as a reliable screening tool in dogs as young as 6 months (Powers *et al.*, 2010). When compared directly, the OFA underestimates the susceptibility to OA compared with PennHIP® (Powers *et al.*, 2010). The Norberg angle, dorsal acetabular slope, and dorsolateral subluxation view are other objective methods of evaluating HD (Gatineau *et al.*, 2012; Verhoeven *et al.*, 2012).

Nonsurgical management

Nonsurgical management involves a multimodal approach including activity modification, rehabilitation, and pain management, maintenance of a lean body condition, pharmacological modulation of joint disease, and regenerative and complementary medicine.

A systematic review of the veterinary literature regarding nonsurgical management of HD found high levels of evidence in support of weight management through dietary restriction, parenteral administration of polysulfated glycosaminoglycans (PSGAGs), and adipose-derived stem cell therapy (Kirkby & Lewis, 2012). Additional techniques that have been shown to be effective include acupuncture, extracorporeal shock wave therapy (ESWT), and omega-3 fatty acid supplementation (Roush *et al.*, 2010).

At the time of this publication, scientific evaluation of physical rehabilitation, including therapeutic exercise and hydrotherapy, for the management of HD and OA in dogs has not been investigated. However, considering the role of passive joint laxity in the pathogenesis of HD, it is practical to assume that strengthening of the soft tissue support structures of the hip would be beneficial. In fact, German Shepherd Dogs are more likely to develop hip OA at a lower distraction index (less passive laxity) than more well-muscled breeds such as Rottweilers (Gatineau *et al.*, 2012). Initiation of a comprehensive rehabilitation program for a dog with HD will likely prove successful either alone or complementary to surgical intervention.

Surgical management

Joint preservation procedures

Greater degrees of hip laxity correlate with an increased likelihood of secondary OA, but not necessarily clinical disability. There are two surgical procedures that aim to improve the clinical signs associated with coxofemoral laxity in skeletally immature dogs.

Juvenile pubic symphysiodesis

Juvenile pubic symphysiodesis (JPS) causes premature closure of the pubic symphysis. This procedure results in ventral rotation of the dorsal acetabular rim as the remaining growth plates continue to grow. The technique reduces the risk of progression of HD in cases of mild to moderate hip laxity, but is significantly less effective in addressing more severe laxity. In puppies with more severe laxity, the progressive correction of acetabular orientation would fail to capture the femoral head. JPS should be performed before 16 weeks of age to improve hip stability (Patricelli *et al.*, 2002; Bernarde, 2010). Consequently, JPS is recommended in dogs that are unlikely to have any contemporary disability from HD. Dynamic imaging of the hips to demonstrate laxity (e.g., hip distraction with PennHIP®) should guide selection or exclusion of the individual dog as a candidate for JPS.

Triple or double pelvic osteotomy

Triple or double pelvic osteotomy (TPO or DPO) aims to increase dorsal acetabular rim coverage of the femoral head. This is achieved by making two or three osteotomies around the acetabulum, manually rotating the acetabulum over the femoral head, and stabilizing it with a plate and screws (Figure 14.12). It is ideally performed in dogs less than 5–8 months of age with an angle of relocation <25–30 degrees and a quality of Ortolani sign that suggests no erosion of the dorsal acetabular rim. Dogs with clinical lameness are less likely to be optimal candidates for TPO/DPO, but there is understandable reluctance to perform corrective osteotomy on dogs with hip laxity that is an incidental finding on physical examination.

Patients typically bear weight on the surgical leg immediately following surgery. The most common complications with this procedure are implant loosening and pelvic canal narrowing (Whelan *et al.*, 2004; Doornink *et al.*, 2006). The recent use of locking implants has decreased the complication rate with this procedure (Rose *et al.*, 2012). Postoperative exercise restriction is imperative until radiographic evidence of bony union is present, at which time therapy aimed at building muscle mass can be initiated. Range

of motion is typically preserved with this procedure, though gait kinematics reveal a base narrow stance that is usually permanent.

The progression of OA remains possible with both the JPS and TPO procedures, particularly in patients that already have damage to joint ligament or cartilage (Manley *et al.*, 2007; Holsworth *et al.*, 2005) (Figure 14.13).

Salvage procedures

Total hip replacement

Total hip replacement (THR) is routinely used to target lameness caused by HD/OA that is refractory to medical management. Other indications include chronic femoral capital physeal or femoral neck fracture, complicated luxation (e.g., chronic luxation, fracture luxation, or luxation of the previously dysplastic hip), and avascular necrosis of the femoral head. THR involves surgical removal of the patient's acetabulum and femoral head and replacement with a polyethylene cup and metallic stem and head. The expected outcome is restoration of

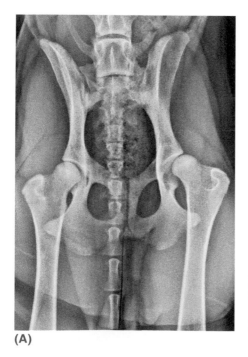

(A)

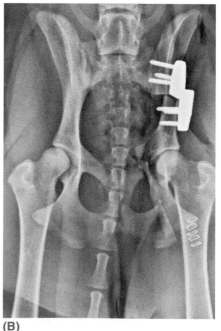

(B)

Figure 14.12 **(A)** Triple pelvic osteotomy aims to increase dorsal acetabular rim coverage of the femoral head by making two or three osteotomies around the acetabulum, manually rotating the acetabulum over the femoral head, and stabilizing it with a plate and screws **(B)**.

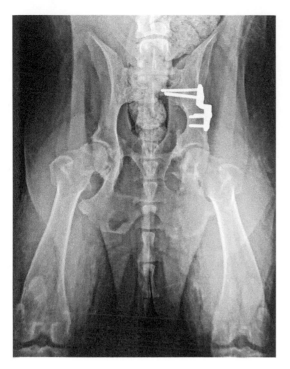

Figure 14.13 Progression of osteoarthritis remains possible with both the JPS and TPO (as shown here) procedures, particularly in patients that already have damage to joint ligament or cartilage.

normal hip function, range of motion, and pelvic and crural muscle bulk. It is unusual that osteoarthritic degeneration will preclude THR. However, there is an increased degree of surgical difficulty in hips with advanced OA. Juvenile dogs with luxation of dysplastic hips (luxoid conformation) can develop rapid remodeling of the femur, notably lateral drift of the proximal medial femoral cortex, which will preclude insertion of a diaphyseal stem. In such cases the window of opportunity for routine THR may be short.

Selection criteria for THR are stringent, and common contraindications to THR include obesity, bacterial pyoderma, other clinically significant orthopedic disease (CCL rupture almost invariably should be addressed prior to consideration for THR), neurological impairment, infective arthritis, immunosuppression, and polyarthropathy. Resolution of some of these conditions is practical and may permit THR at a later date if necessary.

Anchorage of the prosthetic cup and stem is implant-specific and may involve cemented or cementless fixation. In cemented THR, a mantle of acrylic cement is used to bond the implant to bone. Cementless anchorage of the cup can involve press-fit (BioMedtrix and Kyon) or screw home (Innoplant) devices. Cementless fixation of the stem may be simply press-fit, or augmented with locking bolts through the lateral cortex (Kyon and BioMedtrix EBM lateral bolt) or screw home (Innoplant). The initial press-fit should be stable enough to allow osteointegration, which will contribute to the permanent fixation of the implant (Figure 14.14). In selected patients, when using the modular BioMedtrix system, a hybrid fixation—most commonly a cementless cup with a cemented stem—can offer the most durable fixation (Figure 14.15).

The primary advantage of the cemented stem over press-fit cementless systems, is that it offers maximum strength shortly after implantation. It is ideal for patients with more brittle cortical bone, thinner cortices, a cylindrical (rather than conical) proximal femoral diaphysis, and poor-quality trabecular bone (implying increased risk of cementless stem subsidence) as seen typically in the older shepherd breeds. The new BioMedtrix "micro" and "nano" THR systems are fully cemented and specifically address hip disorders in small dogs and cats (Liska, 2010).

Complications of THR are uncommon but include sciatic neuropraxia, prosthetic luxation, femoral fissure/fracture, stem subsidence, periprosthetic infection, aseptic loosening, and implant failure. Aseptic loosening is a biological process initiated by polyethylene wear debris that stimulates macrophage-mediated osteoclastic bone resorption at the implant–bone interface. Debonding of the cement–implant interface, a mechanical deterioration, can also occur (Finkelstein *et al.*, 1991; Edwards *et al.*, 1997).

The early experience with press-fit cementless stems was associated with relatively high rates of subsidence and fissure. Technical refinement in stem implantation and the development of porous ingrowth textures with higher coefficient of friction (Biomedtrix EBM) and augmented fixation (e.g., medial collar, lateral bolt) have all contributed to more consistently successful cementless THR (Zhang *et al.*, 1999; Biemond *et al.*, 2011).

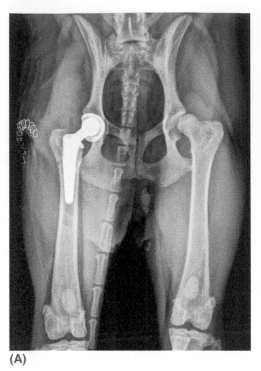
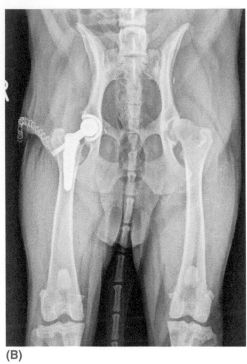

(A) **(B)**

Figure 14.14 (A) BFX press-fit cup with a collard EBM titanium stem. (B) BFX press-fit cup with an EBM titanium stem augmented with a lateral bolt. Both variations to the stem are to decrease the risk of subsidence.

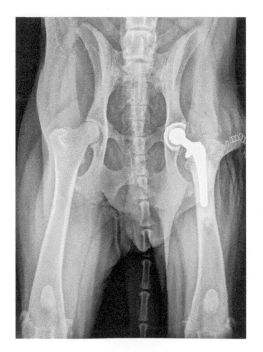

Figure 14.15 Hip replacement using a hybrid hip, which is a combination of a cementless acetabular cup with a cemented stem.

The risk of aseptic and infection-driven loosening is probably greater in cemented fixation. Long-term data are currently not available to document the true life span of these implants (Guerrero & Montavon, 2009; Lascelles *et al.*, 2010; Kidd *et al.* 2016).

Surgical revision with preservation of a functional THR is generally an option to address luxation, subsidence, and femoral fracture. Aseptic loosening, implant failure, and particularly infection do not have an encouraging prognosis for revision, and explantation with conversion to an effective femoral head and neck ostectomy (FHO) may be indicated (Fitzpatrick *et al.*, 2014; Vezzoni *et al.*, 2015; Nesser *et al.*, 2016).

Postoperative management. Most patients will bear weight on the operated limb within 24 hours of surgery. The first 4–6 weeks postsurgery are the most critical. During this time, the joint capsule is healing, and in a cementless hip, osteointegration is taking place. Patients are prone to coxofemoral luxation and subsidence during this time. For most cases, the authors recommend limiting rehabilitation therapy to cryotherapy, laser therapy, and massage during the initial convalescent period. Stretching, manual work, strengthening (land-based and hydrotherapy) can be initiated 1 month following surgery. Off-leash activity is not recommended until 12 weeks following surgery.

Femoral head and neck ostectomy

Femoral head and neck ostectomy is a salvage procedure in which the head and neck of the femur are removed, eliminating the bone-on-bone contact of the worn femoral head and acetabulum (Figure 14.16). This procedure relies on peri-articular fibrosis and muscle to support the body-weight of the patient. There are few perioperative complications, as no implants are present (Dueland *et al.*, 1977). Patients may have a residual gait abnormality,

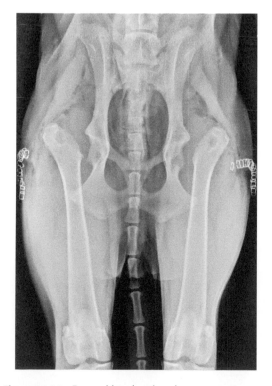

Figure 14.16 Femoral head and neck ostectomy is a salvage procedure in which the head and neck of the femur are removed, eliminating the bone-on-bone contact of the worn femoral head and acetabulum.

but are usually perceived as pain-free by their clients, and can maintain an acceptable level of activity (Off & Matis, 2010).

Postoperative management.   Functional shortening of the limb associated with dorsal displacement of the femur, failure to recover normal muscle mass, and decreased range of hip motion are likely causes of poor outcome with FHO. Most patients will not bear weight on the limb for 3–5 days following surgery. Rehabilitation therapy is imperative for a functional outcome. Long-term administration of analgesic medication and early therapy (5–14 days following surgery) aim to improve comfort and preserve range of motion of the hip (Grisneaux *et al.*, 2003). Once the patient is adequately bearing weight, strength training is initiated. Underwater treadmill therapy can be extremely beneficial and is recommended starting 2–3 weeks following surgery. Swimming tends to be less beneficial in these cases, as patients are often hesitant to fully engage the surgical limb. Recovery is usually longer than that experienced with a THR, typically 16–20 weeks until optimal function is achieved. The most predictable outcome with this procedure is with a thin, well-conditioned patient.

Coxofemoral luxation

Anatomy

The coxofemoral joint derives most of its stability from the round ligament of the femoral head, the joint capsule, and the dorsal acetabular rim. The joint also receives ancillary stabilization from the ventral labrum, surrounding musculature, and the adhesion–cohesion relationship of the joint surfaces and synovial fluid. Disruption of two or more primary stabilizers results in luxation of the hip (Holsworth & DeCamp, 2003).

Pathophysiology

Hip luxation is most often due to a traumatic event, such as vehicular trauma (Bone *et al.*, 1984; Basher *et al.*, 1986; Demko *et al.*, 2006).

This results in disruption of the ligament of the femoral head and joint capsule, with ensuing luxation of the hip. The gluteal and iliopsoas muscle groups act upon the greater and lesser trochanters, causing the femoral head to move in a craniodorsal direction (Basher *et al.*, 1986). Ventral luxation is less common, and is usually a result of a slip or fall causing the stifle to be abruptly abducted. Underlying HD is a predisposing factor for both types of luxation (Herron, 1979).

Diagnosis

The affected patient is often non-weight-bearing, with external rotation of the stifle and adduction of the lower limb. The affected limb appears shorter, with a prominent hard swelling (the greater trochanter) palpable above the coxofemoral joint. Diagnosis is made upon examination and palpation, and is confirmed with radiographs (Figure 14.17). The patient is thoroughly evaluated for concurrent injuries commonly seen with traumatic events.

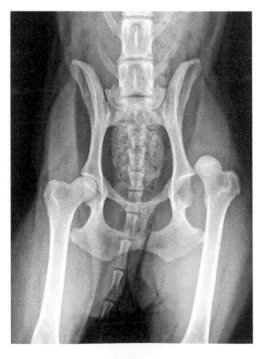

Figure 14.17 Radiograph showing typical appearance of coxofemoral luxation.

Treatment

Treatment options include closed or open reduction. For closed reduction, the patient is placed under general anesthesia and traction maneuvers are employed to replace the head of the femur into the acetabulum. Once in place, the limb is immobilized in an Ehmer sling for 10–14 days (Fox, 1991; McLaughlin, 1995). Commercially available Ehmer slings (Figure 14.18) allow for decreased skin irritation and cutaneous vascular compromise. The ability to open and then reattach the device allows for passive range of motion on the unaffected joints during the convalescent period. Patients with ventral luxation should be placed in hobbles to prevent abduction following reduction.

With closed reduction, hip stability is re-established by joint capsule healing, production of scar tissue, and surrounding musculature. Once the capsule is sealed, the fluid returns to the joint, thus adding additional stability. The ligament of the femoral head never heals. Closed reduction is successful in approximately 50% of first attempts (Bone *et al.*, 1984; Basher *et al.*, 1986; Demko *et al.*, 2006). It is most effective if performed within the first 12–24 hours following the traumatic event. Closed reduction is not an appropriate treatment option if bone fragments are present within the joint, as occurs with avulsion of the ligament.

When closed reduction fails, if immediate weight bearing is necessary, or if there are concurrent orthopedic injuries, surgical intervention is warranted. If the hip joint conformation is normal, open reduction with stabilization is

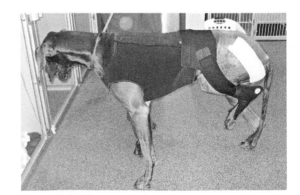

Figure 14.18 Commercially available Ehmer sling.

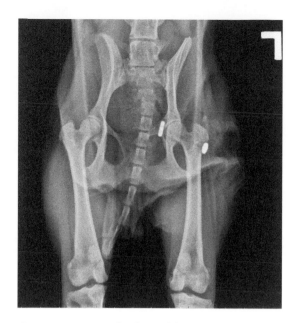

Figure 14.19   Example of one of the most common techniques for repair of hip luxation: reconstruction of the joint capsule with suture and bone anchors, or use of a synthetic material to replace the ligament of the femoral head, termed toggle rod stabilization.

recommended. If the hip is severely dysplastic, a THR or FHO is advised.

Numerous techniques for open reduction and stabilization of the hip have been described. These can be extra-articular or intra-articular repairs. The most common techniques are reconstruction of the joint capsule with suture and bone anchors, or the use of a synthetic material to replace the ligament of the femoral head, termed toggle rod stabilization (Figure 14.19). Both procedures provide immediate stability to the hip. However, long-term stability is achieved from joint capsule healing and periarticular fibrosis, as all synthetic materials will eventually cycle and break.

Postoperative care and prognosis

Limb use following surgical repair is often immediate. However, restricted activity is mandatory for 8–12 weeks following surgery to allow for the joint capsule and surrounding musculature to heal. Rehabilitation therapy, including a home exercise program is strongly encouraged. Initially, static weight-bearing exercises are

introduced along with short-leash walks on even terrain. Hill work and greater intensity strength training is reserved until sufficient healing occurs, usually about 6–8 weeks following repair. The patient can return to full activity level once range of motion of the hip joint and muscle mass of the limb return to normal.

Repeat luxation is the most common complication. Until recently, this rate has been cited as 11–25% (Duff & Bennett, 1982; Bone et al., 1984; Evers et al., 1997; Demko et al., 2006). Advances in suture material have reduced the reluxation rate following toggle rod stabilization to less than 5% (Ash et al., 2012; Kieves et al., 2014).

Cranial cruciate ligament insufficiency

Anatomy

The CCL is composed of two bands, the smaller craniomedial band that is taut in all phases of flexion and extension of the stifle, and the caudolateral band that is taut in extension, but lax in flexion (Figure 14.20). Together, these bands

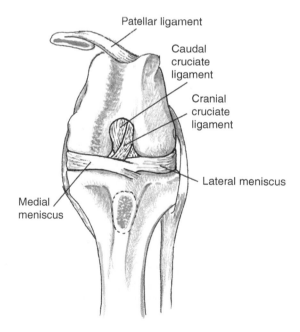

Figure 14.20   The cranial cruciate ligament (CCL) and the caudal cruciate ligament restrict cranial and caudal translation, respectively, of the tibia on the femur. The CCL also resists hyperextension and internal rotation and is the most commonly damaged stifle ligament in dogs. Source: Illustration by Marcia Schlehr.

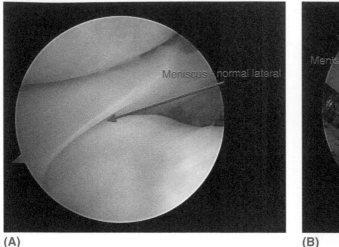
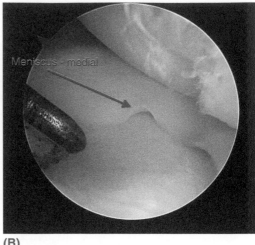

(A)   (B)

Figure 14.21   **(A)** Normal lateral meniscus; note attachment to the tibia and femur. **(B)** Normal medial meniscus. The curled edge is referred to as the "flounce sign" and is highly correlated with a normal meniscus.

limit hyperextension, cranial tibial translation, and internal rotation (Arnoczky & Marshall, 1977). The caudal cruciate is the primary restraint against caudal tibial translation and also helps limit internal rotation of the tibia (Arnoczky & Marshall, 1977; Heffron & Campbell, 1978; Kowaleski *et al.*, 2012). The medial and lateral collateral ligaments serve to limit internal and external rotation.

The menisci are crescent-shaped, cartilaginous tissues that partially divide the articular surfaces of the joint (Figure 14.21). Menisci distribute load during weight bearing and provide structural integrity to the stifle as it undergoes tension and torsion. The menisci also play an important role in joint nutrition and lubrication. Both menisci are anchored to the tibial plateau. The medial meniscus has a firm attachment to the tibia and medial collateral ligament, while the lateral meniscus has a loose attachment to the tibia and an additional attachment to the femur. As a result, the medial meniscus is more vulnerable to injury with cruciate deficiency as it becomes trapped between the condyle and plateau during subluxation.

Kinematics of the cranial cruciate-deficient stifle

While standing, the canine stifle is flexed, resulting in continuous loading of the CCL. This load varies depending on activity level and contraction of various muscle groups. The sloping articular surface of the tibia is called the tibial plateau angle (TPA). TPA reference ranges have been documented in four common canine breeds, although this slope can vary significantly between individual patients (Guastella *et al.*, 2008). When the canine stifle is weight bearing, the tibia is displaced forward, as the femur slides down the slope of the tibia. The steeper the angle present, the more significant the resultant force acting upon the CCL.

Pathophysiology

Traumatic rupture of a healthy CCL is typically caused by hyperextension and excessive internal rotation. More often, CCL injuries occur when normal force is exerted on an abnormal or degenerative joint. Proposed underlying etiologies include biological and biomechanical factors. Biological factors include development, genetics, metabolic function, hormonal influences, infection, immune-mediated processes, and appropriate cellular production and turnover. Biomechanical components include muscular function and forces, alignment, conformation, movement, and joint contacts and pressures (Morgan *et al.*, 2010; Reif *et al.*, 2002). Because cranial cruciate disease is generally degenerative, a patient with a ruptured CCL in has a

50–60% chance of rupturing the opposite CCL (Buote *et al.*, 2009).

Predisposition

Cranial cruciate ligament disease can affect dogs of any breed, sex, or age, although a higher incidence is reported for large-breed and overweight dogs (Duval *et al.*, 1999). Ligament degeneration is also associated with aging, which occurs earlier in large breeds. The Labrador Retriever, Newfoundland, Rottweiler, Mastiff, American Staffordshire Terrier, Akita, Boxer, and Bulldog are overrepresented, supporting the likelihood of a genetic component (Duval *et al.*, 1999). To date, the Newfoundland is the only breed that has identified chromosomal abnormalities associated with cruciate disease (Wilke *et al.*, 2006, 2009). Certain conformation types (an upright stance or marked varus of the pelvic limbs) have an increased incidence of CCL disease. Neutered males and spayed females are also at an increased risk (Duval *et al.*, 1999). Recently, a higher incidence of cruciate disease was seen in female versus male Labrador Retrievers, with an increased incidence in dogs sterilized prior to 1 year of age (Ekenstedt *et al.*, 2017).

Clinical presentation

A rupture due to a traumatic event will initially cause significant stifle effusion, and the patient will be toe-touching to non-weight-bearing lame. In chronic cases, a precipitating event may be associated with an acute notable change in limb use; however, there is often a history of intermittent lameness over a period of several weeks to months. Common findings include the patient sitting with the affected limb extended or positioned laterally rather than flexed and tucked under the body, shifting weight off the affected limb when standing, and displaying stiffness upon rising. Concurrent meniscal injury can cause an audible click when walking or flexing the stifle.

Partial CCL tears typically present with a complaint of a mild weight-bearing lameness following heavy exercise, or stiffness following prolonged periods of rest. Patients with bilateral disease may shift weight back and forth between the pelvic limbs when standing, shift weight to the thoracic limbs, have difficulty or be slow in sitting and rising, and may be exercise intolerant. In some cases, the patient may be unable or unwilling to bear full weight in either pelvic limb, leading to possible misdiagnoses of a neurological condition or hip dysplasia.

Diagnosis

Some dogs with chronic cranial cruciate disease or partial CCL tears do not have significant palpable stifle instability (cranial drawer or tibial thrust test). However, most of these dogs will have significant medial buttress and periarticular thickening of the stifle along with decreased range of motion, particularly flexion. Additional diagnostic tests, such as arthrocentesis, MRI, ultrasound, and/or arthroscopy may be recommended.

Arthroscopy is a minimally invasive technique that allows for live, magnified, high-resolution assessment of the structures within the stifle joint (Figure 14.22). The entire joint can be examined via two or three stab incisions. This not only increases the accuracy of a diagnosis, but also reduces the morbidity and infection rate associated with joint assessment as compared with open arthrotomy (Hoelzler *et al.*, 2004; Pozzi *et al.*, 2008).

Surgical management

Studies have shown surgical intervention to be superior to medical management for CCL disease (Beaulieu & Pozzi, 2016; Hart *et al.*, 2016). Three categories of surgical stabilization exist: intra-articular grafting, extracapsular repair, and corrective osteotomies. The grafting technique has lost popularity, and a study concluded this technique to have inferior results; thus, it will not be covered in detail (Conzemius *et al.*, 2005). It is of note that substantial research is being performed on intra-articular grafting and this method of stabilization may become a viable option for the canine patient in the future. Of the remaining techniques, osteotomies have proven to be superior to extracapsular repair for long-term outcomes (Gordon-Evans *et al.*, 2013; Nelson *et al.*, 2013; Krotscheck *et al.*, 2016).

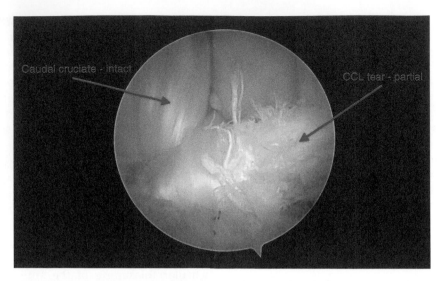

Figure 14.22   Arthroscopic image showing a partial cranial cruciate ligament tear.

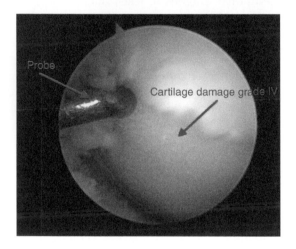

Figure 14.23   Severe cartilage erosion in a dog with cranial cruciate ligament rupture.

The patient's age, size, conformation, activity level, and concurrent medical conditions are considered when selecting the surgical procedure. A thorough evaluation of the joint must be performed at the time of surgery, regardless of the type of stabilization performed (Figure 14.23).

Meniscus

A thorough evaluation of the meniscus with a probe is performed (Thieman *et al.*, 2006; Pozzi *et al.*, 2008; Cook *et al.*, 2010a). Missed meniscal damage is the most common cause of procedural failure in one report (Thieman *et al.*, 2006). The damaged portion of the meniscus is excised, with an attempt to preserve as much of the meniscal rim as possible. If the rim is damaged, a caudal pole hemimeniscectomy or meniscal release is performed. Isolated meniscal lesions are rare in dogs but have been reported in both the medial and lateral menisci (Ridge, 2006; Williams, 2010).

Stabilization techniques

Extracapsular techniques

Variations of extracapsular repair are among the most popular CCL procedures to date. These techniques passively stabilize the stifle by neutralizing cranial drawer via the formation of periarticular fibrosis. The most frequently performed extracapsular technique is the lateral fabellar suture (LFS) repair. This technique involves passing a nonabsorbable synthetic suture external to the joint capsule in either a figure eight or loop pattern around the lateral fabella, and through a hole made in the tibial crest. A knot or a stainless steel crimp clamp is used to hold the suture material taut. Alternatively, two tibial tunnels may be made and the suture passed through these rather than under the patellar tendon. While the suture material will eventually stretch or break, it is meant to provide temporary stabilization to the stifle until the body can form organized scar tissue around the suture material that ultimately provides the long-term, functional stability. The major limitations of this technique are that the monofilament has relatively low tensile strength and a fair amount of creep, and the points of implantation are nonisometric to the cruciate ligament. These factors can lead to joint laxity during the initial 4–8 weeks of healing that may result in either too much scar tissue formation, which decreases functional range of motion of the stifle, or too little scar tissue, which can lead to persistent instability. These limitations become more obvious in large, giant, and active performance dogs.

Several bone anchor and suture combinations are also available for use in extracapsular repair. With these procedures, a bone anchor may be used both in the femur and tibia to anchor mono- or multifilament material. Other systems use only one bone anchor or bone tunnel in the tibia. To date, no clinical comparisons of these various techniques have been published.

The TightRope® CCL technique differs from conventional extracapsular stabilization in that it can be performed in a minimally invasive manner, provides bone-to-bone stabilization, and more accurately mimics the natural orientation of the CCL, using a suture material that is stronger and has less creep than conventional ones (Burgess *et al.*, 2010) (Figure 14.24). Using specific landmarks, bone tunnels are drilled through the femur and tibia. The material is passed through the tunnels and is secured using stainless steel buttons. The procedure relies on the formation of organized scar tissue around the implant for long-term function. Early literature suggests a high level of success with a relative low level of morbidity when compared with osteotomy procedures (Cook *et al.*, 2010b; Christopher & Cook, 2011).

Corrective osteotomies

Tibial plateau leveling osteotomy (TPLO). The TPLO is a common procedure of choice for active, large and giant-breed dogs (Priddy *et al.*, 2003; Lazar *et al.*, 2005; Cook *et al.*, 2010b; Kowaleski *et al.*, 2012). The procedure involves making a curved osteotomy through the upper portion of the tibia (Figure 14.25). The articular

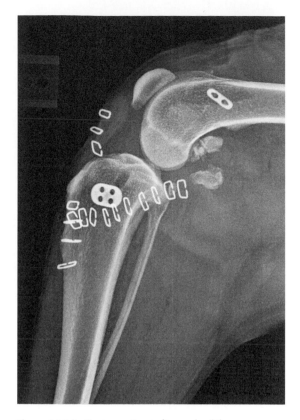

Figure 14.24 Postoperative radiograph of the TightRope® CCL technique.

component of the tibia is rotated to achieve a lower angle of the tibial plateau relative to the long axis of the tibia. The amount of rotation is based upon the tibial plateau angle as measured on preoperative radiographs. After rotation, a plate and screws are applied to hold it in position. This procedure alters the biomechanics of the stifle, placing additional reliance on the caudal cruciate ligament and active muscle stabilizers of the stifle.

This procedure can be used in any size dog with any tibial plateau angle, it has a highly reproducible outcome, and because it relies on bone healing, is easily assessed radiographically. The procedure may also have a slower progression of OA than the LFS procedure (Lazar *et al.*, 2005). Recent prospective, blinded studies have shown the TPLO to have a high success rate with high client satisfaction (93%) when compared with LFS stabilization (Gordon-Evans *et al.*, 2013; Nelson *et al.*, 2013). Force plate analysis has also shown TPLO to be

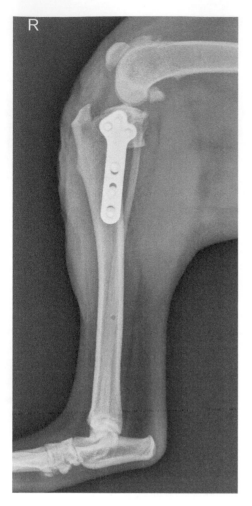

Figure 14.25   The tibial plateau leveling osteotomy is the authors' procedure of choice for active, large, and giant breeds of dogs with a ruptured cranial cruciate ligament.

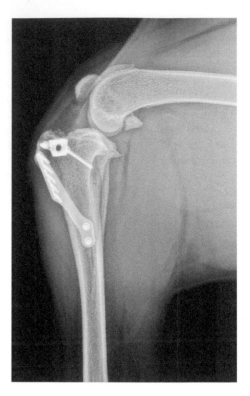

Figure 14.26   Tibial tuberosity advancement involves a linear osteotomy caudal to the tibial tuberosity. The tibial tuberosity is advanced so that the patellar tendon is perpendicular to the tibial plateau.

superior to LFS, with dogs undergoing TPLO returning to normal peak vertical force 1 year following surgery compared with only 85% in dogs undergoing LFS (Nelson *et al.*, 2013). Limitations include cost associated with the procedure compared with other treatment options, the high learning curve for the surgeon, the potential for serious complications, and the lack of suitability in geriatric patients or those with poor bone quality (Priddy *et al.*, 2003; Lazar *et al.*, 2005; Boudrieau, 2009; Christopher & Cook, 2011).

Tibial tuberosity advancement (TTA). The TTA procedure involves a linear osteotomy caudal to the tibial tuberosity (Figure 14.26). The tibial

tuberosity is advanced so that the patellar tendon is perpendicular to the tibial plateau. The advanced portion of bone is held in place with a titanium cage (that acts as a spacer between the two bones) and plate (Kowaleski *et al.*, 2012). A graft may be applied to the space between the bones to promote bone healing. Modifications of the TTA procedure that do not rely on bone plate fixation have been described (Samoy *et al.*, 2015). The procedure relies on neutralizing the tibial thrust by changing the force through the knee to be parallel to the patellar tendon (Kowaleski *et al.*, 2012). TTA provides a biomechanical advantage to the quadriceps muscles, and subsequently stabilizes the stifle. Biomechanical studies suggest that TTA may neutralize the forces exerted on the stifle and preserve the contact mechanics of the stifle better than TPLO (Guerrero *et al.*, 2011; Kim *et al.*, 2009, 2010). However, post-stabilization meniscal tears are reported more commonly with TTA than with TPLO (Lafaver *et al.*,

2007; Stein & Schmoekel, 2008; Christopher & Cook, 2011; Hurt *et al.*, 2011). This procedure is less technically demanding than the TPLO; however, there is still significant risk for surgical error. The TTA is best used in patients with a low tibial plateau angle and no tibial angulation abnormalities (Boudrieau, 2009). There can be issues with preoperative planning for appropriate cage size selection (Cadmus *et al.*, 2011). The advancement of the tibia can change the external appearance of the tibia, particularly in dogs with short hair, which may be a disadvantage in the show ring. The TTA also carries a risk of major complications. Infections of the spacer cage, although uncommon, can be extremely challenging to resolve. Recent research shows that at a trot, the TTA procedure and LFS procedure do not return dogs to normal function at 12 months, while TPLO does when compared with a control population (Krotscheck *et al.*, 2016).

Patellar luxation

Anatomy and pathophysiology

Patellar luxation occurs when one or several structures that comprise the quadriceps mechanism are misaligned, resulting in partial or complete deviation of the patella from the trochlea (L'Eplattenier & Montavon, 2002a; Bevan & Taylor, 2004; Alam *et al.*, 2007). In fact, some have speculated that the condition should actually be termed "femoral trochlear luxation" as the patella will always find its natural position created by the origin and insertion of the quadriceps mechanism, and the distortion of anatomy results in an incorrect position of the trochlea in line with the quadriceps mechanism. The actual bony distortion leading to patellar luxation may be a distortion of the femur or the tibia and it has been speculated that with medial patella luxation asynchronous growth of the distal femoral physis may be a major contributing cause that perpetuates the distortion. As the patella is tracked medially, increased tension develops laterally in the distal femoral physis, which leads to an increase in femoral torsion and distal femoral varus. This increases the forces resulting in medial patellar luxation. In addition, the femoral sulcus does not develop because there is not appropriate retropatellar pressure, and the

medialized forces on the tibial tubercle results in abnormalities in tibial growth.

Medial patellar luxation (MPL) occurs significantly more frequently than lateral patellar luxation in all dogs (Alam *et al.*, 2007). Small breed dogs are most commonly affected by MPL, and the condition is considered heritable in some breeds (Alam *et al.*, 2007). Large-breed dogs are also commonly affected with MPL, with Labrador Retrievers being overrepresented (Gibbons *et al.*, 2006). Patellar luxation occurs bilaterally in 50% of affected dogs, with females affected more commonly than males (L'Eplattenier & Montavon, 2002a; Gibbons *et al.*, 2006; Alam *et al.*, 2007).

Patellar luxation is divided into four grades based on the severity of the luxation (L'Eplattenier & Montavon, 2002a; Bevan & Taylor, 2004) (Table 14.1). MPL predisposes dogs to cranial cruciate ligament rupture (CCLR) and the higher the grade of MPL, the higher the incidence of concurrent CCLR (Campbell *et al.*, 2010). One study found that 40% of dogs with MPL had concurrent CCLR (Campbell *et al.*, 2010).

Diagnosis

Intermittent hopping or skipping and reluctance to jump are typical historical findings in dogs

Table 14.1 Grades of patellar luxation

Grade	Features
I	Patella can be manually luxated but is reduced when released
II	Patella can be manually luxated or it can spontaneously luxate with flexion of the stifle joint. The patella remains luxated until it is manually reduced or when the animal extends the joint and derotates the tibia in the opposite direction of luxation
III	Patella remains luxated most of the time but can be manually reduced with the stifle joint in extension. Flexion and extension of the stifle results in reluxation of the patella
IV	Patella is permanently luxated and cannot be manually repositioned. There may be up to 90 degrees of rotation of the proximal tibial plateau. The femoral trochlear groove is shallow or absent, and there is displacement of the quadriceps muscle group in the direction of luxation

with a grade I–III patellar luxation. Grade IV MPL is generally associated with a significant limb deformity and moderate to severe lameness is common (Alam *et al.*, 2007). An acute exacerbation of lameness in dogs with MPL should raise suspicion for CCLR (Campbell *et al.*, 2010).

Patellar luxation is diagnosed by physical examination. Radiographs are often recommended to assess for degenerative joint disease and to evaluate bony conformation for surgical planning (L'Eplattenier & Montavon, 2002a). Previous recommendations in assessment of a true craniocaudal radiograph have been shown to be inaccurate (Aiken & Barnes, 2014) leading to the suggestion that CT is the gold standard for assessment of femoral and tibial alignment in cases of patella luxation.

Computed tomography is useful in dogs with severe conformational deformities to assist with surgical planning (Towle *et al.*, 2005) (Figure 14.27), and recent increased availability of CT has allowed for validation of techniques to measure femoral and tibial alignment (Barnes *et al.*, 2015; Oxley *et al.* 2013).

Treatment

Nonsurgical management is recommended for animals with grade I and asymptomatic grade II patellar luxation (L'Eplattenier & Montavon, 2002b). The decision to pursue surgery is based upon frequency and severity of lameness, functional limitations, and the opportunity to decrease the likelihood of CCL tears. Several surgical techniques that aim to realign the quadriceps mechanism and decrease the abnormal biomechanical stresses placed on the patella have been developed (Johnson *et al.*, 2001; L'Eplattenier & Montavon, 2002b; Arthurs & Langley-Hobbs, 2006; Swiderski & Palmer, 2007; Langenbach & Marcellin-Little, 2010; Yeadon *et al.*, 2011). Usually several techniques are employed in combination in a single patient.

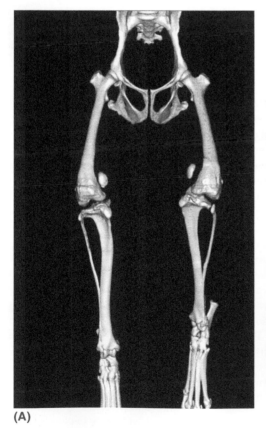

(A)

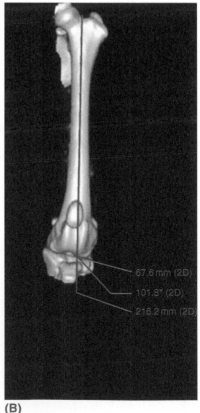

(B)

Figure 14.27   **(A, B)** CT is useful in dogs with severe conformational deformities to assist with surgical planning.

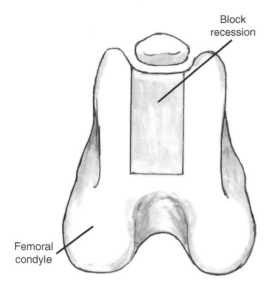

Figure 14.28 Block trochlear recession. Note that the patella is well-seated within the surgically deepened groove. Source: Illustration by Marcia Schlehr.

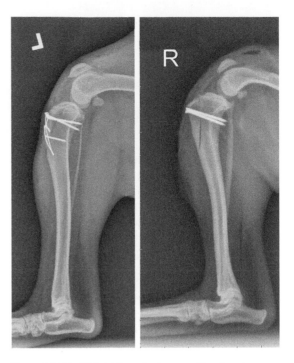

Figure 14.29 Tibial tuberosity transposition involves an osteotomy of the tibial tuberosity and placement of orthopedic implants (K-wires ± cerclage wire) to secure the tuberosity in the transposed location.

Trochleoplasties

Wedge or block trochlear recession can be performed to deepen the sulcus and so provide more effective buttressing to the patella (Johnson *et al.*, 2001; L'Eplattenier & Montavon, 2002b) (Figure 14.28). However, there are no good studies detailing what the trochlear depth should be (as a guideline, the surgeon should aim to have one third of the height of the patella and two thirds the length of the patella in the groove) and both techniques involve some degree of violation to the joint surface. Techniques that do not preserve the articular cartilage such as abrasion arthroplasty should be avoided.

Tibial tuberosity transposition

Deepening the trochlear sulcus will do nothing to realign the quadriceps mechanism and so some form of tibial or femoral osteotomy is also required. Internal rotation of the tibia is common in dogs with MPL (external rotation with lateral patellar luxation). Transposition of the tibial tuberosity by several millimeters has been shown to significantly decrease the incidence of reluxation following surgical correction (Arthurs & Langley-Hobbs, 2006). This procedure involves an osteotomy of the

tibial tuberosity and placement of orthopedic implants (K-wires ± cerclage wire) to secure the tuberosity in the transposed location (L'Eplattenier & Montavon, 2002b) (Figure 14.29). Rates of reluxation can be high after tibial tubercle transposition, especially in grades III and IV (Arthurs & Langley-Hobbs, 2006; Cashmore *et al.*, 2014), and often the anatomic distal femoral lateral angle (aDFLA) will be exaggerated (excessive femoral varus). Tibial osteotomy does not address this primary cause, so consideration should be given to femoral osteotomy in cases of excessive femoral varus (aDFLA of greater than 104 degrees) (Barnes *et al.*, 2015).

Distal femoral osteotomy

The normal range of aDFLA is between 94 and 98 degrees (Barnes *et al.*, 2015). Patients with higher grades of luxation (III and IV) with excessive varus should be treated by distal femoral osteotomy (DFO). Recent advances in CT and the better assessment of femoral torsion means that DFO can also be used to address femoral torsion at the same time. Although undoubtedly more invasive than a simple tibial tubercle transposition, a DFO has a reportedly low complication rate and good long-term outcomes (Brower *et al.*, 2017).

Antirotational suture

A lateral fabellar-tibial suture can be placed to reduce internal tibial rotation. This is the same technique used for the extracapsular repair of CCL tears, and is commonly employed in dogs that have concurrent MPL and CCL tears (L'Eplattenier & Montavon, 2002b).

Soft tissue reconstruction

Surgical release of the tight tissues and imbrication of the loose tissues can be performed along with selected procedures to help maintain the patella within the trochlear groove (L'Eplattenier & Montavon, 2002b).

Concurrent MPL and CCLR

Medial patellar luxation has been shown to predispose animals to rupture of the CCL (Campbell *et al.*, 2010). When the two conditions are diagnosed concurrently, surgical treatment is designed to address both biomechanical deficiencies (L'Eplattenier & Montavon, 2002b; Langenbach & Marcellin-Little, 2010; Yeadon *et al.*, 2011). In addition to antirotational suture (extracapsular stabilization), modifications of the TPLO and TTA procedures have been shown to effectively treat concurrent MPL/CCLR (Langenbach & Marcellin-Little, 2010; Yeadon *et al.*, 2011).

Superficial digital flexor tendon luxation

Anatomy

The superficial digital flexor is one component of the common calcanean tendon. Originating on the lateral supracondylar tuberosity of the femur, it has two insertions onto the lateral and medial surfaces of the calcaneus, before continuing distally to the phalanges (Dyce *et al.*, 1996).

The calcaneal bursa lies deep to the superficial digital flexor tendon at the level of the tuber calcaneus.

Pathophysiology

Luxation of the superficial digital flexor tendon can be seen in either the medial or lateral direction; however lateral luxation is more common due in part to the less well-defined medial retinaculum (Mauterer *et al.*, 1993). Following retinacular tearing, fibrosis of the torn retinaculum and secondary bursitis may develop.

The high prevalence in Shetland Sheepdogs and Collies suggests a hereditary basis (Gough & Thomas, 2004). Pedigree analysis suggests an autosomal recessive method of inheritance (Solanti *et al.*, 2002). Proposed risk factors for superficial digital flexor tendon luxation include obesity (Bernard, 1977; McNicholas *et al.*, 2000), trauma (Bennett & Campbell, 1979), and conformational abnormality (Solanti *et al.*, 2002).

Clinical presentation

Patients present with intermittent or continuous, low-grade, uni- or bilateral pelvic limb lameness, usually before 1.5 years of age (Solanti *et al.*, 2002). Findings include swelling present on either side of the calcaneus as well as a distinct popping of the superficial digital flexor tendon as it luxates when the tarsus is flexed. Discomfort is present on direct palpation of the tuber calcaneus. Patients with accompanying bursitis may have swelling over the tuber calcaneus.

Diagnostics

Radiography, ultrasound, and MRI may be used to confirm physical exam findings and to rule out concomitant impairments.

Treatment

The torn retinaculum is imbricated with nonabsorbable suture and in some cases may require alternative anchoring such as screws or bone tunnels. A 6% recurrence rate requiring a second surgery has been reported (Bernard, 1977; Mauterer *et al.*, 1993; Reinke & Mughannam, 1993; Hoscheit, 1994). Chronic tendonitis and bursitis can decrease the likelihood of a good surgical outcome (Raes *et al.*, 2011). Nonsurgical management can yield adequate function, especially in less active patients.

Postoperative care

Immobilization of the tarsus was traditionally recommended for 2–4 weeks after surgery (Piermattei *et al.*, 2006). Rehabilitation therapy in these patients focuses on maintenance of range of motion as well as static and dynamic weight-bearing exercises to regain strength in the postsurgical limb. Treatment modalities in addition to manual and exercise therapy include ultrasound and laser therapy.

Case Study 14.2   Traumatic Achilles tendon rupture at the level of the mid-tendon

Signalment: 1.5-y.o. M/N, Labrador Retriever, high-activity companion that chases balls, plays Frisbee.

Presenting complaint: Acute grade IV/V right pelvic limb lameness with a dropped tarsus after getting foot stuck in a fireplace vent

Physical examination: Plantigrade stance in the right pelvic limb. Palpation reveals moderate soft tissue swelling at the level of the gastrocnemius with a palpable void of tendon at the level of the mid-tibia. Remainder of orthopedic exam unremarkable (Figure 14.30).

Diagnostics: Radiographs: orthogonal views of right and left tarsi reveal mild soft tissue swelling in the distal 3–4 cm of the right common calcaneal tendon (1 cm thickness right vs. 8 mm thickness left). No osseous changes at calcaneus (Figure 14.31).

Surgical treatment: Superficial digital flexor and gastrocnemius tendons severed 3 cm proximal to the tuber calcaneus. Tendons individually apposed

using 0 Prolene® in a three loop-pulley pattern. Tendon sheath closed with 3-0 PDS® and infused with platelet-rich plasma (PRP-Angel System® set at 7% hematocrit, 1.5 mL). Transarticular external fixator with hinge applied following repair to immobilize tarsus at 160 degrees of extension (Figure 14.32).

Postoperative care: Patient discharged 1 day postop with fixator in locked out position. Clients instructed to provide brief leash walks for first 14 days (Figure 14.33).

Rehabilitation therapy: Weekly therapy recommended for 12 weeks minimum.

Week 2-4: Manual therapies including PROM of affected limb joints, excluding tarsus, joint compressions, cross frictional massage over length of Achilles, and passive limb stretching. Pulsed ultrasound over repair site, and laser therapy of affected region and *compensatory* regions.

Therapeutic exercise goal: Early limb use to encourage proper healing. Initial exercises include weight shifting, cookie stretches, and low front feet up, ensuring weight bearing on the surgical limb. On-leash deliberate walking exercise begins with 5–10-minute walks up to 2–3 times a day if well tolerated, with 3–5-minute intervals added weekly.

Week 4-8: Resistance damper is applied to fixator to allow for controlled, increasingly dynamic motion at tarsus. Continuation of rehabilitation therapies, with partial tarsus ROM, and advanced therapeutic exercise plan to progress tendon loading.

Exercise: Diagonal thoracic limb lifts eventually progresses to the opposite pelvic limb lifts. Backwards walking and pivoting a radius initiated,

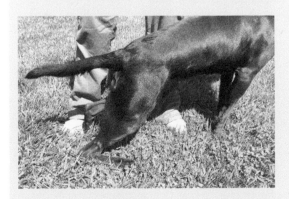

Figure 14.30   Plantigrade stance in the right pelvic limb.

(Continued)

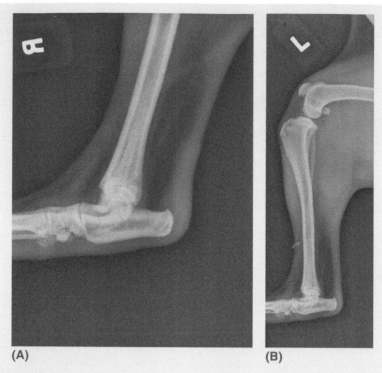

(A) (B)

Figure 14.31 Radiographs of (**A**) right and (**B**) left tarsi revealing mild soft tissue swelling in the distal part of the right common calcaneal tendon.

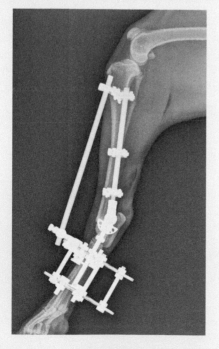

Figure 14.32 Static transarticular external fixator with cross bar.

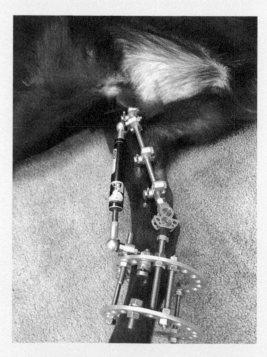

Figure 14.33 Hinged transarticular external fixator with damper.

then sit-to-stand repetitions on flat ground with brief tugging. Walking times increase with start of gentle hills in week 6.

Week 8-12: External fixator removed; Therapaw® (nonthermoplast) support brace in place when not confined or resting. Manual therapies progress to complete ROM for gentle passive flexor tendon stretching. Hill walking increased, with gradually incorporated side hill, circles, and backwards walking. Balance disc work added, increasing repetitions and difficulty. Brace is somewhat cumbersome so exercises are modified. Hydrotherapy introduced at 8 weeks, and client can remove brace for massage and stretching at home.

Week 12-16: Brace is downgraded to remove support straps, and used during lengthy walks or when excitable. Hydrotherapy continues; 45–60-minute walks and hiking in brace, shorter walks without brace, and light trotting and loping allowed for short durations. Therapeutic exercises performed without brace.

Week 16: Transition to off-leash work over next 2 weeks while in brace.

Week 20: Transition to full activity without brace.

Achilles tendon injuries

Anatomy

The Achilles tendon is made up of three components: the gastrocnemius tendon, the common calcaneal tendon (the combined tendons of the biceps femoris, gracilis, and semitendinosus), and the superficial digital flexor tendon (Dyce *et al.*, 1996). The blood flow to the common calcaneal tendon arises predominantly from the caudal saphenous artery. The midbody of the tendon has the poorest blood supply, while the calcaneal insertion has the most vascularity (Gilbert *et al.*, 2010); however, there are five avascular fibrocartilaginous zones located in the distal tendon (Jopp & Reese, 2009). These fibrocartilaginous zones are thought to be an adaptation to pressure and are not considered pathological (Tillmann & Koch, 1995; Benjamin & Ralphs, 1998).

Pathophysiology

Achilles tendon rupture is a common tendon injury in veterinary medicine. Laceration of the Achilles may occur, and in some cases, a skin lesion may not be evident. More often, avulsion of the gastrocnemius tendon is seen after heavy activity in mature sporting and working breeds. Labrador Retrievers and Doberman Pinschers appear to be overrepresented (Corr *et al.*, 2010).

An underlying degenerative process is suspected; however, the definitive cause is not known. Both human and canine Achilles tendon ruptures tend to occur in the area of the fibrocartilaginous zones, which are thought to be areas of increased stress loading (Tillmann & Koch, 1995; Benjamin & Ralphs, 1998). Some drugs and disease processes such as diabetes, endogenous or exogenous steroids (Hossain *et al.*, 2008), and fluoroquinolones (Lim *et al.*, 2008) have been implicated.

Clinical presentation

Patients with acute gastrocnemius avulsion present non-weight-bearing to toe-touching lame with swelling at the calcaneus. Chronic injuries may present with a weight-bearing plantigrade stance. There may be digital flexion present due to increased stress on the intact superficial digital flexor tendon (Figure 14.34). Palpation may identify a fibrous thickening at the site of injury.

Diagnostics

Radiography may demonstrate soft tissue swelling at the level of the injury with possible avulsion of bone fragments and/or mineralization of the tendon (Figure 14.35). Diagnostic ultrasound can identify partial tears, and be used to monitor healing (Kramer *et al.*, 2001). MRI, commonly used in human Achilles tendon injuries (Schweitzer & Karasick, 2000), is gaining use in veterinary medicine.

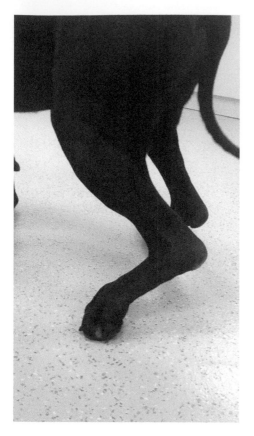

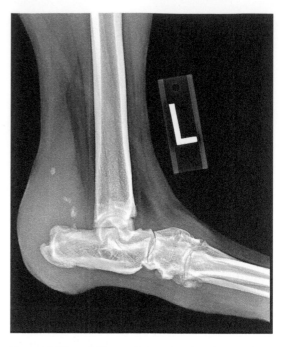

Figure 14.35 Achilles tendon avulsion. Radiography may demonstrate soft tissue swelling at the level of the injury with possible avulsion of bone fragments and/or mineralization of the tendon.

Figure 14.34 This patient with chronic gastrocnemius avulsion presents with a weight-bearing plantigrade stance and digital flexion due to increased stress on the intact superficial digital flexor tendon.

Treatment

Surgical correction is recommended for all Achilles tendon avulsions and lacerations. Primary repair of gastrocnemius tendon avulsions is accomplished via bone tunnels through the calcaneus and specialized suture patterns with nonabsorbable suture. Additional support can be provided with mesh grafts as well as muscle and fascial flaps (Baltzer & Rist, 2009; Morton *et al.*,2015; Katayama, 2016). The repair can be augmented with platelet-rich plasma, which provides high concentrations of growth factors that may increase vascular and fibroblastic proliferation (Hernández-Martínez *et al.*, 2012)

Postoperative immobilization of the joint is essential for several weeks to relive stress on the tendon and allow adequate healing.

Immobilization is performed with the tarsus in an extended position using a cast, splint, external skeletal fixation, or transcalcaneal screw (Nielsen & Pluhar, 2006; Braden, 1974). Alternatively, a hinged tarsal orthotic device can be custom molded following surgery (see Chapter 11) (Figure 14.36). In theory, this allows for a gradual increase in the range of motion of the tarsus following surgical repair. However, our ability to alleviate strain on the Achilles tendon while immobilized is not as one may theorize, in fact, one study failed to demonstrate a difference in maximum strain after immobilization, compared with maximum strain during normal motion in an experimental design (Lister *et al.*, 2009).

Function following surgical repair is generally very good, despite the lack of normal tendon architecture (Kramer *et al.*, 2001).

Tendon injuries with core lesions or incomplete tears can be treated with conservative management. This may include physical rehabilitation and immobilization, as well as the use of orthobiologics (Chen *et al.*, 2012). Ultrasound has been shown to increase tendon healing via

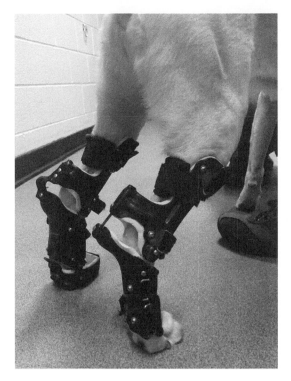

Figure 14.36 Achilles tendon avulsion. Hinged tarsal orthotic devices can be custom molded following surgery.

increased expression of COX-2, TGF-beta 1, collagen I, and collagen II (Kosaka *et al.*, 2011). Mesenchymal stem cell therapy and/or platelet-rich plasma therapy has also shown promising results in improving tendon healing (Chen *et al.*, 2012; Nourissat *et al.*, 2010).

References

Aiken, M. & Barnes, D. 2014. Are the fabellae bisected by the femoral cortices in a true craniocaudal pelvic limb radiograph? *J Small Animal Pract*, 55, 465–470.

Alam, M. R., Lee, J. I., Kang, H. S., Kim, I. S., Park, S. Y., Lee, K. C. & Kim, N. S. 2007. Frequency and distribution of patellar luxation in dogs: 134 cases (2000 to 2005). *Vet Comp Orthop Traumatol*, 20, 59–64.

Arnoczky, S. P. & Marshall, J. L. 1977. The cruciate ligaments of the canine stifle: an anatomical and functional analysis. *Am J Vet Res*, 38, 1807–1814.

Arthurs, G. I. & Langley-HOBBS, S. J. 2006. Complications associated with corrective surgery for patellar luxation in 109 dogs. *Vet Surg*, 35, 559–566.

Ash, K., Rosselli, D., Danielski, A., Farrell, M., Hamilton, M. & Fitzpatrick, N. 2012. Correction of craniodorsal coxofemoral luxation in cats and small breed dogs using a modified Knowles technique with the braided polyblend TightRope systems. *Vet Comp Orthop Traumatol*, 25, 54–60.

Baltzer, W. I. & Rist, P. 2009. Achilles tendon repair in dogs using the semitendinosus muscle: surgical technique and short-term outcome in five dogs. *Vet Surg*, 38, 770–779.

Barnes, D. M., Anderson, A. A., Frost, C. & Barnes, J. 2015. Repeatability and reproducibility of measurements of femoral and tibial alignment using computed tomography multiplanar reconstructions. *Vet Surg*, 44, 85–93.

Basher, A. W. P., Walter, M. C. & Newton, C. D. 1986. Coxofemoral luxation in the dog and cat. *Vet. Surg*, 15, 356–362.

Beaulieu, A. F. & Pozzi, A. 2016. Does physical therapy after a TPLO lead to improvement of the 1-year post-operative peak vertical force? *Veterinary Evidence*, 1(3).

Benjamin, M. & Ralphs, J. R. 1998. Fibrocartilage in tendons and ligaments—an adaptation to compressive load. *J Anat*, 193, 481–494.

Bennett, D. & Campbell, J. R. 1979. Unusual soft tissue orthopaedic problems in the dog. *J Small Anim Pract*, 20, 27–39.

Bernard, M. A. 1977. Superficial digital flexor tendon injury in the dog. *Can Vet J*, 18, 105–107.

Bernarde, A. 2010. Juvenile pubic symphysiodesis and juvenile pubic symphysiodesis associated with pectineus myotomy: short-term outcome in 56 dysplastic puppies. *Vet Surg*, 39, 158–164.

Bevan, J. M. & Taylor, R. A. 2004. Arthroscopic release of the medial femoropatellar ligament for canine medial patellar luxation. *J Am Anim Hosp Assoc*, 40, 321–330.

Biemond, J. E., Aquarius, R., Verdonschot, N. & Buma, P. 2011. Frictional and bone ingrowth properties of engineered surface topographies produced by electron beam technology. *Arch Orthop Trauma Surg*, 131, 711–718.

Bockstahler, B., Krautler, C., Holler, P., Kotschwar, A., Vobornik, A. & Peham, C. 2012. Pelvic limb kinematics and surface electromyography of the vastus lateralis, biceps femoris, and gluteus medius muscle in dogs with hip osteoarthritis. *Vet Surg*, 41, 54–62.

Bone, D. L., Walker, M. & Cantwell, H. D. 1984. Traumatic coxofemoral luxation in dogs results of repair. *Vet Surg*, 13, 263–270.

Boudrieau, R. J. 2009. Tibial plateau leveling osteotomy or tibial tuberosity advancement? *Vet Surg*, 38, 1–22.

Braden, T. D. 1974. Musculotendinous rupture of the Achilles apparatus and repair using internal fixation only. *Vet Med Small Anim Clin*, 69, 729–735.

Breur, G. J. & Blevins, W. E. 1997. Traumatic injury of the iliopsoas muscle in three dogs. *J Am Vet Med Assoc*, 210, 1631–164.

Brower, B. E., Kowaleski, M. P., Peruski, A. M., Dyce, J., Johnson, K. A. & Boudrieau, R. J. 2017. Distal femoral lateral closing wedge osteotomy as a component of comprehensive treatment of medial patellar luxation and distal femoral varus in dogs. *Vet Comp Orthop Traumatol*, 30(1), 20–27.

Buote, N., Fusco, J. & Radasch, R. 2009. Age, tibial plateau angle, sex, and weight as risk factors for contralateral rupture of the cranial cruciate ligament in Labradors. *Vet Surg*, 38, 481–489.

Burgess, R., Elder, S., McLaughlin, R. & Constable, P. 2010. In vitro biomechanical evaluation and comparison of FiberWire, FiberTape, OrthoFiber, and nylon leader line for potential use during extraarticular stabilization of canine cruciate deficient stifles. *Vet Surg*, 39, 208–215.

Cadmus, J. M., Palmer, R. H. & Duncan, C. G. 2011. The effect of preoperative planning method upon the recommended tibial tuberosity advancement cage size. In: *Proceedings of the 38th Annual Conference of the Veterinary Orthopedic Society*, March 5–12, Snowmass, CO, p. 43.

Campbell, C. A., Horstman, C. L., Mason, D. R. & Evans, R. B. 2010. Severity of patellar luxation and frequency of concomitant cranial cruciate ligament rupture in dogs: 162 cases (2004–2007). *J Am Vet Med Assoc*, 236, 887–891.

Cashmore, R. G., Havlicek, M., Perkins, N. R., James, D. R., Fearnside, S. M., Marchevsky, A. M. & Black, A. P. 2014. Major complications and risk factors associated with surgical correction of congenital medial patella luxation in 124 dogs. *Vet Comp Orthop Traumatol*, 27, 263–270.

Chen, L., Dong, S. W., Liu, J. P., Tao, X., Tang, K. L. & XU, J. Z. 2012. Synergy of tendon stem cells and platelet-rich plasma in tendon healing. *J Orthop Res*, 30, 991–997.

Christopher, S. A. & Cook, J. L. 2011. Long-term follow-up of cranial cruciate ligament techniques. In: *Proceedings of the 38th Annual Conference of the Veterinary Orthopedic Society*. March 5–12, Snowmass, CO, p. 55.

Conzemius, M. G., Evans, R. B., Besancon, M. F., Gordon, W. J., Horstman, C. L., Hoefle, W. D., *et al.* 2005. Effect of surgical technique on limb function after surgery for rupture of the cranial cruciate ligament in dogs. *J Am Vet Med Assoc*, 226, 232–236.

Cook, J. L., Kuroki, K., Visco, D., Pelletier, J. P., Schulz, L. & Lafeber, F. P. 2010a. The OARSI histopathology initiative—recommendations for histological assessments of osteoarthritis in the dog. *Osteoarthritis Cartilage*, 18(Suppl. 3), S66–79.

Cook, J. L., Luther, J. K., Beetem, J., Karnes, J. & Cook, C. R. 2010b. Clinical comparison of a novel

extracapsular stabilization procedure and tibial plateau leveling osteotomy for treatment of cranial cruciate ligament deficiency in dogs. *Vet Surg*, 39, 315–323.

Coopman, F., Verhoeven, G., Saunders, J., Duchateau, L. & Van Bree, H. 2008. Prevalence of hip dysplasia, elbow dysplasia and humeral head osteochondrosis in dog breeds in Belgium. *Vet Rec*, 163, 654–658.

Corr, S. A., Draffan, D., Kulendra, E., Carmichael, S. & Brodbelt, D. 2010. Retrospective study of Achilles mechanism disruption in 45 dogs. *Vet Rec*, 167, 407–411.

Dassler, C. 2003. Canine hip dysplasia: diagnosis and nonsurgical treatment. In: Slatter, D. (ed.), *Textbook of Small Animal Surgery*, 3rd edn. Philadelphia, PA: Saunders, pp. 2019–2020.

Demko, J. & McLaughlin, R. 2005. Developmental orthopedic disease. *Vet Clin North Am Small Anim Pract*, 35, 1111–1135.

Demko, J. L., Sidaway, B. K., Thieman, K. M., Fox, D. B., Boyle, C. R. & McLaughlin, R. M. 2006. Toggle rod stabilization for treatment of hip joint luxation in dogs: 62 cases (2000–2005). *J Am Vet Med Assoc*, 229, 984–989.

Doornink, M. T., Nieves, M. A. & Evans, R. 2006. Evaluation of ilial screw loosening after triple pelvic osteotomy in dogs: 227 cases (1991–1999). *J Am Vet Med Assoc*, 229, 535–541.

Dueland, R., Bartel, D. L. & Antonson, E. 1977. Force plate technique for canine gait analysis: preliminary report on total hip and excision arthroplasty [proceedings]. *Bull Hosp Joint Dis*, 38, 35–36.

Duff, S. R. & Bennett, D. 1982. Hip luxation in small animals: an evaluation of some methods of treatment. *Vet Rec*, 111, 140–143.

Duval, J. M., Budsberg, S. C., Flo, G. L. & Sammarco, J. L. 1999. Breed, sex, and body weight as risk factors for rupture of the cranial cruciate ligament in young dogs. *J Am Vet Med Assoc*, 215, 811–814.

Dyce, K. M., Sack, W. O. & Wensing, C. J. G. 1996. The locomotor apparatus. In: *Textbook of Veterinary Anatomy*, 2nd edn. Philadelphia, PA: WB Saunders, pp. 31–98.

Edwards, M. R., Egger, E. L. & Schwarz, P. D. 1997. Aseptic loosening of the femoral implant after cemented total hip arthroplasty in dogs: 11 cases in 10 dogs (1991–1995). *J Am Vet Med Assoc*, 211, 580–586.

Ekenstedt, K. J., Minor, K. M, Rendahl, A. K., & Conzemius, M. G. 2017. DNM1 mutation status, sex, and sterilization status of a cohort of Labrador Retrievers with and without cranial cruciate ligament rupture. *Canine Genet Epidemiol*, epub ahead of print.

Evans, H. E. 1993. *Miller's Anatomy of the Dog*, 3rd edn. Philadelphia, PA: W. B. Saunders Company.

Evers, P., Johnston, G. R., Wallace, L. J., Lipowitz, A. J. & King, V. L. 1997. Long-term results of treatment of traumatic coxofemoral joint dislocation in dogs: 64 cases (1973–1992). *J Am Vet Med Assoc*, 210, 59–64.

Finkelstein, J. A., Anderson, G. I., Richards, R. R. & Waddell, J. P. 1991. Polyethylene synovitis following canine total hip arthroplasty. Histomorphometric analysis. *J Arthroplasty*, 6(Suppl.), S91–96.

Fitzpatrick, N., Law, A. Y., Bielecki, M. & Girling, S. 2014. Cementless total hip replacement in 20 juveniles using BFX™ arthroplasty. *Vet Surg*, 43(6), 715–725.

Fox, S. M. 1991. Coxofemoral luxations in dogs. *Compend Contin Educ Pract Vet*, 13, 1175–1196.

Gatineau, M., Dupuis, J., Beauregard, G., Charette, B., Breton, L., Beauchamp, G. & D'anjou, M. A. 2012. Palpation and dorsal acetabular rim radiographic projection for early detection of canine hip dysplasia: a prospective study. *Vet Surg*, 41, 42–53.

Gibbons, S. E., Macias, C., Tonzing, M. A., Pinchbeck, G. L. & McKee, W. M. 2006. Patellar luxation in 70 large breed dogs. *J Small Anim Pract*, 47, 3–9.

Gilbert, P. J., Shmon, C. L., Linn, K. A. & Singh, B. 2010. Macroscopic and microvascular blood supply of the canine common calcaneal tendon. *Vet Comp Orthop Traumatol*, 23, 81–86.

Gordon-Evans, W. J., Griffon, D. J., Bubb, C, Knap, K. M., Sullivan, M. & Evans, R. B. 2013. Comparison of lateral fabellar suture and tibial plateau leveling osteotomy techniques for treatment of dogs with cranial cruciate ligament disease. *J Am Vet Med Assoc*, 243, 675–680.

Gough, A. & Thomas, A. 2004. *Breed Predispositions in the Dog and Cat*. Ames, IA: Blackwell Publishing, pp. 87, 142.

Grisneaux, E., Dupuis, J., Pibarot, P., Bonneau, N. H., Charette, B. & Blais, D. 2003. Effects of postoperative administration of ketoprofen or carprofen on short- and long-term results of femoral head and neck excision in dogs. *J Am Vet Med Assoc*, 223, 1006–1012.

Guastella, D. B., Fox, D. B. & Cook, J. L. 2008. Tibial plateau angle in four common canine breeds with cranial cruciate ligament rupture, and its relationship to meniscal tears. *Vet Comp Orthop Traumatol*, 21, 125–128.

Guerrero, T. G. & Montavon, P. M. 2009. Zurich cementless total hip replacement: retrospective evaluation of 2nd generation implants in 60 dogs. *Vet Surg*, 38, 70–80.

Guerrero, T. G., Pozzi, A., Dunbar, N., Kipfer, N., Haessig, M., Beth Horodyski, M. & Montavon, P. M. 2011. Effect of tibial tuberosity advancement on the contact mechanics and the alignment of the patellofemoral and femorotibial joints. *Vet Surg*, 40, 839–848.

Hart, J. L., May, K. D., Kieves, N. R., Mich, P. M., Goh, C. S., Palmer, R. H. & Duerr, F. M. 2016. Comparison of owner satisfaction between stifle joint orthoses and tibial plateau leveling osteotomy for the management of cranial cruciate ligament disease in dogs. *J Am Vet Med Assoc*, 249(4), 391–398.

Heffron, L. E. & Campbell, J. R. 1978. Morphology, histology and functional anatomy of the canine cranial cruciate ligament. *Vet Rec*, 102, 280–283.

Hernández-Martínez, J. C., Vásquez, C. R., Ceja, C. B., Fuentes, C. C., Sesma, J. F. & Benítez, A. G. 2012. Comparative study on animal model of acute Achilles tendon rupture with surgical treatment using platelet-rich plasma. *Acta Ortop Mex*, 26, 170–173.

Herron, M. R. 1979. Coxofemoral luxation in small animals. *J Vet Orthoped*, 1, 30.

Hoelzler, M. G., Millis, D. L., Francis, D. A. & Weigel, J. P. 2004. Results of arthroscopic versus open arthrotomy for surgical management of cranial cruciate ligament deficiency in dogs. *Vet Surg*, 33, 146–153.

Holsworth, I. G. & Decamp, C. E. 2003. Coxofemoral luxation. In: Slatter, D. (ed.), *Textbook of Small Animal Surgery*, 3rd edn. Philadelphia, PA: W.B. Saunders, p. 2002.

Holsworth, I. G., Schulz, K. S., Kass, P. H., Scherrer, W. E., Beale, B. S., Cook, J. L. & Hornof, W. J. 2005. Comparison of arthroscopic and radiographic abnormalities in the hip joints of juvenile dogs with hip dysplasia. *J Am Vet Med Assoc*, 227, 1087–1094.

Hoscheit, L. P. 1994. Luxation of the tendon of the superficial digital flexor muscle in two dogs. *Can Vet J*, 35, 120–121.

Hossain, M. A., Park, J., Choi, S. H. & Kim, G. 2008. Dexamethasone induces apoptosis in proliferative canine tendon cells and chondrocytes. *Vet Comp Orthop Traumatol*, 21, 337–342.

Hurt, R. J., McAbee, K. & Cavanaugh, R. 2011. Incidence and risk factors of postliminary meniscal injury following tibial tuberosity advancement in 116 dogs. In: *Proceedings of the 38th Annual Conference of the Veterinary Orthopedic Society*. March 5–12, Snowmass, CO, p. 44.

Johnson, A. L., Probst, C. W., Decamp, C. E., Rosenstein, D. S., Hauptman, J. G., Weaver, B. T. & Kern, T. L. 2001. Comparison of trochlear block recession and trochlear wedge recession for canine patellar luxation using a cadaver model. *Vet Surg*, 30, 140–150.

Jones, P., Dalziel, S. R., Lamdin, R., Miles-Chan, J. L. & Frampton, C. 2015. Oral non-steroidal anti-inflammatory drugs versus other oral analgesic agents for acute soft tissue injury. *Cochrane Database Syst Rev*, 7, CD007789.

Jopp, I. & Reese, S. 2009. Morphological and biomechanical studies on the common calcaneal tendon in dogs. *Vet Comp Orthop Traumatol*, 22, 119–124.

Katayama, M. 2016. Augmented repair of an achilles tendon rupture using the flexor digitorum lateralis tendon in a toy poodle. *Vet Surg*, 45, 1083–1086.

Kealy, R. D., Lawler, D. F., Ballam, J. M., Mantz, S. L., Biery, D. N., Greeley, E. H., *et al.* 2002. Effects of diet restriction on life span and age-related changes in dogs. *J Am Vet Med Assoc*, 220, 1315–1320.

Kidd, S. W., Preston, C. A. & Moore, G. E. 2016. Complications of porous-coated press-fit cementless total hip replacement in dogs. *Vet Comp Orthop Traumatol*, 29, 402–408.

Kieves, N. R., Lotsikas, P. J., Schulz, K. S. & Canapp, S. O. 2014. Hip toggle stabilization using the TightRope® system in 17 dogs: technique and long-term outcome. *Vet Surg*, 43, 515–522.

Kim, S. E., Pozzi, A., Banks, S. A., Conrad, B. P. & Lewis, D. D. 2009. Effect of tibial tuberosity advancement on femorotibial contact mechanics and stifle kinematics. *Vet Surg*, 38, 33–39.

Kim, S. E., Pozzi, A., Banks, S. A., Conrad, B. P. & Lewis, D. D. 2010. Effect of cranial cruciate ligament deficiency, tibial plateau leveling osteotomy, and tibial tuberosity advancement on contact mechanics and alignment of the stifle in flexion. *Vet Surg*, 39, 363–370.

Kirkby, K. A. & Lewis, D. D. 2012. Canine hip dysplasia: reviewing the evidence for nonsurgical management. *Vet Surg*, 41, 2–9.

Kosaka, T., Masaoka, T. & Yamamoto, K. 2011. Possible molecular mechanism of promotion of repair of acute Achilles tendon rupture by low intensity-pulsed ultrasound treatment in a rat model. *West Indian Med J*, 60, 263–268.

Kowaleski, M. P., Boudrieau, R. J. & Pozzi, A. 2012. Stifle. In: Tobias, K. M. & Johnston, S. A. (eds), *Veterinary Surgery Small Animal*. St. Louis, MO: Elsevier Saunders, pp. 906–998.

Kramer, M., Gerwing, M., Michele, U., Schimke, E. & Kindler, S. 2001. Ultrasonographic examination of injuries to the achilles tendon in dogs and cats. *J Small Anim Pract*, 42, 531–535.

Krotscheck, U., Nelson, S. A., Todhunter, R. J., Stone, M. & Zhang, Z. 2016. Long term functional outcome of tibial tuberosity advancement vs. tibial plateau leveling osteotomy and extracapsular repair in a heterogeneous population of dogs. *Vet Surg*, 45, 261–268.

L'Eplattenier, H. & Montavon, P. 2002a. Patellar luxation in dogs and cats: pathogenesis and diagnosis *Compendium*, 24, 234–239.

L'Eplattenier, H. & Montavon, P. 2002b. Patellar luxation in dogs and cats: Management and prevention. *Compendium*, 24, 292–299.

Lafaver, S., Miller, N. A., Stubbs, W. P., Taylor, R. A. & Boudrieau, R. J. 2007. Tibial tuberosity advancement for stabilization of the canine cranial cruciate ligament-deficient stifle joint: surgical technique, early results, and complications in 101 dogs. *Vet Surg*, 36, 573–586.

Langenbach, A. & Marcellin-Little, D. J. 2010. Management of concurrent patellar luxation and cranial cruciate ligament rupture using modified tibial plateau levelling. *J Small Anim Pract*, 51, 97–103.

Lascelles, B. D., Freire, M., Roe, S. C., Depuy, V., Smith, E. & Marcellin-Little, D. J. 2010. Evaluation of functional outcome after BFX total hip replacement using a pressure sensitive walkway. *Vet Surg*, 39, 71–77.

Lazar, T. P., Berry, C. R., Dehaan, J. J., Peck, J. N. & Correa, M. 2005. Long-term radiographic comparison of tibial plateau leveling osteotomy versus extracapsular stabilization for cranial cruciate ligament rupture in the dog. *Vet Surg*, 34, 133–141.

Lewis, D. D., Shelton, G. D., Piras, A., Dee, J. F., Robins, G. M., Herron, A. J., *et al.* 1997. Gracilis or semitendinosus myopathy in 18 dogs. *J Am Anim Hosp Assoc*, 33, 177–188.

Lim, S., Hossain, M. A., Park, J., Choi, S. H. & Kim, G. 2008. The effects of enrofloxacin on canine tendon cells and chondrocytes proliferation in vitro. *Vet Res Commun*, 32, 243–253.

Liska, W. D. 2010. Micro total hip replacement for dogs and cats: surgical technique and outcomes. *Vet Surg*, 39, 797–810.

Lister, S. A., Renberg, W. C. & Roush J. K. 2009. Efficacy of immobilization of the tarsal joint to alleviate strain on the common calcaneal tendon in dogs. *Am J Vet Res*, 70, 134–140.

Lopez, M. J. 2012. Advances in hip dysplasia. *Vet Surg*, 41, 1.

Manley, P. A., Adams, W. M., Danielson, K. C., Dueland, R. T. & Linn, K. A. 2007. Long-term outcome of juvenile pubic symphysiodesis and triple pelvic osteotomy in dogs with hip dysplasia. *J Am Vet Med Assoc*, 230, 206–210.

Mauterer, J. V., Jr., Prata, R. G., Carberry, C. A. & Schrader, S. C. 1993. Displacement of the tendon of the superficial digital flexor muscle in dogs: 10 cases (1983–1991). *J Am Vet Med Assoc*, 203, 1162–1165.

McLaughlin, R. M., Jr. 1995. Traumatic joint luxations in small animals. *Vet Clin North Am Small Anim Pract*, 25, 1175–1196.

McNicholas, W. T., Jr., Wilkens, B. E. & Barstad, R. D. 2000. Luxation of the superficial digital flexor tendon in a cat. *J Am Anim Hosp Assoc*, 36, 174–176.

Morgan, J. P., Voss, K., Damur, D. M., Guerrero, T., Haessig, M. & Montavon, P. M. 2010. Correlation of radiographic changes after tibial tuberosity advancement in dogs with cranial cruciate-deficient stifles with functional outcome. *Vet Surg*, 39, 425–432.

Morton, M. A., Thomson, D. G., Rayward, R. M., Jimenez-Peláez, M. & Whitelock, R. G. 2015. Repair of chronic rupture of the insertion of the gastrocnemius tendon in the dog using a polyethylene terephthalate implant. Early clinical experience and outcome. *Vet Comp Orthop Traumatol*, 28, 282–287.

Nelson, S. A., Krotscheck, U., Rawlinson, J., Todhunter, R. J., Zhang, Z. & Mohammed, H. 2013. Long-term functional outcome of tibial plateau leveling osteotomy versus extracapsular repair in a heterogenous population of dogs. *Vet Surg*, 42, 38–50.

Nesser, V. E., Kowaleski, M. P. & Boudrieau, R. J. 2016. Severe polyethylene wear requiring revision total hip arthroplasty in three dogs. *Vet Surg*, 45(5), 664–671.

Nielsen, C. & Pluhar, G. E. 2005. Diagnosis and treatment of hind limb muscle strain injuries in 22 dogs. *Vet Comp Orthop Traumatol*, 18, 247–253.

Nielsen, C. & Pluhar, G. E. 2006. Outcome following surgical repair of Achilles tendon rupture and comparison between postoperative tibiotarsal immobilization methods in dogs: 28 cases (1997–2004). *Vet Comp Orthop Traumatol*, 19, 246–249.

Nourissat, G., Diop, A., Maurel, N., Salvat, C., Dumont, S., Pigenet, A., et al. 2010. Mesenchymal stem cell therapy regenerates the native bone-tendon junction after surgical repair in a degenerative rat model. *PLoS One*, 5, e12248.

Off, W. & Matis, U. 2010. Excision arthroplasty of the hip joint in dogs and cats. Clinical, radiographic, and gait analysis findings from the Department of Surgery, Veterinary Faculty of the Ludwig-Maximilians-University of Munich, Germany. 1997. *Vet Comp Orthop Traumatol*, 23, 297–305.

Oxley, B., Gemmill, T. J., Pink, J., Clarke, S., Parry, A., Baines, S. & McKee, W. M. 2013. Precision of a novel computer tomographic method for quantification of femoral varus in dogs and an assessment of the effect of femoral malpositioning. *Vet Surg*, 42, 751–758.

Patricelli, A. J., Dueland, R. T., Adams, W. M., Fialkowski, J. P., Linn, K. A. & Nordheim, E. V. 2002. Juvenile pubic symphysiodesis in dysplastic puppies at 15 and 20 weeks of age. *Vet Surg*, 31, 435–444.

Piermattei, D. L., Flo, G. L. & Decamp, C. E. 2006. *Handbook of Small Animal Orthopedics and Fracture Repair*, 4th edn. St. Louis, MO: Saunders Elsevier, pp. 673–674.

Powers, M. Y., Karbe, G. T., Gregor, T. P., McKelvie, P., Culp, W. T., Fordyce, H. H. & Smith, G. K. 2010. Evaluation of the relationship between Orthopedic Foundation for Animals' hip joint scores and PennHIP distraction index values in dogs. *J Am Vet Med Assoc*, 237, 532–541.

Pozzi, A., Hildreth, B. E., 3rd & Rajala-SCHULTZ, P. J. 2008. Comparison of arthroscopy and arthrotomy for diagnosis of medial meniscal pathology: an ex vivo study. *Vet Surg*, 37, 749–755.

Priddy, N. H., 2nd, Tomlinson, J. L., Dodam, J. R. & Hornbostel, J. E. 2003. Complications with and owner assessment of the outcome of tibial plateau leveling osteotomy for treatment of cranial cruciate ligament rupture in dogs: 193 cases (1997–2001). *J Am Vet Med Assoc*, 222, 1726–1732.

Raes, E. V., Bergman, E. H., van der Veen, H., Vanderperren, K., Van der Vekens, E. & Saunders, J. H. 2011. Comparison of cross-sectional anatomy and computed tomography of the tarsus in horses. *Am J Vet Res*, 72, 1209–1221.

Reif, U., Hulse, D. A. & Hauptman, J. G. 2002. Effect of tibial plateau leveling on stability of the canine cranial cruciate-deficient stifle joint: an in vitro study. *Vet Surg*, 31, 147–154.

Reinke, J. D. & Mughannam, A. J. 1993. Lateral luxation of the superficial digital flexor tendon in 12 dogs. *J Am Anim Hosp Assoc*, 29, 303–309.

Ridge, P. A. 2006. Isolated medial meniscal tear in a Border Collie. *Vet Comp Orthop Traumatol*, 19, 110–112.

Rose, S. A., Bruecker, K. A., Petersen, S. W. & Uddin, N. 2012. Use of locking plate and screws for triple pelvic osteotomy. *Vet Surg*, 41, 114–120.

Roush, J. K., Cross, A. R., Renberg, W. C., Dodd, C. E., Sixby, K. A., Fritsch, D. A., et al. 2010. Evaluation of the effects of dietary supplementation with fish oil omega-3 fatty acids on weight bearing in dogs with osteoarthritis. *J Am Vet Med Assoc*, 236, 67–73.

Runge, J. J., Kelly, S. P., Gregor, T. P., Kotwal, S. & Smith, G. K. 2010. Distraction index as a risk factor for osteoarthritis associated with hip dysplasia in four large dog breeds. *J Small Anim Pract*, 51, 264–269.

Samoy, Y., Verhoeven, G., Bosmans, T., Van Der Vekens, E., DE Bakker, E., Verleyen, P. & Van Ryssen, B. 2015. TTA Rapid: description of the technique and short term clinical trial results of the first 50 cases. *Vet Surg*, 44(4), 474–484.

Schweitzer, M. E. & Karasick, D. 2000. MR imaging of disorders of the Achilles tendon. *AJR Am J Roentgenol*, 175, 613–625.

Smith, G. K., Hill, C. M., Gregor, T. P. & Olson, K. 1998. Reliability of the hip distraction index in two-month-old German shepherd dogs. *J Am Vet Med Assoc*, 212, 1560–1563.

Smith, G. K., Lawler, D. F., Biery, D. N., Powers, M. Y., Shofer, F., Gregor, T. P., et al. 2012. Chronology of hip dysplasia development in a cohort of 48 labrador retrievers followed for life. *Vet Surg*, 41, 20–33.

Solanti, S., Laitinen, O. & Atroshi, F. 2002. Hereditary and clinical characteristics of lateral luxation of the superficial digital flexor tendon in Shetland sheepdogs. *Vet Ther*, 3, 97–103.

Spain, C. V., Scarlett, J. M. & Houpt, K. A. 2004. Long-term risks and benefits of early-age gonadectomy in dogs. *J Am Vet Med Assoc*, 224, 380–387.

Stein, S. & Schmoekel, H. 2008. Short-term and eight to 12 months results of a tibial tuberosity advancement as treatment of canine cranial cruciate ligament damage. *J Small Anim Pract*, 49, 398–404.

Steiss, J. E. 2002. Muscle disorders and rehabilitation in canine athletes. *Vet Clin North Am Small Anim Pract*, 32, 267–85.

Swiderski, J. K. & Palmer, R. H. 2007. Long-term outcome of distal femoral osteotomy for treatment of combined distal femoral varus and medial patellar luxation: 12 cases (1999–2004). *J Am Vet Med Assoc*, 231, 1070–1075.

Taylor, J. & Tangner, C. H. 2007. Acquired muscle contractures in the dog and cat. A review of the literature and case report. *Vet Comp Orthop Traumatol*, 20, 79–85.

Thieman, K. M., Tomlinson, J. L., Fox, D. B., Cook, C. & Cook, J. L. 2006. Effect of meniscal release on rate of subsequent meniscal tears and owner-assessed outcome in dogs with cruciate disease treated with tibial plateau leveling osteotomy. *Vet Surg*, 35, 705–710.

Tillmann, B. & Koch, S. 1995. Functional adaptation processes of gliding tendons. *Sportverletz Sportschaden*, 9, 44–50.

Towle, H. A., Griffon, D. J., Thomas, M. W., Siegel, A. M., Dunning, D. & Johnson, A. 2005. Pre- and postoperative radiographic and computed tomographic evaluation of dogs with medial patellar luxation. *Vet Surg*, 34, 265–272.

Vaughan, L. C. 1979. Muscle and tendon injuries in dogs. *J Small Anim Pract*, 20, 711–736.

Verhoeven, G., Fortrie, R., VAN Ryssen, B. & Coopman, F. 2012. Worldwide screening for canine hip dysplasia: where are we now? *Vet Surg*, 41, 10–19.

Vezzoni, L., Vezzoni, A. & Boudrieau, R. J. 2015. Long-term outcome of zürich cementless total hip arthroplasty in 439 cases. *Vet Surg*, 44(8), 921–929.

Whelan, M. F., McCarthy, R. J., Boudrieau, R. J. & Kraus, K. H. 2004. Increased sacral screw purchase minimizes screw loosening in canine triple pelvic osteotomy. *Vet Surg*, 33, 609–614.

Wilke, V. L., Conzemius, M. G., Kinghorn, B. P., Macrossan, P. E., Cai, W. & Rothschild, M. F. 2006. Inheritance of rupture of the cranial cruciate ligament in Newfoundlands. *J Am Vet Med Assoc*, 228, 61–64.

Wilke, V. L., Zhang, S., Evans, R. B., Conzemius, M. G. & Rothschild, M. F. 2009. Identification of chromosomal regions associated with cranial cruciate ligament rupture in a population of Newfoundlands. *Am J Vet Res*, 70, 1013–1017.

Williams, R. A. 2010. Isolated lateral meniscus tear in a boxer. *Vet Rec*, 167, 419–420.

Witsberger, T. H., Villamil, J. A., Schultz, L. G., Hahn, A. W. & Cook, J. L. 2008. Prevalence of and risk factors for hip dysplasia and cranial cruciate ligament deficiency in dogs. *J Am Vet Med Assoc*, 232, 1818–1824.

Yeadon, R., Fitzpatrick, N. & Kowaleski, M. P. 2011. Tibial tuberosity transposition-advancement for treatment of medial patellar luxation and concomitant cranial cruciate ligament disease in the dog. Surgical technique, radiographic and clinical outcomes. *Vet Comp Orthop Traumatol*, 24, 18–26.

Zhang, Y., Ahn, P. B., Fitzpatrick, D. C., Heiner, A. D., Poggie, R. A. & Brown, T. D. 1999. Interfacial frictional behavior: cancellous bone, cortical bone, and a novel porous tantalum biomaterial. *Journal of Musculoskeletal Research*, 3, 245–251.

15 Evaluation and Rehabilitation Options for Orthopedic Disorders of the Pelvic Limb

Judy C. Coates, MEd, MSPT, CCRT

Summary

A comprehensive evaluation from a physical therapy perspective requires keen observational and manual skills. Assessment of the pelvic limb entails careful examination of the toes, tarsus, stifle, and hip as well as a scan of the spine to rule out referred pain. Elements of the exam include postural evaluation, functional assessment, gait analysis, strength testing, passive range of motion (PROM), flexibility testing, soft tissue palpation, joint play assessment, and special tests. Abnormal findings are used to create a problem list. Interpretation of the history and objective exam are considered in developing an assessment and physical therapy working diagnosis. Functional and measurable goals are established and are used as benchmarks of progress. Finally, a treatment plan is formulated to addresses the stated abnormal findings relative to the preset goals. The plan will include frequency and duration of treatment as well as the specific elements of the treatments. Treatment may include manual techniques such as soft tissue techniques and joint mobilization, modalities such as laser and electrical stimulation, and therapeutic exercise such as proprioceptive and strengthening exercises. Frequent reassessment is necessary to determine the effectiveness of the plan.

Evaluation of the pelvic limb

A rehabilitation orthopedic assessment includes a thorough patient history and a detailed examination. The therapist should be aware of the patient's past medical history, results of imaging, current medications, and treatment to date. Subjectively, the client provides information regarding the mechanism of injury if applicable, aggravating or relieving activities, and observed functional deficits.

Achieving an accurate diagnosis requires a strong knowledge of anatomy, finely tuned manual skills, keen observational skills, and a good understanding of biomechanics. When examining the pelvic limb, it is important to scan the spine and pelvis to rule out referred pain from these proximal segments. A brief

Canine Sports Medicine and Rehabilitation, Second Edition. Edited by Chris Zink and Janet B. Van Dyke.
© 2018 John Wiley & Sons, Inc. Published 2018 by John Wiley & Sons, Inc.

scan will include active range of motion (AROM) of the spine, assessment of pelvic alignment, soft tissue palpation, and joint provocation testing. Additionally, conscious proprioception is tested and gait is observed for possible neurological signs.

Orthopedic examination of the pelvic limb

Organizing the examination

Sequencing of the exam is driven by patient comfort. At the first appointment, building trust is essential. Relaxed, friendly communication with the client will help put the patient at ease. The patient is free to explore the new surroundings while the therapist obtains historical information from the client. This author prefers to begin the exam with the hands-off elements of the evaluation, allowing the patient additional time to gain the trust of the examiner. These elements include observation of posture, functional transfers, strength, and gaiting (see Chapter 2). The hands-on elements of the exam are performed next and include passive range of motion (PROM), flexibility, palpation, joint play, and special tests. The exam can be performed with the patient in lateral recumbency or standing depending on patient preference. Ideally the involved limb is evaluated last.

Posture

Posture is observed in the standing and sitting positions. Observing the patient in standing, the therapist should note foot placement, topline (lordosis or kyphosis), pelvic alignment, head and tail position, balance of weight bearing (weight shift forward or backward, left or right), and any off-weighting of a limb (Figure 15.1). Weight bearing can be classified as non-weight bearing (NWB), toe-touch weight bearing (TTWB), partial weight bearing (PWB), or full weight bearing (FWB). The amount of weight bearing can also be documented with an approximate percentage (i.e., PWB approximately 60%). The patient is observed for the symmetry of the sitting posture, with a normal sit considered *square*. If sitting posture is not

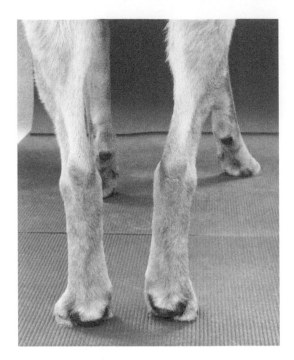

Figure 15.1   Abnormal weight bearing. Dog is offloading the right pelvic limb.

square, joint angulation of the limbs is noted. For example, a patient with a stifle injury will commonly sit with the involved limb in hip abduction and external rotation with decreased stifle and/or tarsal flexion (Figure 15.2).

Function

A functional assessment examines the patient's activities of daily living. The assessment will depend on the patient's job and condition. Therefore, the components included in assessment of a tetraparetic patient will be quite different than those of a postsurgical cranial cruciate ligament (CCL) patient or an agility patient with post-event lameness. Function is assessed by observation of specific activities. Analysis of the movement requires a good understanding of functional anatomy and biomechanics. Elements of a functional exam may include stand-to-sit, sit-to-down, and sternal to lateral recumbency transfers as well as the reverse of each. Proper sequencing, timing, range of motion (ROM), and strength are required to complete each transition appropriately. Pain and weakness will be reflected in compensations.

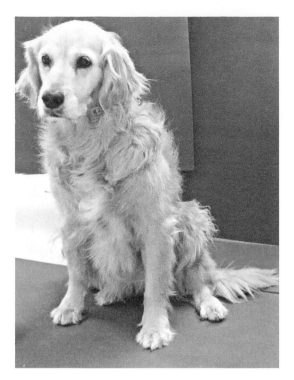

Figure 15.2   Abnormal sitting posture. Dog is sitting with left stifle extended and left pelvic limb abducted.

Gait analysis

The difference between a lameness exam and gait analysis should be noted. The physical therapist evaluates gait with an eye for functional impairments and compensatory movement. The patient is observed in each gait (as appropriate for their current condition), as well as on stairs, inclines, declines, and while moving in circles in both directions. The patient is viewed from the front, the back, and each side. Stance and swing phases of gait are observed for appropriate ROM at each joint, proper muscle firing, and for compensatory movement. For example, if a patient is limited in stifle extension on the right pelvic limb, the ipsilateral swing phase of gait will be decreased. The examiner may note compensatory excessive lumbar side bending to the right in the patient's attempt to lengthen the swing phase. Further evaluation is necessary to determine whether the stifle extension is limited by swelling, muscle, joint, or nerve.

Strength

Strength testing in humans is performed by asking the patient to hold a limb in a specific position against manual resistance. Strength is graded according to the amount of resistance tolerated. Grading is documented on a 0 to 5 scale, representing none, trace, poor, fair, and good or normal. Attempts to design strength testing for the canine patient have been made. One such design uses position and gravity in place of human manual resistance. Grading is categorized as poor, fair or good according to the ability to maintain good posture in the test position. Strength testing is important as the results are used to direct the therapeutic exercise treatment program. For example, if a pelvic limb is graded fair, exercises are chosen that are appropriate for this strength grade. As strength improves, the exercises are changed accordingly.

Canine strength is tested by placing the patient in specific test positions of varying difficulty. Grading the test depends on the patient's ability to maintain a static, symmetrical posture for at least 10 seconds. The therapist makes note of compensatory movement related to weakness or pain. For more on strength testing in the canine patient, see Chapter 13. Information regarding specific muscle function is obtained by palpating individual muscles for intensity of contraction while the test is being performed. Strength tests are performed bilaterally for comparison. For accurate, reproducible testing it is essential that the patient's head be positioned appropriately. In the case of pelvic limb testing, treats are offered such that the head is elevated and retracted in order to shift the weight to the pelvic limbs. Strength grades are defined and documented as poor (inability to maintain the standard test position), fair (ability to maintain the standard test position), and good (ability to maintain the advanced test position).

Testing is initiated on a flat surface, using a three-leg stance position. If the dog is unable to maintain the test position for 10 seconds (compensation is noted), a poor grade is documented and the test session is ended. If this test position is well maintained without compensation for 10 seconds, a fair grade is documented and a more advanced position can be

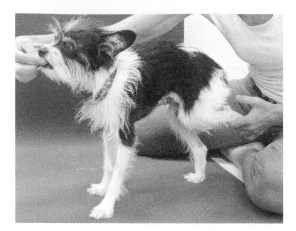

Figure 15.3   Three-legged standing test.

tested. Advanced test positions include diagonal leg lift (see below) and three-leg stance with thoracic limbs elevated on an elbow-height box. If these tests are satisfactory, a good grade is documented. Figure 15.3 shows an example of a three-leg stance assessment.

To test the general strength of the right pelvic limb, the therapist unweights the left pelvic limb by holding the dorsal surface of the pes. (Because dogs will not weight bear on the dorsum of their feet, this keeps them from "cheating" by putting weight on the leg that is being lifted.) The patient's head must be elevated to ensure weight bearing by the pelvic limbs. The therapist will observe the patient's ability to maintain normal alignment of the standing leg. Specific muscles are palpated, including the hamstrings, quadriceps, and gluteals, noting the extent of contraction.

Diagonal leg standing is similarly assessed. This is a more challenging test for the patient who demonstrates good strength on the three-leg stand. The assistant unweights a diagonal pair of legs, encouraging the patient to support full body-weight through the standing limbs (Figure 15.4). To specify pelvic limb assessment, the patient is offered a treat such that the head is elevated and the weight is shifted to the pelvic limbs. The therapist observes alignment, palpates each muscle group, and documents the findings as above. With different head positioning, this test can also be used to assess thoracic limb strength or core stability.

A second test for the dog that passes the fair test is a three-leg stand with the thoracic

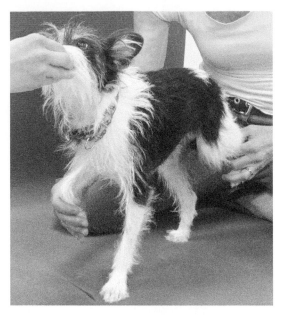

Figure 15.4   Diagonal leg standing test.

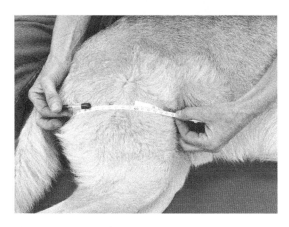

Figure 15.5   Measuring the circumference of the thigh using a Gulick tape.

limbs elevated on an elbow-height box. As with the tests above, the treat should be positioned appropriately, muscles are palpated, and posture is observed for at least 10 seconds.

Because atrophy may be associated with weakness, additional information regarding strength can be obtained with girth measurements. A Gulick tape measure is used to assess the circumference of both thighs (Figure 15.5). This baseline information provides the therapist with a means of monitoring progress. Gulick measurements can be performed in a weight-bearing or non-weight-bearing position.

Because thigh circumference measurements vary according to the test position, the therapist should use the same test position for follow-up measurements.

Passive range of motion

Restricted ROM at one segment often leads to compensatory increased ROM at a related segment. As discussed in Chapter 6, the options for treating hypermobility are fewer and less desirable than the options for treating hypomobility. Therefore, it is important to identify hypomobility in its early stages before resulting compensatory hypermobility occurs. This is accomplished by assessing PROM.

PROM is performed by moving the joint through its available ROM, adding overpressure and determining the end-feel. If a restriction is noted, ROM is measured with a goniometer and compared with the contralateral side. The measurement of the uninjured limb is used as normal for that patient. The end-feel of the restricted joint is determined. This information is used to identify the limiting structure. The therapist can then choose the proper treatment to affect that particular structure. PROM is assessed throughout the toes, tarsus, stifle, and hip. Except for the hip, flexion and extension are the primary motions to be evaluated. At the hip, internal and external rotation and abduction and adduction can be examined. For more detailed descriptions of assessment of PROM, refer to Chapters 5 and 6.

Flexibility

Movement can be limited by muscle tightness; therefore, it is important to assess flexibility and determine whether it is contributing to the loss of motion. Muscle flexibility is assessed by placing the limb in the position that is opposite the action(s) of the muscle being tested. Results are documented as normal or minimally, moderately, or severely restricted. A goniometer can be used to include an objective measurement. This technique is described in detail in Chapter 6. Pelvic limb muscles that should be evaluated include the gluteals, iliopsoas, sartorius, hamstring group (biceps femoris, semimembranosus, semitendinosus, gracilis), sartorius, quadriceps, adductor, pectineus, gastrocnemius/calcanean tendon, and superficial digital flexor (Table 15.1).

Palpation

Palpating for abnormal or painful tissues is performed after PROM and flexibility testing have been completed. For patient comfort, it is important to palpate with the pads rather than the tips of the fingers. In a thorough exam, the therapist assesses muscles, ligaments, tendons, and joint lines for pain, heat, swelling, tone, texture, and trigger points (see Chapter 6). Any abnormality is compared with the contralateral side. Important structures to assess include the gluteal, piriformis, tensor fascia latae, iliopsoas, sartorius, quadriceps, hamstring, gracilis, adductor, pectineus, gastrocnemius, superficial digital

Table 15.1 Flexibility testing

Muscle(s)	Stretched position
Gluteal	Hip and stifle flexion
Iliopsoas	Hip extension and internal rotation
Biceps femoris	Hip flexion and adduction, stifle extension, tarsal flexion
Semimembranosus/semitendinosus	Hip flexion with slight abduction, stifle extension
Gracilis	Hip flexion with abduction, stifle extension
Sartorius/rectus femoris	Hip extension, stifle flexion
Adductor/pectineus	Hip abduction
Quadriceps	Stifle flexion
Gastrocnemius/calcaneal tendon	Stifle extension, tarsal flexion
Superficial digital flexor	Stifle extension, tarsal flexion, digital extension

flexor, deep digital flexor, and cranial tibial muscles, as well as the sacrotuberous ligament, stifle medial collateral ligament (MCL) and lateral collateral ligament (LCL), popliteal lymph node, patellar ligament, parapatellar region, stifle joint line, possible medial buttress, calcaneal tendon, long digital extensor tendon, tarsal MCL and LCL, sesamoids, and digital joints.

Joint play

It is beyond the scope of this text to train the reader to perform arthrokinematic assessment glides, as they require hands-on training. These glides are used to assess for normal joint play movement at each joint. Normal arthrokinematic motion is required for normal osteokinematic motion to occur. If a restriction is noted, it is documented on a 0 to 6 scale. The reader is referred to Chapter 5 for a detailed description of joint play assessment. Table 15.2 provides a list of the most commonly used assessment glides for the pelvic limb. Figure 15.6 shows an example of a cranial glide of the tibia on the stabilized femur.

Table 15.2   Pelvic limb joint play assessment

Joint	Assessment glides/traction
Coxofemoral joint	Distraction
Tibiofemoral joint	Caudal, cranial, distraction
Talocrural joint	Caudal, cranial, distraction
Phalangeal joints	Dorsal, ventral, distraction

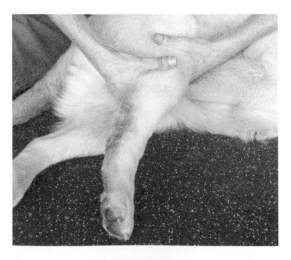

Figure 15.6   Cranial glide of the tibia on a stabilized femur.

Special tests

In addition to the special tests described for each joint in Chapters 5 and 13, the physical therapist might use the following tests.

McMurray test

The McMurray test is a human evaluative technique used to assess for meniscal tears. The action of this test is designed to compress a potential meniscal tear, with a positive result indicated by pain, a springy end-feel, and/or an audible clunk. To test the medial meniscus, the therapist starts with the stifle in flexion. The stabilizing hand is on the stifle, palpating the joint line, and the other hand grasps the tarsal–metatarsal region. The distal hand is used to externally rotate the tibia. While maintaining tibial external rotation, the proximal hand applies a valgus stress to the stifle as the joint is moved into extension. This test can be reversed for testing of the lateral meniscus.

Long digital extensor subluxation

Long digital extensor tendon subluxation is tested by palpating the tendon of origin while flexing and extending the stifle. This disorder can be mistaken for patellar luxation, as the patient will present with an intermittent skipping gait.

Superficial digital flexor tendon luxation

Integrity of the support structures of the superficial digital flexor tendon is tested by flexing the tarsus while palpating the tuber calcaneus. A positive test reveals a popping or sliding of the tendon to the medial or lateral aspect of the tuber depending which retinaculum has been stretched or ruptured.

Treatment options for disorders of the pelvic limb

The physical therapist's approach to treating commonly diagnosed pelvic limb disorders in canine patients begins with the understanding that the goal of physical therapy is to maximize function. Normal musculoskeletal function requires normal ROM, flexibility, strength, and muscle recruitment in the absence of pain. Rehabilitation treatment techniques address one or more of the following conditions: pain (inflammation), hypomobility, hypermobility, and weakness or altered muscle recruitment. There are many options for addressing each of these conditions, thus skilled treatment lies in the nuance of introducing and discharging the most efficient treatment techniques according to the stage of recovery and the individual response. Keys to successful outcomes are:

(1) The ability to extrapolate the *why* behind the abnormal findings
(2) The art of configuring the most effective treatment elements for the particular stage of recovery and patient needs
(3) The skillful delivery of manual techniques, therapeutic exercise and modalities
(4) The ability to change or advance the treatment plan in accordance with patient response to ongoing reassessment
(5) Client education and home exercise program design.

Prior to initiating treatment, a problem list is developed consisting of the abnormal findings uncovered in the examination. A working diagnosis is determined and clearly stated functional goals are established. Treatment is directed toward resolving the issues on the problem list as they relate to the functional goals and the working diagnosis. Success is measured by achieving objective progress towards the goals.

As mentioned in Chapter 13, physical therapy treatment employs the use of manual techniques, therapeutic exercise, and modalities. Initially pain should be addressed, allowing the patient to tolerate progression of the treatment plan. Pain reduction may involve medical management, modalities, or increasing ROM and/or flexibility. Because the ultimate goal is to maximize function, the therapist should walk the fine line of increasing the difficulty of exercise without increasing pain and inflammation. Speed of recovery often depends on the efficiency with which the therapist initiates and discharges elements of the treatment. A reassessment at each visit is necessary to determine the appropriate blend of modalities, manual work, and therapeutic exercise for the

Table 15.3   Therapeutic exercise variables

Amount of weight bearing	Non-, partial and full weight bearing
Type of contraction	Isometric, concentric, eccentric
Treatment plane	Sagittal, frontal, transverse
Effect of gravity	Assisted, neutral, resisted
Surface	Flat, unstable, uneven, inclined, declined
Resistance	None, weights, therapy band
Intensity, frequency and duration	Number of repetitions, how often, for how long

patient on that particular day. Every element of the treatment plan must be justified for the patient at the specific time of treatment.

As pain and mobility issues are resolved, therapeutic exercise becomes the primary focus. Important considerations for initiating and progressing a strengthening program are listed in Table 15.3.

Rather than offering treatment protocols for the pelvic limb conditions listed below, it is the author's intent to highlight the clinical findings and treatment rationale from a physical therapy perspective. With this information, the therapist can create an individualized treatment plan on a per case basis. Detailed techniques and exercises will be provided for the first diagnosis only. Thereafter, additional techniques specific to each disorder will be mentioned.

Hip dysplasia

This commonly diagnosed, multifactorial disease is well described in Chapter 14. The techniques for applying manual therapies, physical modalities, therapeutic exercises, and aquatic therapy are described in detail in the respective chapters earlier in this text.

Common findings on physical therapist's evaluation

- Tenderness to palpation of hip musculature
- Overactive (hypertonic) pectineus muscle
- Decreased/painful hip extension
- Decreased flexibility—iliopsoas, pectineus
- Atrophy of gluteals and thigh muscles
- Altered transfers and gait

- Adults may appear slow to rise from lateral recumbency or sitting, using the forelimbs to pull themselves into the standing position. During gait, diminished stride length and stance time is noted on the involved side(s)
- Transfers, gait, and activity may be painful
- Puppies may require multiple attempts to get from sit to stand and display poor muscle control in transitioning between gaits
- Coxofemoral joint laxity (puppies)
- Positive hip subluxation test(s) (puppies).

Treatment goals—adult

- Decrease pain
- Decrease hypertonicity of pectineus
- Maintain/improve ROM
- Increase flexibility—iliopsoas, pectineus
- Increase strength—gluteals and thigh
- Increase joint proprioception
- Improve core stabilization
- Manage weight
- Develop home exercise program (HEP).

Treatment

Treatment options will depend on patient age, current level of function and extent of arthritis.

Treatment rationale

- Puppy: slow the progression of growth and weight gain, modify activities, and strengthen hip stabilizers and core musculature. Address pain, if present.
- Adult: address pain, modify activities, address weight management, strengthen hip stabilizers and core musculature, and maintain/improve ROM and flexibility.

A multimodal approach to the osteoarthritic patient should be established and frequently re-evaluated. Human research emphasizes the importance of skilled manual work, suggesting that it is more effective than exercise in treating hip function and pain (Hoeksma et al., 2004). The authors of this study correlate high intra-articular pressure due to restriction of the joint capsule in osteoarthritis, with pain intensity and reduced hip ROM. Their study found that manual therapy (manipulation and stretching) aimed at increasing the elasticity of the joint capsule and surrounding muscles was most effective in reducing pain and increasing ROM. Additional research in humans has shown that aquatic therapy had some short-term benefits for the osteoarthritic patient but no long-term effects were demonstrated (Bartels et al., 2007). Therefore, aquatic therapy may be best utilized in the early stages of rehabilitation. An individualized approach to treatment of this common condition should include frequent modification as the animal progresses through the treatment process.

Treatment by goal

See the chapters covering modalities (Chapter 7), manual therapy (Chapter 6) and therapeutic exercise (Chapter 8) for details regarding implementation of the following treatments.

Pain management

- Laser
- Heat
- Joint compressions at hip performed in slight hip abduction and flexion
- Grade I and II coxofemoral joint distraction
- Transcutaneous electrical neuromuscular stimulation (TENS).

Decrease hypertonicity of pectineus

- Ischemic compression.

Maintain/improve range of motion

- PROM: all motions with emphasis on hip extension as tolerated
- Soft tissue mobilization (STM): to promote circulation; increase ROM restricted by soft tissues with particular attention to the gluteals, quadriceps, hamstrings, and paraspinals; and address trigger points and myofascial restrictions
- Joint mobilization: grade III coxofemoral joint distraction traction.

Increase flexibility

- Passive stretch: iliopsoas and pectineus
- STM: cross-fiber and effleurage to iliopsoas and pectineus.

Increase strength

- Neuromuscular electrical stimulation (NMES): gluteals, quadriceps, hamstrings
- Therapeutic exercise: gluteals, quadriceps, hamstrings, core stabilization
- Starting with low-level, low-impact exercises for short periods of time (such as partial sit-to-stands or isometric therapy band exercises), increasing intensity of the exercise as tolerated
- Aquatic therapy (see Chapter 9).

Increase joint proprioception

- Joint compressions: emphasis on the hip joint in non-weight-bearing and weight-bearing positions
- Proprioception exercises: wobble board exercises or walking over ground poles, increasing the difficulty level as strength permits.

Reach functional goals per individual patient's needs

Rehabilitation programs vary greatly according to the specific needs and goals of the individual patient and the patient's response to therapy. Long-term functional goals are broken down into their integral components and addressed in small increments. For instance, if the long-term goal is to walk up four steps to get into the house, the therapist should consider the amount of ROM and the particular muscle flexibility required at each joint to accomplish the task. Additionally, the specific muscular demands of key muscle groups should be analyzed and addressed. In this case, the gluteals and quadriceps must contract concentrically as the patient lifts the body-weight onto a step. Accordingly, the therapist will design a program that emphasizes concentric use of these muscles in an environment that is less challenging. An example would be sit-to-stand exercises on level ground with the assistance of NMES, followed by sit-to-stand exercises on an incline, followed by walking uphill and performing small step-ups.

Weight management

This is a common issue with this patient group. Techniques for weight management are discussed in Chapter 4.

Home program

Client education will include lifestyle management information such as weight management and activity counseling (no jumping up, no standing up on pelvic limbs, no jogging until growth plates have closed, and minimizing stair climbing). Other recommendations would include providing a soft surface for sleeping and creating surfaces with traction (carpeting) to prevent falls.

An HEP is designed for each patient. Pictures and written instructions of the HEP are provided for the client. It is extremely important for the therapist to not only instruct the client in the home program, but to observe them practicing the program while still in the rehabilitation facility.

Femoral head ostectomy

Common findings on physical therapist's evaluation

- Atrophy throughout the gluteal muscles, hamstrings, and quadriceps
- Decreased and painful hip extension PROM
- Decreased flexibility (iliopsoas, sartorius, hamstrings)
- Altered gait (PWB, decreased stance phase of gait, difficulty with circle walking).

Treatment rationale

- Encourage immediate postoperative weight bearing
- Emphasize hip extension ROM, proprioceptive training, and hip and core strengthening.

Treatment goals

- Decrease pain
- Promote weight bearing
- Increase hip PROM
- Improve proprioception
- Increase strength of hip musculature
- Increase core stabilization.

Treatment by goal

- Decrease pain: as for hip dysplasia

Case Study 15.1　Hip pain with secondary muscle impairments

Signalment: 6-y.o. F/S Golden Retriever.

Presenting complaint: Right pelvic limb (RPL) lameness; refuses to jump into car or onto bed.

Evaluation: Physical exam WNL except:
　Gait: Shortened stride length and stance time of RPL on moderate incline and clockwise circles; patient stops frequently to sit down.
　Transfers: Appears mildly painful and slow with sit-to-stand and recumbent-to-sit.
　Atrophy: Minimal to moderate R gluteals and thigh muscles.
　Palpation: Tender R middle gluteal and pectineus muscles
　PROM: R hip extension 135.
　Flexibility: Moderate tightness of the iliopsoas, pectineus, sartorius, and medial hamstrings.
　Strength: Fair grade with three-leg stand test with inadequate contraction of gluteals, quadriceps, and hamstrings; poor grade with diagonal leg lift.
　Joint play: Grade 2+ R coxofemoral hip traction.

Assessment: right hip pain, restriction, and weakness likely due to early-onset R hip osteoarthritis.

Problem list:

- Decreased R hip extension
- Tenderness at middle gluteal and pectineus
- Tight R iliopsoas and pectineus
- Weak R gluteals, quadriceps, and hamstrings
- Weight-bearing sensitive
- Decreased endurance.

Goals:

- Improved symmetry in gait in 6 weeks
- Symmetrical sit-to-stand transfers in 6 weeks
- Ability to walk up 10 stairs with minimal difficulty in 8 weeks
- Return to 1-hour hikes in 10 weeks.

Treatment:

(1)　Modalities:
　　- Laser to R gluteal region, coxofemoral joint region and pectineus.
(2)　Manual therapy:
　　- Grade III coxofemoral joint distractions
　　- Passive stretch of R iliopsoas, pectineus, sartorius, and medial hamstrings muscles with simultaneous STM of the muscle
　　- STM throughout hip and thigh
　　- Gentle hip extension PROM.
(3)　Therapeutic exercise:
　　- Hip strengthening (gluteals, biceps femoris, quadriceps)
　　- Emphasize underwater treadmill for first 2–3 weeks, and then progress to land-based exercise
　　- Include isometric, concentric, and eccentric exercises, gradually increasing the level of difficulty, frequency, and intensity.
(4)　HEP:
　　- Instruct client in gentle PROM and stretching exercises as well as a detailed progressive strengthening program
　　- Initiate core stabilization as tolerated.

- Promote weight bearing. For example:
  - Joint compressions (weight-bearing and NWB positions)
  - Weight-shifting exercises
  - Slow walking
  - Cavaletti walking
- Increase hip extension PROM: PROM into hip extension with STM of the rectus femoris, sartorius, and iliopsoas
- Improve proprioception. For example:
  - Standing perturbations
  - Ladder walking
  - Wobble board, fit disc, cushion with the pelvic limbs on the piece of equipment
- Increase strength of hip musculature. For example:
  - NMES
  - Three-leg stands
  - Therapy band exercises

- Backward walking
- Side stepping
- Incline and zigzag walking
- Step-ups.

Patellar luxation: grades I–II medial luxation; nonsurgical

Common findings on physical therapist's evaluation

- Abnormal patellar stability test
- Skipping gait and/or kicking leg into hip and stifle extension
- Thigh atrophy
- Compensatory tightness of sartorius, quadriceps, hamstrings, and hip flexors
- Compensatory posture (increased flexion of lumbosacral, coxofemoral, and stifle joints).

Treatment rationale

Treatment should emphasize stretching of the medial soft tissues and strengthening of the lateral musculature in an effort to redirect the pull on the patella.

Treatment goals

- Decrease pain
- Increase flexibility of the medial soft tissues (medial quadriceps, medial hamstrings, adductors, sartorius, iliopsoas)
- Increase strength of the lateral thigh musculature
- Normalize gait
- Develop HEP.

Treatment by goal

Pain management

As for hip dysplasia.

Increase flexibility

- Passive stretch and STM of the sartorius, medial quadriceps, medial hamstrings, adductor, and iliopsoas with manual stabilization of the patella
- Passive stretch and STM of the patellar ligament and musculotendinous junction of quadriceps, mobilizing tissues laterally.

Increase strength

- Lateral thigh musculature (e.g., side stepping on flat and elevated surfaces).

Home exercise program

The client is instructed in performing the stretching and strengthening exercises.

Cranial cruciate ligament insufficiency

Disruption of the CCL is a very common canine orthopedic injury. The mechanism of injury can be either acute or chronic. Typically, CCL tears are treated surgically; however, increasing numbers of clients are opting for conservative management due to health and financial concerns. The success of conservative management depends on the extent of the tear and whether or not the meniscus is involved.

Case Study 15.2   Medial patellar maltracking with secondary muscle impairments

Signalment: 2-y.o. F/N Jack Russell Terrier; agility competitor

Presenting complaint: Left pelvic limb (LPL) hiking gait lameness; hesitant to jump into car or onto bed.

Evaluation: Physical exam WNL except for:
  Special tests: Positive patellar stability test (grade I–II medial laxity).
  Gait: Intermittent skipping noted particularly with clockwise and counter-clockwise walking and in transitions from trot to canter.
  Atrophy: Minimal to moderate at L quadriceps and hamstrings; Gulick measurement: left thigh 24.5 cm; right thigh 25 cm.
  Flexibility: Moderate tightness of L semimembranosus, gracilis, and sartorius.

Assessment: Patellar maltracking (medially) with associated flexibility and strength issues. Treatment will focus on stretching the medial stifle musculature and strengthening the lateral musculature.

Problem list:

- Patellar maltracking
- Skipping gait
- Atrophy/weakness L thigh
- Tight L semimembranosus and gracilis.

Goal: Normal gait within 6 weeks.

Treatment:

(1) Manual therapy:
  - Passive stretch with STM at semimembranosus, gracilis, and adductors
  - Passive stretch of the sartorius with manual patellar stabilization
  - STM with lateral strokes to the patellar ligament and the musculotendinous junction of the quadriceps.
(2) Therapeutic exercise: Progressive strengthening exercises of the hip abductors such as side stepping in varying degrees of front-end elevation.
(3) HEP: Instruct client in treatment described above.

Stifle joint biology and biomechanics are key contributors to CCL disease and should be addressed in rehabilitation. Specifically, joint biology is addressed with modalities to decrease pain, promote tissue healing, and reduce inflammation and swelling. Laser, TENS, and grade I–II joint compressions are effective tools for achieving these goals. Biomechanical concerns regarding joint stability are addressed with therapeutic exercises to strengthen the dynamic stabilizers of the stifle and the core stabilizers. Retraining the proprioceptive feedback loop is essential after disruption of a ligament.

Treatment goals for surgical and nonsurgical CCL rehabilitation are generally quite similar with the exception of important differences during the early stages of rehabilitation. With osteotomies, early treatment must allow for proper bone healing by promoting weight bearing in the sagittal plane, and promoting healing with the use of modalities and activity restriction. Early rehabilitation of the nonsurgical case will depend on the acuity of the injury. Therapeutic exercise can be accelerated so long as pain and inflammation are not increased.

Nonsurgical rehabilitation

Common findings on physical therapist's evaluation

- Positive cranial drawer and/or cranial tibial thrust test
- NWB to PWB gait
- Abnormal sitting posture (hip abducted and stifle partially extended)
- Swelling
- ROM limited and painful at end range stifle flexion and extension
- Compensatory tightness of gastrocnemius, hamstrings, sartorius, and iliopsoas
- Disuse atrophy throughout the involved pelvic limb.

Treatment goals

- Decrease pain and inflammation
- Normalize ROM
- Normalize flexibility
- Enhance proprioceptive awareness
- Achieve FWB gait
- Strengthen quadriceps, hamstrings, and gluteals

- Promote core stabilization
- Develop HEP.

Treatment rationale

A nonsurgical, partially torn CCL warrants particular attention to reflexive training of the hamstrings with advanced proprioceptive work. In so doing, the hamstrings can help to substitute for the dysfunctional CCL.

Treatment by goal

Decrease pain and inflammation.   Use ice, laser, NMES, TENS, joint compressions, and STM.

Normalize ROM.   Grade III stifle joint distraction, grade III–IV caudal glide of the talus, PROM (emphasis on stifle flexion and extension and tarsal flexion), walking over high cavaletti poles performed at mid-tibial height

Normalize flexibility.   Muscle stretching with simultaneous STM of the muscle being stretched (hamstrings, gastrocnemius, sartorius, iliopsoas).

Achieve FWB gait.   Examples of progressive exercises are:

- Joint compressions (NWB and weight-bearing positions)
- Weight-shifting exercises
- Low cavaletti walking
- Slow walking with head elevated
- Circle walking (involved leg to the inside)
- Three-leg stands; lifting the uninvolved pelvic limb; head must be elevated
- Balance activities such as placing thoracic limbs on a wobble board.

Muscle strengthening.   Initial use of NMES for muscle re-education of the quadriceps, gluteals, and hamstrings performed in NWB or weight-bearing positions. Example exercises:

- Gluteals, quadriceps, and hamstring muscles: sit-to-stand transfers while facing uphill, backward walking up an incline, and unilateral step-ups onto a block

- Core stabilization: diagonal leg lifts with and without perturbations, side sit-ups, and weave pole walking
- Reflexive hamstring training: perturbations with the involved limb on a fit disc with the thoracic limbs elevated, and backward walking on a foam mattress
- Advanced proprioceptive training: walking backwards over a ladder, side stepping over cavaletti poles, and standing on a physioball.

Home exercise program:

- Per stage of recovery
- Weight management
- Modified activity.

Surgical rehabilitation

The initial stages of postoperative rehabilitation will focus on controlling swelling, encouraging ROM, promoting weight bearing, initiating muscle re-education, and educating the client regarding activity modification. Protecting the joint for proper bone healing must be emphasized with osteotomies. Preventing falls or slips is important and can be avoided with the use of non-skid throw rugs or mats for stable footing. Crate confinement when unsupervised is suggested.

Common findings on physical therapist's evaluation

- NWB to PWB gait
- Sitting with hip abducted and stifle partially extended
- Swelling
- ROM limited and painful at end range stifle flexion and extension
- Compensatory tightness of gastrocnemius, hamstrings, sartorius, and iliopsoas
- Disuse atrophy.

Treatment rationale

This depends on the type of surgery performed. For example, a primary concern post osteotomy is activity modification that ensures good bone healing. Human research supports the use of NMES in the early stages of rehabilitation as a means of preventing muscle atrophy and

weakness (Hasegawa *et al.*, 2011). The early use of eccentric muscle contractions (as compared to a standard strengthening protocol) was shown to increase quadriceps and gluteus maximus muscle mass and function over a 1-year period of time (Gerber *et al.*, 2009). Additionally, the use of perturbation exercises has been shown to enhance recovery by improving coordinated muscle activity (Chmielewski *et al.*, 2005; Risberg *et al.*, 2007).

Treatment goals

These are the same as those of nonsurgical rehabilitation:

- Decrease pain and inflammation
- Normalize ROM
- Normalize flexibility
- Achieve FWB
- Strengthen thigh, gluteal, and core musculature
- Develop HEP.

Treatment by goal

These are the same as the nonsurgical goals with the exception of greater activity restrictions for bone healing.

Gastrocnemius avulsion/calcaneal tendon injury

A gastrocnemius avulsion is often the result of an acute event; however, chronic degenerative calcaneal tendinopathy is common. The classification of calcaneal tendon lesions according to Meutstege (1993) is shown in Table 15.4.

Common findings on physical therapist's evaluation

Partial rupture

- Standing posture reveals tarsal hyperflexion
- PWB/antalgic gait with shortened stance phase
- Tenderness to palpation of the calcaneal tendon
- Thickened calcaneal tendon
- Pain with stretch of the gastrocnemius.

Table 15.4   Classification of Achilles injuries

Type	Pathological change	Clinical signs
I	Complete tendon rupture	Plantigrade stance; palpable tendon defect
IIa	Musculotendinous rupture	Increased tarsal flexion; inflammation at musculotendinous junction
IIb	Tendon rupture with paratenon intact	Increased tarsal flexion; tense paratenon palpable
IIc	Gastrocnemius tendon avulsion, with intact superficial digital flexor	Increased tarsal flexion; excessive flexion of digits
III	Tendinosis and/or peritendinitis	Normal stance; thickened Achilles tendon

Gastrocnemius rupture with intact superficial digital flexor

- Plantigrade stance, with stifle extension, and flexion of the two proximal phalangeal joints
- Toe-down weight bearing to PWB.

Complete rupture

- Non-weight bearing.

Treatment rationale

Efforts are focused on soft tissue nutrition and managing the delicate balance between protecting the tendon and minimizing the damaging effects of immobilization. Gentle tensile force is used to promote collagen fiber realignment and healing and to minimize adhesion formation (Lake *et al.*, 2009). In human medicine, there has been a shift toward earlier postsurgical mobilization in an effort to increase blood supply, improve ROM, and decrease atrophy (Sorrenti, 2006). Animal studies have shown that early motion can safely begin at the end of fibroplasia or about 14–21 days postoperatively (Sivacolundhu *et al.*, 2001). Gentle eccentric exercises are introduced in the subacute phase of healing (Cook *et al.*, 2002; Pull & Ransonb, 2007). Gently increase ROM and gradually progress muscle strengthening.

Treatment by goal

Decrease pain and swelling

- Ice, laser, NMES, TENS, joint compressions, and STM.

Promote soft tissue nutrition

- Massage gastrocnemius muscle belly with strokes toward the tendon for increased circulation.

Promote fiber realignment

- Gentle friction massage
- Gentle PROM into tarsal flexion.

Minimize adhesion formation

- Gentle friction massage.

Gradually increase ROM

- Progressive tarsal PROM
- Progressive AROM exercises such as walking and sit-to-stands.

Gradually increase muscle strengthening

- In the subacute phase of healing, initiate eccentric exercises such as backward walking, and progress to backward walking downhill
- Progressive gastrocnemius strengthening (concentrically) such as step-ups and uphill walking.

Conclusion

In conclusion, the effectiveness of a rehabilitation program depends on several key components. First, a skilled and thorough evaluation should be performed. A solid understanding of anatomy and biomechanics is required for accurate interpretation of the data. Creative problem solving will direct the treatment plan. Successful treatment is based on knowledge of soft tissue physiology and joint mechanics, superb manual skills, a solid understanding of modalities and their effect, and a methodical approach to therapeutic exercise. Constant re-evaluation and modification of the treatment plan is necessary to maximize the efficiency of recovery.

References

Bartels, E. M., Lund, H., Hagen, K. B., Dagfinrud, H., Christensen, R. & Danneskiold-Samsoe, B. 2007. *Aquatic Exercise for the Treatment of Knee and Hip Osteoarthritis (Review).* Chichester: John Wiley & Sons, Ltd.

Chmielewski, T. L., Hurd, W. J., Rudolph, K. S., Axe, M. J. & Snyder-Mackler, L. 2005. Perturbation training improves knee kinematics and reduces muscle co-contraction after complete unilateral anterior cruciate ligament rupture. *Phys Ther,* 85, 740–9; discussion 750–754.

Cook, J. L., Khan, K. M. & Purdam, C. 2002. Achilles tendinopathy. *Man Ther,* 7, 121–130.

Gerber, J. P., Marcus, R. L., Dibble, L. E., Greis, P. E., Burks, R. T. & Lastayo, P. C. 2009. Effects of early progressive eccentric exercise on muscle size and function after anterior cruciate ligament reconstruction: a 1-year follow-up study of a randomized clinical trial. *Phys Ther,* 89, 51–59.

Hasegawa, S., Kobayashi, M., Arai, R., Tamaki, A., Nakamura, T. & Moritani, T. 2011. Effect of early implementation of electrical muscle stimulation to prevent muscle atrophy and weakness in patients after anterior cruciate ligament reconstruction. *J Electromyogr Kinesiol,* 21, 622–630.

Hoeksma, H. L., Dekker, J., Ronday, H. K., Heering, A., Van Der Lubbe, N., Vel, C., *et al.* 2004. Comparison of manual therapy and exercise therapy in osteoarthritis of the hip: a randomized clinical trial. *Arthritis Rheum,* 51, 722–729.

Lake, S. P., Miller, K. S., Elliott, D. M. & Soslowsky, L. J. 2009. Effect of fiber distribution and realignment on the nonlinear and inhomogeneous mechanical properties of human supraspinatus tendon under longitudinal tensile loading. *J Orthop Res,* 27, 1596–1602.

Meutstege, F. J. 1993. The classification of canine Achilles' tendon lesions. *Vet Comp Ortho Traumatol,* 6, 53–55.

Pull, M. R. & Ransonb, C. 2007. Eccentric muscle actions: Implications for injury prevention and rehabilitation. *Physical Therapy in Sport,* 8, 88–97.

Risberg, M. A., Holm, I., Myklebust, G. & Engebretsen, L. 2007. Neuromuscular training versus strength training during first 6 months after anterior cruciate ligament reconstruction: a randomized clinical trial. *Phys Ther,* 87, 737–750.

Sivacolundhu, R. K., Marchevsky, A. M., Read, R. A. & Eger, C. 2001. Achilles mechanism reconstruction in four dogs. *Vet Comp Ortho Traumatol,* 14, 25–31.

Sorrenti, S. J. 2006. Achilles tendon rupture: effect of early mobilization in rehabilitation after surgical repair. *Foot Ankle Int,* 27, 407–410.

16 Biological Therapies in Canine Sports Medicine

Samuel P. Franklin, MS, DVM, PhD, DACVS-SA, DACVSMR,
Antonio Pozzi, DVM, MS, DECVS, DACVS, DACVSMR,
and Frank Steffen, DECVN

Summary

Orthobiologics have emerged as new treatment options in human and animal athletes. Musculoskeletal disorders such as tendinopathies, desmopathies, and osteoarthritis are common in competition and working dogs because of stresses induced by their repetitive activities. Several therapies, such as anti-inflammatory drugs, corticosteroids, shockwave therapy, and surgery have been used to treat these disorders, but variable levels of evidence and success have been reported. Tendon and ligament healing potential is limited, especially in chronic injuries, which are commonly seen in athletes. Therefore, novel regenerative treatment approaches are of great interest in sports medicine. There are two goals of this chapter. First, the definitions and proposed mechanisms of action for different orthobiologics are reviewed; second, the clinical applications and the evidence for efficacy of these novel treatments are discussed. The chapter focuses on two major topics. Platelet-rich plasma is reviewed in detail, as this is the most commonly used orthobiologic in veterinary medicine. Stem cell applications are also presented, focusing on musculoskeletal and spinal injuries. The chapter is not intended to provide a thorough review of the literature on these topics, but aims to introduce the sports medicine and rehabilitation therapist to the growing area of regenerative medicine.

Platelet-rich plasma

Definition

There is no universally accepted definition of what constitutes a plasma that is "platelet-rich" (PRP) but the most lenient definition is that the platelet concentration need only exceed that in the whole blood from which the PRP is prepared (Arnoczky & Shebani-Rad, 2013). The proposed mechanism by which PRP may be beneficial is the provision of anabolic growth factors to injured tissues of the musculoskeletal system, stored within the platelet alpha-granules, which may mitigate inflammation and initiate anabolic processes and tissue regeneration. Many different growth factors are contained in these alpha-granules, but those most commonly cited to facilitate tissue healing include vascular endothelial growth factor (VEGF), platelet-derived growth factors (PDGF), and transforming growth factor beta (TGF-β). Several of the applications for which PRP have been used, but not necessarily demonstrated to be efficacious, include injection into injured tendons, muscles, and ligaments, placement in fractures to facilitate bone healing, and intra-articular injection for symptomatic management of osteoarthritis.

Characteristics

Concentration of platelets is typically the characteristic of PRP that is most scrutinized. However, eliminating erythrocytes is also a potential goal of PRP preparation because erythrocytes are inflammatory stimuli when extravascular, and have been shown to significantly increase cell death of human fibroblast-like synoviocytes *in vitro* (Braun *et al.*, 2014). In addition, some investigators contend that removal of leukocytes is also a desired objective of PRP preparation because the concentrations of inflammatory cytokines correlates with leukocyte concentration in human PRP (Sundman *et al.*, 2011). The ideal PRP may be a function of platelet, erythrocyte, and leukocyte concentrations (or their ratio), and the optimal PRP likely varies for different medical conditions (Arnoczky & Shebani-Rad, 2013). As a result, clinicians should know the characteristics of the PRP they use and the evidence supporting the use of that particular type of PRP for a specific ailment. Classification systems have been devised to categorize the numerous different PRP compositions to enable comparison and summary of the evidence supporting their clinical use. These classification systems are based on the cellular composition of the PRP (platelets, leukocytes, erythrocytes) and if or how platelets in the PRP are intentionally activated (DeLong *et al.*, 2012; Dohan Ehrenfest *et al.*, 2014).

The goal of PRP therapy is to provide anabolic growth factors. This requires platelet activation, fusion of the alpha-granule with the external platelet membrane, and release of the growth factors into the extracellular environment. One mechanism of *in vivo* platelet activation is contact and interaction with collagen, which is a common component of musculoskeletal tissues. Accordingly, PRP is often injected without intentional exogenous activation, in which case the clinician depends on activation to occur *in vivo* at the site of tissue injury. This practice may allow a more extended release of growth factors if activation occurs over time *in vivo* (Harrison *et al.*, 2011; Arnoczky & Shebani-Rad, 2013). However, suboptimal activation could occur *in vivo*. As a result, some authors recommend that intentional exogenous activation be performed prior to PRP application to assure that platelets are activated. Numerous studies using human, equine, and canine PRPs have compared different activators including soluble collagen, calcium-based products, and thrombin (Fufa *et al.*, 2008; Harrison *et al.*, 2011; Silva *et al.*, 2012; Textor & Tablin, 2012). There are some differences among studies but all demonstrate that use of these substances increases platelet activation and growth factor release in comparison to samples that are not activated. As a result, an additional component of PRP classification schemes is what, if any, intentional exogenous activation has been performed.

Although not part of classification schemes, the volume of blood used in PRP preparation and the volume of PRP are relevant when comparing different PRP products and systems. The volume of blood used in PRP preparation is germane because acquisition of larger volumes of blood from small dogs can be unappealing, and hence preparation of an effective PRP with a smaller blood volume is desirable. However, having the ability to process a large volume of blood is also appealing because the easiest way to prepare PRP with a high concentration of platelets is to begin with more platelets, which is achieved by using a larger volume of blood. In turn, consideration of both the minimum and maximum volumes of blood that can be processed is pertinent to PRP preparation. Similarly, the final volume of PRP and total number of platelets in the PRP should be quantified rather than just evaluating the final platelet concentration. A PRP with a high platelet concentration, but a small volume of PRP, may not provide more platelets than a larger volume of PRP with a lower platelet concentration. The ideal final volume of PRP is influenced by the volume that can be delivered to a site of injury and whether any aliquots of PRP are to be frozen for future use. In the latter case, production of a larger volume of PRP might be preferable.

Preparation

Platelet-rich plasma can be prepared from canine blood with basic laboratory supplies and specific centrifugation protocols (Perazzi *et al.*, 2013). Blood is collected and usually, but not always, anticoagulated. Acid citrate dextrose-A is the most commonly used anticoagulant although sodium citrate and citrate phosphate dextrose-A can also be used (Franklin *et al.*, 2015). These are the only two anticoagulants that have been shown to support the metabolic needs of platelets. Use of heparin is less common, and ethylene-diamine tetracetic acid (EDTA) should not be used (Marx, 2001). Centrifugation with a soft spin (190–1000 g, depending on the protocol and the centrifuge; Perazzi *et al.*, 2013; Silva *et al.*, 2013; Franklin *et al.*, 2015), is performed to separate the contents with red blood cells at the bottom, plasma at the top, and the buffy coat at the interface. Depending upon the centrifugation protocol, the canine platelets are in the deeper portion of the plasma and the buffy coat. Accordingly, the deeper portion of the plasma, and potentially some portion of the buffy coat, are collected to obtain a PRP. If a double centrifugation is performed, all of the plasma and some portion of the buffy coat is transferred to another tube and a faster spin is performed to pellet all cellular components, including the platelets, within platelet-poor plasma (PPP) (Figures 16.1 and 16.2). The final volume of the desired PRP is determined, any excess volume of PPP is removed and discarded, and the pellet is suspended in the remaining volume of PPP to produce the final PRP (Figures 16.1 and 16.2).

The location of the platelets relative to the plasma layer and buffy coat is the most important concept to understand. If one retrieves only the plasma layer and either very little or none of the buffy coat, the platelet concentration will be relatively low and the leukocyte concentration will also be low. With increasing retrieval of the buffy coat, the platelet concentration will increase but so will the leukocyte concentration. Retrieval of much of the buffy coat results in extremely high platelet and leukocyte concentrations. Importantly, unpublished data from one author's (SF) lab confirm that the platelets are more superficially located within the preparation than the leukocytes, which would be expected based upon their smaller size in comparison to the leukocytes. This means that it is feasible to obtain relatively high platelet concentrations with low or negligible leukocyte concentrations if one can select this fraction of the plasma and buffy coat— something that is simple in principle but can be challenging to execute.

Although preparation of PRP can be done using basic supplies, many practitioners in human and veterinary medicine elect to use commercially available centrifugation or filtration-based PRP concentrating systems because

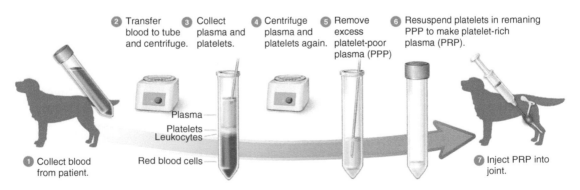

Figure 16.1   Double-spin platelet-rich plasma (PRP) preparation protocol.

2 Transfer blood to tube and centrifuge.   3 Collect plasma and platelets.   4 Centrifuge plasma and platelets again.   5 Remove excess platelet-poor plasma (PPP)   6 Resuspend platelets in remaning PPP to make platelet-rich plasma (PRP).

Plasma
Platelets
Leukocytes
Red blood cells

1 Collect blood from patient.

7 Inject PRP into joint.

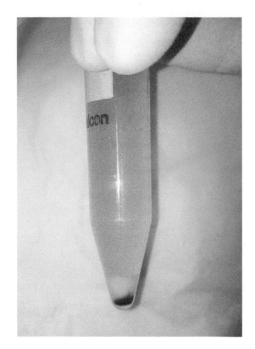

Figure 16.2   Platelet pellet after a second centrifugation in a double-spin platelet-rich plasma preparation protocol.

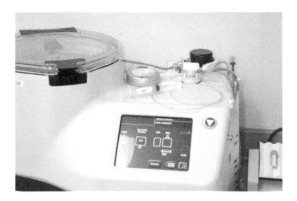

Figure 16.3   Platelet-rich plasma (PRP) preparation machine that can provide automated separation of the blood into separate fractions including platelet-poor plasma, PRP, and the red blood cell pellet.

they are convenient and require less time and hands-on work (Figure 16.3). In addition, these commercially available point-of-care systems might facilitate maintenance of sterility and could potentially produce a more consistent PRP product, although this has not been demonstrated.

Commercially available PRP preparation systems

Most PRP systems were designed and manufactured for preparing PRP from human blood. However, the cellular elements in human blood differ from those in canine blood in characteristics such as size, density, and sedimentation rate. Hence, characteristics of PRP acquired using a given system with human blood are not necessarily representative of the PRP that is acquired using the same system with canine blood. Therefore, it is important that data from dogs are considered. Fortunately, there are now several studies characterizing PRPs made with canine blood (Thoesen *et al.*, 2006; Stief *et al.*, 2011; Carr *et al.*, 2015; Franklin *et al.*, 2015; Frye *et al.*, 2016). Of these, one author (SF) completed a 15-dog cross-over study assessing the characteristics of PRP made with five different PRP systems (Franklin *et al.*, 2015). The degree of platelet concentration varied from platelet reduction in one system to an average increase of five-fold over baseline with another system. Similarly, three systems produced a PRP with negligible hematocrit while the PRP from two systems consistently had a notable hematocrit. Lastly, some systems produced leukocyte-rich PRP while other produced a leuko-reduced PRP.

Growth factor concentrations (TGF-β1, PDGF-BB) were also quantified in these PRPs. As with human PRPs, there were moderate correlations between the platelet concentration and the anabolic growth factor concentrations (Sundman *et al.*, 2011). However, the greatest variable influencing growth factor concentration was intentional activation of the PRP. This became apparent as one of the PRP systems included a calcium chloride activator that was used during the PRP preparation. Although the platelet concentration in this PRP was moderate, it had significantly higher TGF-β1 and PDGF-BB concentrations than all other PRPs. Further investigation with one of the other PRP preparations confirmed that platelets in such a PRP preparation are not activated during the PRP preparation process. Like platelets in human and equine PRPs, these platelets were capable of activation, and growth factor release was dramatically increased once the PRP was mixed with either calcium chloride or thrombin, with thrombin producing the most robust activation and greatest release of anabolic growth factors (Franklin *et al.*, 2017a) (Figure 16.4). Importantly, assessment of frozen samples of this particular PRP showed that the anabolic growth factor concentrations from the frozen sample were similar to those obtained with calcium chloride activation, thus raising the question of whether frozen and thawed PRP samples might be

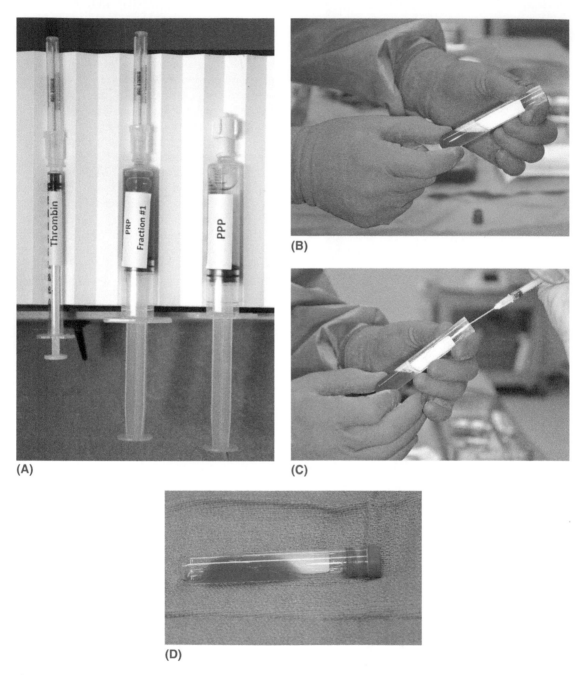

(A)

(B)

(C)

(D)

Figure 16.4 (**A**) Resultant platelet-poor plasma, platelet-rich plasma (PRP), and calcium/thrombin mixture that can be used to activate the PRP and form a platelet-rich fibrin gel. (**B**) Platelet-rich plasma placed in a sterile glass tube for intraoperative activation and formation of a platelet-rich fibrin gel. (**C**) Injection of bovine thrombin and calcium chloride into a sterile glass tube of platelet-rich plasma to form a platelet-rich fibrin gel. (**D**) A platelet-rich fibrin gel is formed by activating platelet-rich plasma with thrombin/calcium chloride.

used clinically. This is one reason that the final volume of PRP produced is possibly clinically relevant.

The findings of these studies assessing multiple canine PRPs underscore that the term PRP is not specific. Rather, PRPs make up a diverse array of biological blood-derived products with varying characteristics with regard to cellular composition and growth factor delivery. It is important that the specific characteristics of a PRP are considered, and in the context of a specific medical condition, when evaluating the efficacy data for a particular PRP and its potential clinical benefit.

Efficacy data

Tendon injury: surgical application

A series of three experiments using platelet-rich fibrin constructs were performed to assess the suitability of PRP for treating tendon defects in dogs. The first of the studies confirmed that substantial TGF-β1 was eluted from the activated PRP fibrin membrane that was created by activation of PRP with calcium chloride coupled with a simultaneous and additional centrifugation (Visser *et al.*, 2010a). In the second experiment, it was demonstrated that canine tenocytes demonstrated greater proliferation *in vitro* when supplemented with the growth factor-rich eluent from this PRP fibrin membrane (Visser *et al.*, 2010b). In the third study, the central third of the patellar tendon was excised from both stifles in eight dogs and the PRP fibrin membrane was sutured into the defect of one tendon (Visser *et al.*, 2011). Dogs were sacrificed at 4 ($n = 4$) and 8 weeks ($n = 4$). The rate and quality of tissue healing was not improved with use of the PRP fibrin membrane. However, the total volume of fibrous repair tissue was significantly greater in the group treated with the PRP membrane. The authors of this study concluded that use of the platelet-rich fibrin membrane may not be indicated for augmenting the repair of tendons that have been injured acutely and are healthy in all other aspects. However, since the PRP fibrin membrane increased the volume of healing tissue, a PRP fibrin membrane could be beneficial if an increased volume of tissue is considered desirable.

Tendinopathy: percutaneous injection

Percutaneous injection to treat tendon injuries is highly pertinent to canine sports medicine given the frequency of supraspinatus, common calcaneal, and iliopsoas tendon injuries in competitive dogs. However, the only data regarding PRP for such applications are from one case series evaluating the benefits of a single ultrasound-guided injection of a leukocyte-rich PRP in 10 dogs with supraspinatus tendinopathy (Ho *et al.*, 2015). Subjective client-assessed lameness improved in 40% of dogs. However, the caregiver placebo effect has previously been documented to be approximately (or slightly greater than) 40% in veterinary medicine (Conzemius & Evans, 2012). Tendon heterogeneity and echogenicity based upon ultrasonography were improved in six of the 10 dogs. Force plate assessments at 6 weeks post injection did not demonstrate any improvement in treated dogs (Ho *et al.*, 2015). Accordingly, there are insufficient data to demonstrate that percutaneous PRP injections are effective in treating tendinous injury in dogs, and further study is needed to ascertain whether PRP is useful for such conditions.

Bone healing

A recent review and meta-analysis of all preclinical animal studies concluded that the evidence suggests that PRP confers several beneficial effects on animal long bone models (Gianakos *et al.*, 2015). However, these conclusions were based largely on data from species other than dogs. The author (SF) is aware of only three studies assessing the effects of PRP on long bone healing in dogs. One study compared the benefit of an uncharacterized, calcium-activated PRP in conjunction with calcium phosphate granules (as a bone filler) in an ulnar defect model in dogs (Rabillard *et al.*, 2009). Although control dogs treated with autogenous cancellous bone graft healed uneventfully, dogs treated with the granules, with or without adjunctive PRP, did not have successful bone healing. Conversely, another study assessed use of a PRP (moderate platelet concentration and calcium activation) in a heterogeneous population of dogs in whom a mid-diaphyseal defect in the radius had been created and stabilized with external skeletal fixation (Souza *et al.*, 2012). Dogs treated with PRP had significantly greater healing scores based upon radiography. This prospective, randomized study provides good evidence of the benefit of PRP use on bone healing. One characteristic of the study, however, that was unclear is whether all the dogs studied were of the same age. This is relevant because the author (SF) recently completed a prospective, randomized clinical trial assessing the effects of PRP on bone healing in 60 dogs treated by tibial plateau leveling osteotomy (Franklin *et al.*, 2017b). The PRP had a high platelet concentration, neutral leukocyte concentration, no erythrocytes, and was activated with calcium chloride and thrombin to form a gel that was placed in the osteotomy at the time of surgery (Figure 16.4). Bone healing was assessed using radiography, ultrasonography, and MRI. With basic statistical testing, it appeared that PRP provided a small, but statistically significant, benefit. However, multivariate analysis demonstrated that the small differences in healing scores were attributable to variations in individual dog age rather than to use of PRP. Accordingly, there is limited and variable evidence regarding benefit of PRP on long bone healing in dogs.

Osteoarthritis (intra-articular injections)

In 2013, three studies were published providing initial data regarding efficacy of different PRP preparations in treating naturally occurring disease in dogs. The author (SF) performed a blinded, prospective, randomized study comparing the efficacy of intra-articular use of a leuko-reduced PRP with the use of hyaluronan and corticosteroid for treatment of elbow osteoarthritis (OA) in 10 dogs (Franklin & Cook, 2013). Significant improvements were identified in both treatment groups based on client and veterinarian assessments using subjective outcomes measures. Some improvements were greater in the PRP treatment group but the study did not include force plate data, so only limited conclusions can be drawn.

Fahie and colleagues (2013) performed a prospective, randomized, controlled study comparing the efficacy of filtered platelet therapy with saline injection for treatment of OA in 20 dogs. This product is not technically a PRP because it suspends the cellular components in saline

rather than plasma. However, it is considered similar to PRP in concept and probable mechanism of action. The solution contains a mild increase in platelet concentration and is leukocyte-rich with a hematocrit of approximately 22%. The study included objective force plate data for half the dogs in addition to using validated subjective outcome measures for all dogs. The results demonstrated significant improvements in objective and subjective outcomes over a 12-week follow-up period with intra-articular use of the product. Interestingly, the nine dogs in the control group were injected at study end and showed significant improvement based upon force plate data after receiving treatment.

Yet another group published results from a prospective, randomized study assessing the effects of three PRP injections after intra-articular stabilization for treatment of cranial cruciate ligament (CCL) rupture in 10 dogs (Silva *et al.*, 2013). Peak vertical force and vertical impulse measured using a force plate improved from preoperative to day 90 post surgery for the six dogs treated with PRP; no such improvement was noted for the four dogs in the control group. Likewise, force plate data indicated significantly greater weight bearing with the affected limb for dogs treated by PRP compared with the affected limb of control dogs at day 90 post surgery.

More recently, three *in vivo* studies in research dogs have been performed. One study induced OA in the stifle of 12 dogs by partial CCL transection and complete medial meniscal release (Cook *et al.*, 2015). Dogs were randomized to receive five injections of either saline or a leuko-reduced PRP. Comfortable range of motion was better maintained in the treatment group. Based upon objective, kinetic pressure mat data, weight bearing was significantly better (by about 10%) at weeks 5, 12, and 18 following treatment with PRP in comparison to the saline sham-treated group. Blinded histological scoring of the CCL was significantly better in the treatment group. A follow-up investigation compared the efficacy of the same PRP with oral carprofen or arthroscopic saline lavage for managing experimentally induced injury of the CCL in dogs (Bozynski *et al.*, 2016). Both arthroscopic lavage- and PRP-treated dogs had less lameness, pain, and stifle effusion and greater subjective function than dogs treated with carprofen. Dogs receiving PRP demonstrated the greatest benefit. PRP was also associated with the lowest severity of pathological changes in the CCL based upon follow-up arthroscopic assessment.

A third study was performed in which 24 dogs had experimental transection of the CCL to induce instability, lameness, and OA (Yun et al., 2016). Dogs were randomized to receive sham treatment, PRP, adipose-derived mesenchymal stem cells (MSCs), or PRP plus MSCs. Dogs in the PRP group demonstrated significantly greater improvement than sham-treated dogs based upon lameness scores. They also had significant improvement in comparison to saline-treated dogs based on mechanical testing of articular cartilage, cartilage thickness, histology, and biochemical composition of the cartilage.

The consistency of positive results from these six prospective, randomized, blinded, and controlled studies are encouraging, suggesting that intra-articular PRP is beneficial in dogs. Three of the studies included kinetic assessments of weight bearing using force plate or pressure mat data. All six studies demonstrated positive effects on either subjective, objective, or both types of outcome measures. However, there are still notable limitations to the conclusions that can be drawn. The conditions treated in each study were different. Furthermore, three of the studies were done in research dogs with experimentally induced pathological changes. This latter point is particularly pertinent to the studies involving dogs with induced CCL injury, which differs from naturally occurring disease. There are not yet any published studies evaluating the use of PRP for managing naturally occurring partial CCL rupture. Finally, it should be noted that the total number of dogs receiving PRP in the six studies assessing intra-articular injection was just 48. As a result, there remains a need for large (>50) randomized controlled trials with kinetic (force plate or pressure mat) data to assess the use of PRP in dogs with naturally occurring disease.

Other blood-derived biological treatments

Autologous conditioned serum

Autologous conditioned serum (ACS), also known as interleukin receptor antagonist protein (IRAP), is prepared by incubating whole blood in a device with glass or borosilicate beads at 37 °C for 7–24 hours. Leukocytes adhere to the beads and are activated during this incubation and can release high concentrations of interleukin 1 receptor antagonist (IL-1ra). The blood is then centrifuged and the serum fraction containing the high concentration of IL-1ra is collected for intra-articular injection in patients with OA. This is potentially beneficial for patients with OA because IL-1β is the most important inflammatory cytokine in the catabolic process of OA and cartilage destruction. Blocking the effects of IL-1β could mitigate progression of this disease process. Randomized studies in people and horses provide variable evidence of efficacy with some positive results (Frisbie, 2015). There are two published studies in dogs demonstrating that ACS in this species contains high concentrations of IL-1ra, as well as increased concentrations of IL-1β to some degree (Huggins et al., 2015; Sawyere et al., 2016). However, there are no studies at this time reporting the efficacy of ACS for the treatment of OA in dogs.

Autologous protein solution

Autologous protein solution (APS) is a blood-derived product that is similar to both PRP and ACS. Blood is first processed in a commercial device to make PRP. The PRP is transferred to another device and filtered through polyacrylamide beads, desiccating the PRP and providing concentrated leukocyte, platelets, and plasma proteins (Bertone et al., 2014). With human blood this process results in the concentration of anabolic and anti-inflammatory cytokines and lower concentrations of catabolic cytokines (Woodell-May et al., 2011). No studies have assessed the cellular, growth factor, or cytokine composition of APS made from the blood of dogs. However, there has been one randomized, controlled clinical trial of APS in horses and one in dogs with OA of the stifle or elbow (Bertone et al., 2014; Wanstrath et al., 2016). Results of the canine study were mixed; dogs treated with APS were significantly more lame 2 weeks following injection based upon kinetic force plate data but better at 12 weeks following injection. Control dogs treated with saline did not show any improvement based upon kinetic data. Future studies will add to our understanding of the utility of this biological treatment.

Case Study 16.1   Flexor enthesiopathy

Signalment: 9-y.o. M/C Border Collie, 25 kg.

History: Patient had past history of agility training, and presented for an intermittent right thoracic limb lameness that started 3 years prior to presentation without evidence of trauma. At that time, an intra-articular (shoulder) injection of cortisone was performed, with no evidence of improvement. In addition, arthroscopy of the right elbow was done, with a report of synovitis. Rehabilitation therapy was initiated with good initial results.·

Clinical examination: Patient showed 2/4 right thoracic limb lameness, worse at trot. Muscle atrophy detected in the affected limb. Patient reacted at flexion and extension of the elbow (mild pain), but showed more severe pain at pin-point palpation over the medial humeral epicondyle.

Imaging: Radiographs and CT scan of both elbows were unremarkable. MRI was performed to evaluate the soft tissue structures of the right elbow (Figure 16.5).

Radiographic diagnosis was enthesiopathy of the origin of the flexor musculature at the medial epicondyle.

A transverse ultrasonographic image distal to the medial epicondyle was obtained during the intralesional injection of autologous conditioned plasma (ACP), with the same diagnosis (Figure 16.6).

Comments: Based on the diagnosis of flexor enthesiopathy at the origin from the medial humeral epicondyle, an intralesional injection with ACP was performed under ultrasound guidance. The dog was re-evaluated 6 weeks after the injection and the lameness was significantly improved.

Flexor enthesiopathy has been reported as a primary injury or concurrently with other elbow pathologies such as fragmented coronoid process. The flexor enthesiopathy can be diagnosed with radiography, scintigraphy, CT, MRI, and arthroscopy. The advantage of MRI and ultrasound is the potential for earlier diagnosis should mineralization not be evident radiographically (de Bakker *et al.*, 2013).

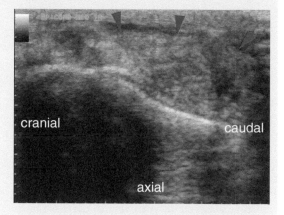

Figure 16.6 Transverse ultrasonographic image distal to the medial epicondyle during an intralesional injection of autologous conditioned plasma, revealing that the origin of the flexor musculature at the medial epicondyle (red arrow heads) is mildly thickened. The organization of the musculature is reduced and the echogenicity heterogeneously reduced.

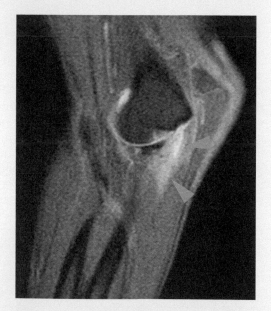

Figure 16.5 T1 turbo spin echo sequence with spectral presaturation with inversion recovery for fat saturation in a sagittal plane after i.v. injection of gadolinium. The origin of the flexor musculature at the medial epicondyle (gray arrow heads) is mildly thickened and undergoing contrast enhancement.

Stem cells

Definitions and sources

The use of MSC therapies in veterinary patients is a field that is evolving rapidly, both experimentally and clinically. MSCs have received increasing attention due to the potential of augmenting healing of muscles, tendons, ligaments, and bone. However, the lack of strict regulations has led to the proliferation of commercially available products and therapies that have either not been tested or have not demonstrated efficacy. Many questions remain unanswered, including the best tissue source, best method of collection and preparation, ideal cell numbers, and best administration technique. A summary of the sources of various stem cell types, and their effects, clinical uses, and limitations is provided in Table 16.1.

Stem cells are defined based on their ability to differentiate into a wide range of cells and to self-renew. Stem cells can be classified in different ways, although the classification based on the source may be the most relevant for the clinician. Embryonic stem cells are derived from embryos at a developmental stage; induced pluripotent cells are engineered by manipulating the expression of certain genes; adult stem cells, applicable to clinical uses, are undifferentiated multipotent cells, found throughout the body after embryonic development. Their function is to repair tissue and replenish senescent cells. Among the adult stem cells, MSCs have the important advantage of being more readily available and easy to obtain compared with embryonic and fetal stem cells. Sources of MSCs include fetal tissue such as umbilical cord, and blood and adult tissues such as bone marrow, skin, adipose tissue, synovium, periosteum, and dental pulp. Because tumor formation has been reported after application of embryonic stem cells, potential adverse effects include stem cell-induced carcinogenesis and tissue formation. However, multipotent MSCs used in most studies are in a more committed cell stage and have far more limited differentiation potential than totipotent embryonic stem cells. As a result, there is no published evidence demonstrating carcinogenesis of multipotent MSC in either *in vitro* or *in vivo* models (Hernigou *et al.*, 2013).

MSCs are undifferentiated cells that have unique characteristics as they can (1) move during angiogenesis; (2) differentiate into specialized cell types (e.g., chondrocyte, osteocyte); (3) proliferate and regenerate; and (4) release immune regulators and growth factors. More specifically, MSCs are defined based on their ability to differentiate *in vitro* into osteoblasts, adipocytes, or chondroblasts, adhere to plastic, and express specific genes. The first application of MSC-based therapy in veterinary medicine was performed in horses using bone marrow aspirate for treating suspensory ligament desmitis. Bone marrow is an attractive source for MSCs, although only a very small cellular fraction corresponds to MSCs (<0.001%). For this reason, culture expansion techniques over

Table 16.1 Comparison of stem cells from different sources: their effects, uses, and limitations

	Hematopoietic stem cells	Embryonic stem cells	Mesenchymal (adult) stem cells
Source	Bone marrow (autologous or allogeneic)	Blastocysts/early embryo (allogeneic)	Bone marrow, fat, cord blood (autologous or allogeneic)
Potency	Multipotent	Pluripotent	Multilineage differentiation
Beneficial effects	Transplantation of healthy cells in diseased individual	Source of biological material for various cell restorative treatments	Anti-inflammatory; anti-apoptotic; differentiation into cartilage, muscle, bone, nerve cells
Clinical uses	Neoplastic disorders of blood and bone marrow; autoimmune disease; skeletal dysplasia; mucopolysaccharidosis	Potential for tissue regeneration	Regeneration of several tissues, e.g., tendons, neurons, chondrocytes, cornea
Limitations	Potential for graft versus host reaction	Risk for tumor formation Ethical concerns Legal restrictions	Difficult to identify, isolate, maintain, and culture

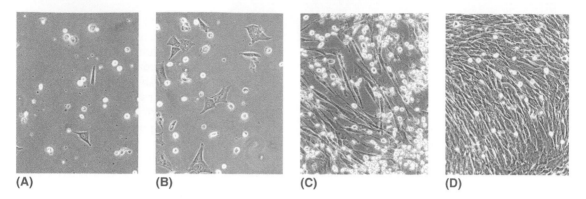

Figure 16.7   Maturation during culture of bone marrow-derived mesenchymal stem cells including: (**A**) cells on the day of culture, (**B**) after several days of culture, (**C**) after 10–14 days of culture, and (**D**) at 4 weeks of culture.

3–6 weeks are used to increase the total number of MSCs (Crovace *et al.*, 2010) (Figure 16.7).

Adipose tissue can also be used as a source of MCSs for the culture expansion technique (Guercio *et al.*, 2012). Several studies have characterized adipose-derived MSCs (AD-MSCs) and evaluated their ability to differentiate into chondrogenic, osteogenic, and adipogenic lines (Neupane *et al.*, 2008; Guercio *et al.*, 2012, 2013). A recent study compared bone marrow MSCs (BM-MSCs) with AD-MSCs and concluded that higher isolation success and proliferation rates were found with adipose tissue (Russell *et al.*, 2016). In contrast, another study showed that BM-MSCs may have greater osteogenic potential than AD-MSCs when obtained from young dogs (Alves *et al.*, 2014).

Another strategy to isolate MSCs is by enzymatic digestion followed by filtration and centrifugation of adipose tissue. This process results in the stromal vascular fraction, a mixture of cells, which is injected, without cell culture, into the patient. This approach has the advantage of providing cells more quickly as culture is not required so it can be prepared patient-side. The benefits of adipose tissue for cell isolation include more abundant tissue, accessibility, and potentially higher MSC populations. However, only a small percentage of the cells derived from adipose tissue digestion are MSC, with a maximum of 7.7% of cells meeting the most lenient definition of MSCs (Sullivan *et al.*, 2016). The stromal vascular fraction has been compared with bone marrow aspirate for the amount of tissue harvested, the ease of harvest, and the cellular content in each

sampled tissue. Although the highest cell number in average was found in bone marrow, the adipose stromal vascular fraction yielded more consistent results, supporting the authors' conclusion of recommending the falciform ligament as the first choice for harvest (Sullivan *et al.*, 2016).

Mechanism of action

Despite the large number of experimental studies, the mechanism of action of MSCs is still unclear. MSCs are identified by specific properties that relate to their potential therapeutic action. MSCs have demonstrated the ability to migrate to sites of injury and inflammation (Maerz *et al.*, 2017). The tissue trauma induces increased expression of inflammatory cytokines and chemokines and initiates the mobilization of marrow-derived cells. MSCs migrate to injured tissue to participate in regenerative and/or immunomodulatory pathways. The original hypothesis was that MSCs would regenerate tissue based on the ability of the MSCs to differentiate into the host tissue. Meniscus regeneration is often used as an example for a MSC-based treatment aiming at tissue regeneration (Horie *et al.*, 2012). Limited results from animal studies would suggest a potential for using intra-articular injection of MSCs for the regeneration of meniscus. However, it should be considered that spontaneous meniscal regeneration has been observed following meniscectomy.

A recent paradigm shift has emerged suggesting that MSCs may act on the local environment by secreting cytokines, growth factors, and extracellular matrix molecules that act either on themselves (autocrine actions) or on neighboring cells (paracrine actions) (Mei *et al.*, 2017). Given their ability to modulate host immune responses, MSCs have been proposed as a potential cellular therapy for autoimmune disease such as rheumatoid arthritis. In the treatment of OA, it has been suggested that MSCs may have a positive effect via the secretion of bioactive trophic factors to exert potent anti-inflammatory and immunomodulatory effects (Zhang *et al.*, 2016).

Most likely MSCs repair tissue by multiple interactions that include secretion of paracrine factors to enhance regeneration of injured cells, and stimulation of proliferation and differentiation of the stem-like progenitor cells found in most tissue. In the case of OA, for example, MSC-based treatments may enhance repair and regeneration ability by the modulation of the local T cell-mediated immunological response and by enhancing the potential for tissue regeneration.

Osteoarthritis

Stem cell therapy is an emerging option for OA treatment in dogs. The standard therapies for OA involve palliation of pain using a multimodal approach including NSAIDs, analgesics, weight loss, exercise moderation, and physical therapy. This approach offers symptomatic relief in some cases, but provides no disease-modifying effect. The MSC-based treatment of OA aims at decreasing the catabolic activity while enhancing cartilage regeneration.

A recent experimental study using a canine CCL transection model for developing OA evaluated the synergistic effect of PRP and adipose-derived MSC in 24 Beagles (Yun *et al.*, 2016). The combination of PRP and MSCs is attractive because PRP provides growth factors and may enhance and promote cellular engraftment, resulting in a synergistic effect. The dogs were divided into four groups treated with PRP, MSCs, a combination of PRP and MSCs, and a control group with intra-articular saline injection. The animals were treated with one injection per week for 4 weeks

and followed for 2 months. Outcomes included lameness scoring for evaluating function and focal compression strength, articular extracellular matrix compositions, histopathology, and real-time polymerase chain reaction (PCR) for assessment of the treatment effect on cartilage. Following treatment, the lameness scores were significantly improved at 2 and 3 months in the PRP and combined PRP and MSC groups, but no difference was found between PRP and MSC.

Naturally occurring hip OA has been the focus of clinical trials using AD-MSCs (Vilar *et al.*, 2013, 2014; Cuervo *et al.*, 2014) and stromal vascular fraction (Black *et al.*, 2007; Marx *et al.*, 2014). One of the studies used injection of MSCs at acupuncture points (Marx *et al.*, 2014), while the other studies delivered MSCs intra-articularly. These studies consistently showed improved outcomes in the dogs treated with MSCs with no adverse effects reported, providing preliminary evidence of a biological effect of MSCs in dogs with OA. Similar results were obtained in dogs with elbow OA (Black *et al.*, 2008; Guercio *et al.*, 2012). It is important to point out that force plate analysis, considered the gold standard in objective gait analysis, was performed in only two of the available canine OA studies and that a randomized design was applied in only one study (Cuervo *et al.*, 2014).

A prospective, randomized, masked, placebo-controlled, multicenter clinical trial investigated the effect of a single dose of allogeneic AD-MSCs, delivered intra-articularly to either one or two joints in 74 dogs (Harman *et al.*, 2016). The primary outcome measure was a client-based questionnaire, in addition to evaluation by the veterinarian. AD-MSC treatment was shown to be safe and efficacious in comparison to the placebo. AD-MSC treatment resulted in a significant improvement in client- and veterinarian-based outcomes. Similar results have been obtained by one author (AP) in a prospective, randomized, double-blind, placebo-controlled study investigating the effect of allogeneic umbilical-cord-derived MSCs as an intra-articular treatment for elbow OA (trial in progress). The group treated with MSC experienced significantly more improvement in client-based outcomes in comparison to the group that received placebo.

Ligament and tendon injuries

Despite the advances in nonsurgical and surgical techniques, treatment of tendinopathies, desmitis, and chronic tears remain a challenge in people and animals. Reasons for the high failure rate include the limited potential for healing (in chronic injuries) and the development of scar tissue with lower mechanical properties than the original tissue. Stem cells have been evaluated for treatment of tendinopathies for their potential for restarting the healing process by differentiating into tenocytes and releasing growth factors and cytokines. BM-MSCs have been evaluated in horses with superficial flexor tendon injuries, demonstrating a significant decrease in re-injury after return to competition (Godwin et al., 2012).

A recent study in dogs investigated the use of autologous bone marrow aspirate concentrate or AD-MSCs with PRP combination and a rehabilitation therapy protocol for the treatment of partial CCL rupture (Canapp et al., 2016b). Dogs presenting with an early partial CCL rupture (n = 36) were diagnosed and treated with a single intra-articular injection of either bone marrow aspirate concentrate or AD-MSCs with PRP. Outcome measures included client-based questionnaire (n = 12), veterinary evaluation, and objective gait analysis (n = 11). Of the 12 questionnaires that were returned, seven of the eight performance dogs had returned to full activity. The same authors described the outcomes for 55 dogs with supraspinatus tendinopathy treated with adipose-derived progenitor cells and PRP therapy (Canapp et al., 2016a). After ultrasound-guided injection, 25 of 55 dogs were rechecked with objective gait analysis. At 90 days following injection, 88% of cases had no significant difference in total pressure index percentage between the treated and the contralateral limb. All cases showed improvement in fiber pattern at ultrasonographic recheck.

Additional data are needed before making any conclusion on the effect of MSCs in the treatment of tendinopathies in dogs. Interestingly, in human patients, despite some promising clinical reports, no sufficient evidence is found to support MSC treatment for tendinopathies (Pas et al., 2017) at this point. Additional veterinary studies are needed, with the inclusion of standardized protocols, control groups, and randomized design.

Intervertebral disc disease

Currently available treatments for intervertebral disc disease (IVDD) in dogs focus on alleviation of pain and include anti-inflammatory/analgesic medication, physiotherapy, and various surgical procedures. All those treatment modalities may resolve neurological deficits and reduce pain but they do not lead to repair of the degenerated disc. In fact, long-term medication may be necessary with resultant side effects, and surgical treatments can result in various complications including implant failure, adjacent segment disease, and recurrence of IVDD. The problems described above and the inability to solve them with current conservative and surgical approaches, have led to a growing consensus of the need to develop new therapies based on the methods of regenerative medicine and tissue engineering.

Because there are relatively few cells in the degenerated disc and cell viability is impaired, stimulation of the remaining cells to proliferate and to produce matrix is challenging. Cell-based therapies may overcome this problem. Thus far, cell-based treatment strategies have used chondrocyte-like cells (CLCs), MSCs, and notochordal cells.

Autologous transplantation of CLCs has been used successfully in an experimental canine model (Ganey et al., 2009). After expansion of disc chondrocytes in culture and return into the disc by injection, transplanted cells remained viable and produced extracellular matrix. While clinical results in dogs are not available, this procedure has been used in human patients. People receiving autologous CLC transplantation experienced a greater reduction in pain after 2 years and had a higher intervertebral disc (IVD) fluid content on MRI than the control group (Hohaus et al., 2008). CLC transplantation has its limitations because, practically, these cells can only be obtained from herniated discs in low numbers and with a reduction of their chondrogenic potential as they have already undergone degenerative alterations.

Currently, the use of MSCs is emerging as a leading cellular treatment for several diseases, since they can be isolated from several tissues including bone marrow, adipose tissue, muscle, placenta, and umbilical cord blood. Depending on their environment, MSCs can differentiate into various cell types, such as osteoblasts, myocytes, neural cells, adipocytes, and chondrocytes. Besides their ability to maintain viability and to proliferate after transplantation, MSCs have immunosuppressive properties and secrete growth/trophic factors that support regenerative processes. The combination of these properties makes MSCs highly suitable for strategies to regenerate IVDs. Consequently, a large body of *in vitro* studies and experimental investigations based upon injury models in laboratory animals has been accumulated in the last decade with impressive results. An experimental study reported a significant delay in disc degeneration in Beagles treated with MSC compared with the control group 12 weeks after injection, as evaluated using MRI (Hiyama *et al.*, 2008). This work constitutes a valuable amount of knowledge but still lacks the evidence that MSC delivery is also successful in spontaneously occurring IVD degeneration.

Recently, human patients with lumbar IVDD treated with intradiscal bone marrow-derived MSC injections reported diminished pain and disability at the 12-month follow-up. The disc water content on MRI was significantly elevated (Orozco *et al.*, 2011). Another recent human study documented an improvement of one modified Pfirrmann grade (increased T2 signal of nucleus pulposus) along with clinical improvement at the 1-year follow-up in 8/20 patients after percutaneous injection of MSCs (Pettine *et al.*, 2016). One conclusion from these studies was that functional improvement of patients was more evident than morphological improvement demonstrated by way of MRI. Functional improvement was mainly attributed to the immunomodulatory properties of MSCs, leading to reduction of local inflammation. However, based upon clinical benefit and increased water signal on MRI alone it cannot be stated that MSC treatment is able to regenerate nucleus pulposus tissue. Histological and immunophenotypic studies would be necessary to determine survival, proliferation, and differentiation of MSCs into functional nucleus pulposus cells. To date, only indirect methods are available to demonstrate effectiveness of the transplanted cells in the clinical situation.

A first clinical canine study was recently presented using a model of working German Shepherd Dogs with spontaneously degenerated lumbosacral discs that were treated with intradiscal injections of autologous bone marrow-derived MSCs in combination with dorsal laminectomy (Steffen *et al.*, 2017) (Figure 16.8).

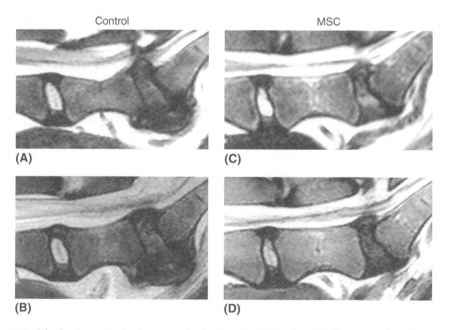

Figure 16.8 MRI of the lumbar spine in dogs treated with intradiscal injection of saline (control) and mesenchymal stem cells (MSCs). The L6–L7 and L7–S1 intervertebral disc are shown on the left and right in each image, respectively. **(A)** Preoperative and **(B)** postoperative MRI of the control dog. **(C)** Preoperative and **(D)** postoperative MRI of a dog treated with MSCs. Note the progressive degeneration in the MSC-treated dog compared to the unaltered degeneration status in the control dog. The untreated L6–L7 discs in both dogs represent the signal behavior of healthy discs.

The results of this study showed that intradiscal injection of autologous MSCs was well tolerated without side effects, but did not have clear regenerative benefits as evaluated by way of disc height and disc volumetric measurements. In addition, this treatment did not result in a different clinical score compared with controls. Moreover, on the basis of Pfirrmann scoring, disc degeneration progressed more in the MSC group, suggesting that the injection procedure itself can enhance degenerative mechanisms within the IVD.

Taken together, these results highlight the potential of cell-based strategies to regenerate IVDs. However, further efforts are needed to translate *in vitro* and experimental research into clinical practice. An interdisciplinary approach including expertise from biology, tissue engineering, biomechanics, and surgery is required. Currently, methods including micro-carriers and growth factors to enhance regenerative effects of MSC are being evaluated in clinical canine studies to pave the way to future clinical applications of these procedures.

Case Study 16.2   Sprain of medial carpal collateral ligament

Signalment: 6-y.o. M/I mixed breed (Border Collie and German Shepherd); 35 kg.

History: Patient first presented April 2015 for right thoracic limb lameness that began 6 months before presentation. The onset of lameness was not associated with a specific event such as trauma, although patient often played Frisbee with client. Patient was very active, typically walking several hours every day with client. At the time of first evaluation patient was too aggressive for a complete orthopedic examination and diagnosis could not be obtained. Patient received Rimadyl® for 10 days and a recommendation of leash walks and rest for 6 weeks. Patient presented 18 months after initial onset of clinical signs because of progressive worsening of lameness.

Clinical examination: Patient showed a 2/4 right thoracic lameness, worse at trot. Patient reacted at flexion and extension of the elbow (mild pain), but showed more severe pain on pin-point palpation over the medial humeral epicondyle.

Imaging: A CT scan of both elbows was unremarkable. MRI of the right carpus was performed to evaluate soft tissue structures (Figures 16.9 and 16.10). Imaging diagnosis was strain of the medial carpal collateral ligament.

Comments: Carpal injuries are common in active dogs. In this case, the ligament sprain diagnosed with MRI was treated with an intralesional injection of autologous conditioned plasma and an orthosis for 3 months. It is important to emphasize that earlier and more accurate diagnosis of desmitis may offer more potential for healing. Chronic tendinitis and desmitis are therapeutic challenges because of the

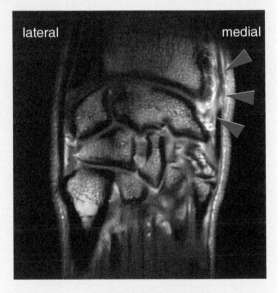

Figure 16.9   T1 turbo spin echo sequence in a dorsal orientation after i.v. injection of gadolinium of a carpal MRI examination. Mild soft tissue swelling (red arrowheads). undergoing contrast enhancement is noted in the area of the straight part of the medial carpal collateral ligament that is separated from the oblique part by the tendon of the abductor pollicis longus muscle. Fibers of both parts of the medial collateral ligament are maintained but their organization is reduced and they show contrast enhancement.

limited healing capacity of the tendon. In contrast, acute desmitis and tendinitis may be treated with early modification of the exercise regimen and use of orthobiologics with greater potential for healing and return to normal activity.

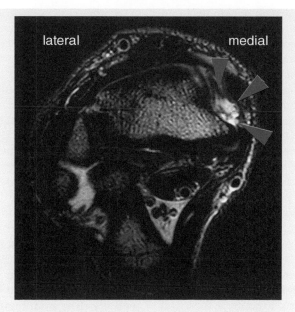

Figure 16.10 Turbo spin echo sequence with spectral presaturation with inversion recovery for fat saturation in a transverse plane after i.v. injection of gadolinium. Both parts of the medial carpal collateral ligament (red arrowheads), divided by the tendon of the abductor pollicis longus muscle, are mildly thickened and show contrast enhancement.

Spinal cord injuries

Spinal cord injury (SCI) may result in permanent motor and sensory dysfunction. Therefore, there is significant interest in regenerative therapies aimed at the biological repair of injured nervous tissue. Dogs with clinical SCIs represent a feasible large-animal model for translational studies on spinal cord regeneration in humans. Specifically, dogs with SCI due to IVD herniations have been used in several studies exploiting promising laboratory interventions for the benefit of both paraplegic people and dogs. The types of these treatments have ranged from acute neuroprotective strategies to pharmacological interventions in chronic SCI to cell-based therapies.

Two acute neuroprotective studies have recently been completed using the clinical dog model. In the first study, a metalloproteinase inhibitor (GM6001) in dimethyl sulfoxide (DMSO) was injected subcutaneously in dogs with both complete and incomplete acute injuries. A randomized, placebo-controlled study design was used with two control groups receiving either saline injections or DMSO alone. Improved functional recovery was observed for dogs with complete SCI receiving either GM6001 in DMSO or DMSO alone, suggesting that DMSO

was likely the mechanism by which improvement was enhanced (Levine *et al.*, 2014). A second study was a multicenter, placebo-controlled, prospective, randomized clinical trial evaluating the effects of polyethylene glycol (PEG) and methylprednisolone sodium succinate (MPSS) on outcome in dogs with acute and complete SCI. The study failed to detect a treatment effect of either PEG or MPSS at 12 weeks after injury, and the study was terminated after interim analysis (Olby *et al.*, 2014).

Cell-based treatments of chronic and complete SCI have recently been reported. A randomized, double-blinded trial evaluated the effects of intraspinal olfactory ensheathing cell (OEC) transplantation on locomotor outcome in dogs with sensorimotor complete thoracolumbar injuries of longer than 3 months' duration. Dogs received intraparenchymal injections of OECs. Outcome measures included kinematic assessment of thoracic limb–pelvic limb coordination, lateral stability, somatosensory-evoked potentials, transcranial magnetic motor-evoked potentials, and bladder compliance. A significant treatment effect was observed in the OEC group for limb coordination but the remaining parameters did not indicate restoration of long tract function. It was concluded that OECs are efficacious to restore motor function that is not under brain control, but used alone are unlikely to restore meaningful return of complex functions such as balance or continence (Granger *et al.*, 2012).

MSCs and neural crest stem cells are promising cell types for treatment of SCI. Beneficial effects include immunomodulation, regulation of a regenerative permissive environment, promotion of axonal growth, and remyelination. MSCs were shown to be safe and possibly beneficial in several canine SCI experimental and clinical studies (McMahill *et al.*, 2015). Intraspinal injections of various types of autologous and allogenic MSCs in dogs with experimentally induced SCI revealed that different MSC groups showed significant improvements in locomotion at 8 weeks after transplantation. This recovery was accompanied by increased numbers of surviving neurons and neurofilament-positive fibers in the lesion site. Compared to controls, the lesion sizes were smaller, and fewer microglia and reactive astrocytes were found in the spinal cord epicenter of all MSC groups. The data suggested that transplantation of MSCs promotes functional recovery after SCI. Furthermore, application of umbilical cord-derived MSCs led to more nerve regeneration and neuroprotection and less inflammation compared with other types of MSCs (Ryu *et al.*, 2012).

Percutaneous transplantation of human umbilical cord-derived MSCs has been reported in a clinical case. In a paraplegic dog without nociception, suspected to have fibrocartilaginous embolic myelopathy at the level of L3, treatment resulted in restoration of ambulatory function (Chung *et al.*, 2013). However, the dog did not regain nociception which raises the possibility that the clinical improvement was the result of activation of local spinal circuitries and plasticity (spinal walking) and not necessarily associated with treatment.

To summarize the status of spinal cord regeneration in dogs, at the time of writing, clinical applications of treatment protocols are not yet available. Functional recovery after SCI is complex and dependent on the inherent plasticity of the tissue and its responses and local environmental effects. It is likely that multimodal efforts including differentiation of transplanted cells into relevant cell types (neurons, glial cells), regulation of scar formation, prevention of cyst formation, and secretion of neurotrophic and other factors to promote matrix repair and regeneration are necessary to result in restoration of spinal cord function.

Regulation of orthobiologics

Regulation of biological therapies is an important aspect of practicing regenerative medicine. In the United States, the Center for Veterinary Medicine (CVM) at the Food and Drug Administration (FDA) is the regulatory body overseeing the use of drugs. It is the authors' understanding that most animal cell-based products, such as cultured stem cell therapies, stromal vascular fraction, and, potentially, bone marrow aspirate concentrate, are considered to be drugs. It is less clear whether PRP, ACS, and APS are considered to be drugs. It is also not entirely clear what regulation exists for animal cell-based therapies. Presumably any animal cell-based therapies, if considered drugs, are subject to existing regulation for animal drugs. However, this is not entirely clear as the FDA has also issued *Guidance for Industry Cell-Based Products for Animal Use #218* that specifically states that this document provides guidance and does "not establish legally enforceable responsibilities." A full discussion regarding the regulation and approval of regenerative medicine therapies is beyond the scope of this chapter. However, potential users of cell-based products are encouraged to educate themselves on the regulatory process and the current status of any products they intend to use and should direct inquiries to the CVM at the FDA.

References

Alves, E. G., Serakides, R., Boeloni, J. N., Rosado, I. R., Ocarino, N. M., Oliveira, H. P., *et al.* 2014. Comparison of the osteogenic potential of mesenchymal stem cells from the bone marrow and adipose tissue of young dogs. *BMC Vet Res*, 10, 190.

Arnoczky, S. P. & Shebani-Rad, S. 2013. The basic science of platelet-rich plasma (PRP): what clinicians need to know. *Sports Med Arthrosc*, 21(4), 180–185.

Bertone, A. L., Ishihara, A., Zekas, L. J., Wellman, M. L., Lewis, K. B., Schwarze, R. A., *et al.* 2014. Evaluation of a single intra-articular injection of autologous protein solution for treatment of osteoarthritis in horses. *Am J Vet Res*, 75(2), 141–151.

Black, L. L., Gaynor, J., Gahring, D., Adams, C., Aron, D., Harman, S., *et al.* 2007. Effect of adipose-derived mesenchymal stem and regenerative cells on lameness in dogs with chronic osteoarthritis of the coxofemoral joints: a randomized, double-blinded, multicenter, controlled trial. *Vet Ther*, 8(4), 272–284.

Black, L. L., Gaynor, J., Adams, C., Dhupa, S., Sams, A. E., Taylor, R., *et al.* 2008. Effect of intraarticular injection of autologous adipose-derived mesenchymal stem and regenerative cells on clinical signs of chronic osteoarthritis of the elbow joint in dogs. *Vet Ther*, 9(3), 192–200.

Bozynski, C. C., Stannard, J. P., Smith, P., Hanypsiak, B. T., Kuroki, K., Stoker, A., *et al.* 2016. Acute management of anterior cruciate ligament injuries using novel canine models. *J Knee Surg*, 29(7), 594–603.

Braun, H. J., Kim, H. J., Chu, C. R. & Dragoo, J. L. 2014. The effect of platelet-rich plasma formulations and blood products on human synoviocytes: implications for intra-articular injury and therapy. *Am J Sports Med*, 42(5), 1204–1210.

Canapp, S. O., Jr., Canapp, D. A., Ibrahim, V., Carr, B. J., Cox, C. & Barrett, J. G. 2016a. The use of adipose-derived progenitor cells and platelet-rich plasma combination for the treatment of supraspinatus tendinopathy in 55 dogs: a retrospective study. *Front Vet Sci*, 9(3), 61.

Canapp, S. O., Jr., Leasure, C. S., Cox, C., Ibrahim, V. & Carr, B. J. 2016b. Partial cranial cruciate ligament tears treated with stem cell and platelet-rich plasma combination therapy in 36 dogs: a retrospective study. *Front Vet Sci*, 14(3), 112.

Carr, B. J., Canapp, S. O., Jr., Mason, D. R, Cox, C. & Hess, T. 2015. Canine platelet-rich plasma systems: a prospective analysis. *Front Vet Sci*, 2, 73.

Chung, H. W., Park, S. A., Lee, J. H., Chung, D. J., Yang, W. J, Kang, E. H., *et al.* 2013. Percutaneous transplantation of human umbilical cord-derived mesenchymal stem cells in a dog suspected to have fibrocartilaginous embolic myelopathy. *J Vet Sci*, 14(4), 495–497.

Conzemius, M. G. & Evans, R. B. 2012. Caregiver placebo effect for dogs with lameness from osteoarthritis. *J Am Vet Med Assoc*, 241(10), 1314–1319.

Cook, J. L., Smith, P. A., Bozynski, C. C., Kuroki, K., Cook, C. R., Stoker, A. M. & Pfeiffer, F. M. 2015. Multiple injections of leukoreduced platelet rich plasma reduce pain and functional impairment in a canine model of ACL and meniscal deficiency. *J Orthop Res*, 34(4), 607–615.

Crovace, A., Lacitignola, L., Rossi, G. & Francioso, E. 2010. Histological and immunohistochemical evaluation of autologous cultured bone marrow mesenchymal stem cells and bone marrow mononucleated cells in collagenase-induced tendinitis of equine superficial digital flexor tendon. *Vet Med Int*, 2010, 250978.

Cuervo, B., Rubio, M., Sopena, J., Dominguez, J. M., Vilar, J., Morales, M., *et al.* 2014. Hip osteoarthritis in dogs: a randomized study using mesenchymal stem cells from adipose tissue and plasma rich in growth factors. *Int J Mol Sci*, 15(8), 13437–13460.

de Bakker, E., Gielen, I., Saunders, J. H., Polis, I., Vermerire, S., Peremans, K., et al. 2013. Primary and concomitant flexor enthesopathy of the canine elbow. *Vet Comp Orthop Traumatol*, 26(6), 425–434.

DeLong, J. M., Russell, R. P. & Mazzocca, A. D. 2012. Platelet-rich plasma: the PAW classification system. *Arthroscopy*, 28(7), 998–1009.

Dohan Ehrenfest, D. M., Andia, I., Zumstein, M. A., Zhang, C. Q., Pinto, N. R. & Bielecki, T. 2014. Classification of platelet concentrates (platelet-rich plasma-PRP, platelet-rich fibrin-PRF) for topical and infiltrative use in orthopedic and sports medicine: current consensus, clinical implications and perspectives. *Muscles Ligaments Tendons J*, 4(1), 3–9.

Fahie, M. A., Ortolano, G. A., Guercio, V., Schaffer, J. A., Johnston, G., Au, J., *et al.* 2013. A randomized controlled trial of the efficacy of autologous platelet therapy for the treatment of osteoarthritis in dogs. *J Am Vet Med Assoc*, 243(9), 1291–1297.

Franklin, S. P. & Cook, J. L. 2013. Autologous conditioned plasma versus hyaluronan plus corticosteroid for treatment of chronic elbow osteoarthritis in dogs. *Can Vet J*, 54(9), 881–884.

Franklin, S. P., Garner, B. C. & Cook, J. L. 2015. Characteristics of canine platelet-rich plasma prepared with five commercially available systems. *Am J Vet Res*, 76(9), 822–827.

Franklin, S. P., Birdwhistell, K. E., Strelchik, A., Garner, B. C. & Brainard, B. M. 2017a. Influence of cellular composition and exogenous activation on growth factor and cytokine concentrations in canine platelet-rich plasmas. *Front Vet Sci*, 4, 40.

Franklin, S. P., Burke, E. E. & Holmes, S. P. 2017b. The effect of platelet-rich plasma on osseous healing in dogs undergoing high tibial osteotomy. *PLoS One*, 12(5), e0177597.

Frisbie, D. D. 2015. Autologous-conditioned serum: evidence for use in the knee. *J Knee Surg*, 28(1), 63–66.

Frye, C. W., Enders, A., Brooks, M. B., Struble A. M. & Wakshlag, J. J. 2016. Assessment of canine autologous platelet-rich plasma produced with a commercial centrifugation and platelet recovery kit. *Vet Comp Orthop Traumatol*, 29(1), 14–19.

Fufa, D., Shealy, B., Jacobson, M., Kevy, S. & Murray, M. M. 2008. Activation of platelet-rich plasma using soluble type I collagen. *J Oral Maxillofac Surg*, 66(4), 684–690.

Ganey, T., Hutton, W. C., Moseley, T., Hedrick, M. & Meisel, H. J. 2009. Intervertebral disc repair using adipose tissue-derived stem and regenerative cells: experiments in a canine model. *Spine*, 34, 2297–2304.

Gianakos, A., Zambrana, L., Savage-Elliott, I., Lane, J. M. & Kennedy, J. G. 2015. Platelet-rich plasma in the animal long-bone model: an analysis of basic science evidence. *Orthopedics*, 38(12), e1079–1090.

Godwin, E. E., Young, N. J., Dudhia, J., Beamish, I. C. & Smith, R. K. 2012. Implantation of bone marrow-derived mesenchymal stem cells demonstrates improved outcome in horses with overstrain injury of the superficial digital flexor tendon. *Equine Vet J*, 44(1), 25–32.

Granger, N., Blamires, H., Franklin, R. J. & Jeffery, N. D. 2012. Autologous olfactory mucosal cell transplants in clinical spinal cord injury: a randomized double-blinded trial in a canine translational model. *Brain*, 135, 3227–3237.

Guercio, A., Di Marco, P., Casella, S., Cannella, V., Russotto, L., Purpari, G., *et al.* 2012. Production of canine mesenchymal stem cells from adipose tissue and their application in dogs with chronic osteoarthritis of the humeroradial joints. *Cell Biol Int*, 36, 189–194.

Guercio, A., Di Bella, S., Casella, S., Di Marco, P., Russo, C. & Piccione, G. 2013. Canine mesenchymal stem cells (MSCs): characterization in relation to donor age and adipose tissue-harvesting site. *Cell Biol Int*, 37(8), 789–798.

Harman, R., Carlson, K., Gaynor, J., Gustafson, S., Dhupa, S., Clement, K., *et al.* 2016. A prospective, randomized, masked, and placebo-controlled efficacy study of intraarticular allogeneic adipose stem cells for the treatment of osteoarthritis in dogs. *Front Vet Sci*, 3, 81.

Harrison, S., Vavken, P., Kevy, S., Jacobson, M., Zurakowski, D. & Murray, M. M. 2011. Platelet activation by collagen provides sustained release of anabolic cytokines. *Am J Sports Med*, 39(4), 729–734.

Hernigou, P., Flouzat Lachaniette, C. H., Poignard, A., Chevalier, N. & Rouard, H. 2013. Cancer risk is not increased in patients treated with autologous bone marrow cell concentrate. *J Bone Joint Surg Am*, 195, 2215–2221.

Hiyama, A., Mochida, J., Iwashina, T., Omi, H., Watanabe, T., Serigano, K., *et al.* 2008. Transplantation of mesenchymal stem cells in a canine disc degeneration model. *J Orthop Res*, 26, 589–600.

Ho, L. K., Baltzer, W. I., Nemanic, S. & Stieger-Vanegas, S. M. 2015. Single ultrasound-guided platelet-rich plasma injection for treatment of supraspinatus tendinopathy in dogs. *Can Vet J*, 56(8), 845–849.

Hohaus, C., Ganey, T. M., Minkus, Y. & Meisel, H. J. 2008. Cell transplantation in lumbar spine disc degeneration disease. *Eur Spine J*, 17(Suppl. 4), 492–503.

Horie, M., Driscoll, M. D., Sampson, H. W., Sekiya, I., Caroom, C. T., Prockop, D. J. & Thomas, D. B. 2012. Implantation of allogenic synovial stem cells promotes meniscal regeneration in a rabbit meniscal defect model. *J Bone Joint Surg Am*, 94, 701–712.

Huggins, S. S., Suchodolski, J. S., Bearden, R. N., Steiner, J. M. & Saunders, W. B. 2015. Serum concentrations of canine interleukin-1 receptor antagonist protein in healthy dogs after incubation using an autologous serum processing system. *Res Vet Sci*, 101, 28–33.

Levine, J. M., Cohen, N. D., Heller, M., Fajt, V. R., Levine, G. J., Trivedi, A. A., *et al.* 2014. Efficacy of a metalloproteinase inhibitor in spinal cord injured dogs. *PLoS One*, 9(5), e96408.

Maerz, T., Fleischer, M., Newton, M. D., Davidson, A., Salisbury, M., Altman, P., *et al.* 2017. Acute mobilization and migration of bone marrow-derived stem cells following anterior cruciate ligament rupture. *Osteoarthritis Cartilage*, 25(8), 1335–1344.

Marx, C., Silveira, M. D., Selbach, I., da Silva, A. S., Braga, L. M., Camassola, M. & Nardi, N. B. 2014. Acupoint injection of autologous stromal vascular fraction and allogeneic adipose-derived stem cells to treat hip dysplasia in dogs. *Stem Cells Int*, 2014, 391274.

Marx, R. E. 2001. Platelet-rich plasma (PRP): what is PRP and what is not PRP? *Implant Dent*, 10(4), 225–228.

McMahill, B. G., Borjesson, D. L., Sieber-Blum, M., Nolat, J. A. & Sturges, B. K. 2015. Stem cells in canine spinal cord injury—promise for regenerative therapy in a large animal model of human disease. *Stem Cell Rev and Rep*, 11, 180–193.

Mei, L., Shen, B., Ling, P., Liu, S., Xue, J., Liu, F., *et al.* 2017. Culture-expanded allogenic adipose tissue-derived stem cells attenuate cartilage degeneration in an experimental rat osteoarthritis model. *PLoS One*, 12(4), e0176107.

Neupane, M., Chang, C. C., Kiupel, M. & Yuzbasiyan-Gurkan, V. 2008. Isolation and characterization of canine adipose-derived mesenchymal stem cells. *Tissue Eng Part A*, 14(6), 1007–1015.

Olby, N. J., Muguet, A. C., Lim, J. H., Davidian, M., Mariani, C. L., Freeman, A. C., *et al.* 2014. A placebo-controlled, prospective, randomized clinical trial of polyethylene glycol and methylprednisolone sodium succinate in dogs with intervertebral disk herniation. *J Vet Intern Med*, 30, 206–214.

Orozco, L., Soler, R., Morera, C., Alberca, M., Sanchez, A. & Garcia-Sancho, J. 2011. Intervertebral disc repair by autologous mesenchymal bone marrow cells: a pilot study. *Transplantation*, 92, 822–828.

Pas, H. I. M. F. L., Moen, M. H., Haisma, H. J. & Winters, M. 2017. No evidence for the use of stem cell therapy for tendon disorders: a systematic review. *Br J Sports Med*, 51(13), 996–1002.

Perazzi, A., Busetto, R., Martinello, T., Drigo, M., Pasotto, D., Cian, F., et al. 2013. Description of a double centrifugation tube method for concentrating canine platelets. *BMC Vet Res*, 9, 146.

Pettine, K., Suzuki, R., Sand, T. & Murphy, M. 2016. Treatment of discogenic back pain with autologous bone marrow concentrate injection with minimum two year follow-up. *Int Orthop*, 40, 135–140.

Rabillard, M., Grand, J. G., Dalibert, E., Fellah, B., Gauthier, O. & Niebauer, G. W. 2009. Effects of autologous platelet rich plasma gel and calcium phosphate biomaterials on bone healing in an ulnar ostectomy model in dogs. *Vet Comp Orthop Traumatol*, 22(6), 460–466.

Russell, K. A., Chow, N. H., Dukoff, D., Gibson, T. W., LaMarre, J., Betts, D. H. & Koch, T. G. 2016. Characterization and immunomodulatory effects of canine adipose tissue- and bone marrow-derived mesenchymal stromal cells. *PLoS One*, 11(12), e0167442.

Ryu, H. H., Kang, B. J., Park, S. S., Kim, Y., Sung, G. J., Woo, H. M., et al. 2012. Comparison of mesenchymal stem cells derived from fat, bone marrow, Wharton's jelly, and umbilical cord blood for treating spinal cord injuries in dogs. *J Vet Med Sci*, 74(12), 1617–1630.

Sawyere, D. M., Lanz, O. I., Dahlgren, L. A., Barry, S. L., Nichols, A. C. & Werre, S. R. 2016. Cytokine and growth factor concentrations in canine autologous conditioned serum. *Vet Surg*, 45(5), 582–586.

Silva, R. F., Carmona, J. U. & Rezende, C. M. 2012. Comparison of the effect of calcium gluconate and batroxobin on the release of transforming growth factor beta 1 in canine platelet concentrates. *BMC Vet Res*, 8, 121.

Silva, R. F., Carmona, J. U. & Rezende, C. M. 2013. Intra-articular injections of autologous platelet concentrates in dogs with surgical reparation of cranial cruciate ligament rupture: a pilot study. *Vet Comp Orthop Traumatol*, 26(4), 285–290.

Souza, T. F., Andrade, A. L., Ferreira, G. T., Sakamoto, S. S., Albuquerque, V. B., Bonfim, S. R., et al. 2012. Healing and expression of growth factors (TGF-beta and PDGF) in canine radial ostectomy gap containing platelet-rich plasma. *Vet Comp Orthop Traumatol*, 25(6), 445–452.

Steffen, F., Smolders, L., Bertolo, A., Roentgen, A. & Stoyanov, J. 2017. Bone marrow-derived mesenchymal stem cells as autologous therapy in dogs with naturally occurring intervertebral disc disease:

feasibility, safety and preliminary results. *Tissue Eng Part C Methods*, doi: 10.1089/ten (epub ahead of print).

Stief, M., Gottschalk, J., Ionita, J. C., Einspanier, A., Oechtering, G. & Böttcher, P. 2011. Concentration of platelets and growth factors in canine autologous conditioned plasma. *Vet Comp Orthop Traumatol*, 24(2), 122–125.

Sullivan, M. O., Gordon-Evans, W. J., Fredericks, L. P., Kiefer, K., Conzemius, M. G. & Griffon, D. J. 2016. Comparison of mesenchymal stem cell surface markers from bone marrow aspirates and adipose stromal vascular fraction sites. *Front Vet Sci*, 15, 2:82.

Sundman, E. A., Cole, B. J. & Fortier, L. A. 2011. Growth factor and catabolic cytokine concentrations are influenced by the cellular composition of platelet-rich plasma. *Am J Sports Med*, 39(10), 2135–2140.

Textor, J. A. & Tablin, F. 2012. Activation of equine platelet-rich plasma: comparison of methods and characterization of equine autologous thrombin. *Vet Surg*, 41(7), 784–794.

Thoesen, M. S., Berg-Foels, W. S., Stokol, T., Rassnick, K. M., Jacobson, M. S., Kevy, S. V. & Todhunter, R. J. 2006. Use of a centrifugation-based, point-of-care device for production of canine autologous bone marrow and platelet concentrates. *Am J Vet Res*, 67(10), 1655–1661.

Vilar, J. M., Morales, M., Santana, A., Spinella, G., Rubio, M., Cuervo, B., et al. 2013. Controlled, blinded force platform analysis of the effect of intraarticular injection of autologous adipose-derived mesenchymal stem cells associated to PRGF-Endoret in osteoarthritic dogs. *BMC Vet Res*, 9, 131.

Vilar, J. M., Batista, M., Morales, M., Santana, A., Cuervo, B., Rubio, M., et al. 2014. Assessment of the effect of intraarticular injection of autologous adipose-derived mesenchymal stem cells in osteoarthritic dogs using a double blinded force platform analysis. *BMC Vet Res*, 10, 143.

Visser, L. C., Arnoczky, S. P., Caballero, O. & Egerbacher, M. 2010a. Platelet-rich fibrin constructs elute higher concentrations of transforming growth factor-beta1 and increase tendon cell proliferation over time when compared to blood clots: a comparative in vitro analysis. *Vet Surg*, 39(7), 811–817.

Visser, L. C., Arnoczky, S. P., Caballero, O., Kern, A., Ratcliffe, A. & Gardner, K. L. 2010b. Growth factor-rich plasma increases tendon cell proliferation and matrix synthesis on a synthetic scaffold: an in vitro study. *Tissue Eng Part A*, 16(3), 1021–1029.

Visser, L. C., Arnoczky, S. P., Caballero, O. & Gardner, K. L. 2011. Evaluation of the use of an autologous platelet-rich fibrin membrane to enhance tendon healing in dogs. *Am J Vet Res*, 72(5), 699–705.

Wanstrath, A. W., Hettlich, B. F., Su, L., Smith, A., Zekas, L. J., Allen, M. J. & Bertone, A. L. 2016. Evaluation of a single intra-articular injection of autologous protein solution for treatment of osteoarthritis in a canine population. *Vet Surg*, 45(6), 764–774.

Woodell-May, J., Matuska, A., Oyster, M., Welch, Z., O'Shaughnessey, K. & Hoeppner, J. 2011. Autologous protein solution inhibits MMP-13 production by IL-1beta and TNFalpha-stimulated human articular chondrocytes. *J Orthop Res*, 29(9), 1320–1326.

Yun, S., Ku, S. K. & Kwon, Y. S. 2016. Adipose-derived mesenchymal stem cells and platelet-rich plasma synergistically ameliorate the surgical-induced osteoarthritis in Beagle dogs. *J Orthop Surg Res*, 11, 9.

Zhang, Q., Chen, Y., Wang, Q., Fang, C., Sun, Y., Yuan, T., *et al.* 2016. Effect of bone marrow-derived stem cells on chondrocytes from patients with osteoarthritis. *Mol Med Rep*, 13(2), 1795–1800.

17 Diagnosis of and Treatment Options for Disorders of the Spine

H. Steven Steinberg, VMD, DACVIM (Neurology), CCRT, CVA, and
Joan R. Coates, DVM, MS, DACVIM (Neurology)

Summary

Almost all of the attention directed toward disorders of the spine involves its role in protecting the spinal cord. Certainly, damage to the spinal cord can be devastating but the demands placed upon the canine athlete highlight the functional aspects of the spine as a structure independent of the nervous tissue it protects. The spine is the scaffold that integrates the propulsive forces of the entire animal. Besides propulsion, the spine maintains the dog's head in its most versatile position while preserving energy expenditure in doing so. The vertebrae are similar but change in conformation determined by their position and function in relation to the rest of the body. The forces placed upon the various components of the individual vertebrae have been studied in discourses on phylogeny and the effects of bone density studies as they relate to pathology in humans have been examined. The soft tissue structures of the spine include ligaments, tendons, muscles, joint capsules, and the intervertebral discs. Although poorly studied, they all add flexibility, strength, and protective forces to many movements. Degenerative, traumatic, pathological, and congenital malformations impact normal function but have not been studied in a scientific manner in the performance of the canine athlete. Surgical and nonsurgical considerations might vary depending upon the type of performance of a particular canine athlete, and our standards of care should be re-evaluated in light of the demands anticipated.

Role of the spine in normal gait

The requirements that determine the anatomy of the spine are diverse and complex. The spine must support the head and the abdominal contents, allow for propulsion while co-ordinating limb movement, and be flexible to a limited extent, all the while protecting an extremely delicate structure, the spinal cord (Figure 17.1).

Most veterinary descriptions of the spine are about mechanical failures of the spine that result in spinal cord injury. The canine athlete is

---

Canine Sports Medicine and Rehabilitation, Second Edition. Edited by Chris Zink and Janet B. Van Dyke.
© 2018 John Wiley & Sons, Inc. Published 2018 by John Wiley & Sons, Inc.

so dependent upon the spine working properly that the structural functions assigned the vertebrae and the associated soft tissue cannot be ignored. Although there is a large body of literature about the workings of the canine spine, the focus has been almost exclusively toward applications for spinal conditions in humans.

This chapter concentrates on the functions of the spine specifically. Spinal cord conditions will be discussed in general terms. Detailed descriptions of spinal pathology affecting the

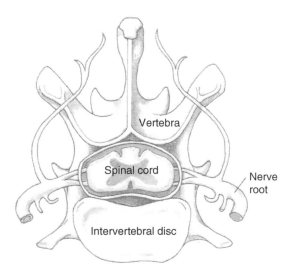

Figure 17.1 Cross-section through the spine showing the relationship between the vertebra, intervertebral disc, nerve roots, and spinal cord. Source: Illustration by Marcia Schlehr.

spinal cord and spinal cord diseases are readily available in numerous veterinary publications (Birchard, 2006; Dewey, 2008; Jaggy, 2010).

Interactions of the head, thoracic limbs, and pelvic limbs

The head

The head in upright, bipedal primates is a rather large, heavy structure, the weight of which is carried by a stack of relatively thin vertebrae. It is interesting to note that in bipeds where the head is not suspended from the body, the thoracic dorsal spines are small. In the dog the head is cantilevered away from the body and needs to be suspended by structures over the thoracic limbs. This arrangement requires that the thoracic limbs carry more weight than the pelvic limbs. Numerous spinal components are necessary to support this load efficiently. The nuchal ligament is a thick band of elastic fibers that help support the head with the least expenditure of energy. The nuchal ligament extends cranially to a large spinous process of the second cervical vertebra (the axis) and attaches caudally to the most dorsal portions of the dorsal spines of the first few thoracic vertebrae (Figure 17.2). The fibers of the nuchal ligament actually can be followed caudally into the ligaments that attach to the dorsal prominence of each dorsal spine

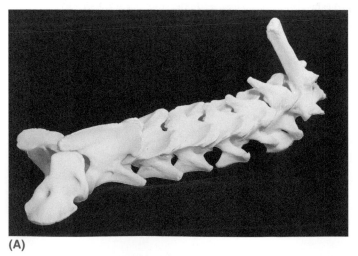

(A)

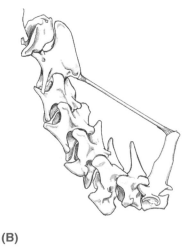

(B)

Figure 17.2 Photograph **(A)** and line drawing **(B)** of the cervical spine demonstrating the variations in conformation and the large dorsal thoracic spine needed to support the head. Source: (B) Illustration by Marcia Schlehr.

of each vertebral body. This ligamentous continuation of the nuchal ligament is called the supraspinous ligament. The thoracic spines are attached to each other by way of the interspinous ligament. The interspinous ligaments allow the force of the weight of the head to dissipate through the dog's body but still maintain a level of flexibility. These nonmuscular components form a very efficient system where muscular energy is conserved. The cervical vertebrae are large and proportional to the weight of the head. The forces required to suspend the head are complemented by absorption of compressive forces placed upon the cervical intervertebral discs.

The first and second cervical vertebrae have rather unique conformations that serve two significant purposes. The nuchal ligament is attached to the second cervical vertebra's large and wide dorsal spine so that the forces required to keep the head in various positions are dissipated over a large surface. Fan-shaped muscles, predominately the splenius, attach to the nuchal crest of the caudal skull and, like the nuchal ligament, arise from the cranial thoracic vertebrae's dorsal spines. This conformation also acts as a cantilever allowing the head to rotate and be supported by the compressive forces placed upon the atlanto-occipital joint (Figure 17.3).

The joints and articular facets of the cervical vertebrae C3–C7 are quite large and play a significant role in controlling fine movement of the head and neck in three planes. Their role in support of the neck is unknown but they may play a minor role, as their removal does not significantly affect the biomechanics of the neck (Crisco *et al.*, 1990).

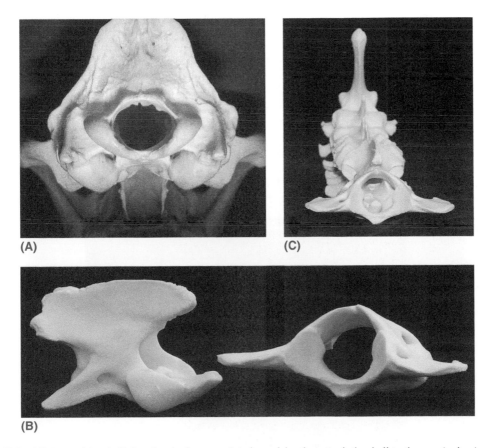

Figure 17.3 **(A)** Base of the skull showing the large occipital condyles that attach the skull to the cervical spine and the broad nuchal crest that is an important muscular attachment. **(B)** The first (atlas) and second (axis) cervical vertebrae disconnected to demonstrate how C2 fits into and joins C1. **(C)** An end-on view of the most rostral cervical spine demonstrating the C1–C2 articulation and the large atlanto-occipital joint.

The head initiates all purposeful movement, not only by determining the proposed activity through mentation, but also by determining the position that the body occupies in space through the vestibular apparatus within the skull. "Where the head goes, the body must follow" is a common phrase among rehabilitation therapists. It is understood that head position and movement initiates the next body movement and allows for appropriate body mechanics. Visual and olfactory input as well as reflex modification are important but are not critical for the vestibular system to perform its duties although they may be critical for developing training routines. A better understanding of how the neural feedback loops initiate, maintain, and protect propulsion and in this case, related spinal structures, is critical to attain peak performance.

The thoracic limbs

The thoracic limbs play a major role in maintaining the head's normal positions in space. The most cranial thoracic vertebrae with their large dorsal spines form the anchor that allows the head to be suspended at some distance from the body (Figure 17.4). These cranial thoracic vertebrae are supported directly by the thoracic limbs. The weight of this entire unit is supported by the thoracic limbs and it is often noted that this represents 60% of the body-weight of the animal. Considering the tremendous variation in conformation that exists from breed to breed and from individual to individual this would have to be a very rough estimate.

The thoracic limb has no bony or ligamentous attachment to the spine. The extrinsic thoracic limb muscular apparatus attaches the thoracic limb to the thoracic body wall allowing for freedom of movement that permits extreme changes in direction while protecting the spinal column's rigidity throughout the area of the rib cage.

The pelvic limbs

The pelvic limbs are responsible for carrying the weight of the caudal portion of the body. The pelvic limbs interact with the body in a completely different manner from the thoracic limbs (Figure 17.5). The coxofemoral joint transmits forces to the caudal spine through the sacroiliac joint. Although the box-like structure formed by the pelvis has less flexibility than the muscular attachment of the thoracic limb to the body wall, there is significant rotational advantage afforded by the range of motion of the ball and socket joints. This also allows the pelvic limbs to move far forward under the body, producing significant forward propulsion. When turning, a great deal of the actual body movement has been committed by the trajectory of the head, and the actions of the forelimbs and thoracic cavity. The

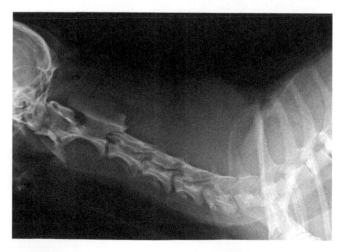

Figure 17.4   Lateral view of the cervical and rostral thoracic vertebrae demonstrating the functional anatomy described in the text.

limited flexibility of the spine allows for fluid movement once propulsion is initiated.

The tail, like the head, is cantilevered from the body. The apparatus necessary to carry this weight is not extensive but the tail has a role in balance and fine movement that has been extremely well documented in the cat (Walker *et al.*, 1998). Although not as well studied, the canine tail also serves to help with balance during locomotion (Wada *et al.*, 1993).

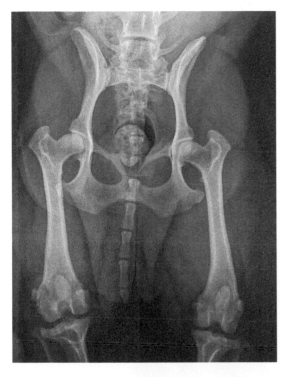

Figure 17.5   Ventrodorsal radiograph of the pelvis and femurs showing the box-like nature of the pelvis and the ball and socket joints of the femurs.

Conformational considerations

Each vertebra interlocks with the adjacent vertebra cranial and caudal to it. Except for the first and second cervical vertebrae (Figure 17.3B), the components of each individual vertebra are similar but each varies as the morphology of that site is determined by its functional requirements (Figure 17.6).

The first few thoracic vertebrae have the tallest dorsal spines, as they are the scaffold that carries the weight of the head. These forces are transmitted through the vertebral joint, muscle, and ligamentous structures. The arch of the thoracolumbar spine is greatest usually at the point at which the 10th thoracic and 11th thoracic dorsal spines meet. At this site, the dorsal spines acutely reverse direction from a caudal sweep (T10) to a dorsal sweep (T11). The anticlinal vertebra is the one where this change occurs and is usually, but not always, T11.

A fibrous ring, the fibrous annulus, which is composed of strong cross fibers that firmly attach one vertebra to another, interconnects the vertebral bodies. The central portion of this ring is filled with a gelatinous substance, the nucleus pulposus, a remnant of the phylogenetically primitive notochord. The nucleus pulposus absorbs forces created between the vertebral endplates and dynamically transfers those forces to the surrounding fibrous ring in response to dorsoventral and lateral movements of the spine. We do not usually appreciate the dynamic nature of these structures as they are often viewed through still-motion studies such as radiography, CT, and MRI. With motion the gel becomes compressed at the side of narrowing of the disc space and expanded at

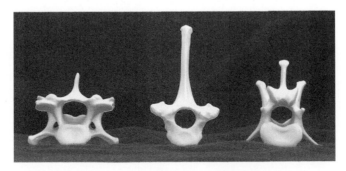

Figure 17.6   From left to right, the cervical, thoracic, and lumbar vertebra showing the tremendous variation in conformation in the same animal.

the side that widens as the spine routinely and regularly changes from one angle to another through all gaits. Faster gaits will also involve greater changes in dorsoventral movements as the pelvis is alternately tilted to gain more distance with each stride. This spinal flexibility is dramatically demonstrated in the canter, trot, and gallop gaits.

An interspinous ligament stabilizes the dorsal spines of the vertebrae. The articular surfaces, which are extensions of the dorsal lamina of each vertebra, form joints with the vertebrae, both cranial and caudal. The cranial articular surface is ventral to the caudal articular surface of the vertebra cranial to it (Figure 17.7). All of these intervertebral articulations allow for a significant but limited motion that permits the spine to bend in all planes. The sacral vertebrae are fused and have the least flexibility in any plane. The thoracic wall and the rib attachments limit the amount of mobility of the thoracic vertebrae (Figure 17.8).

The chest wall, which consists of the interconnecting vertebrae, ribs, and associated soft tissue, forms a stable element and serves to anchor the more flexible and mobile cervical and lumbar regions of the spine. The increased mobility at the cervicothoracic, thoracolumbar, and lumbosacral junctions in comparison to other spinal segments is quite significant. The forces produced at these junctures are most likely responsible for a higher degree of degeneration at these sites.

The atlanto-occipital and atlanto-axial joints are unique and allow for tremendous freedom of movement of the skull. This is critical so that the special senses are able to harness information from the widest possible area. Head mobility is extremely important, too, as the mouth is the dog's main means of defense. The occipital condyles are extremely large and allow for considerable dorsoventral range of motion of the head. The odontoid process bound to the floor of the atlas and the joints formed by the articular surface of the atlas and axis permit considerable rotation of the head in relation to the neck (Figure 17.3).

The muscles that act upon the spine are too extensive and numerous to enumerate in this book. These are classified as intrinsic muscles

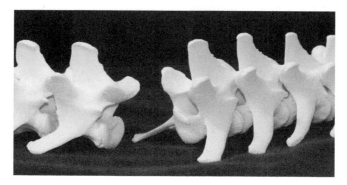

Figure 17.7　Several lumbar vertebrae showing how they articulate and the appearance of the joint surfaces when disarticulated.

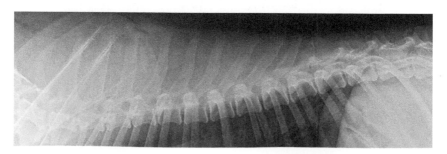

Figure 17.8　Lateral radiograph of the thoracic spine showing the ribs and chest wall that give it its rigidity.

such as the multifidus musculature, which help with the stability of the spine, and extrinsic muscles such as the iliopsoas muscle, which help in more complex motions allowing for positioning within the axial or appendicular skeleton. One overriding factor that should be kept in mind is that all of these activities occur while the spinal cord remains protected.

Very little attention has been paid to the extreme conformational variation that occurs among breeds and individuals within a specific breed (Figure 17.9). Small dogs have large cervical spinal canals with what seems to be relatively thinner dorsal lamina for their size. The relative sizes of the spinal canal going from L4 caudally to the sacral vertebrae can vary tremendously. Sacralization of the last lumbar vertebra and lumbarization of the first sacral vertebra are very common. The tremendous variation evident in different canine spines makes it difficult to provide generalizations about function. Breeding desirable conformations and using appropriate training regimens have to be considered in light of these variations, when considering the canine athlete. These are likely to be conformations that are advantageous for competition and competitive longevity.

Forces that affect the spine

It is quite obvious that the spine can rotate on one axis and move in all planes and in more than one plane at the same time at different points along its length. Although these motions are critical for day-to-day activities, very little information is available about the actual forces involved and the limits necessary to protect spinal structures, including the spinal cord, from damage.

A biomechanical evaluation of L3–L4 in canine cadavers (Figure 17.10), where most extrinsic soft tissue structures had been removed from the vertebrae, has been performed (Smith & Walter, 1988). Excision of the supraspinous and interspinous ligaments yielded a decrease in stiffness in flexion, an increase in the range of motion of the interspace, and a decrease in the ultimate flexion bending strength by 62%. Panjabi and colleagues (1988) studied the *in vivo* effects of transecting the supraspinous and interspinous ligaments in the cervical spine at C4–C5. In the cervical spine, this injury caused a decreased range of motion. It is, of course, hard to compare the two studies as one study involved cadavers with most soft tissues removed and the other was on live dogs.

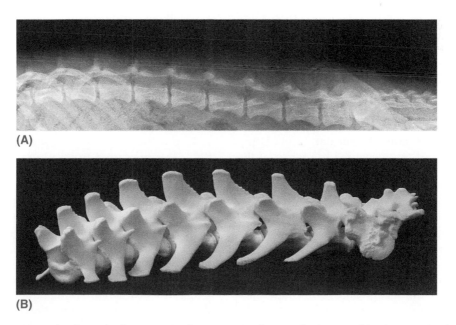

(A)

(B)

Figure 17.9 (A) Lateral radiograph of a normal lumbar spine. (B) Photograph of a normal lumbar spinal column with the sacrum attached.

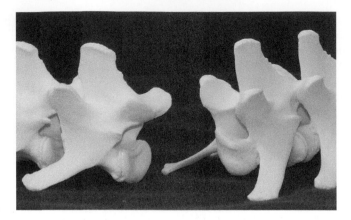

Figure 17.10   Lumbar vertebrae 3 and 4 demonstrating the structures that adjoin the two vertebrae.

There are numerous articles examining the forces placed upon the articular facets and intervertebral discs of the canine lumbar spine. These studies were intended to study the effects that these forces might have upon the human spine and many conclusions were found to be applicable to both species.

Wood and colleagues (1992) found that while walking, the canine's L2–L3 vertebrae became 2–3 degrees more kyphotic compared with the standing position and the average excursion between opposing facets was 3.4±1.3 mm. Although it is well recognized that these motions and their limits protect the spine from excessive flexion and torsion and help to stabilize the spine, the actual forces involved have not received much attention. Buttermann and colleagues (1992) were the first to measure actual loads on the facet joint *in vivo*. They determined the load on the articular joint surface of the L3 cranial articular facet. Using strain gauges, they measured the forces of the right L3 articular surface of five mongrel dogs in various positions and performing various activities. They verified their findings using two *in vitro* studies. A Newton (N) is an internationally accepted unit of force that by definition is the force necessary to provide a 1 kg mass with an acceleration of 1 m/s.

Their results demonstrated the relative forces placed upon the facets under varying conditions. For the following data, only the right L3 cranial facet was measured in five animals, and the forces found were:

- While sitting:10–65 N
- While lying, 0–45 N
- When flexing the head to get a treat from between the thoracic limbs while standing: 0–65 N
- Sitting while having the thoracic limbs held in the air and then turning (torsion) to the left: 0–40 N (this activity unloads the forces on the right facet)
- Sitting while having the thoracic limbs held in the air and then turning (torsion) to the right: 65–130 N
- Walking while having the thoracic limbs held off the ground: 65–140 N
- Climbing stairs: 105–170 N
- Decending stairs: 100–120 N
- Right turning: 45–135 N
- Left turning: 0–80 N
- Sit to stand: 65–110 N.

To put these numbers in some perspective, the forces measured from a human prosthetic hip while walking are 800–2200 N. Comparing the force per unit area of the human coxofemoral joint, the measurement would convert to 1–6 MPa (megapascals). Since the facet joint is considerably smaller, the forces over the L3 articular surface convert to a maximum of 2 MPa. A megapascal is $10^6 N/M^2$. It is worth noting that although the joint forces on the cartilaginous structures in humans and dogs are in the same range per unit area, the cartilage in the dog is considerably thinner. Although we do not usually consider joint function in terms of

Newtons and megapascals, the relationships give us starting points to consider improving our treatment and training outcomes and considerations for the causes of spinal degeneration.

In the study by Butterman and colleagues (1992), there was considerable variability between individuals. The authors believe this was due to differences in the anatomy, in muscle mass and distribution, in motion patterns, and in the individual animal's motivation to perform the tasks. It is interesting to note that the variations between individual dogs, which affected the results of this study, are reflected frequently in the training of dogs to complete tasks and to successfully compete. These individual variations require our attention if we are going to train the successful athlete or competitor.

Several other interesting points were noted. The force on the joint surface remained virtually constant regardless of the speed with which the subject was walking. The results were similar to the findings of *in vitro* studies. The caudal portion of the joint surface was rarely loaded unless there was extreme extension of the spine or the intervertebral disc had been compromised.

Breit followed up on this study by comparing the facet geometry of the canine thoracolumbar spine using three distinct groups of dogs (Breit, 2002). He divided 140 dogs into three groups: large, chondrodystrophic, and small breeds. His findings enhance the concerns we must share about the variations between individuals. Torsional strain between vertebrae is determined by the transverse distance between the articular surfaces (Figure 17.11). In small-breed and chondrodystrophic dogs the transverse distance was very consistent when adjustments were made for size. In these cases, the facets consisted of lateral and ventral components that made the joint surfaces rather flat. In all large breeds the transverse distance was considerably less, adjusted for size, and these joints were completely different in conformation. All of the large breeds had a caudal facet component that made their articular joints virtually ball and socket joints. This design is able to handle the much greater forces that their greater mass absorbs. Interestingly, none of the small breeds had caudal facet components but some chondrodystrophic breeds did. The increased stability of this conformation should be a desirable trait that could be heritable.

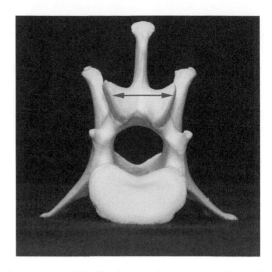

Figure 17.11   Third lumbar vertebra. Arrow indicates the transverse distance between the joint surfaces, which plays a major role in many of the force measurements referenced.

Lastly, there are several studies using the dog as a model evaluating the mechanical properties of the intervertebral disc. Most of these have been *in vitro* studies and most have looked at the mid-lumbar vertebrae. However, routine intervertebral disc failure leading to spinal cord compression is not nearly as common in the mid-lumbar spine as in the thoracolumbar region.

Zimmerman and colleagues (1992) determined mechanical properties of the canine intervertebral disc at two sites, L2–L3 and L5–L6. Compressive stiffness varied at each site, from 717.8 N/mm at the L2–L3 interspace to 949.0 N/mm at the L5–L6 interspace. Torsional stiffness also varied in each case. At the L2–L3 interspace it was 1.04 Nm/degree, and 1.72 Nm/degree at L5–L6. Axial or compressive stress on the intervertebral disc at L2–L3 was 14.03 MPa, and 16.30 MPa at L5–L6. Adjusting for size, these are similar to those seen in people and the differences reflect the fact that the caudal lumbar spine plays a greater role in spinal stabilization. Interestingly, the torsional stress measured in the dog at both sites was considerably higher than in people, at 30.8 MPa for L2–L3 and 26.17 MPa for L5–L6.

Unfortunately, information from studies using the dog spine as a model for understanding and treating human spinal conditions has not been incorporated into specific requirements for canine athletes. These studies have, however, dramatically illuminated the differences in breeds and among individual dogs within breeds.

The sum of these studies clearly demonstrates that specifics about spinal conformation can be measured, and through genetics, specific training, and attention to detailed anatomy, better functioning spines are possible.

Congenital predispositions

Malformations

Spinal anomalies are usually considered incidental findings. Additional ribs and absence of ribs, as well as additional lumbar vertebrae, are probably the most common vertebral anomalies. Occasionally a lack of a transverse spine is noted and on occasion the anticlinal vertebra is not T11 but one of the neighboring vertebrae.

Spina bifida

Spina bifida is an uncommon malformation of the spine that is frequently an incidental finding. Spina bifida is an interruption of or incomplete fusion of the dorsal spinal arches. This can occur at several vertebral sites but is most often recognized at the level of the sacrum and sometimes involves L7. Spina bifida is most common in the screw-tailed breeds: Boston Terriers, French Bulldogs, English Bulldogs, and others. This malformation is sometimes associated with incomplete formation of the neural tube causing dysplasia of the spinal cord and protrusions of the meninges and occasionally also the spinal cord. Dogs in which the sacral segments of the spinal cord are malformed are often presented for a lack of urinary and/or fecal control.

Caudal occipital malformation syndrome

Caudal occipital malformation syndrome has been described (Churcher & Child, 2000; Rusbridge et al., 2000; Rusbridge & Knowler, 2003). In this condition there is crowding of the cerebellum within the caudal fossa of the skull. This malformation often leads to a fluid-filled

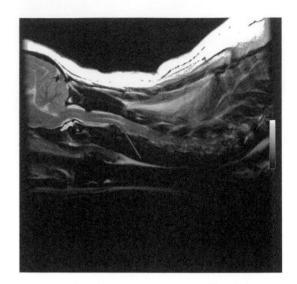

Figure 17.12   Lateral MRI of a Cavalier King Charles Spaniel with caudal occipital malformation syndrome (COMS). Note the syrinx in the center of the spinal cord (arrow). The white color denotes fluid as this is a T2 image.

tubular structure, a syrinx, forming within the cervical spinal cord and in many cases hydrocephalus (Figure 17.12). Flow dynamics and the Venturi effect are suspected to be responsible for the syrinx formation. These fluid-filled tubes can occur when the dogs are very young or can develop as the dog ages. Affected dogs often present with neck pain and tetraparesis, frequently affecting the thoracic limbs to a greater extent than the pelvic limbs. A peculiar obsessive scratching of the neck area is a common occurrence. This disease is more prevalent in certain toy breeds such as the Cavalier King Charles Spaniel and Brussels Griffon, although it has also been described in other breeds.

Atlanto-axial instability

The second cervical vertebra, C2, is held in place by several ligamentous structures. The bony projection, the odontoid process or dens, of C2 attaches to the ventral floor of C1 and allows for rotation of the head within limits in each direction. Dogs who have atlanto-axial subluxations usually have a hypoplastic dens or aplasia of the dens. This condition occurs most commonly in toy and miniature breeds, and in most cases clinical signs occur when the dogs are young. The spine of C2 is displaced caudally at an angle, leading one to conclude that the nuchal ligament is what is giving the C2 subluxation its characteristic radiographic appearance (Figure 17.13).

Hemi or block vertebra

Hemi or block vertebrae are usually incidental findings seen on radiography involving the mid-thoracic vertebrae in the screw-tailed breeds (French Bulldogs, English Bulldogs, Pugs, and others). These vertebrae are mal-formed and can have quite an anomalous con-formation (Figure 17.14). They can be wedge-shaped or fused and often cause an

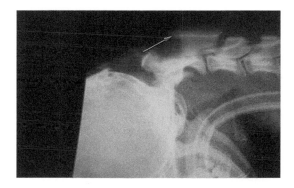

Figure 17.13   Lateral radiograph of an atlanto-axial subluxation. Notice the tilt (arrow) of C2 away from C1 and the odontoid process (dens) riding up into the spinal canal.

extreme angle to the spine. The vertebrae are foreshortened and cause crowding of the ribs. The spinal alignments often are severe but the dogs usually do not manifest clinical signs of spinal cord dysfunction.

Congenital stenosis

Within the spinal column there are two abrupt transitions of spinal mobility that probably have the greatest forces placed upon them. Advanced imaging of these areas in individuals with con-genital stenosis seem to expose a smaller spinal canal than is normal for the diameter of their spinal cord and associated nerve roots (Fourie & Kirberger, 1999; Drost *et al.*, 2002; da Costa *et al.*, 2006). These changes are present from a very early age. At the level of C6–T1 many large- and giant-breed dogs seem to have very little addi-tional space around their spinal cords. A similar loss of spinal canal volume is seen in many dif-ferent breeds of dogs at the area between L5 and S1. If the spinal canal is pathologically narrowed in younger animals, clinical signs usually occur before 1 year of age. These relatively stenotic spinal canals predispose affected animals to spi-nal cord compression. In large breeds that have stenosis in the caudal cervical spinal canal, abnormal gaits and postural deficits can be seen in dogs as young as 12 weeks of age. Although several names describe caudal cervical spinal cord impingement, stenosis of the spinal canal underlies these pathological conditions.

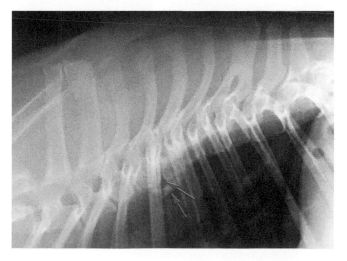

Figure 17.14   Lateral thoracic radiograph demonstrating hemi or blocked vertebral abnormalities in this French Bulldog. These vertebral changes were an incidental finding. Note the common bunching of the ribs (arrows).

Likewise, we can, on rare occasions, see dogs less than 1 year of age with severe signs from lumbosacral nerve root entrapment. More typically, these dogs develop nerve root entrapment at various adult ages determined by the encroachment caused by degeneration and proliferations of the surrounding ligamentous and sometimes bony structures that further compromise an already stenotic spinal canal.

Many of these conditions are highlighted by dynamic advanced imaging (Figure 17.15). These conditions are often overlooked when only static representations are evaluated (Jones & Inzana, 2000).

Breed-specific intervertebral disc disease

When Hansen first described disc degeneration, he made a distinction between the chondrodystrophic breeds and non-chondrodystrophic breeds (Hansen, 1951). The degeneration that occurs in both groups of dogs is actually quite similar, the difference being that in chondrodystrophic breeds disc degeneration usually starts before 1 year of age. The degeneration has a genetic predisposition in the chondrodystrophic breeds and virtually all of the discs deteriorate. The collagen components of the nucleus pulposus and annulus fibrosus change. This has a fairly complex epidemiological/genetic distri-

bution as the specific genetic mutation that is associated with chondrodysplasia is not found in the Beagle, yet their discs deteriorate in a similar manner and time frame as those of chondrodystrophic breeds. Likewise, although Jack Russell Terriers are chondrodystrophic, they seem to have a rather low incidence of intervertebral disc disease.

An excellent review of intervertebral disc degeneration by Bergknut (2011) is available online.

Degenerative and stress-related conditions of the spine

Spondylosis deformans and diffuse idiopathic skeletal hyperostosis

Spondylosis deformans and diffuse idiopathic skeletal hyperostosis (DISH) are different diseases. These conditions are often confused but have been shown to be quite distinct in people (Resnick, 1985).

Spondylosis is very common bony production at the ventral endplates of the vertebrae, seen as simple prominences to actual bony fusions without evidence of inflammation (Figure 17.16). There is very little evidence that spinal cord or nerve root pathology occurs as a result of this condition.

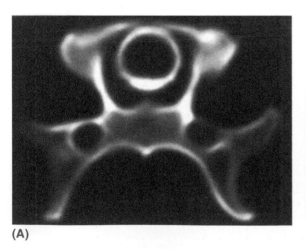

(A)

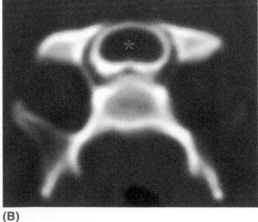

(B)

Figure 17.15   **(A)** Transverse CT with contrast of a normal C6 vertebra. Note the large amount of space surrounding the spinal cord. **(B)** Transverse CT with contrast of the C6 vertebra. Note that there no room around the spinal cord and the spinal cord appears flattened (asterisk). Both figures are at approximately the same level of the spine and both dogs' heads were positioned similarly. The dog in **(B)** had significant clinical signs.

DISH describes excessive ossification of the spine that occurs along the juncture of the ventral longitudinal ligament. This poorly understood ossification can occur at numerous places where ligament, tendon, or muscle attach to bone (entheses) but is most often appreciated on the spine. DISH can readily be distinguished from spondylosis in that there is significant bony production with DISH along the entire length of the vertebral body, intervertebral spaces, and contiguous vertebrae that follows the course of the ventral longitudinal ligament (Figure 17.17).

The causes of these conditions are unknown and neither condition has a strong association with intervertebral disc disease. Both conditions can occur concurrently.

Kranenburg and colleagues (2011) have published a retrospective study of 2041 dogs outlining the variations and breed specificity of these conditions in the canine. There is a strong potential for DISH having a genetic predisposition as the prevalence in the canine purebred population is 3.8%, but 40.6% in the Boxer breed (Hansen, 1951; Kranenburg *et al.*, 2010). DISH is easy to diagnose radiographically, and the inherent decreased spinal flexibility can be clinically significant, affecting gait, posture, and performance.

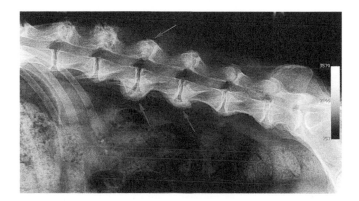

Figure 17.16   Lateral radiograph of the lumbar spine. The exostoses of the vertebral bodies (arrows) are spondylosis. They arise from the ventral ridges of bone cranial and caudal to the disc space. These changes are common and most often are said to be incidental findings. Note also the tremendous degeneration of the articular facets in this dog. Whether either of these changes would cause serious limitations in the active dog is not known.

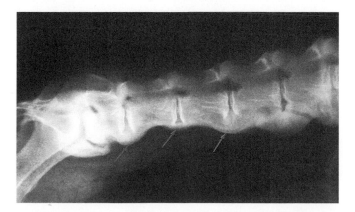

Figure 17.17   Lateral radiograph of the lumbar spine demonstrating severe diffuse idiopathic skeletal hypersotosis (DISH) (arrows). Although this condition is not supposed to be associated with intervertebral disc disease, this dog had multiple disc prolapses. This dog was only 2 years old at the time of these radiographs and was extremely limited by this condition. These multiple bony changes resulted in the dog being euthanized at 4 years of age.

Trauma

Spinal fractures are the result of the load exceeding the bone's strength (Figure 17.18). Luxations of the vertebrae without fractures occur when external forces exceed the strength of the soft tissues holding the vertebrae in place (Figure 17.19). Combinations of both types of spinal injuries are common. In everyday veterinary practice, the vast majority of these fractures/luxations occur from severe external trauma that is most often from automobile-induced injuries. Second to this external injury is weakening of the spinal structures through internal processes such as neoplasia or infection or rarely osteoporosis. Fractures related to these internal complications are generally grouped together as pathological fractures (Figure 17.20).

In the canine athlete, the injury most likely to cause a spinal fracture is a misstep while moving at speed or an accident involving the equipment necessary for the activity being performed. Muscle damage and joint capsule tears involving the paraspinal soft tissue are very likely to occur with or without bony lesions but have been very poorly documented. Localized pain secondary to soft tissue paraspinal injury is gathering more and more attention, but these types of injuries related to spinal soft tissue structures have not been studied in any well-organized manner.

At the junction of a very flexible spine to a rather inflexible spine there is a greater chance of exceeding the ultimate force of the bony structures or joints. The vast majority of spinal fractures occur at the thoracolumbar junction or at the lumbosacral junction (Feeny & Oliver, 1980; Zotti *et al.*, 2011). Complete dislocations without fractures, growth plate luxations in the young dog (Figure 17.18), and body and facet fractures all occur at these same sites. With the advent of CT, multiple smaller fractures that were not evident with radiographs alone are now appreciated. Although cervical spinal fractures are much less frequently reported, it may simply be that they are more likely incompatible

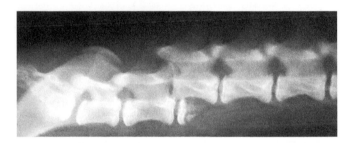

Figure 17.18   Lateral radiograph of a spinal fracture through the endplate of a young dog due to an automobile injury. Notice that there is also a fracture fragment from the body of the vertebra.

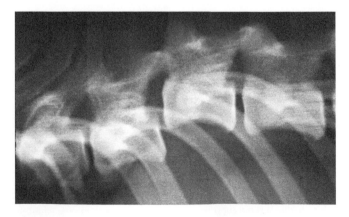

Figure 17.19   Lateral radiograph demonstrating a dislocation without any fracture due to running at speed into a tree. Some such radiographs will demonstrate fractures with advanced imaging.

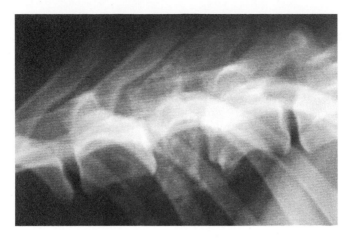

Figure 17.20 Lateral radiograph of a pathological fracture of the thoracic spine. Although there is significant destruction of the entire vertebra, many of these dogs present with acute onset of symptoms rather than having a slow, progressive course as we frequently expect with neoplasia.

with life as they can catastrophically affect respiration.

The biomechanical parameters that determine the likelihood of a spinal fracture are well known and a great deal of the work defining these has been done in rodents (Kranenburg *et al.*, 2010). The ultimate breaking force of a bony structure is a simple measure of its strength. The ultimate displacement of a bony structure is the reciprocal of its brittleness. The work-to-failure measurement defines the ability of a bony structure to absorb energy. All three of these biomechanical modalities can be improved upon, but bone remodeling must occur at a rate that keeps up with the forces placed upon it. The ability to resorb and replace bone in response to stress-related injuries is well documented in younger dogs but less well studied in adult dogs. The potential for bone repair in relation to age in dogs is not known.

Genetic factors may have significance in determining susceptibility to bony fractures. There seems to be a strong correlation between bone mineral density (BMD) and bone strength. Certain strains of rats have a higher BMD and are less prone to fractures (Turner, 2002). A study of twins found that BMD was genetically based, and the genetic association was particularly strong within the spine for BMD specifically (Pocock *et al.*, 1987).

Nutrition is also a significant factor in maintaining normal BMD and therefore preventing

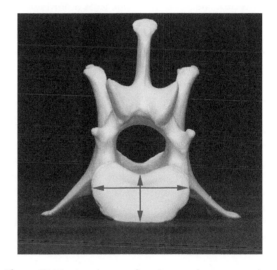

Figure 17.21 Lumbar vertebra. Arrows demonstrate the measurements used by Slijper to determine the moment of resistance.

potential fractures. Dogs maintained on a low calcium diet had a decrease in their BMD. Bone strength measured in the L2 vertebra, femoral neck, and mid-femur was reduced in dogs fed calcium-restricted diets (Motoie *et al.*, 1995).

In 1946, E. J. Slijper in his seminal work defined the moment of resistance (MoR) as a way to determine the spine's ability to resist bending. The MoR is calculated by multiplying the transverse diameter of the vertebra by the square of the height of the caudal surface of each vertebra (Figure 17.21). Zotti and colleagues (2011) determined that the MoR is similar across various breed conformations. They also confirmed, by taking the BMD into account, that most fractures occur between T9 and L7, as has been determined clinically by retrospective studies. The vertebral column's chief structural function is to resist dorsal and lateral bending. Ventral bending is resisted predominately by the abdominal musculature. This knowledge should direct appropriate physical training based on the anticipated functional results. Soft tissue elements are critical support structures. Muscular development and ligamentous strength can decrease the forces placed upon the spine. This may limit bony vertebral strength and development, yet still be protective. The exact combination of bony development and soft tissue development is unknown and would be specific for the movements being attempted. Obviously, special attention needs to be given to core strength specifically to protect the T9–L7 region (Zotti et al., 2011).

Repetitive motion conditions

In the canine athlete, practice and competition has been directed to learning a complicated and often forceful set of movements that can cause damage as the work-to-failure ability of the soft tissues or bones cannot absorb the repeated stresses that occur without significant healing, remodeling, and recovery. Dogs that do not have obvious spinal cord issues have been characterized as having sore backs or sore necks. With the wide availability of CT, degenerative bony conditions can be described in detail, yet these changes often are not correlated to performance.

Soft tissue damage to the paraspinal structures and joints in many cases may be the source of spinal pain or poor performance. These changes often can be appreciated with MRI but few studies have evaluated this potential source of spinal pain.

Repetitive stress to bones creates failures in the bone matrix known as microfractures (Frost, 1960; Lee et al., 2003). These microfractures accumulate and are known to decrease the stiffness of the bone and its ability to absorb additional stress (Burr et al., 1998). Healing of microfractures starts with resorp-

tion of the surrounding bone matrix and may decrease the ability of the bone to handle additional stress until healing is complete (Carter & Hayes, 1977). Microfractures are cumulative and their ability to repair is decreased with age in people. The association of bone failure and microfractures is not linear with the stress placed upon the bone. The ability of the bone to withstand compressive forces is also dependent upon the bone volume fraction (bone volume/total volume) of the structure being tested. Microfractures only start to accumulate when there is a stiffness loss in the bone of approximately 15% (Burr et al., 1997). Dogs whose microfractures were prevented from healing by pharmacological methods (Flora et al., 1981) or endocrine manipulation (Norrdin et al., 1990) developed pathological fractures. Compressive strength was decreased in the lumbar and thoracic vertebrae even though the bone volume was normal. Hasegawa and colleagues (1995) determined that surgical damage to the intervertebral discs in dogs also increased the accumulation of microfractures within the vertebrae.

Several important considerations come out of these studies. Developing strong bones necessary to handle the stresses placed upon them should be part of the training procedures to produce long-lasting successful canine athletes. Strong soft tissue components involving core strength can protect forces placed on the bones and joints. Attention to bone and soft tissue strength should be directed to vertebrae T9–L7 specifically. Adequate time between rigorous activities has to be a consideration. There is a period of time when bones are particularly prone to stress once the microfractures have occurred and the remodeling process further decreases bone strength, as bone resorption is the initial step in healing. Whether these changes in bone strength and remodeling forces are responsible for so-called sore backs or are in fact responsible for any of the osteoarthritic changes noted in spinal studies, is an area that requires further investigation. In addition, there are numerous circumstances where intervertebral disc degeneration is diagnosed with conventional radiography or advanced imaging. In those cases, even when there are no overt neurological deficits, the biomechanics of the spine are compromised (Burr et al., 1997).

Common compressive spinal cord conditions

Age-related conditions

Age-related degenerative conditions of the spine are common and often are unrecognized and underdiagnosed. Conditions include enlargement of the articular processes, proliferation of the dorsal longitudinal ligament, proliferation of the yellow ligaments that connect the neural arches, and bulging of the intervertebral disc. These space-occupying changes may encroach upon an already limited space surrounding the spinal cord in predisposed breeds (Burbidge *et al.*, 1999). The lower cervical spine and lumbosacral region are most commonly affected.

Spinal cord and nerve root compressions are often accompanied by denervation and muscle atrophy. In the thoracic limb, the triceps muscle group is most commonly affected. The elbows tend to flex more than necessary during the walk as the antagonist muscles, the triceps group, do not resist the agonists, the elbow flexors. In the pelvic limbs, the biceps femoris and cranial tibial muscles are often affected. These dogs tend to stand base-wide and do not flex their stifles during gaits used in propulsion. In most cases, nerve root entrapments of the cauda equine significantly decrease tail strength and movement. Spinal cord or nerve root compression at both of these sites is extremely common in older dogs but the severity of gait alterations is variable as certain individuals are more prone to the degenerative changes described (Figure 17.15).

Bulging of the annulus fibrosus into the spinal canal in older dogs has been incriminated often as a source of spinal cord compression. However, the dynamics of this pathology have not been studied and it is often difficult or impossible to prove that the bulging disc alone is the cause of any dysfunction or pain (Mayhew *et al.*, 2002).

A well-documented nerve root entrapment or foraminal stenosis has been reported in dogs with lumbosacral stenosis. It is difficult to diagnose as the dogs present with intermittent lameness. Avalanche rescue dogs may be more prone to this condition although other breeds have been diagnosed (Godde & Steffen, 2007) (Figures 17.22 and 17.23). It has been noted that

larger dogs have a cranial articular process that, with degeneration and osteophyte formation, is likely to impinge on the L7 nerve root and/or ganglion. Furthermore, the decreased impact surface provided by the L7 endplate makes larger dogs more prone to osteophyte formation. Breit and Kunzel (2001) noted that these changes are likely to be more significant in the athletic canine.

Intervertebral disc disease

Dogs of any breed can have intervertebral disk degeneration with similar pathological processes as described above (Bergknut, 2011). Conventional radiography for the diagnosis of intervertebral disk disease has been replaced with advanced imaging procedures. Unfortunately, the study of the dynamic nature of intervertebral disc

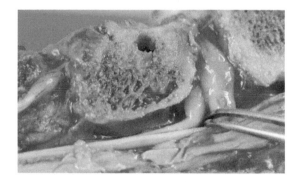

Figure 17.22   Nerve root entrapment or foraminal stenosis. A swollen nerve root can be seen at the end of the forceps.

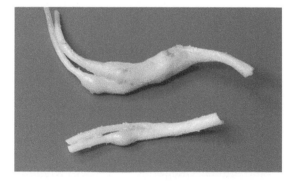

Figure 17.23   Entrapped nerve roots removed from the spinal cord demonstrating swelling and discoloration, likely a result of inflammation.

pathology has been limited. When looking at static evaluations of intervertebral disc disease, it is common to find a poor association between the extent of the clinical signs and the disease determined by imaging, particularly when the clinical signs are limited (Adams *et al.*, 1995). It is reasonable to assume that dynamic studies will determine potential and actual compressive conditions with greater accuracy in the future.

Video fluoroscopy and kinematic studies allow one to appreciate the forces involved and the dynamic ranges of not only the intervertebral discs but the spinal cord as well (Medical Legal Art, 2009). A general overview of intervertebral disc disease in the dog is available elsewhere (Coates, 2000).

Trauma

The most common traumatic injury to the spinal cord is acute intervertebral disc herniation. The second most common is blunt trauma to the spine that is most often the result of an automobile-related injury. The treatment protocols are similar, based predominately on an accurate diagnosis and neurological evaluation.

In the veterinary literature, traumatic injuries to the spine are most often assigned severity based upon the spinal cord damage imposed by that injury. Very little attention has been given to ligamentous, muscular, and paraspinal structural damage that leads to decreased performance in the absence of neurological deficits. Although rest, rehabilitation modalities, core strengthening, and stretching would seem to be therapeutic, there is little hard evidence promoting any one treatment course or program. Based on the previous discussion and the type of activity being performed, special attention needs to be directed to prevention and rehabilitation in the area from T9 to L7 across breed conformations (Kranenburg *et al.*, 2011).

Neoplastic disease

Neoplasms of the vertebrae themselves fall within similar categories as seen elsewhere in the body. Primary bone tumors such as osteosarcoma can affect the vertebrae. They do not seem to be as aggressive as those affecting the

long bones. Histiocytic sarcomas, lymphosarcomas, hemangiosarcomas, and multiple myelomas are common soft tissue neoplasms that often affect the vertebrae. CT and MRI each have their own advantages and disadvantages and at times both are necessary to make an accurate diagnosis. Treatment is based on a histopathological diagnosis. The biological behavior of these neoplasms and the results of various combinations of treatments are becoming better understood.

Treatment protocols for neoplasms within the spinal canal involving the spinal cord are based on whether the neoplasm is causing compression and/or invading the neural tissue and whether it is primary or metastatic. Routine surveys of the chest and abdomen for metastatic disease are part of a thorough evaluation. Surgical decompression, tumor resection or biopsy, radiation therapy, and/or chemotherapy all have their successes and failures. It is difficult to guide a decision based upon the lack of statistically relevant studies.

Common noncompressive spinal cord conditions

Vascular disease of the spinal cord

Vascular anomalies have been reported in the dog but they are extremely rare. In one review only eight cases could be found (Westworth & Sturges, 2010).

Hematomyelia is a poorly understood condition that describes hemorrhage within the spinal cord. In dogs, hematomyelia is often secondary to trauma, and may be due to release of vasoactive substances causing vascular collapse or primary hemorrhage alone. Experiments with injections of blood into rat spinal cords do not seem to simulate the total liquefaction of the spinal cord that is the hallmark of hematomyelia (Leep Hunderfund & Wijdicks, 2009). In most cases, the cranial and caudal dissemination of the spinal cord hemorrhage and destruction occurs at or near the time of injury and at the trauma site. There have been circumstances where the process of hematomyelia begins days after the initial trauma.

The most common spinal cord vascular event is a spinal cord embolic phenomenon called

Case Study 17.1   Acute onset tetraparesis

Signalment: 12-y.o. M/N Australian Shepherd presented as acute asymmetrical, severely tetraparetic emergency.

History: Patient is an active swimmer. Was swimming in the client's pool when he cried out and was taken from the water by clients.

Examination: Patient bright and alert and not in significant discomfort. Paresis very lateralized to the right, involving right pelvic limb and left pelvic limb to a much greater degree than left forelimb although all four limbs were weaker than expected and patient unable to stand.

Neurological examination:

- Bright and alert
- All cranial nerve reflexes WNL
- Tetraparetic with right side weaker than left
- Knuckling of feet evident in both pelvic limbs but neither thoracic limb
- Right-sided sympathetic palsy: Horner's syndrome
- Increased tone in both thoracic limbs
- Stretch reflexes present and symmetrical in all four limbs
- Response to noxious stimuli symmetrical and appropriate in the pelvic limbs including perception and withdrawal
- Perception of noxious stimuli present in thoracic limbs but withdrawal diminished.

Neuroanatomical localization: C6 to T2.

Discussion: The acute nature of this incident makes an infarction or intervertebral disc prolapse most likely. Although the patient did not seem to be in any discomfort, he did resist movement of his head and neck to the left. The decrease in the withdrawal response and the lateralization of these clinical signs would make one consider a lesion, most likely localized to the left side of the cervical intumescence. The Horner's syndrome is more commonly seen with acute spinal cord disease, with severe spinal cord compression or intramedullary disease.

The acute nature and severity of the clinical signs would make one want to obtain a specific diagnosis.

Outcome: This patient had an osteosarcoma of the second thoracic vertebra (Figure 17.24). This was an unexpected outcome as the signs were acute and the dog was not in very much pain. The localization was slightly more caudal than would have been expected and there was likely a shift of soft tissue (neoplasm) that occurred while swimming. There was no obvious pathological fracture. The neoplasm was surgically removed and was followed with chemotherapy.

Osteosarcoma of the axial skeleton is often not as aggressive as the same neoplasm affecting the limbs. The author (HSS) has followed one dog for 4 years and two dogs for more than 2 years, all with histological diagnoses. All had surgical decompression and follow-up chemotherapy.

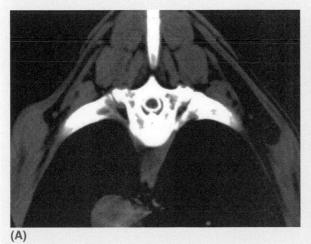
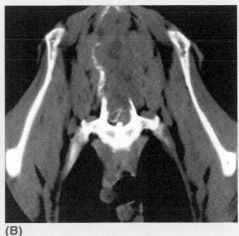

(A)   **(B)**

Figure 17.24   **(A)** CT with contrast showing the spine at the level of T1 of a dog that became acutely tetraparetic while swimming. **(B)** CT with contrast showing T2 of the same dog. Although his signs were acute it is obvious that this osteosarcoma caused destruction of the vertebra over some period of time.

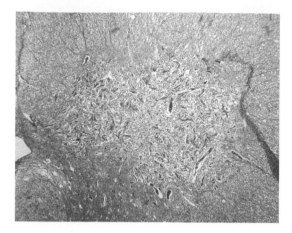

Figure 17.25 Tissue section from a dog's spinal cord showing gray matter destruction from a fibrocartilaginous embolus. The area with a diffuse light pattern has been damaged by a lack of perfusion.

fibrocartilaginous embolization (FCE). Although the origin of the fibrocartilage is unknown, it is suspected that the source is the nucleus pulposus. More than 40 years after this condition was first described, we still do not have a clear understanding of how the material gets into the arterial vasculature of the spinal cord (Zaki & Prata, 1976). Dogs with suspected FCE usually recover adequate function so autopsy material is very uncommon (Figure 17.25). The hallmark of this disease is an acute onset of spinal cord dysfunction, usually during activity. The signs are often asymmetrical, rapidly progressive, and usually not associated with hyperpathia (De Risio & Platt, 2010). Transient hyperalgesia at the onset of the signs is common but short in duration. Most dogs return to normal function over a 6–8-week period dependent upon the amount and location of the ischemic damage. Intact pain sensation and signs of motor recovery within 2 weeks after onset of signs indicate a favorable outcome.

Degenerative conditions of the spinal cord

Sporadic and rare degenerative conditions of the spinal cord have been recorded over many decades. Consideration should be given to these disorders based on clinical signs, typical young age of onset, and breed predilection. The classification scheme for the degenerative spinal cord disorders of animals is further described in Table 17.1. Breed predispositions suggest that many of these disorders have an inherited basis. Initial clinical signs often are worse in the pelvic limbs but then progress to involve the thoracic limbs and possibly the brainstem and forebrain. Definitive diagnosis of these diseases is usually determined by histopathology of the affected tissues. Degenerative spinal cord disorders involving myelinopathy and axonopathy are classified based on their histopathological features. Canine degenerative myelopathy, the most common degenerative spinal cord disorder, is covered in the next section. A more extensive list of these degenerative conditions and the breeds they affect can be found in the *Handbook of Veterinary Neurology* (Lornez *et al.*, 2010).

Degenerative myelopathy

History, signalment, and epidemiology

Canine degenerative myelopathy (DM) was first described by Averill in 1973 as an insidious, progressive, general proprioceptive ataxia and upper motor neuron (UMN) spastic paresis of the pelvic limbs ultimately leading to paraplegia and necessitating euthanasia. The earliest clinical signs begin when dogs are at least 8 years or older with a mean age of onset at 9 years. There is no sex predilection. The pathological features of DM include axonal degeneration with secondary demyelination and astroglial proliferation (sclerosis) in all spinal cord funiculi, but consistently most severe in the dorsal portion of the lateral funiculus and in the dorsal columns of the middle to lower thoracic region (Averill, 1973; Griffiths & Duncan, 1975; Braund & Vandevelde, 1978; March *et al.*, 2009). Neuronal cell body degeneration or loss in the ventral horn of the spinal cord is not a prominent histopathological finding but does occur in terminal disease (Ogawa *et al.*, 2014).

In 1975, Griffiths and Duncan published a series of cases with similar clinical signs and histological changes in the white matter. They also reported hyporeflexia and nerve root involvement, and they termed the condition chronic degenerative radiculomyelopathy. Recent histopathological studies of dogs in the late disease stage with lower motor neuron (LMN) signs have documented denervation

Table 17.1   Classification of myelin, axonal, and neuronal disorders of the central nervous system (CNS) (spinal cord) and peripheral nervous system (PNS)

Neuroanatomic pathology	Specific description
CNS—Encephalopathy/encephalomyelopathy	
Myelinopathy	Hypomyelination
	Dysmyelination: leukodystrophy, myelinolytic disorders
	Leukomyelopathy
	Leukoencephalomyelopathy
Spongy degeneration	Myelin vacuolation
	Neuronal vacuolation
Axonopathy: Wallerian degeneration, distal axonopathy (dying-back neuropathy), segmental degeneration	Central axonopathy
	Central–peripheral axonopathy
	Central–peripheral distal axonopathy
Neuroaxonal dystrophy	Axonal transport disorder
Multisystem degeneration	Axonopathy, neuronopathy, and neuropathy
PNS—Neuropathy	
Neuronopathy: degeneration and loss of neurons, neurofibrillary accumulations in neurons	Motor neuronopathy
	Sensory neuronopathy
Myelinopathy	Segmental demyelination
	Hypomyelination
Axonopathy	Sensory–motor neuropathy: distal sensorimotor, central–peripheral distal axonopathy
	Sensory neuropathy
	Metabolic neuropathy
	Autonomic neuropathy

atrophy in muscle, nerve fiber loss with axonal degeneration, and secondary myelin loss in myelinated fibers of the peripheral nerves (Awano *et al.*, 2009; Shelton *et al.*, 2012). Studies conducted on the thoracic intercostal muscles and associated thoracic motor and sensory neurons of dogs with DM indicate that there are significant atrophic changes in these muscles at defined disease stages but there is no apparent degeneration of the associated motor neurons (Morgan *et al.*, 2013, 2014). However, significant sensory neuron degeneration did precede any evidence of motor neuron pathology (Morgan *et al.*, 2014). The clinical spectrum of DM has now been broadened to involve both the UMN and LMN systems and is considered a multisystem disease involving the central and peripheral motor and sensory axons (Coates & Wininger, 2010; Johnston *et al.*, 2001).

Since most of the dogs in the initial reports were German Shepherd Dogs, the disease also was called German Shepherd Dog myelopathy (Braund & Vandevelde, 1978). However, in those same earlier reports, other breeds were represented (Averill, 1973; Braund & Vandevelde, 1978). Canine DM is now recognized as a common problem in a number of pure breeds and mixed breeds with an overall prevalence of 0.19% (Coates *et al.*, 2007; Zeng *et al.*, 2014).

Pathophysiology

The cause underlying canine DM has been enigmatic for many years. In 2009, Awano and collegues identified a c.118G >A transition in the *SOD1* gene that predicted an E40K missense underlying canine DM. In this initial study, there was a highly significant association between homozygosity for the *SOD1:c.118A* allele and the DM phenotype in Pembroke Welsh Corgis and also in four other dog breeds: Boxer, Chesapeake Bay Retriever, German Shepherd Dog, and Rhodesian Ridgeback. Mutations in the *SOD1* gene are known to cause some forms of familial amyotrophic lateral sclerosis (ALS or Lou Gehrig's disease) in humans. ALS, the most common adult motor neuron disease, is characterized by loss of motor neurons causing stiffness and slowing of muscle movements, difficulty speaking and swallowing, muscle atrophy, and severe weakness.

Not all *SOD1:c.118A* homozygote dogs develop clinical signs. Initially DM appeared to be an autosomal recessive disease with incomplete penetrance, whereas most human *SOD1* mutations in human ALS are autosomal dominant. Thus, homozygosity for the E40K mutation in *SOD1* is a major risk factor for canine DM. The DM-associated *SOD1:c.118A* allele has been detected in over 100 different dog breeds and mixed breeds; thus is widespread in the canine population (Zeng *et al.*, 2014). The mutant allele appears to be very common in some breeds (Zeng *et al.*, 2014) and DM is considered a recognized health issue by the breed club health committees (see the AKC Canine Health Foundation website: http://akcchf.org/). More recently, DM has also been histopathologically confirmed in a few heterozygous dogs (Zeng *et al.*, 2014). The occurrence of DM in a heterozygote seems plausible since most human *SOD1* mutations cause dominant ALS. Nonetheless, the age at onset for many dogs has exceeded the mean life expectancy of dogs, indicating that DM has an age-related, incomplete penetrant mode of inheritance. Recently, Ivansson and colleagues (2016) reported a modifier locus within the SP110 nuclear body protein (*SP110*) on canine chromosome 25 that affects risk and age of onset of DM in Pembroke Welsh Corgis *SOD1:c.118A* homozygotes and is associated with altered changes and expression in the gene isoform of SP110 that may be relevant to disease progression.

A second *SOD1* mutation (c.52A>T), predicting a T18S missense mutation that was homozygous, has been identified in an affected Bernese Mountain Dog (Wininger *et al.*, 2011). This mutant allele appears to be restricted to the Bernese Mountain Dog breed but is less common than the *c.118A* allele (Zeng *et al.*, 2014). In addition, a few *c.52T+c.118A* compound heterozygous Bernese Mountain Dogs with DM have been identified (Pfahler *et al.*, 2014; Zeng *et al.*, 2014). This finding serves as a reminder that direct DNA tests indicate the presence or absence of disease-causing alleles but cannot be used to rule out a diagnosis because other sequence variants in the same gene or in a different gene might produce a similar disease phenotype.

Clinical spectrum

Dogs with DM follow a stereotypical pattern of clinical signs that initially begins with an asymmetrical UMN pelvic limb paresis and general proprioceptive ataxia, which progresses to LMN paraparesis and then spreads to involve the thoracic limbs and brainstem. The homogeneous progression represents degeneration of the sensory and upper and lower motor neurons. Clinical presentation has been categorized into four clinical disease stages (Coates & Wininger, 2010). Clinical signs emerge as an asymmetrical spastic paraparesis and general proprioceptive ataxia (stage 1), progressing to nonambulatory paraparesis/paraplegia with pelvic limb LMN signs within 1 year from disease onset (stage 2). Neurological deficits progress to include thoracic limb weakness (stage 3) followed by flaccid tetraplegia, generalized muscle atrophy, and brainstem dysfunction (stage 4) (Coates *et al.*, 2007; Awano *et al.*, 2009; Coates & Wininger, 2010; Shelton *et al.*, 2012; Ogawa *et al.*, 2014). As LMN signs become more profound in terminal disease, dogs often have difficulty swallowing and barking and lose respiratory function (Awano *et al.*, 2009; Ogawa *et al.*, 2014).

Early disease (upper motor neuron signs)

The earliest clinical signs of DM are general proprioceptive ataxia and mild spastic paresis in the pelvic limbs. Worn nails and the appearance of asymmetrical pelvic limb lameness are common. At disease onset, asymmetry of signs and spinal reflex abnormalities consistent with UMN paresis (T3–L3 spinal cord segments) are commonly reported. Patellar reflexes may be normal or exaggerated to clonus; however, hyporeflexia early in the course of the disease has also been reported (Griffiths & Duncan, 1975).

Involvement of the dorsal roots of the femoral nerve may inhibit sensory impulses from stretch receptors located in the quadriceps muscle. Flexor (withdrawal) reflexes may also be normal or show crossed extension (suggestive of chronic UMN dysfunction). Often within 12 months from time of disease onset, patients progress to nonambulatory paraparesis (Kanazono et al., 2013). Clients usually elect euthanasia when their dogs can no longer support weight in their pelvic limbs. Clients can care for smaller dog breeds over a longer time (Matthews & de Lahunta, 1985; Coates et al., 2007). The median disease duration prior to euthanasia in the Pembroke Welsh Corgi was 19 months (Coates et al., 2007).

Late disease (lower motor neuron signs)

If the DM-affected patient is not euthanized early, clinical signs will progress to LMN paraplegia and ascend to affect the thoracic limbs within 18–24 months. LMN signs emerge as hyporeflexia of the patellar and withdrawal reflexes, flaccid paralysis, and widespread muscle atrophy beginning in the pelvic limbs as the patient becomes nonambulatory (Matthews & de Lahunta, 1985; Awano et al., 2009). The paresis becomes more symmetrical and progresses to flaccid tetraplegia. Widespread and severe loss of muscle mass occurs in the axial and appendicular musculature. Most previous reports attributed loss of muscle mass to disuse, but flaccidity in patients with protracted disease suggests denervation. Cranial nerve signs include dysphagia and inability to bark. The hypoventilation as a result of respiratory muscle dysfunction results in hypoxemia in later stages of DM (Oyake et al., 2016). Onset of urinary and fecal incontinence will vary with individual dogs but frequently develops near the development of nonambulatory paraparesis.

Diagnosis

Accurate antemortem diagnosis is based on pattern recognition of the progression of clinical signs supported by inclusionary and exclusionary diagnostic testing. A careful neurological examination is fundamental to developing a diagnostic approach. Lack of paraspinal hyperesthesia is a key clinical feature of DM that distinguishes it from compressive myelopathies. An antemortem diagnosis of canine DM is based on ruling out spinal cord compressive diseases. A presumptive diagnosis of DM often is made based on lack of clinically relevant compressive myelopathy as determined by MRI. If MRI is unavailable, CT/myelography also can be performed. Often, imaging reveals disc protrusions that can confound a diagnosis of DM. Ultimately, the clinician must be guided by clinical experience to evaluate for rapidity of disease progression, presence of paraspinal hyperesthesia, and amount of spinal cord compression to account for the significance of the compressive myelopathy.

Electrodiagnostic testing is useful for detecting evidence of neuromuscular disease. Early in the progression of DM, when UMN signs predominate, electromyography (EMG) and nerve conduction studies are within normal limits. Later in the disease course with the emergence of LMN signs, EMG reveals multifocal spontaneous activity, fibrillation potentials, and positive sharp waves in the appendicular musculature. Recordings of compound muscle action potentials (M waves) from stimulation of mixed nerves have shown decreases in amplitudes consistent with axonopathy, and temporal dispersion and decreased motor nerve conduction velocities that also signify demyelination (Awano et al., 2009).

A DNA test based on the SOD1 mutation is commercially available and can assist in the diagnosis of DM. Dogs homozygous for the mutation are at risk for developing DM and will contribute one chromosome with the mutant allele to all of their offspring. The heterozygotes are DM carriers and are less likely to develop clinical DM but could pass on a chromosome with the mutant allele to half of their offspring. The normal homozygotes are unlikely to develop DM and will provide all of their offspring with a protective normal allele. A test result of "at risk" can support a presumptive diagnosis of DM in light of typical clinical signs and normal findings on neuroimaging and cerebrospinal fluid analysis. The SOD1 DNA test is of potential use to dog breeders wishing to reduce the incidence of DM in the breed or line.

Management overview

The efficacy of pharmacotherapies including drugs and nutritional supplements for canine DM have been based on empirical observation with a lack of evidence-based medicine approaches. The long-term prognosis of DM is poor. To date, no prospective studies have established whether exercise has a beneficial effect in DM-affected dogs. Kathmann and colleagues (2006) reported survival data from 22 DM-affected dogs that received varying degrees of physiotherapy. Dogs that received intensive physiotherapy had significantly longer survival times (mean = 255 days) compared with dogs that received moderate (mean = 130 days) or no (mean = 55 days) physiotherapy. The physiotherapy regimen consisted of active and passive exercises without taking into account disease stage or UMN/LMN signs. Although study limitations included lack of randomization and definitive diagnosis, a small group size, and bias from client perception, results warrant further investigation into the efficacy of rehabilitation in DM-affected dogs. Caution must be taken when rehabilitation, especially therapeutic exercise, is considered as these dogs can be easily exhausted and return on effort, without care, can be counterproductive.

After the discovery of mutations in the *SOD1* gene, DM is being now recognized as a naturally occurring, progressive, adult-onset neurodegenerative disease that has many similarities to human ALS and may serve as an important, novel disease model for therapy development. A spontaneous canine disease model offers a ready clinical population on which therapies can be evaluated in a setting closely mimicking human clinical trials. This approach has proven successful in developing cancer chemotherapies in canine patients, which have then been applied to humans. We propose that canine DM will serve as a potentially useful intermediate-sized model of ALS, which could be valuable for temporal studies of disease progression and evaluation of ALS- and DM-targeted new therapeutic/diagnostic regimens.

In face of inevitable gradual progression, regardless of various therapeutic modalities, it is important to realize the emotional support a client can provide to maintain quality of life for their pet. As a DM-affected dog progresses through the disease stages, the client encounters the challenges of at-home management and providing appropriate daily care for their dog. Ultimately, the client will need to make the decision for humane euthanasia, which often is guided with assistance from their veterinarian.

Case Study 17.2   Degenerative myelopathy

Signalment: 9-y.o. M/N German Shepherd Dog with progressive asymmetrical incoordination of the pelvic limbs.

History: Toenails dragging for about 1 month. Difficulty rising from sit and down positions.

Examination: Patient bright and alert. Incoordination and worn nails evident in both pelvic limbs.

Neurological examination:

- Bright and alert
- Cranial nerves WNL
- General proprioceptive ataxia present in both pelvic limbs. Worse left
- Foot placement deficits evident in both pelvic limbs. Worse left
- Hopping responses reduced in both pelvic limbs
- Stretch reflexes present and symmetrical in all four limbs

- Response to noxious stimuli symmetrical and appropriate in pelvic limbs
- Crossed-extensor reflex elicited on left when flexor reflex performed on right
- No spinal hyperesthesia.

Neuroanatomic localization: T3 to L3.

Discussion: Chronic progressive presentation and absence of paraspinal hyperesthesia establishes a unique list of differentials. This patient manifested paraparesis with intact spinal reflexes, typical for upper motor neuron signs in the pelvic limbs. This provides localization cranial to the lumbosacral intumescence (cranial to L3). Thoracic limb function was normal, placing the lesion caudal to the cervicothoracic intumescence (caudal to T3). A key finding is the lack of paraspinal hyperesthesia, ruling out involvement of pain-sensitive tissues (e.g., nerve root, disc, periosteum, joint, muscle). A neoplastic mass within the spinal cord is very plausible because of lesion asymmetry. The lack of spinal hyperesthesia would be consistent since there are no nociceptive fibers in the spinal cord tissue. Hansen type II intervertebral disc protrusion is a common spinal cord disorder in older dogs. Due to the progressive and insidious nature of a disc protrusion, spinal hyperesthesia may or may not be a clinical sign. Degenerative conditions, such as degenerative myelopathy should also be considered a differential in patients with progressive paraparesis. It is important to perform thorough cross-sectional imaging of the spine to diagnose extradural compression or intramedullary disease. A presumptive diagnosis of degenerative myelopathy is based on ruling out these causes of acquired myelopathy, which may be treatable. Degenerative myelopathy can only be definitively diagnosed based on microscopic examination of the spinal cord tissue.

Outcome: The DNA test for the *SOD1* mutation was homozygous (at risk) for the mutant allele. Since the test result only reveals a risk factor, the client wanted to rule out a treatable cause. A spinal MRI from T3 to the sacrum was performed and revealed a mild disc protrusion at the lumbosacral disc space. Since there were no supportive clinical signs of degenerative lumbosacral stenosis, the most likely presumptive diagnosis was degenerative myelopathy.

The client opted to have the patient monitored monthly by her veterinarian and pursued physical rehabilitation including underwater treadmill therapy, cavaletti, cone weaving, and ROM exercises. Six months after diagnosis, patellar and flexor reflexes became reduced. The patient also was becoming more fatigued with exercises. It was opted to continue only with the underwater treadmill therapy and focus on massage and passive ROM exercises.

The patient became nonambulatory paraparetic 10 months after diagnosis and muscle wasting was evident in the pelvic limbs. The patient developed urinary incontinence. A cart to support the pelvic limbs was recommended to enhance mobility. However, the client felt her dog's desire and attitude was diminishing and she opted for euthanasia.

Surgical and nonsurgical options for spinal cord conditions

Surgical considerations

Almost all surgical interventions of the spine involve decompression of the spinal cord and/or stabilization of the spine for realignment and preventing further impingement of the neural tissues.

In those cases where spinal cord integrity is presumed intact, determined by the animal's response to noxious stimuli, the results are often favorable. This is true even though a wide choice of surgical procedures has been recommended. There is a tremendous amount of plasticity in the neural tissues and, even in the face of significant permanent spinal cord damage, an acceptable recovery can occur.

Successful outcome is related to the rapidity of the spinal cord compromise and the amount and chronicity of the spinal cord compression. This was first clearly demonstrated by the balloon compression experiments performed by Tarlov in the 1950s (Tarlov, 1954). These variables do not determine successful outcomes based on absolutes and many dogs have recovered full function unexpectedly when given time.

An issue that has not been given adequate attention is determining prognosis in the recovery process of the canine athlete or working dog. These dogs depend upon complete recovery to an extreme level of performance. One author's (HSS) experience with determining prognosis in working dogs has been complicated by the fact that the dog whose performance is greater than that of the standard pet may not recover enough function to perform at their original level. Will a spinal surgery absorb the shock of a dog hitting the flyball box? Will the dog be able to handle the turn? It is difficult to assure a police officer that his canine partner will be completely dependable when the officer's life is on the line.

Monitoring the changes in range of motion (ROM) of experimentally produced surgical injury to the cervical spines of mongrel dogs produced interesting results (Panjabi *et al.*, 1988). A sham surgery that consisted of a skin incision and reflecting of the paraspinal musculature and periosteum was compared with:

(1) Cutting of the supra- and infraspinous ligaments at C4–C5
(2) C4 laminectomy
(3) C4 laminectomy and facetectomy.

ROM was compared at the levels of C3–C4, C4–C5, and C5–C6. For injuries (1) and (2), for about 2 weeks the ROM was increased compared with the sham procedure. For injury (3), the ROM was actually decreased for about 6–8 weeks. The differences in ROM were only appreciated during the healing phase, but were significant. At 25 weeks, all animals exhibited the same ROM as the sham control. This study provides some guideline as to when to expect complete recovery as well as the ROM changes as the animals heal and return to presurgical limits. A similar study concluded that ROM returns to presurgical levels in all injury studies when evaluating flexion–extension, lateral movement, and rotation after 6 months of healing (Crisco et al., 1990). ROM does not equate with strength but return of strength in the face of full ROM might mean that spinal surgery may not limit a canine athlete's ability to compete. More scientific information on how to get the best return to normal function is sorely needed.

Conservative therapy

Very little scientific evidence is available about the treatment or prevention of spinal injuries in the canine athlete.

Cage confinement with spinal injuries treated conservatively is still very popular but has changed dramatically from the 12 weeks common in the 1970s to the 2–4 weeks currently recommended. This kind of extreme confinement is very often successful when the patient is recovering from an acute episode of spinal discomfort. Pain medication is used judiciously and walks are for defecation and urination only. Many physical therapists believe that cage confinement is likely to be detrimental because experience in people suggests that early therapy works best. Animals whose spinal cords have been experimentally transected make the best recovery when rehabilitation is immediate (Chau et al., 1998). Whether there is a best middle ground for these two extremes is currently unexplored territory. Anecdotal recommendations abound.

Once dogs are beyond the acute phase, individual patients take to their exercise programs differently. Usually by week 8, patients can start training for their particular event. The goal is to keep the exercises below full exertion for at least 12 weeks. There is no standard protocol for retraining, as often we do not know whether the back pain is from bone, disc, muscle, joint, or ligament.

This really is no different than the standard treatment for sciatica in people. The specific cause of this particular condition is poorly understood, yet stretching and strengthening done slowly usually works. These conservative therapies are usually applied after the acute episode subsides.

New approaches to spinal cord rehabilitation

It has been known for almost half century that non-primates are less dependent than primates on intracranial centers to walk (Grillner, 1975; Kiehn, 2006). The typical hemiplegia seen in severe intracranial stroke victims is virtually unheard of in dogs. There is significant evidence that the dog does not have separate right brain and left brain functions as occurs in humans (Springer & Deutsch, 2001). With extensive hemispheric damage, the dog quickly learns to compensate. The locomotion generators that are located within the spinal cord to pattern each limb specifically and in concert with the other limbs are well developed in the dog (Handa et al., 1986). The reflex arcs so eloquently described by Sherrington modify this locomotion so that it is appropriate to the environment without having to draw much cortical attention. Grillner (1975) has extensively reviewed the history of these discoveries. An animal with a complete spinal cord transection at T13 not only walks very well on the treadmill but can adjust its speed to that of the changing treadmill. This animal has formed new connections within its spinal cord. Afferent neurons that originally were part of the reflex pathway now initiate movement by way of new connections to the pattern generators (Cote & Gossard, 2004). Turbes (1997) showed that virtually any neural information that spans the gap of a spinal cord defect could initiate good movement. These discoveries are not new but the massive locomotion literature has had very little impact on the way we treat the canine spinal patient.

By encouraging new connections and retraining lost motions, the plasticity of the canine spinal cord is likely to outperform any recovery expected in humans. It behooves us to look into this rich literature. Getting spinal-transected animals to walk on a treadmill works best under a series of prescribed circumstances and these are most definitely considerations that should bear fruit for us working with the spine and its functions in the canine athlete.

Webliography

Bergknut, N. 2011. Intervertebral disc degeneration in dogs. https://pub.epsilon.slu.se/2427/1/bergknut_n_110113.pdf.

Medical Legal Art. 2009. Cervical spine and intervertebral disc anatomy—female version. *YouTube*. www.youtube.com/watch?v=RMZ0dSJUzTg&feature=fvsr.Both websites accessed October 2017.

References

Adams, W., Daniel, G., Pardo, A. & Selcer, R. 1995. Magnetic resonance imaging of the caudal lumbar and lumbosacral spine in 13 dogs (1990–1993). *Vet Radiol Ultrasound*, 36, 3–13.

Averill, D. R., Jr. 1973. Degenerative myelopathy in the aging German Shepherd dog: clinical and pathologic findings. *J Am Vet Med Assoc*, 162, 1045–1051.

Awano, T., Johnson, G. S., Wade, C. M., Katz, M. I.., Johnson, G. C., Taylor, J. F., *et al.* 2009. Genome-wide association analysis reveals a SOD1 mutation in canine degenerative myelopathy that resembles amyotrophic lateral sclerosis. *Proc Natl Acad Sci USA*, 106, 2794–2799.

Birchard, S. 2006. Disorders of the spinal cord. In: Birchard, S. & Sherding, R. (eds), *Saunder's Manual of Small Animal Practice*, 3rd edn. St. Louis, MO: Saunders-Elsevier, pp. 1294–1303.

Braund, K. G. & Vandevelde, M. 1978. German Shepherd dog myelopathy—a morphologic and morphometric study. *Am J Vet Res*, 39, 1309–1315.

Breit, S. 2002. Functional adaptations of facet geometry in the canine thoracolumbar and lumbar spine (Th10-L6). *Ann Anat*, 184, 379–385.

Breit, S. & Kunzel, W. 2001. Breed specific osteological features of the canine lumbosacral junction. *Ann Anat*, 183, 151–157.

Burbidge, H. M., Pfeiffer, D. U. & Guilford, W. G. 1999. Presence of cervical vertebral malformation in Dobermann puppies and the effects of diet and growth rate. *Aust Vet J*, 77, 814–818.

Burr, D. B., Forwood, M. R., Fyhrie, D. P., Martin, R. B., Schaffler, M. B. & Turner, C. H. 1997. Bone microdamage and skeletal fragility in osteoporotic and stress fractures. *J Bone Miner Res*, 12, 6–15.

Burr, D. B., Turner, C. H., Naick, P., Forwood, M. R., Ambrosius, W., Hasan, M. S. & Pidaparti, R. 1998. Does microdamage accumulation affect the mechanical properties of bone? *J Biomech*, 31, 337–345.

Buttermann, G. R., Schendel, M. J., Kahmann, R. D., Lewis, J. L. & Bradford, D. S. 1992. In vivo facet joint loading of the canine lumbar spine. *Spine*, 17, 81–92.

Carter, D. R. & Hayes, W. C. 1977. The compressive behavior of bone as a two-phase porous structure. *J Bone Joint Surg Am*, 59, 954–962.

Chau, C., Barbeau, H. & Rossignol, S. 1998. Early locomotor training with clonidine in spinal cats. *J Neurophysiol*, 79, 392–409.

Churcher, R. K. & Child, G. 2000. Chiari 1/syringomyelia complex in a King Charles Spaniel. *Aust Vet J*, 78, 92–95.

Coates, J. R. 2000. Intervertebral disk disease. *Vet Clin North Am Small Anim Pract*, 30, 77–110, vi.

Coates, J. R. & Wininger, F. A. 2010. Canine degenerative myelopathy. *Vet Clin North Am Small Anim Pract*, 40, 929–950.

Coates, J. R., March, P. A., Oglesbee, M., Ruaux, C. G., Olby, N. J., Berghaus, R. D., *et al.* 2007. Clinical characterization of a familial degenerative myelopathy in Pembroke Welsh Corgi dogs. *J Vet Intern Med*, 21, 1323–1331.

Cote, M. P. & Gossard, J. P. 2004. Step training-dependent plasticity in spinal cutaneous pathways. *J Neurosci*, 24, 11317–11327.

Crisco, J. J., Panjabi, M. M., Wang, E., Price, M. A. & Pelker, R. R. 1990. The injured canine cervical spine after six months of healing. An in vitro three-dimensional study. Spine, 15, 1047–1052.

da Costa, R. C., Parent, J., Dobson, H., Holmberg, D. & Partlow, G. 2006. Comparison of magnetic resonance imaging and myelography in 18 Doberman pinscher dogs with cervical spondylomyelopathy. *Vet Radiol Ultrasound*, 47, 523–531.

De Risio, L. & Platt, S. R. 2010. Fibrocartilaginous embolic myelopathy in small animals. *Vet Clin North Am Small Anim Pract*, 40, 859–869.

Dewey, C. W. 2008. *A Practical Guide to Canine and Feline Neuology*, 2nd edn. Ames, IA: John Wiley & Sons, Inc.

Drost, W. T., Lehenbauer, T. W. & Reeves, J. 2002. Mensuration of cervical vertebral ratios in Doberman pinschers and Great Danes. *Vet Radiol Ultrasound*, 43, 124–131.

Feeny, D. A. & Oliver, J. E. 1980. Blunt spinal trauma in the dog and cat: insight into radiographic lesions. *J Am Anim Hosp Assoc*, 16, 885–890.

Flora, L., Hassing, G. S., Cloyd, G. G., Bevan, J. A., Parfitt, A. M. & Villanueva, A. R. 1981. The long-term skeletal effects of EHDP in dogs. *Metab Bone Dis Relat Res*, 3, 289–300.

Fourie, S. L. & Kirberger, R. M. 1999. Relationship of cervical spinal cord diameter to vertebral dimensions: a radiographic study of normal dogs. *Vet Radiol Ultrasound*, 40, 137–143.

Frost, H. M. 1960. Presence of microscopic cracks in vivo in bone. *Henry Ford Hosp Med Bull*, 8, 25–35.

Godde, T. & Steffen, F. 2007. Surgical treatment of lumbosacral foraminal stenosis using a lateral approach in twenty dogs with degenerative lumbosacral stenosis. *Vet Surg*, 36, 705–713.

Griffiths, I. R. & Duncan, I. D. 1975. Chronic degenerative radiculomyelopathy in the dog. *J Small Anim Pract*, 16, 461–471.

Grillner, S. 1975. Locomotion in vertebrates: central mechanisms and reflex interaction. *Physiol Rev*, 55, 247–304.

Handa, Y., Naito, A., Watanabe, S., Komatsu, S. & Shimizu, Y. 1986. Functional recovery of locomotive behavior in the adult spinal dog. *Tohoku J Exp Med*, 148, 373–384.

Hansen, H. J. 1951. A pathologic-anatomical interpretation of disc degeneration in dogs. *Acta Orthop Scand*, 20, 280–293.

Hasegawa, K., Turner, C. H., Chen, J. & Burr, D. B. 1995. Effect of disc lesion on microdamage accumulation in lumbar vertebrae under cyclic compression loading. *Clin Orthop Relat Res*, 311, 190–198.

Ivansson, E. L., Megquier, K., Kozyrev, S. V., Muren, E., Baranowska-Korberg, I., Swofford, R., *et al.* 2016. Variants within the SP110 nuclear body protein modify risk of canine degenerative myelopathy. *Proc Natl Acad Sci USA*, 113, E3091–E3100.

Jaggy, A. 2010. *Atlas and Textbook of Small Animal Neurology*. Hannover, Germany: Schlutersche, pp. 334–360.

Johnston, P. E., Knox, K., Gettinby, G. & Griffiths, I. R. 2001. Serum alpha-tocopherol concentrations in German shepherd dogs with chronic degenerative radiculomyelopathy. *Vet Rec*, 148, 403–407.

Jones, J. C. & Inzana, K. D. 2000. Subclinical CT abnormalities in the lumbosacral spine of older large-breed dogs. *Vet Radiol Ultrasound*, 41, 19–26.

Kanazono, S., Pithua, P., Johnson, G. C., Gilliam, S. N., Johnson, G. S., O'brien, D. P. & Coates, J. R. 2013. Clinical progression of canine degenerative myelopathy. American College of Veterinary Internal Medicine Annual Forum. Seattle, WA June 16–18, 2013. *J Vet Int Med*, 24(3), 699.

Kathmann, I., Cizinauskas, S., Doherr, M. G., Steffen, F. & Jaggy, A. 2006. Daily controlled physiotherapy increases survival time in dogs with suspected degenerative myelopathy. *J Vet Intern Med*, 20, 927–932.

Kiehn, O. 2006. Locomotor circuits in the mammalian spinal cord. *Annu Rev Neurosci*, 29, 279–306.

Kranenburg, H. C., Westerveld, L. A., Verlaan, J. J., Oner, F. C., Dhert, W. J., Voorhout, G., *et al.* 2010. The dog as an animal model for DISH? *Eur Spine J*, 19, 1325–1329.

Kranenburg, H. C., Voorhout, G., Grinwis, G. C., Hazewinkel, H. A. & Meij, B. P. 2011. Diffuse idiopathic skeletal hyperostosis (DISH) and spondylosis deformans in purebred dogs: a retrospective radiographic study. *Vet J*, 190, e84–90.

Lee, T. C., Mohsin, S., Taylor, D., Parkesh, R., Gunnlaugsson, T., O'brien, F. J., *et al.* 2003. Detecting microdamage in bone. *J Anat*, 203, 161–172.

Leep Hunderfund, A. N. & Wijdicks, E. F. 2009. Intramedullary spinal cord hemorrhage (hematomyelia). *Rev Neurol Dis*, 6, E54–E61.

Lornez, M., Coates, J. C. & Kent, M. 2010. *Handbook of Veterinary Neurology*, 5th edn. St. Louis, MO: Saunders, pp. 432–440.

March, P. A., Coates, J. R., Abyad, R. J., Williams, D. A., O'brien, D. P., Olby, N. J., *et al.* 2009. Degenerative myelopathy in 18 Pembroke Welsh Corgi dogs. *Vet Pathol*, 46, 241–250.

Matthews, N. S. & de Lahunta, A. 1985. Degenerative myelopathy in an adult miniature poodle. *J Am Vet Med Assoc*, 186, 1213–1215.

Mayhew, P. D., Kapatkin, A. S., Wortman, J. A. & Vite, C. H. 2002. Association of cauda equina compression on magnetic resonance images and clinical signs in dogs with degenerative lumbosacral stenosis. *J Am Anim Hosp Assoc*, 38, 555–562.

Morgan, B. R., Coates, J. R., Johnson, G. C., Bujnak, A. C. & Katz, M. L. 2013. Characterization of intercostal muscle pathology in canine degenerative myelopathy: a disease model for amyotrophic lateral sclerosis. *J Neurosci Res*, 91, 1639–1650.

Morgan, B. R., Coates, J. R., Johnson, G. C., Shelton, G. D. & Katz, M. L. 2014. Characterization of thoracic motor and sensory neurons and spinal nerve roots in canine degenerative myelopathy, a potential disease model of amyotrophic lateral sclerosis. *J Neurosci Res*, 92, 531–541.

Motoie, H., Nakamura, T., O'uchi, N., Nishikawa, H., Kanoh, H., Abe, T. & Kawashima, H. 1995. Effects of the bisphosphonate YM175 on bone mineral density, strength, structure, and turnover in ovariectomized beagles on concomitant dietary calcium restriction. *J Bone Miner Res*, 10, 910–920.

Norrdin, R., Robinson, H., Powers, B. & Histand, B. 1990. Evaluation of microdamage in canine trabecular bone in hyperadrenocorticism and radiation injury. In: *22nd International Workshop on Hard Tissue Biology*, Sun Valley, Idaho.

Ogawa, M., Uchida, K., Yamato, O., Inaba, M., Uddin, M. M. & Nakayama, H. 2014. Neuronal loss and decreased GLT-1 expression observed in the spinal cord of pembroke welsh corgi dogs with canine degenerative myelopathy. *Vet Path*, 51, 591–602.

Oyake, K., Kobatake, Y., Shibata, S., Sakai, H., Saito, M., Yamato, O., *et al.* 2016. Changes in respiratory function in Pembroke Welsh Corgi dogs with degenerative myelopathy. *J Vet Med Sci*, 78, 1323–1327.

Panjabi, M. M., Pelker, R., Crisco, J. J., Thibodeau, L. & Yamamoto, I. 1988. Biomechanics of healing of posterior cervical spinal injuries in a canine model. *Spine*, 13, 803–807.

Pfahler, S. L., Bachmann, N., Fechler, C., Lempp, C., Baumgartner, W. & Disti, O. 2014. Degenerative myelopathy in a SOD1 compound heterozygous Bernese Mountain dog. *Animal Genetics*, 45, 309–310.

Pocock, N. A., Eisman, J. A., Hopper, J. L., Yeates, M. G., Sambrook, P. N. & Eberl, S. 1987. Genetic determinants of bone mass in adults. A twin study. *J Clin Invest*, 80, 706–710.

Resnick, D. 1985. Degenerative diseases of the vertebral column. *Radiology*, 156, 3–14.

Rusbridge, C. & Knowler, S. P. 2003. Hereditary aspects of occipital bone hypoplasia and syringomyelia (Chiari type I malformation) in cavalier King Charles spaniels. *Vet Rec*, 153, 107–112.

Rusbridge, C., MacSweeny, J. E., Davies, J. V., Chandler, K., Fitzmaurice, S. N., Dennis, R., *et al.* 2000. Syringohydromyelia in Cavalier King Charles spaniels. *J Am Anim Hosp Assoc*, 36, 34–41.

Shelton, G. D., Johnson, G. C., O'BRIEN, D. P., Katz, M. L., Pesayco, J. P., Chang, B. J., *et al.* 2012. Degenerative myelopathy associated with a missense mutation in the superoxide dismutase 1 (SOD1) gene progresses to peripheral neuropathy in Pembroke Welsh corgis and boxers. *J Neurol Sci*, 318(1–2), 55–64.

Slijper, E. J. 1946. *Comparative Biological-Anatomical Investigations on the Vertebral Column and Spinal Musculature of Mammals.* Cornell University, NY: North-Holland Publishing Co.

Smith, G. K. & Walter, M. C. 1988. Spinal decompressive procedures and dorsal compartment injuries: comparative biomechanical study in canine cadavers. *Am J Vet Res*, 49, 266–273.

Springer, S. & Deutsch, G. 2001. *Left Brain, Right Brain: Perspectives from Cognitive Neuroscience*, 5th edn. New York, NY: W. H. Freeman and Company.

Tarlov, I. M. 1954. Spinal cord compression studies. III. Time limits for recovery after gradual compression in dogs. *AMA Arch Neurol Psychiatry*, 71, 588–597.

Turbes, C. C. 1997. Peripheral nerve (PNS) spinal cord anastomoses bridging spinal cord transection—enhancement of central neurons (CNS) axonal regeneration. *Biomed Sci Instrum*, 33, 326–331.

Turner, C. H. 2002. Biomechanics of bone: determinants of skeletal fragility and bone quality. *Osteoporos Int*, 13, 97–104.

Wada, N., Hori, H. & Tokuriki, M. 1993. Electromyographic and kinematic studies of tail movements in dogs during treadmill locomotion. *J Morphol*, 217, 105–113.

Walker, C., Vierck, C. J., Jr. & Ritz, L. A. 1998. Balance in the cat: role of the tail and effects of sacrocaudal transection. *Behav Brain Res*, 91, 41–47.

Westworth, D. R. & Sturges, B. K. 2010. Congenital spinal malformations in small animals. *Vet Clin North Am Small Anim Pract*, 40, 951–981.

Wininger, F. A., Zeng, R., Johnson, G. S., Katz, M. L., Johnson, G. C., Bush, W. W., *et al.* 2011. Degenerative myelopathy in a Bernese Mountain Dog with a novel SOD1 missense mutation. *J Vet Intern Med*, 25, 1166–1170.

Wood, K. B., Schendel, M. J., Pashman, R. S., Buttermann, G. R., Lewis, J. L., Ogilvie, J. W. & Bradford, D. S. 1992. In vivo analysis of canine intervertebral and facet motion. *Spine*, 17, 1180–1186.

Zaki, F. A. & Prata, R. G. 1976. Necrotizing myelopathy secondary to embolization of herniated intervertebral disk material in the dog. *J Am Vet Med Assoc*, 169, 222–228.

Zeng, R., Coates, J. R., Johnson, G. C., Hansen, L., Awano, T., Kolicheski, A., *et al.* 2014. Breed distribution of SOD1 alleles previously associated with canine degenerative myelopathy. *J Vet Int Med*, 28, 515–521.

Zimmerman, M. C., Vuono-Hawkins, M., Parsons, J. R., Carter, F. M., Gutteling, E., Lee, C. K. & Langrana, N. A. 1992. The mechanical properties of the canine lumbar disc and motion segment. *Spine*, 17, 213–220.

Zotti, A., Gianesella, M., Gasparinetti, N., Zanetti, E. & Cozzi, B. 2011. A preliminary investigation of the relationship between the "moment of resistance" of the canine spine, and the frequency of traumatic vertebral lesions at different spinal levels. *Res Vet Sci*, 90, 179–184.

18 Rehabilitation for Geriatric Patients

Rosemary J. LoGiudice, DVM, DACVSMR, CCRT, CVA, CVSMT, FCoAC, and Lisa Starr, DVM, CCRP, CVA, CVSMT

Summary

Quality of life—it is what people want for their dogs, and it is something that rehabilitation therapists can help to provide, especially for aging dogs. Aging is not a disease; it is a complex process that occurs at the genomic, cellular, and organ level—a process that appropriately selected rehabilitation therapies can help manage. Each organ system experiences senescence, or decreased function and degeneration, with aging. Many factors contribute to how an animal ages, and aging tables are readily available that can be used as guidelines while considering these factors. In human geriatric practice, there is no set age at which patients are considered geriatric. Rather, this decision is determined by the individual patient's condition. In veterinary medicine, helping to recognize and manage the factors that may contribute to an animal's aging process is an important role that the rehabilitation therapist should play as part of a patient's health-care team. Factors affecting the older dog, in addition to chronological age, that are crucial to evaluate when prescribing appropriate rehabilitation plans include weight, existing diseases or physiological conditions, sensory deficits, musculoskeletal conditions, and abnormalities resulting in mobility and incontinence issues, as well as neuromuscular, neurological, and cognitive deficits. The rehabilitation therapist must understand the client's goals for the patient to be able to determine whether the goals are possible to achieve, and how to best develop the rehabilitation plan to achieve these goals. Geriatric patients respond to traditional therapies differently than younger athletic dogs. Choosing eccentric versus concentric exercises for an individual patient, for example, is key. A multimodal therapy plan including pain management is often necessary to allow the patient to achieve success.

Defining and identifying the geriatric patient: chronology and size

The 2012 Demographic Survey of US Pet Ownership reported that 33.2% of the canine population was aged 6–10 years old (up from 29.8% reported in 2006) and 14.7% was aged 11 years and older (up from 14.1% reported in 2006) (AVMA, 2012). Extrapolating from Table 18.1, between 14.7% and 47.9% of the pet population is moving into the second half of their life span. Understanding aging is important so that adjustments can be made to accommodate for physiological changes that occur in older patients.

According to the Senior Care Guidelines Task Force of the American Animal Hospital Association (AAHA, 2005), dogs are considered senior (geriatric) when they are in the last 25% of their breed's life expectancy. Clients have easy access to many sources of aging tables, so it is important for the rehabilitation therapist to be well versed on current information about aging (PetPlace, 2015). It is generally accepted that smaller breeds of dogs have a longer life span and are considered geriatric at an older age than larger breeds of dogs. While not listing specific breeds, the information in Table 18.1 is a generally accepted guideline reference for determining when dogs of different breed sizes may be considered geriatric, although a life expectancy study of 299,555 dogs insured in Japan (Inoue et al., 2015) indicated that dogs weighing less than 5 kg had a slightly shorter life expectancy than dogs in the 5-10 kg group. Note that in this study, in contrast to previously reported canine longevity studies, the category of dog breeds weighing less than 10 kg was further divided into toy breeds (body weight <5 kg) and small breeds (5–10 kg). The authors indicate that further research is needed to identify why toy breeds had a shorter life expectancy than small breeds.

Table 18.1 Ages at which dogs may be considered geriatric

Dog size	Body weight	Age (mean ± SD)
Small	0–10 kg (0–20 lbs)	11.48 ± 1.86
Medium	10–20 kg (21–50 lbs)	10.19 ± 1.56
Large	20–40 kg (51–90 lbs)	8.85 ± 1.38
Giant	>40 kg (>90 lbs)	7.46 ± 1.27

Source: Adapted from Goldston (1995)

The Inoue study provided the following subcategories of life expectancy according to bodyweight: 13.8 years for <5 kg, 14.2 years for 5–10 kg, 13.6 years for 10–20 kg, 12.5 years for 20–40 kg, and 10.6 years for the >40 kg group (Inoue et al., 2015). If one applies the calculation for determining when a dog is considered geriatric (in the last 25% of their life expectancy), the geriatric ages are as follows: 10.35 years for <5 kg, 10.65 years for 5–10 kg, 10.2 years for 10–20 kg, 9.375 years for 20–40 kg, and 7.95 years for dogs in the >40 kg group.

There are many factors that are being studied to identify relationships between breed size and life span. Since there are considerably more factors to the aging process than chronology, a working knowledge of the various physiological changes that occur is critical to providing appropriate rehabilitation therapy. Senescence (from the Latin, senescere, which means to grow old) can refer to individual cellular aging and deterioration, aging, deterioration, and decreased function of individual organ systems, or aging of the entire organism. Mechanisms by which to change the rate of senescence is a topic of much discussion and research. One study seemed to show that senescence begins at an earlier age in giant breeds (>50 kg) than in smaller dog breeds. Once senescence begins, aging progresses more rapidly (Kraus et al., 2013).

According to Cornelia Kraus, an evolutionary biologist at the University of Gottingen in Germany, a review of data from more than 56,000 dogs including 74 different breeds showed that dogs lose about 1 month of life expectancy for each increase of 4.4 pounds (2.0 kg) (Kraus et al., 2013). Differences in insulin-like growth factor 1 (IGF-1) between breed groups has been reported as a factor in growth, aging, and senescence (Sutter, et al., 2007; Kraus et al., 2013; Inoue et al., 2015). A study by Fick et al. (2012) revealed peripheral blood mononuclear cell (PBMC) telomere length to be a statistically significant (p <0.0001) predictor of average life span among 15 breeds tested, indicating that telomeres play a role in determining the average canine life span. This study may also reveal information as to why our canine companions live a shorter overall life than people: dogs lose telomeric DNA approximately 10-fold faster than humans, which is similar to the ratio of average life spans between humans and canines. Life span and aging among breeds of dogs are dynamic areas of research with interest for both canine and human health and wellbeing.

Geriatric is an approximate, and can be a relative, term. How our clients think of their dogs in terms of aging is important because the rehabilitation therapist may recommend specific therapies and conditioning modalities for geriatric dogs, but if the client does not consider their dog to be geriatric, they might not comply. A survey by VetSTREET in 2014 indicated that clients, veterinarians and other veterinary professionals think differently about when a pet is considered senior or geriatric (Seymour, 2014). According to the article, "regardless of size, veterinary professionals considered dogs senior earlier than dog owners: 5 to 7 years old was the answer among 79 percent of professionals, while most dog owners (57 percent) believed that 7 to 9 years was more accurate." Clients and veterinary professionals both believed that larger/giant-breed dogs are considered senior at a younger age than were small and medium dogs, but at different ages. Veterinary professionals who participated in the VetSTREET survey (213 respondents) considered small, medium and large dogs to be senior at around 7 years of age, and giant breed dogs were considered to be senior around 5 years of age. Readers of VetSTREET who participated in the survey (1896 respondents) considered small breeds to be seniors at around the age of 11, with medium breeds around age 9, and large and giant breeds around age 7.

What about the use of the term geriatric versus senior? Does using one term or the other affect how clients view what rehabilitation therapists are recommending? In the same survey by VetSTREET, veterinary professionals used the term *geriatric* for dogs at around 9 years of age (with small and medium dogs around 11 and large and giant breeds around 9 and 7 years old, respectively), while clients were more likely to consider dogs around 11 years old to be geriatric (with small dogs considered geriatric at 13 years, medium dogs at 11–13 years, and giant breeds close to 9 years). Only 3% of the clients indicated that they would be offended if the veterinary professional referred to their pet as senior, but 11% indicated that they would be offended if their pet were referred to as geriatric.

It is, therefore, important for the rehabilitation therapist to be specific when discussing geriatric and/or senior recommendations with the client. Whatever term is used, and senior may be more readily accepted, therapists must be specific about what recommendations they make to meet the special needs of the senior dog while working to meet the goals of the client.

The market for geriatric rehabilitation

Clients have established a very close bond with their dogs by the time they become geriatric and often view them as part of the family. Geriatric patients may end up having a long-term relationship with physical rehabilitation facilities. The 2012 AVMA US Pet Ownership Survey indicated that 66.7% of dog owners considered their dogs to be family members (up from 53.5% in the 2006 survey), 32.6% viewed them as pets or companions (down from 45.1% in 2006), and 0.7% viewed them as property (down from 1.3% in 2006) (AVMA, 2012). Those viewing dogs as family may be willing to invest more time and money to ensure maintenance of a good quality of life and to foster longevity.

Client concerns for the geriatric patient

Client concerns for their geriatric dog can include reduced mobility (trouble rising, difficulty walking on smooth surfaces such as hard wood or tile floors, inability to use the stairs and get in or out of the car, and decreased willingness to go on walks), increased pain, urinary or fecal incontinence, changing appetite, and decreased mental alertness or interaction with the family. The goal for rehabilitation therapists is to work with the client and the patient to improve functional ability in the home environment, to improve quality of life and interaction with the client and to assist the client to manage the patient's compromised function (Figure 18.1).

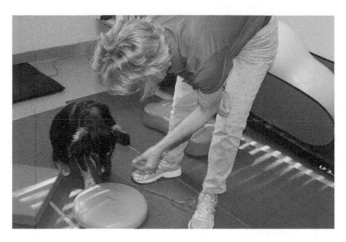

Figure 18.1   A rehabilitation therapist can improve the quality of life of a geriatric dog by challenging the dog with new, but safe, ways to strengthen supporting musculature, such as standing on a disc.

Rehabilitation objectives for the geriatric patient include managing pain, improving mobility and strength, providing appropriate assistive devices to promote independent ambulation, and modifying the patient's home environment to provide adequate traction, bedding, and obstacle-free space for ambulation.

Conditions commonly affecting the geriatric patient

Susceptibility to disease increases with age as the body's ability to respond to stress and maintain homeostasis declines. Graying of a dog's muzzle with age is a common occurrence (Figure 18.2). A 2016 study indicates that anxiety may contribute to premature graying of the muzzles of young dogs (King *et al.*, 2016). Cellular metabolism releases reactive oxygen species that cause free radical or oxidative damage. Oxidative damage reduces mitochondrial function, which affects the normal mechanisms of cell differentiation and apoptosis (Johnson *et al.*, 1999). In the case of cancer, it is suspected that normal apoptosis (programmed, orderly cell death) is interrupted, and rapidly dividing cells or cells with mutations propagate (Guyton & Hall, 2011).

Physical rehabilitation in geriatric patients often must be tailored to accommodate for

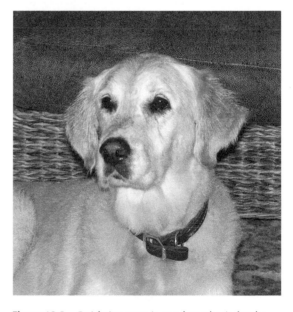

Figure 18.2   Oxidative stress is one hypothesis for the graying of the coat that occurs in most older dogs.

medical issues to avoid compromising the patient's condition when providing treatment. Older patients can have issues with lethargy, weakness, wound healing, change in quality of hair coat, urinary habits, body weight, and general immune resistance to infection (Strasser *et al.*, 2000). Proper diagnosis of conditions that contribute to these issues is important to allow patients to tolerate and receive treatment and to protect them from exposure to other patients in the physical rehabilitation environment.

Recommended management of the geriatric patient

Frequent examinations (at least every 6 months), including complete blood count, serum biochemistry, thyroid panel, urinalysis, and fecal flotation are recommended for geriatric patients (Hoskins, 2003). A comprehensive physical examination should include evaluation of dental health and mammary glands, and a digital rectal examination in addition to evaluating muscle mass and body condition score. Any new masses should be documented and aspirated (if indicated) by the primary care veterinarian. When discussing patient history with client, nutrition and behavioral issues should be reviewed. Thoracic radiographs may be considered as well as an electrocardiogram, intraocular pressure, and blood pressure evaluation. Practices may consider providing discounted rehabilitation packages, making frequent visits more affordable as well as providing hospice services for terminal patients. Training support staff to provide client education and nursing care for geriatric patients

creates an outlet for clients to express concerns. Maintaining a spreadsheet to monitor body weight, body condition score, muscle mass, and pain scores is appropriate to provide objective assessments of how the patient is progressing over time.

Common conditions of geriatric dogs that may affect rehabilitation therapy

Musculoskeletal changes

Many clients with senior dogs notice a loss of muscle mass, or muscle atrophy (Figure 18.3). As the body ages, lean body mass including muscle, bone, and cartilage declines (Metzger, 2005). Muscle atrophy may be secondary to loss of muscle fibers themselves, reduced oxygenation of the muscles, or fibrosis developing within the muscles (Goldston, 1995). Neurogenic muscle atrophy occurs more rapidly than disuse atrophy due to poor innervation of the muscles. Conditions causing neurogenic atrophy include intervertebral disc disease, fibrocartilaginous embolism, or more peripheral conditions such as diffuse lower motor neuron disease. It is extremely important to differentiate between muscle atrophy that is due to a disease process versus loss of muscle mass in

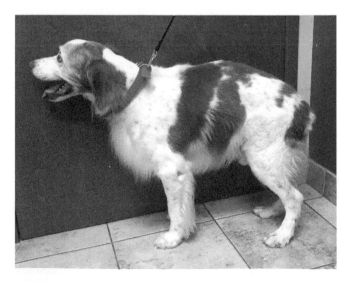

Figure 18.3 Geriatric dog with muscle atrophy demonstrating postural changes including of mild kyphosis and reduced extension of the pelvic limbs.

association with aging, without an underlying disease condition (sarcopenia) (Freeman, 2012). Identifying the cause of muscle atrophy plays an important role in determining appropriate exercises, especially in choosing concentric or eccentric exercises (see the therapeutic exercise discussion later in this chapter).

Muscle atrophy leads to loss of strength in the tendons, which leads to decreased support for the joints to counteract weight-bearing forces. This, in turn, leads to increased stress on the bone and cartilage. Studies have shown a decline in the number of chondrocytes of aging patients due to cell senescence and decreased ability to respond to growth factors. Additionally, the water content of the cartilage declines with age, all leading to thinning of the cartilage layer (Martin & Buckwalter, 2003; Loeser, 2010). Age-related thinning of cartilage and increased stress on the joints due to loss of muscle strength predispose the geriatric patient to eburnation of subchondral bone and the onset of osteoarthritis, one of the most common musculoskeletal conditions seen in geriatric patients.

While we do not recognize osteoporosis as a common condition in dogs, their bones can become more brittle with age due to infiltration of fat into the bone marrow and thinning of the cortex (Beaglehole *et al.*, 2001).

Arthritis/degenerative joint disease

Arthritis or degenerative joint disease (DJD) is a common problem of geriatric rehabilitation patients, often secondary to a congenital condition such as elbow or hip dysplasia, an injury, or excessive wear and tear. Symptoms include discomfort, lameness, restricted mobility, and muscle atrophy. Muscle atrophy may be present due to disuse secondary to pain from orthopedic causes such as DJD or an injury.

Pain from arthritis, synovitis, and DJD leads to a decreased desire to move and be active. This decreased activity can contribute to weight gain, and loss of lean body mass. Rehabilitation therapies can help decrease pain, and encourage weight loss, appropriate nervous system function, joint movement, and muscular strength.

Hydrotherapy sessions may be beneficial in improving strength and mobility. An exercise program, passive range of motion (PROM), and

massage can be taught as a home program or can be performed regularly in the practice. Laser therapy, spinal manipulative therapy (chiropractic), acupuncture, and other modalities may be useful in pain management.

Hip joint osteoarthritis is common in geriatric patients. The pain caused by the changes in the joint and periarticular tissues due to osteoarthritis leads to decreased range of motion (ROM), which results in functional shortening and decreased flexibility of the hip joint stabilizer muscles, such as the pectineus. With decreased ROM all hip joint muscles are less active and atrophy. The rehabilitation therapist has many therapeutic exercise options that can be used to address these issues.

Specific exercises such as backwards walking and side-stepping are very beneficial to help strengthen the pectineus, biceps femoris, and gluteal muscles that often atrophy or become weakened in older patients, especially those with hip joint and lumbar spine arthritis.

Behavioral and cognitive changes

Behavioral issues may develop in geriatric patients, including decreased interaction with the client other people and animals, house-soiling, altered sleep cycles, restlessness, disorientation, anxiety, altered appetite, vocalization, and aggression. Each of these issues might have other causes, or they might be signs of cognitive dysfunction syndrome (CDS) (Hoskins, 2003).

CDS is a progressive neurodegenerative disorder associated with cognitive and behavioral changes. Therapy for CDS has included antioxidant therapy, fatty acid supplementation, mitochondrial cofactor supplementation, phosphatidylserine, *Ginkgo biloba* (a monoamine oxidase (MAO)-A and MAO-B inhibitor) that increases dopamine levels and protects neurons against apoptosis, and drug therapy with selegiline (an MAO-B inhibitor) (Landsberg, 2006). Araujo and colleagues (2008) showed improvement in short-term memory in aged Beagles using phosphatidylserine, *Ginkgo biloba*, vitamin E, and pyridoxine.

Cognitive decline is seen along with several neurodegenerative changes in the brain in geriatric dogs. Documented changes in the brain include oxidative stress, deposition of beta-amyloid plaques (as seen in human patients with Alzheimer's disease), DNA fragmentation or damage, and changes in intracellular signaling leading to a loss of neurotrophic factors (Dimakopoulos & Mayer, 2002). Because dogs can naturally develop cognitive dysfunction, and they develop brain beta-amyloid deposition with cognitive deficits, they are being studied as a possible model for Alzheimer's disease research (Bosch et al., 2012; Davis & Head, 2014). Grossly, cortical atrophy and increased ventricular volume have been noted in the aged canine brain, along with reduced neurogenesis in the hippocampus, which is responsible for learning and memory (Head, 2011).

Metabolic changes

Metabolic changes in the geriatric patient include decreased metabolic rate and immune compromise (Goldston, 1995). Maintenance energy requirements in older dogs decline by approximately 20% as compared with young adult dogs. Senior diets are commonly restricted in calories due to reduced caloric needs in an attempt to prevent weight gain. However, they should provide an increased percentage of highly digestible protein, with a total composition of at least 25% protein (Laflamme, 2005). According to Larsen and Farcas, in 2014 there had been no studies that indicate that geriatric dogs have any decrease in digestive efficiency or nutrient absorption as compared with young adult dogs. While some functional effects of canine aging, such as diminished hydrochloric acid production and bile acid secretion, have been noted, these have little overall significance, much the same as in humans. The changes that have been documented in aged dogs in the function of the salivary glands, small intestine, liver, and pancreas likely reflect the general organ degeneration association with aging (senescence) and may not be clinically relevant as dogs have significant digestive functional reserves (Larsen & Farcas, 2014).

Case Study 18.1   Geriatric patient with obesity and compromised mobility

Signalment: 11-y.o. M/N Labrador Retriever; 117 lbs.

History: Progressive pelvic limb weakness over several years. Difficulty rising and going up stairs (fear of climbing stairs worsened after slipping on stairs several months ago). Diminished endurance on long walks; swims in local pond when possible. Atopy, hypothyroid.

Receiving Carprofen™ p.o. o.d., levothyroxine p.o. b.i.d., glucosamine/chondroitin/ASU p.o. o.d., omega-3 fatty acid p.o. o.d., diphenhydramine p.o. b.i.d., and chlorpheniramine p.o. b.i.d. Recently began polysulfated glycosaminoglycan (PSGAG) injections.

Referral radiographs: Left stifle lateral view: significant DJD; right stifle lateral view: moderate DJD; VD pelvis, frog-leg positioning: irregularity of left femoral head, narrowing of coxofemoral joint spaces, left greater than right.

Client's goals: Slow progression of arthritis, enable patient to accompany client on walks, and provide best possible quality of life.

Physical examination: BAR; WNL except: significantly overweight—body condition score 7–8/9; panting throughout exam; lacking appropriate abdominal muscle tone.

Rehabilitation examination:
Posture: Front end loading, moderate lumbar lordosis, pelvis rotated ventral-cranial; pelvic limb conformation very upright, tarsi and stifles lack appropriate angulation.

Sit: Sits with both pelvic limbs extended cranially.

Gait: Slides rear feet rather than lifting them at walk; circumducts with external rotation of both hip joints; minimal flexion of stifles and tarsi.

Neurological exam: WNL except patellar reflexes diminished (left worse than right); proprioception greatly delayed for both rear feet, with left worse than the right, correcting each after approximately 3–5 seconds (repeatable).

Transitions: From sternal to stand: pulls forequarters up then pushes up with both pelvic limbs while pulling himself forward; immediately transitions from a sit to sternal—not staying in sit for more than a few seconds.

Palpation: Triceps muscles very tight bilaterally, mild resistance (muscular) to full thoracic limb extension bilaterally, slight resistance to full thoracic limb flexion bilaterally, tension noted on palpation of biceps tendons bilaterally; decreased muscle tone and mass of quadriceps and hamstring muscle groups bilaterally; no crepitus of hip or stifle joints; Sensitivity to palpation at T7 and L–S junction with heat palpable at L–S; hypomobile thoracic and lumbar spine. Slight positive tibial thrust tests bilaterally, negative cranial drawer tests bilaterally.

Gulick girthometry: Initial measurements: Left and right pelvic limbs (mid-femur) = 46 cm, proximal to patella = 37 cm, mid-tibia (distal to tibial crest) = 18 cm. Left and right thoracic limbs distal humerus = 23 cm. Abdominal girth = 84 cm.

Diagnosis: Lumbosacral disease, spondylosis, osteoarthritis/DJD in bilateral stifles and hip joints, obesity-induced/aggravated musculoskeletal strain and weakness.

Assessment and rehabilitation plan:
Primary objectives:

(1) *Weight loss and weight management:* Decrease treats by half; substitute commercial treats with dried fruit chips, baby carrots, raw green beans; decrease calories by 1/3 and replace the volume of food reduced with 2× that volume of plain, canned pumpkin.
(2) *Pain and inflammation management:* Continue current omega-3 and glucosamine/chondroitin supplements; consider adding methylsulfonylmethane (MSM). Provide protocol for continuing injectable PSGAGs. NSAIDs as prescribed by rDVM with follow-up bloodwork by rDVM. Recommended laser therapy, spinal manipulative therapy, PROM, therapeutic massage (including instruction for home therapeutic massage).
(3) *Improve mobility and neuromuscular function:* Gait retraining. Once inflammation and pain are managed, continue periodic veterinary spinal manipulative therapy, PROM, and massage; add therapeutic exercises, increase length of daily leash walks as tolerated, and begin hydrotherapy via underwater treadmill

to enable gait retraining. Consider carpeting stairs to improve traction.
(4) *Maintain and improve strength and mobility:* improve posture/topline and core muscle strength and flexibility. If doing well, increase home exercise and underwater treadmill programs.

Re-evaluate every 4 weeks as indicated.
Therapeutic exercises:

(1) Sit-to-stands—initially, patient unable to hold a sit, but gradually (within 2 months of therapy) became able to do so
(2) Rhythmic stabilization
(3) Standing leg lifts—three-legged stands initially
(4) Standing with front feet on balance disc: weight shifting and rhythmic stabilization
(5) Tummy tickles to encourage dorsiflexion of lordotic spine
(6) Cookie stretches
(7) Cavalettis—starting at 5 cm high
(8) Side-stepping added after 12 weeks
(9) Backwards walking—progressed to backwards step-ups after 16 weeks.

Case summary:
Measurements after 6 months of rehabilitation therapy: Left and right pelvic limbs (mid-femur) = 53 cm; proximal to patella = 39 cm; mid-tibia (distal to tibial crest) = 19 cm; left and right thoracic limbs distal humerus = 23 cm; abdominal girth = 75 cm.
    NOTE: the limb circumferences remained constant at the 6-month values, while the patient's weight continued to decrease.

Weight: Initial = 117 lbs (girth = 84 cm)
At 4 months of rehabilitation = 103 lbs (girth = 76 cm)
At 6 months of rehabilitation = 99 lbs (girth = 75 cm)
At 12 months of rehabilitation = 96.6 lbs (girth = 74 cm)

Clients were very compliant, implementing diet changes and the therapy plan. Patient lost 26 lbs, regained mobility, was able to resume longer walks, and had improved quality of life.

Obesity

Obesity is exacerbated by some of the medical issues that can be common to the senior/geriatric dog, such as those that lead to decreased mobility and activity. The concern

about obesity is not only the mechanical stresses that the extra weight places on an obese animal's musculoskeletal frame, but also because adipose tissue produces adipokines, including leptin, a hormone that promotes the release of inflammatory mediators such as tumor necrosis factor alpha (TNF-α), interleukin (IL)-1β, IL-6, and C-reactive protein (Laflamme, 2005; Wakshlag *et al.*, 2011), which signal inflammatory responses in peripheral tissues. Increased inflammation in the body plus concussive forces on the joints due to carrying more body mass predispose obese patients to more severe osteoarthritis.

A study published in 2002 showed that food-restricted dogs had longer median life spans and delayed onset of chronic disease (Kealy *et al.*, 2002). Weight reduction (11–18% of body weight) decreased pelvic limb lameness in dogs with radiographic evidence of hip osteoarthritis in one study, while another showed weight loss (6.10–8.85% of bodyweight), decreased lameness, and improved kinetic gait analysis scores in dogs with radiographic evidence of elbow or hip osteoarthritis (Impellizeri *et al.*, 2000; Marshall *et al.*, 2010). Yet another study showed intensive physiotherapy in addition to caloric restriction provided improved weight loss, mobility, and ground reaction forces in dogs with osteoarthritis over caloric restriction alone (Mlacnik *et al.*, 2006).

Designing and facilitating weight loss and weight management and exercise plans for overweight seniors can be one of the most important and rewarding functions of a rehabilitation therapist in providing and maintaining their patient's best possible quality of life.

Hypothyroidism

Hypothyroid patients suffering from either primary or secondary hypothyroidism can develop skin issues including seborrhea, hyperpigmentation, secondary pyoderma, recurrent bacterial dermatitis, and otitis externa/ceruminous otitis (Ettinger & Feldman, 2010). These issues can impede treatment choices, including the use of electrical stimulation over compromised skin or the ability to use hydrotherapy.

Hypothyroidism should be considered in patients exhibiting muscle atrophy, lethargy, weight gain, exercise intolerance, or neurological signs such as weakness, diffuse peripheral neuropathy, knuckling, ataxia, seizures, vestibular signs, or facial nerve paralysis (Ettinger & Feldman, 2010) (Figure 18.4).

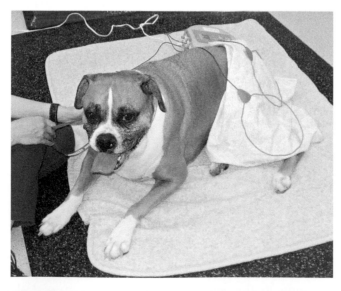

Figure 18.4   Hypothyroid patient receiving postoperative treatment for cranial cruciate ligament rupture. The client complained that the dog panted frequently. Dog is overweight due to decreased metabolism without modification of food intake.

Hyperadrenocorticism

Hyperadrenocorticism (Cushing's disease) is the result of pituitary-dependent, adrenocortical, or iatrogenically induced excess cortisol in the blood. Cushing's patients can exhibit skin changes such as hyperpigmentation and calcinosis cutis. They are predisposed to weight gait and obesity, ascites, weakness, muscle wasting, panting, and decreased pulmonary compliance (Ettinger & Feldman, 2010). Respiratory distress may be increased by excitement or exercise.

Hypoadrenocorticism

Hypoadrenocorticism (Addison's disease) is characterized by a lack of mineralocorticoid and glucocorticoid secretion, and is often due to an immune-mediated destruction of the adrenal gland. Lethargy, depression, and weakness are the most common clinical signs affecting the Addison's patient. Weight loss, and shaking or shivering may be additional clinical signs, and seizures may occur from hypoglycemia (Ettinger & Felman, 2010). If a geriatric patient has underlying Addison's disease, the effects of Addison's may, for example, compound the weakness that they may experience due to sarcopenia, so it presents an additional challenge to the rehabilitation therapist. Addison's patients should be monitored for response to stress during visits to the rehabilitation facility and may need additional glucocorticoid supplementation.

Diabetes mellitus

Patients with diabetes mellitus may present for signs of peripheral neuropathy such as scuffing, dropped tarsi (aplantigrade stance is more common in cats), or other issues related to weakness (Figure 18.5). Diabetic neuropathy is less common in dogs than in cats, and usually is seen in dogs that have been diabetic for 5 years or longer (Ettinger & Feldman, 2010). Secondary complications of diabetes mellitus include cataracts and poor wound healing. Adequate diabetic control is necessary when treating these patients to ensure that progress with therapy is not hindered.

Immune compromise

Immune compromise may be secondary to diseases such as neoplasia, iatrogenic drug

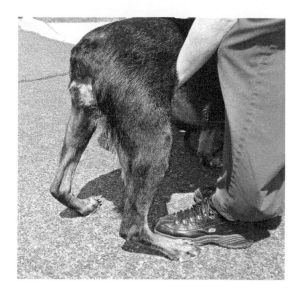

Figure 18.5   Geriatric patient with muscular weakness resulting in dropped tarsi.

suppression, or resistant infections. Routine screening with lab work and urine cultures should be pursued, and these patients should receive appropriate antibiotic therapy if warranted.

Neoplasia

In a 2011 study of canine mortality as recorded in the Veterinary Medical Database (VMDB) between 1984 and 2004, neoplastic processes were the leading cause of death overall among adult dogs (Fleming *et al.*, 2011). Monitoring for rapid weight loss, muscle wasting, cachexia, dyspnea, peripheral lymphadenopathy, or enlargement of the abdomen is recommended. Many of the modalities used in physical rehabilitation are contraindicated over areas of malignant tumors as they increase regional blood flow. Patients receiving chemotherapy should be monitored for nadirs in white blood cell counts, which may warrant postponing therapies such as hydrotherapy until their blood counts stabilize.

Pain relating to cancer and its treatment has been categorized for people in a three-stage analgesic pyramid by the World Health Organization (Fox, 2012; WHO, 2017) This may be helpful for the rehabilitation therapist in determining appropriate pain management measures to allow the cancer patient to regain the best possible mobility.

Cardiopulmonary disease

The stability of the cardiovascular system should be evaluated in the geriatric rehabilitation patient. Cardiopulmonary changes in elderly patients include declining cardiac output, decreased elasticity with concurrent fibrosis of the pulmonary tissue, and decreased cough reflexes. Pulmonary secretions often have increased viscosity, leading to difficulty expelling air and reduced resistance to respiratory disease (Goldston, 1995).

Cardiovascular and respiratory conditions more commonly encountered in geriatric patients include endocardiosis, cardiomyopathy, arrhythmias, pulmonary fibrosis, laryngeal paralysis, neoplasia, pneumonia, and bronchitis. Symptoms of coughing, abdominal swelling (due to ascites), exercise intolerance, syncope, dyspnea, or cyanosis are all indications of potential cardiac disease.

Dogs with laryngeal paralysis may present with stridor, respiratory distress, or changes in their bark. Loss of function of the recurrent laryngeal nerve, which innervates the muscles that abduct the arytenoid cartilages, results in upper airway obstruction. Caution should be used with these patients during therapeutic exercise sessions and when in the underwater treadmill to avoid compromising air exchange secondary to exertion or excitement.

Parenchymal pulmonary conditions that might be encountered in geriatric rehabilitation patients include pulmonary fibrosis, pneumonia, or neoplasia. Pulmonary fibrosis is an interstitial lung disease overrepresented in West Highland White Terriers (Norris *et al.*, 2005). Exercise intolerance, coughing, and dyspnea are the most common clinical signs. Pneumonia often has an infectious (viral or bacterial) origin, and can be incited by aspiration. Chronic bronchitis, most commonly seen in older small-breed dogs, is characterized by exercise intolerance and a slowly progressive cough.

Renal disease

Chronic renal disease is commonly encountered in older patients. Renal blood flow and the reserve of healthy renal glomeruli decline with age (Goldston, 1995). Patients with compromised renal reserves are more sensitive to insults such as dehydration and should not be overworked in the physical rehabilitation environment.

Urinary and fecal incontinence

Urinary and fecal incontinence may occur secondary to resistant urinary tract infections, neuropathies, reduced sphincter control, or hormonal imbalance. Neurological conditions, especially of the caudal lumbosacral plexus (including lumbosacral stenosis) often have side effects of decreased urinary and anal sphincter control. Sanitary concerns should be addressed in these patients when determining appropriate treatments. Many rehabilitation facilities will not allow incontinent patients in the underwater treadmill or pool. These patients should be evaluated for urine scald or irritation of the perineal area. Clients can be taught how to express the urinary bladder or stimulate bowel movements (e.g., cotton swabbing the rectum) to maintain a sanitary elimination schedule.

Incontinence can be a primary reason for clients to have a geriatric dog euthanized (AHA, 2006) If continence can be improved, a dog's quality of life can be changed significantly. Therapies to improve continence often address improving neuromuscular function relating to the caudal lumbosacral plexus, including veterinary spinal manipulative therapy, acupuncture (see Chapter 22), and laser therapy (see Chapter 7).

Animals unable to completely empty their bladders are more prone to urinary tract infections. Regular urinalyses and urine cultures should be performed to evaluate appropriate antibiotics to treat urinary tract infections while aiming to prevent the development of antibiotic resistance. It is prudent to avoid putting patients with resistant urinary tract infections in the underwater treadmill or therapy pool.

Neurological and neuromuscular conditions

A study of the mortality of dogs in North America published in 2011 revealed that diseases of the nervous system were the leading organ system cause of death in older dogs, and their frequency increased with age (Fleming *et al.*, 2011). Neurological conditions encountered in geriatric patients include vascular events, vestibular disease, neoplasia, seizures, and degenerative issues. Degenerative neurological conditions commonly seen include chronic intervertebral disc disease, degenerative myelopathy (see Chapter 17), and degenerative lumbosacral stenosis. Laryngeal paralysis had been thought to be idiopathic, but polyneuropathy, hypothyroidism, and neoplasia should also be considered when patients present with signs of this condition. In addition, studies have documented a polyneuropathy initially presenting with laryngeal paralysis and esophageal dysfunction and progressing to pelvic limb weakness and loss of muscle mass, referred to as geriatric-onset laryngeal paralysis and polyneuropathy (GOLPP) (Stanley *et al.*, 2010; Thieman *et al.*, 2010; Stanley, 2012).

Mechanoreceptors innervated by large myelinated nerve fibers provide input necessary for proprioception. The muscle spindle is a stretch-sensitive mechanoreceptor that provides input on joint position and facilitates coordinated movement. With aging, muscle spindle cells become less sensitive, joint and tendon mechanoreceptor volume declines, myelinated nerve fibers decline, tactile sensitivity decreases at a greater rate in distal extremities, and nerve conduction velocity slows in the advanced elderly, presumably all contributing to a decline in proprioception (Shaffer & Harrison, 2007) (Figure 18.6).

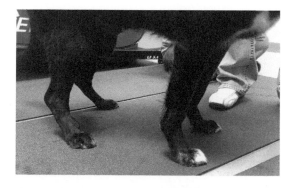

Figure 18.6 Geriatric patient displaying dropped tarsi and carpal hyperextension from muscle weakness due to neurogenic muscle atrophy.

Aging patients experience sensory losses, including decreased vision and hearing, leading to lack of awareness of their environment. These sensory deficits require the rehabilitation therapist to carefully create appropriate physical therapies. Deaf patients will be limited in their ability to respond to verbal commands or comforting words during treatment. When doing therapeutic exercise with deaf patients, the patient's sense of smell or sight can be used for motivation. Blind patients may be tentative in accepting treatment and will respond better to a soothing touch and verbal reassurance. These patients will be unable to effectively perform exercises that require visual input, such as stepping over cavaletti poles.

Coordination and proprioception decline in older patients, leading to ataxia. Combined lack of proprioception, loss of muscle strength, and postural instability contribute to falls in elderly humans. Awareness of joint movement (kinesthesia) and where the body is in space (joint position sense) contribute to proprioception, which, along with sensory factors such as vision and vestibular input, is important for maintaining balance.

Megaesophagus in an older dog is acquired esophageal weakness. This is most often idiopathic but can also be secondary to a neuropathy, myopathy, or junctionopathy. Most patients present for regurgitation, and a common complication of the disease is aspiration pneumonia. Treatment of an existing underlying disease such as myasthenia gravis, hypothyroidism, or hypoadrenocorticism can be beneficial in controlling megaesophagus, so a diagnostic work-up should be recommended in patients with regurgitation. Over two-thirds of the dogs studied for GOLPP, formerly known as idiopathic laryngeal paralysis, had esophageal dysfunction with the laryngeal paralysis (Stanley, 2012).

Degenerative lumbosacral stenosis

Patients with degenerative lumbosacral stenosis often present with a combination of orthopedic and neurological signs such as caudal lumbar pain, being slow to rise and climb stairs, decreased tail wag, and sometimes fecal or urinary incontinence. Large-breed dogs, such as Labrador

Case Study 18.2 Geriatric patient with compromised mobility

Signalment: 12-y.o. M/N Labrador Retriever; 87 lbs.

History: Referred with presumptive diagnosis of degenerative myelopathy. Client informed patient would be non-ambulatory within 6 months. Eight months earlier, patient's gait started to change with pelvic limbs slightly weak; patient will get on the couch, but climbs up rather than jumping; patient's toenails drag on sidewalk. One week prior to referral, after swimming for about 20 minutes, patient's pelvic limbs splayed out and seemed weak.

Currently receiving fish oil, meloxicam, tramadol, famotidine, plus monthly heartworm (oral) and flea/tick (topical) prevention.

Referral radiographs: V/D and lateral views of pelvis/lumbar spine unremarkable, consistent for breed and age. Very slight flattening of femoral heads (L > R) and very slight roughening of the caudal endplate of L6.

Client's goals: Provide best possible mobility for as long as possible.

Physical examination: BAR, WNL except BCS 5–6/9.

Rehabilitation examination:
Posture: Slight kyphosis of lumbar spine and tucking of pelvis, tail held down; stands base wide behind with slight decreased extension of both tarsi and stifles. Occasionally knuckles on left rear foot, but immediately self-corrects. Slightly more wear of left rear toenails.

Gait: Toes in and abducts/externally rotates both elbow joints; circumducts both pelvic limbs from coxofemoral joints; first steps after getting up are very base wide. Knuckled over less than 10% of his strides; holds pelvis to right with left pelvic limb under midline; tail held slightly to right and down; pelvic limbs occasionally cross over.

Palpation: Pain on palpation L3–S1 and SI joint; slight heat over L3–L6 and SI joint; mild decreased flexion both carpi; mild resistance to full flexion of coxofemoral joints—firm end-feel, consistent with tight hip extensor muscles.

Gulick girthometry: Initial measurements: left and right mid-thigh = 35 cm; left mid-tibia = 21 cm; right mid-tibia = 22 cm.

Neurological exam: Patellar and cranial tibial reflexes bilaterally diminished; proprioception both pelvic limbs very slightly diminished (approximately 1 second).

Diagnosis: Lumbosacral disease and degenerative myelopathy.

Assessment and rehabilitation plan:
Primary objectives:

(1) *Pain and inflammation management:* Therapeutic massage, acupuncture, veterinary spinal manipulative therapy, and therapeutic laser.
(2) *Moderate weight loss and weight management:* Goal weight 82 lbs. Discuss optimal diet with client.
(3) *Improve and maintain mobility and neuromuscular function:* Therapeutic exercises, VSMT, and underwater treadmill; mobility harness to assist the patient's walking and with positioning/stability during therapeutic exercises.
(4) *Improve and maintain overall strength, including core muscle strength and flexibility, and endurance:* Therapeutic exercises and underwater treadmill.
(5) *Medications and supplements:* Continue medications prescribed by rDVM.

Reassess patient response to treatment in 4 weeks.

Therapeutic exercises:

(1) Corrected, guided sit-to-stands
(2) Single leg lifts. Goal: work up to diagonal leg lifts
(3) Balance disc and balance board—front feet on with weight shifting and rhythmic stabilization
(4) Thoracic antebrachii on a large inflated peanut; progress to front feet on peanut
(5) Cavalettis—5 cm high
(6) Sitting back extensions
(7) Tummy tickles
(8) Backwards walking and side-stepping.

Case summary:
Six-month measurements: Left mid-thigh = 37 cm; right mid-thigh = 36.5 cm; left mid-tibia = 22 cm; right mid-tibia = 22.5 cm.

Patient responded well to therapy, improving in mobility and activity. After 12 months of therapy, client pleased with the patient's improvement, walking 20–30 minutes without difficulty; weight maintained at 80–81 lbs.

Retrievers and German Shepherds have a higher incidence of this disease, which may require advanced imaging such as CT or MRI for diagnosis (Hoskins, 2003). Surgical correction is often indicated for these patients, but mild cases may be managed conservatively with pain management and rehabilitation including controlled exercise and hydrotherapy (Worth *et al.*, 2009).

Polyneuropathies

Peripheral neurological conditions secondary to polyneuropathy are characterized by signs including weakness, knuckling, muscle atrophy, hyporeflexia, change in bark, and stridorous breathing (Hoskins, 2003). Affected patients should be screened for hypothyroidism, myasthenia gravis, and laryngeal paralysis within a comprehensive work-up, with possible referral to a neurologist.

Diffuse lower motor neuron dysfunction

Among the differential diagnoses that should be considered for dogs that present with absent limb reflexes and sudden-onset pelvic limb weakness that may progress to immobility, the four most commonly seen are: acute idiopathic polyradiculoneuritis (coonhound paralysis), tick paralysis, botulism, and acute myasthenia gravis (Troxel, 2014). Determining the underlying cause is key to implementing appropriate treatment prior to developing and instituting an appropriate rehabilitation therapeutic prescription.

Seizures

Differential diagnoses for seizures in a geriatric patient include metabolic imbalances (e.g., encephalopathy from hepatic disease or hypoglycemia from diabetes mellitus), toxic insults, neoplastic or inflammatory processes in the brain, and vascular events such as infarction (Hoskins, 2003). Knowing the underlying cause of seizures is essential in determining prognosis for the patient and how well they may tolerate modalities and exercises.

Nutritional evaluation

A nutritional assessment should include evaluation of the patient's body weight, body condition score (grade 1–9), and muscle mass in addition to discussing diet (including supplements and treats). As noted earlier, metabolic energy requirements decline with age, so geriatric patients may require fewer calories in their diet. If caloric content is restricted, it is important to ensure that good-quality, highly digestible ingredients are still present in the diet (in particular proteins and fats). A higher protein diet may be warranted. It is important to encourage maintenance of a lean body condition, and diet recommendations should be geared toward achieving optimal body weight.

Quality of life assessment

When evaluating quality of life, the concept of whether the patient is having more good days than bad is often used. Assessments of pain, appetite, mobility, independence, interest and interaction with other people and pets, general cleanliness, and hydration status are important. The HHHHHMM Scale adapted by Villalobos and Kaplan (2007) can be used to assist clients struggling with quality of life decisions (Table 18.2). While this scale can be used as a guideline, the therapist should assist clients in evaluating these parameters to help improve comfort, mobility, and happiness, if possible.

Therapeutic options for geriatric patients

Pain management

Multimodal pain management is a critical component of the rehabilitation protocol in achieving client compliance and patient cooperation. The Colorado State University College of Veterinary Medicine and Biomedical Sciences produced a pain scale (Hellyer *et al.*, 2006) that the International Veterinary Academy of Pain Management has adopted as the standard for acute pain scoring (Table 18.3). Validated chronic pain scales still need to be developed in dogs. See Chapter 19 for a discussion of multimodal pain management options for rehabilitation patients.

Supplements and nutraceuticals

Supplements can augment pain management and improve the health of the tissues in the

Table 18.2   The HHHHHMM quality of life scale

Score*	Criterion
1–10	*Hurt*—Adequate pain control, including breathing ability, is first and foremost on the scale. Is the patient's pain successfully managed? Is oxygen necessary?
1–10	*Hunger*—Is the patient eating enough? Does hand feeding help? Does the patient require a feeding tube?
1–10	*Hydration*—Is the patient dehydrated? For patients not drinking enough, use subcutaneous fluids once or twice daily to supplement fluid intake
1–10	*Hygiene*—The patient should be brushed and cleaned, particularly after elimination. Avoid pressure sores and keep all wounds clean
1–10	*Happiness*—Does the patient express joy and interest? Is the patient responsive to things around it (family, toys, etc.)? Is the patient depressed, lonely, anxious, bored, or afraid? Can the patient's bed be close to the family activities and not be isolated?
1–10	*Mobility*—Can the patient get up without assistance? Does the patient need human or mechanical help (e.g., a cart)? Does the patient feel like going for a walk? Is the patient having seizures or stumbling? (Some caregivers feel euthanasia is preferable to amputation, yet an animal that has limited mobility but is still alert and responsive can have a good quality of life as long as caregivers are committed to helping the patient)
1–10	*More Good Days than Bad*—When bad days outnumber good days, quality of life might be compromised. When a healthy human–animal bond is no longer possible, the caregiver must be made aware the end is near. The decision needs to be made if the patient is suffering. If death comes peacefully and painlessly, that is okay
Total	A total over 35 out of 70 points represents an acceptable quality of life based on the parameters reviewed in this scale

*1 is poor, 10 is good.
Source: Adapted from Villalobos & Kaplan (2007)

body. Long-chain omega-3 polyunsaturated fatty acids (PUFAs) including eicosapentaenoic acid (EPA) and docosahexaenoic acid (DHA) decrease production of proinflammatory mediators such as IL-1 and IL-6 and decrease expression of mRNA for inflammatory mediators including MMP-13, MMP-3, COX-2, 5-lipoxygenase, TNF-α, IL-1α, and IL-1β (Curtis *et al.*, 2002; LeBlanc *et al.*, 2008). In addition, long-chain omega-3 PUFAs improve kidney, gastrointestinal, cardiopulmonary, nervous system, immune system, and cognitive functions as well as skin health, and aid in diabetes mellitus and cancer treatment (Bauer, 2011; Chandler, 2015). Improved mean peak vertical force and subjective lameness scores were noted in 82% of osteoarthritic dogs fed a diet containing omega-3 fatty acids in one study (Roush *et al.*, 2010). Consideration should be given to antioxidants and chondroprotective agents such as polysulfated glycosaminoglycans (PSGAGs), and possibly glucosamine, and chondroitin sulfate for osteoarthritis. PSGAGs reduce the production of degradative enzymes such as metalloproteinases. In addition to improving the health of cartilage, chondroprotective agents can help decrease discomfort associated with osteoarthritis (Taylor *et al.*, 2004; Laflamme, 2005).

Physical modalities

Laser therapy is an excellent tool for decreasing pain and reducing inflammation (Alves, 2013). Laser therapy is indicated for DJD, intervertebral disc disease, muscle strains and sprains, and wound healing. Refer to Chapter 7 for more information on laser, thermotherapy, and other physical modalities.

Acupuncture, spinal manipulative therapy, and massage

Table 18.4 offers commonly used acupuncture points in geriatric patients. See Chapters 6 and 22 for more details on the use of acupuncture, spinal manipulative therapy, and massage in canine patients (Figure 18.7).

Table 18.3   Adaptation of the Colorado State University acute pain scale

Pain score	Dog's posture	Psychological and behavioral	Response to palpation	Body tension
0		• Comfortable at rest • Happy, content • Interested in surroundings	• Not tender to palpation	Minimal
1		• Content to slightly unsettled or restless • Distracted easily by surroundings	• Reacts by looking around, flinching, or whimpering	Mild
2		• Uncomfortable at rest • Whimpers, cries, licks painful area • Droopy ears, worried facial expression • Reluctant to respond • Not eager to interact with surroundings	• Flinches, whimpers, cries, or guards/pulls away	Mild to moderate
3		• Unsettled, crying, groaning, biting/chewing painful area • Limps, shifts weight • Unwilling to move	• Increased breathing • Cries, growls • Bites or pulls away	Moderate
4		• Constant groaning or screaming • Biting/chewing painful area • Unwilling to move • Potentially unresponsive to surroundings • Difficult to distract from pain	• Cries at gentle palpation • Might react aggressively	Moderate to severe

Source: Adapted from Hellyer and colleagues (2006). Illustrations by Marcia Schlehr

Table 18.4   Useful acupuncture points in geriatric patients to address aging issues and senility

Acupuncture point	Traditional Chinese medicine indication	Western medicine indication
ST36	Master point for gastrointestinal (GI) tract and abdomen Strengthens stomach and spleen Tonifies qi (pelvic limb "3-mile point")	Digestion Generalized weakness Pelvic limb weakness Chronic illness
LI10	Thoracic limb "3-mile point" (analogous to ST36 in the pelvic limb) Tonifies qi	Thoracic limb lameness, paresis, paralysis Elbow pain Generalized weakness
SP6	Master point for caudal abdomen and urogenital system (3 Yin crossing/meeting point of spleen, liver, and kidney channels Tonifies spleen and kidneys Tonifies qi, blood, and yin	Diarrhea Pelvic limb paresis or paralysis Sleep disorders *Contraindicated* during pregnancy
GV20	Quiets spirit and shen	Anxiety, seizures, sleep disorders
PC6	Master point for chest/cranial abdomen Calms shen Moves qi and heat	Cardiac disorders Nausea Seizures, anxiety Vestibular disorders, vertigo Thoracic limb pain, paresis, or paralysis
BL17	Influential point for blood Back shu association point for diaphragm Tonifies blood and yin Clears heat	Immunostimulation Supports blood flow Fatigue Cough, dyspnea
LIV3	Shu-stream point (Earth) Yuan source point Moves liver qi stagnation	Liver, gallbladder, urogenital, and GI disorders Pelvic limb paresis or paralysis General painful conditions

Source: Adapted from Xie & Preast (2007); diagrams of acupuncture point locations are given in this reference

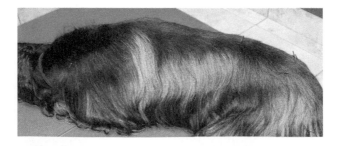

Figure 18.7   Acupuncture is a valuable tool for pain management and nervous system stimulation in patients with degenerative lumbosacral stenosis or thoracolumbar intervertebral disc disease as in this case. It is very relaxing for many patients due to the release of endorphins that occurs.

Improving mobility

After pain has been managed, the next step in the physical rehabilitation plan is to improve mobility, as it is critical for quality of life. Increasing daily exercise in moderation will start to improve cardiovascular fitness, endurance, neuromuscular function, muscular strength, and flexibility, as well as joint ROM.

Biological therapies, including stem cell and platelet-rich plasma (PRP) therapies, are potentially valuable modalities for improving mobility and function. See Chapter 16 for information regarding biological therapies.

Some geriatric patients may need assistance with mobility, for walking, rising, or maneuvering in their home environment. Frequent nail trims and keeping the hair between the foot pads and on the bottom of the foot short can aid traction on slippery floors. Yoga mats or runners can be placed over slippery floors. Skid-resistant dog socks, foot waxes, or sprays promoting traction are available to help prevent slipping. Canine-specific booties are helpful in winter to prevent snow from forming ice between the foot pads and to prevent salt from irritating them (Figure 18.8).

After traction has been addressed, strength and ability to rise independently should be evaluated. Patients with severe DJD may lack pain-free ROM in the affected joints, inhibiting ability to transition into a standing position. Muscle atrophy from sarcopenia or from pain-related inactivity may contribute to weakness,

incoordination, and inability or difficulty rising. Patients needing assistance rising benefit from devices that aid elevation from the floor such as slings under the belly, chest harnesses, harnesses that lift under the pelvis, or harnesses that combine lifting and support under the chest and the pelvis. These devices also provide balance support for ambulation. Patient needs, including a consideration of the environment as well as client abilities and needs, ease of use, and patient comfort all should be considered when recommending and selecting an appropriate harness or sling (Figure 18.9).

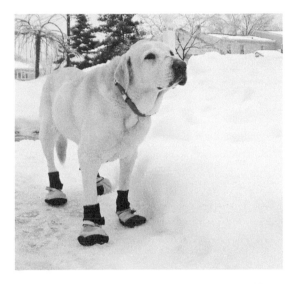

Figure 18.8   Boots can provide protection from cold temperatures as well as increased traction in wintery climates.

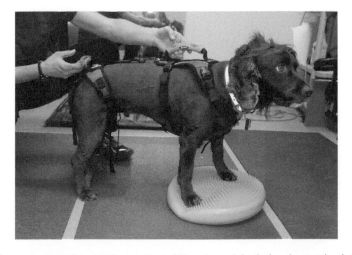

Figure 18.9   Patient demonstrating a harness that assists in lifting through both the chest and pelvis.

Carts

Wheelchairs or carts provide mobility for patients with severe paresis or plegia. Carts allow patients to maintain an exercise schedule, to interact with clients and other pets, and to eliminate in a more sanitary manner if they cannot support themselves independently (Figure 18.10).

Passive range of motion

Passive range of motion therapy assists in maintaining comfort and mobility. It is important for

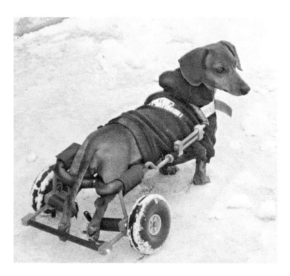

Figure 18.10 Carts can provide improved mobility and quality of life for patients with paresis due to neurological injury.

patients that are recumbent or restricted in joint motion secondary to neurological or orthopedic conditions to maintain joint lubrication and mechanoreceptor stimulation. PROM improves extensibility of the soft tissues such as muscle and the joint capsule to prevent adhesions from forming in restricted joints (Figure 18.11). See Chapters 5 and 6 for information on how to properly perform PROM therapy.

Improving strength

After pain management and mobility are addressed, the next step in the physical rehabilitation plan is to promote increased strength and muscle mass in the geriatric patient. Increased muscle mass will help maintain comfort by acting as a shock absorber for concussive forces and provide more padding for recumbent patients. Muscle has a higher metabolic rate than fat and will help to maintain a leaner body weight in these patients.

Therapeutic exercises

Therapeutic exercises for the geriatric patient may focus on improving coordination, proprioception, and strengthening of the antigravity and stabilizer muscles (see Chapter 8). Eccentric exercises, where the muscle is contracting and lengthening while being loaded, promote greater gain in muscle mass as compared with concentric exercises (Millis & Levine, 2014). However, sarcopenia and its associated reduced

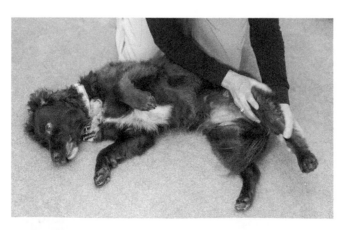

Figure 18.11 Passive range of motion for dogs with restricted mobility can decrease pain, improve lubrication of the joints, and decrease stiffness.

muscle regeneration capability may result in muscle injury before the muscle can adapt (Gault & Willems, 2013). As a result, focusing on concentric exercises may be more appropriate for geriatric patients, especially in the early stages of geriatric rehabilitation therapy. Senior dogs may need additional stabilization and assistance during exercise sessions. Using a well-fitting harness can be beneficial (Figure 18.12).

Rhythmic stabilization, joint compressions, and gait patterning are important basic exercises. Cookie stretches and spinal flexion can be helpful in improving flexibility and comfort in stiff patients (Figure 18.13). Extensor muscles (the muscles of posture, the antigravity mus-

cles) often weaken in geriatric patients, resulting in a shuffling gait. Seated trunk extensions help improve core muscle strength and flexibility and can be used to begin to position the patient to correctly transition to a stand (Figure 18.14). Sit-to-stand exercises (similar to squats for people) can be performed assisted and initially done with the patient sitting on a raised surface when necessary. These exercises improve thoracic limb extensor muscle strength. They should be performed without the patient stepping forward so that it does not pull itself up into a stand by using the thoracic limbs.

Walking over cavaletti poles helps to improve proprioception and coordination (presuming the patient does not have visual

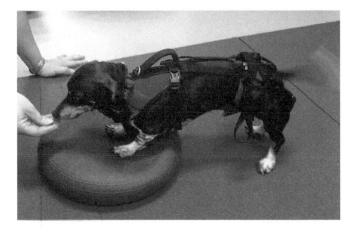

Figure 18.12 A geriatric patient wearing a harness during exercises to allow the therapist to easily provide stabilization as needed.

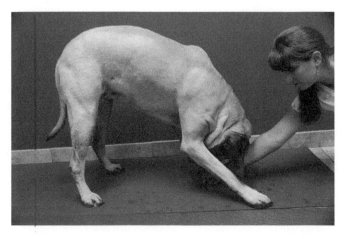

Figure 18.13 Therapeutic exercises such as cookie stretches and spinal flexion can improve spinal flexibility and balance.

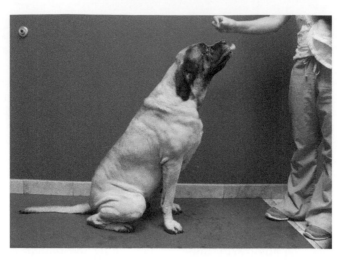

Figure 18.14   Seated trunk extensions help to improve posture and topline, engaging the core muscles and helping the dog to position itself correctly to extend the pelvic limbs, transitioning from sit to stand.

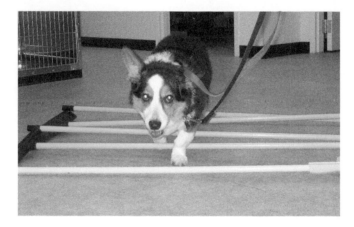

Figure 18.15   Cavaletti exercises can improve balance and proprioception in geriatric patients with weakness in the muscles of posture and locomotion as well as core muscles, such as the iliopsoas, abdominals, and paraspinals.

deficits) (Figure 18.15). Simple items can be used for home therapy cavalettis such as broom sticks, downspouts, or serpentined garden hose, while softer foam poles may prevent tripping in a weak patient that scuffs its feet or drags its toes.

Geriatric patients often have difficulty maintaining traction when trying to stand and/or walk. They may experience pelvic limbs suddenly abducting or slipping caudally. Backward walking can help strengthen the hamstring muscles, especially the biceps femoris, as well as the gluteal muscles, and side-stepping can address weak adductor muscles such as the pectineus, especially in patients with pelvic limb weakness secondary to neurological conditions or DJD.

Exercises such as rocker board and weaving around cones improve balance and lateral stability for patients that are prone to falling. Focusing on abdominal muscle strength with core exercises such as crunches, side sit-ups, tummy tickles, cookie stretches, and leg lifts is helpful in improving topline and maintaining best possible posture, especially in lordotic patients. Carefully supported leg lift exercises, beginning with the therapist lifting just one of the patient's legs and progressing to diagonal leg lifts if possible, can help to improve balance and core muscle strength. It is extremely important to provide a geriatric patient adequate breaks and rest periods during exercise sessions (Figure 18.16).

Hydrotherapy

Hydrotherapy provides buoyancy, decreasing concussive forces on potentially painful or arthritic joints (see Chapter 9). Prior screening for medical conditions is important to ensure that the geriatric patient will be able to tolerate the warmth and moisture of the water as well as the stress and exertion encountered with hydrotherapy. Providing shorter hydrotherapy sessions with more breaks may be beneficial for a weakened geriatric patient. The buoyancy of the water may allow the therapist to perform standing therapeutic exercises such as rhythmic stabilization, joint compressions, and pattern-ing for patients that are too weak to stand independently or those with severely compromised mobility (Figure 18.17).

Neuromuscular electrical stimulation

Targeted muscle strengthening with neuromuscular electrical stimulation (NMES) can assist patients with severe muscle atrophy. In weakened patients, NMES activates muscles that can be targeted later with therapeutic exercise. NMES can be done two to three times a week at the clinic for patients with mild to moderate muscle atrophy, or taught to capable clients so that it can be done three to five times a week at home for patients with neurogenic or severe muscle atrophy.

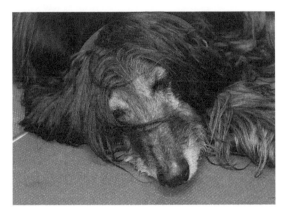

Figure 18.16   A geriatric pelvic limb amputee with a prosthetic enjoys a rest period during a therapeutic exercise session.

Bedding and decubital ulcers

Patients with muscle atrophy as well as recumbent patients with thin body condition and poor muscle mass are at greatest risk for pressure sores or decubital ulcers. Comfortable padding helps keep these patients warm and protects their skin (Figure 18.18). Frequent turning (every 2–4 hours) should be employed if patients are unable or unwilling to do so on their own so as to prevent atelectasis and excessive pressure on bony points.

Patients with decubital ulcers should not enter the underwater treadmill or therapy pool without a waterproof seal over the wound.

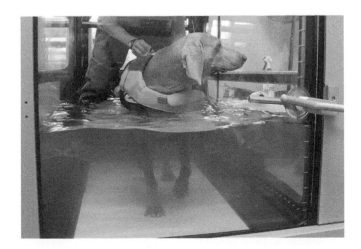

Figure 18.17   Geriatric patients benefit from the hydrostatic and cardiovascular benefits of aerobic exercise in a lower impact hydrotherapy environment.

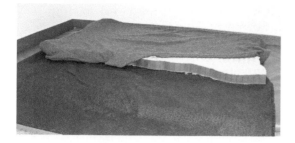

Figure 18.18   Providing soft bedding that is supportive of prominent bony protuberances, while easy to rise from, is helpful in maintaining mobility and preventing decubital ulcers in geriatric patients.

The decubital ulcer should be cultured to determine appropriate antibiotic therapy, pressure should be relieved if possible, and the wound should be cleaned regularly. Topical therapy may be used in addition to oral antibiotics and laser therapy to promote local blood supply and wound healing.

Hospice care

End of life issues are very difficult for clients. The rehabilitation therapist can be an important source of education on pain management, nutrition, and nursing care issues for terminal or recumbent patients. Teaching clients to keep these patients well padded, hydrated, adequately fed, and to express their urinary bladder and bowels is often indicated. Laser therapy for pain management and wound healing, massage, and PROM to maintain flexibility and comfort in the joints are all beneficial (Bjordal *et al.*, 2003). Discussing parameters that detract from an acceptable quality of life is encouraged early in the relationship with clients with hospice patients so they can remain more objective. Encouraging clients to write down how much they are willing to assist their dog and what level of dysfunction or loss of independence they are willing to accept can be a valuable reference once decisions about end of life are necessary.

Marketing to clients with geriatric dog

Clients with geriatric patients can be contacted to educate them about the services that the rehabilitation professional can provide. Clients that purchase NSAIDs, thyroid supplementation, urinary incontinence medication, chemotherapy, or medications prescribed for cognitive dysfunction, or even clients with geriatric patients (based on age) are good candidates to receive educational materials about geriatric wellness or hospice programs offered by the rehabilitation practice.

Webliography

AAHA. 2005. *Senior Care Guidelines for Dogs and Cats.* https://www.aaha.org/professional/resources/senior_care.aspx.

AHA. 2016. Euthanasia: making the decision. American Humane Association. http://www.americanhumane.org/fact-sheet/euthanasia-making-the-decision/.

AVMA. 2012. *U.S. Pet Ownership and Demographics Sourcebook.* https://www.avma.org/kb/resources/statistics/pages/market-research-statistics-us-pet-ownership-demographics-sourcebook.aspx.

Hellyer, P. W., Uhrig, S. R. & Robinson, N. G. 2006. Colorado State University, Veterinary Medical Center, Canine Acute Pain Scale v.2. http://www.vasg.org/pdfs/CSU_Acute_Pain_Scale_Canine.pdf.

PetPlace. 2015. When is a dog considered senior? http://www.petplace.com/article/dogs/keeping-your-dog-healthy/senior-dog-care/when-is-a-dog-considered-senior.

Seymour, K. 2014. Aging pets: senior, geriatric and what it all means to experts and readers. http://www.vetstreet.com/our-pet-experts/aging-pets-senior-geriatric-and-what-it-all-means-to-experts-and-readers.

WHO, 2017. World Health Organization cancer pain ladder for adults. http://www.who.int/cancer/palliative/painladder/en/. All websites accessed October 2017.

References

Alves, A. C., Vieira, R., Leal-Junior, E., dos Santos, S., Ligeiro, A. P., Albertini, R., *et al.* 2013. Effect of low-level therapy on the expression of inflammatory mediators and on neutrophils and macrophages in acute joint inflammation. *Arthritis Res Ther*, 15(5), R116.

Araujo, J. A., Landsberg, G. M., Milgram, N. W. & Miolo, A. 2008. Improvement of short-term memory performance in aged beagles by a nutraceutical supplement containing phosphatidylserine, Ginkgo biloba, vitamin E, and pyridoxine. *Can Vet J*, 49(4), 379–385.

Bauer, J. E. 2011. Therapeutic use of fish oils in companion animals. *J Am Vet Med Assoc*, 239(11), 1441–1451.

Beaglehole, R., Lunenfeld, B. & Kalache, A. 2001. *Men, Ageing and Health: Achieving Health across the Life Span*. Geneva: World Health Organization, p. 63.

Bjordal, J. M., Couppe, C., Chow, R. T., Tuner, J. & Ljunggren, E. A. 2003. A systematic review of low level laser therapy with location-specific doses for pain from chronic joint disorders. *Aust J Physiother*, 49, 107–116.

Bosch, N. M., Pugliese, M., Gimeno-BAYON, J., Jose RODRIGUEZ, M. & Mahy, N. 2012. Dogs with cognitive dysfunction syndrome: a natural model of Alzheimer's disease. *Curr Alzheimer Res*, 9(3), 298–314.

Chandler, M. L. 2015. Top 5 therapeutic uses of omega-3 fatty acids. *Clinicians Brief*, Feb.

Curtis, C. L., Rees, S. G., Little, C. B., Flannery, C. R., Hughes, C. E., Wilson, C., et al. 2002. Pathologic indicators of degradation and inflammation in human osteoarthritic cartilage are abrogated by exposure to n-3 fatty acids. *Arthritis Rheum*, 46, 1544–1553.

Davis, P. R. & Head, E. 2014. Prevention approaches in a preclinical canine model of Alzheimer's disease: benefits and challenges. *Front Pharmacol*, 5, 47.

Dimakopoulos, A. C. & Mayer, R. J. 2002. Aspects of neurodegeneration in the canine brain. *J Nutr*, 132, 1579S–1582S.

Ettinger, S. J. & Feldman, E. C. 2010. *Textbook of Veterinary Internal Medicine*, 7th Edn. St. Louis, MO: Saunders.

Fick, L. J., Fick, G. H., Li, Z., Cao, E., Bao, B., Heffelfinger, D., et al. 2012. Telomere length correlates with life span of dog breeds. *Cell Rep*, 2(6), 1530–1536.

Fleming, J. M., Creevy, K. E. & Promislow, D. E. 2011. Mortality in North American dogs from 1984 to 2004: an investigation into age-, size-, and breed-related causes of death. *J Vet Intern Med*, 25, 187–198.

Fox, S. M. 2012. Painful decisions for senior pets. *Vet Clin North Am Small Anim Pract*, 42, 727–748.

Freeman, L. M. 2012. Cachexia and sarcopenia: emerging syndromes of importance in dogs and cats. *J Vet Intern Med*, 26(1), 3–17.

Gault, M. L. & Willems, M. E. T. 2013. Aging, functional capacity and eccentric exercise training. *Aging Dis*, 4(6), 351–363.

Goldston, R. T. 1995. Introduction and overview of geriatrics. In: Goldston, R.T. & Hoskins, J.D. (eds), *Geriatrics and Gerontology of the Dog and Cat*, 1st edn. Philadelphia, PA: W. B. Saunders, pp. 1–9.

Guyton, A. C. & Hall, J. E. 2011. *Textbook of Medical Physiology*, 12th edn. Philadelphia, PA: Saunders/Elsevier.

Head, E. 2011. Neurobiology of the aging dog. *Age*, 33, 485–496.

Hoskins, J. D. 2003. *Geriatrics and Gerontology of the Dog and Cat*, 2nd edn. Philadelphia, PA: Saunders.

Impellizeri, J. A., Tetrick, M. A. & Muir, P. 2000. Effect of weight reduction on clinical signs of lameness in dogs with hip osteoarthritis. *J Am Vet Med Assoc*, 216, 1089–1091.

Inoue, M., Hasegawa, A., Hosoi, Y. & Sugiura, K. 2015. A current life table and causes of death for insured dogs in Japan. *Prev Vet Med*, 120, 210–218.

Johnson, F. B., Sinclair, D. A. & Guarente, L. 1999. Molecular biology of aging. *Cell*, 96, 291–302.

Kealy, R. D., Lawler, D. F., Ballam, J. M., Mantz, S. L., Biery, D. N., Greeley, E. H., et al. 2002. Effects of diet restriction on life span and age-related changes in dogs. *J Am Vet Med Assoc*, 220, 1315–1320.

King, C., Smith, T. J., Grandin, T. & Borchelt, P. 2016. Anxiety and impulsivity: factors associated with premature graying in young dogs. *Appl Anim Behav Sci*, 185, 78–85.

Kraus, C., Pavard, S. & Promislow, D. E. L. 2013. The size-life span trade-off decomposed: why large dogs die young. *Am Nat*, 181(4), 492–505.

LaFlamme, D. P. 2005. Nutrition for aging cats and dogs and the importance of body condition. *Vet Clin North Am Small Anim Pract*, 35, 713–742.

Landsberg, G. 2006. Therapeutic options for cognitive decline in senior pets. *J Am Anim Hosp Assoc*, 42, 407–413.

Larsen, J. A. & Farcas, A. 2014. Nutrition of aging dogs. *Vet Clin North Am Small Anim Pract*, 44(4), 741–759.

LeBlanc, C. J., Horohov, D. W., Bauer, J. E., Hosgood, G. & Mauldin, G. E. 2008. Effects of dietary supplementation with fish oil on in vivo production of inflammatory mediators in clinically normal dogs. *Am J Vet Res*, 69, 486–493.

Loeser, R. F. 2010. Age-related changes in the musculoskeletal system and the development of osteoarthritis. *Clin Geriatr Med*, 26, 371–386.

Marshall, W. G., Hazewinkel, H. A., Mullen, D., DE Meyer, G., Baert, K. & Carmichael, S. 2010. The effect of weight loss on lameness in obese dogs with osteoarthritis. *Vet Res Commun*, 34, 241–253.

Martin, J. A. & Buckwalter, J. A. 2003. The role of chondrocyte senescence in the pathogenesis of osteoarthritis and in limiting cartilage repair. *J Bone Joint Surg Am*, 85, 106–110.

Metzger, F. L. 2005. Senior and geriatric care programs for veterinarians. *Vet Clin North Am Small Anim Pract*, 35, 743–753.

Millis, D. & Levine, D, 2014. *Canine Rehabilitation and Physical Therapy*, 2nd edn. Philadelphia, PA: Elsevier, p. 117.

Mlacnik, E., Bockstahler, B. A., Muller, M., Tetrick, M. A., Nap, R. C. & Zentek, J. 2006. Effects of caloric restriction and a moderate or intense physiotherapy program for treatment of lameness in overweight dogs with osteoarthritis. *J Am Vet Med Assoc*, 229, 1756–1760.

Norris, A. J., Naydan, D. K. & Wilson, D. W. 2005. Interstitial lung disease in West Highland White Terriers. *Vet Pathol*, 42, 35–41.

Roush, J. K., Cross, A. R., Renberg, W. C., Dodd, C. E., Sixby, K. A., Fritsch, D. A., *et al.* 2010. Evaluation of the effects of dietary supplementation with fish oil omega-3 fatty acids on weight bearing in dogs with osteoarthritis. *J Am Vet Med Assoc*, 236, 67–73.

Shaffer, S. W. & Harrison, A. L. 2007. Aging of the somatosensory system: a translational perspective. *Phys Ther*, 87, 193–207.

Stanley, B. J. 2012. Evaluating the lar-par patient—more to swallow than realized? ACVS Proceedings 2012, pp. 255–258.

Stanley, B. J., Hauptman, J. G., Fritz, M. C., Rosenstein, D. S. & Kinns, J. 2010. Esophageal dysfunction in dogs with idiopathic laryngeal paralysis: a controlled cohort study. *Vet Surg*, 39, 139–149.

Strasser, A., Teltscher, A., May, B., Sanders, C. & Niedermuller, H. 2000. Age-associated changes in the immune system of German shepherd dogs. *J Vet Med A Physiol Pathol Clin Med*, 47, 181–192.

Sutter, N. B., Bustamante, C. D., Chase, K., Gray, M. M., Zhao, K., Zhu, L., *et al.* 2007. A single IGF-1 allele is a major determinant of small size in dogs. *Science*, 316, 112–115.

Taylor, R. A., Millis, D. L., Levine, D., Adamson, C. P., Bevan, J. & Marcellin-LITTLE, D. 2004. Physical rehabilitation for geriatric and arthritic patients. In: Millis, D.L., Levine, D. & Taylor, R.A. (eds), *Canine Rehabilitation and Physical Therapy*. St. Louis, MO: Saunders-Elsevier, pp. 411–425.

Thieman, K. M., Krahwinkel, D. J., Sims, M. H. & Shelton, G. D. 2010. Histopathological confirmation of polyneuropathy in 11 dogs with laryngeal paralysis. *J Am Anim Hosp Assoc*, 46, 161–167.

Troxel, M. 2014. Diffuse lower motor neuron dysfunction in dogs. *Clinicians Brief*, 75–79.

Villalobos, A. & Kaplan, L. 2007. *Canine and Feline Geriatric Oncology: Honoring the Human-Animal Bond*. Ames, IA: Blackwell Publishing.

Wakshlag, J. J., Stuble, A. M., Levine, C. B., Bushey, J. J., LaFlamme, D. P. & Long, G. M. 2011. The effects of weight loss on adipokines and markers of inflammation. *Br J Nutr*, 106, S11–S14.

Worth, A. J., Thompson, D. J. & Hartman, A. C. 2009. Degenerative lumbosacral stenosis in working dogs: current concepts and review. *N Z Vet J*, 57, 319–330.

Xie, H. & Preast, V. 2007. *Xie's Veterinary Acupuncture*. Ames, IA: Blackwell Publishing.

19 The Prevention and Management of Pain in Canine Patients

Mark E. Epstein, DVM, DABVP (C/F), CVPP

Summary

Undermanaged acute and chronic pain can lead to a cascade of negative physiological, medical, and emotional consequences. Therefore, the imperative for the proper recognition, assessment, prevention, and treatment of pain is not only an ethical one but a physiological and medical one as well. Fortunately, there are a great many pain management tools available to the veterinarian to mitigate these effects and improve not only patient comfort, but overall recovery and quality (and in some cases, length) of life. Unfortunately, it can be a challenge indeed to know which treatment plan can best—and most safely—meet the needs of our patients, a matter made more difficult for veterinarians since animals cannot self-report their pain. This chapter is a succinct overview of the multimodal approach to the prevention and treatment of pain in dogs, utilizing evidence-based veterinary medicine insofar as possible, and a consensus of expert opinion otherwise. Drug classes and modalities discussed include: NSAIDs, opioids, alpha-2 agonists, locoregional anesthesia, subanesthetic ketamine, and a variety of other pain-modifying analgesic drugs in common use (e.g., gabapentin, amantadine, acetaminophen, tramadol, and others). This chapter also includes tips for practical clinical use, with an emphasis on safe and responsible use of the various drug classes. In addition, descriptions of other drugs possibly on the horizon for veterinary use (some based on utility in human medicine) are included. Lastly, evidence-based approaches to managing postsurgical and varieties of chronic pain (osteoarthritis, osteosarcoma, and noninflammatory) are described, with sample cases to illustrate.

Introduction

This chapter explores the fundamentals of acute and chronic pain management in dogs. The reader is directed to more comprehensive resources for discussions of pain neurobiology, neuropharmacology, and most drug doses. An emphasis is placed on practical and evidence-based approaches, with attention to safe and responsible drug use.

Canine Sports Medicine and Rehabilitation, Second Edition. Edited by Chris Zink and Janet B. Van Dyke.
© 2018 John Wiley & Sons, Inc. Published 2018 by John Wiley & Sons, Inc.

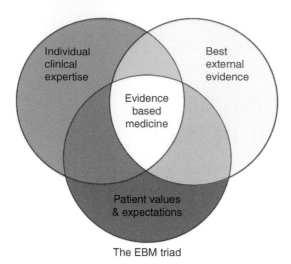

The EBM triad

Figure 19.1 Evidence, experience and client expectations must all be addressed in pain management.

It is important to be mindful that there is relatively little evidence-based veterinary medicine (EBVM); thus, guidance with regard to complex clinical choices is in short supply. It is both the blessing and the curse of contemporary medicine that there exists an impressive array of tools in the pain management toolbox.

What drug(s) shall we use? In what order? In which combinations? For which type of pain? At what dose? For how long? For these and many other variables there are no simple answers in the veterinary literature. The competing values of a best evidence approach, personal experience, and client values (preferences) will always be in dynamic tension (Sackett *et al.*, 1996) (Figure 19.1).

Pain is further complicated for veterinarians as our patients are nonverbal, mirroring the challenge in human medicine with nonverbal subpopulations: neonates (Schechter, 1989), the cognitively impaired (Cook *et al.*, 1999), and the elderly (Lovheim *et al.*, 2006). In verbal patients, pain is what the patient says it is; in nonverbal patients, pain is what *we* say it is.

These collective challenges were recently addressed by two industry expert panels and their recommendations published in separate comprehensive manuscripts to which the reader is referred: the 2015 *AAHA/AAFP Pain Management Guidelines* (Epstein *et al.*, 2015), and the *WSAVA Global Pain Council's Guidelines for Recognition, Assessment, and Treatment of Pain* (Matthews *et al.*, 2014). Clinicians often limit

pain medications for fear of adverse drug effects (ADEs) or interactions (Belshaw *et al.*, 2016). Yet we must *also* consider the harm to the patient if pain is inadequately managed. We have an ethical obligation to minimize pain in our patients, and to recognize negative medical, physiological, emotional, and even cognitive consequences—the multidimensional negative experiences—that are a direct result of undermanaged pain.

Pain elicits a cascade of debilitating neurohormonal effects that includes hypertension, catabolism, immunosuppression, and worse. With undermanaged pain, surgical patients heal and recover more slowly, and may develop chronic pain states and even severe, life-threatening complications (Anand & Hickey, 1992). Chronic pain in humans is associated with cognitive impairment including learning and memory (Kreitler *et al.*, 2007), and is comorbid with clinical depression. For dogs, in the extreme, underrecognized, underattended, undermanaged pain can become a criterion for euthanasia.

We know much about optimal pain management in animals, but what we think we know is dwarfed by what we do not. Literature must be read critically, and any recommendations about protocols, including those in this chapter, must be considered analytically, with an open mind towards the viewpoints of others and a commitment to continued learning.

Multimodal approach to pain management

The principle is simple: relying upon one modality or drug requires higher doses and/or more frequent and/or prolonged administration to achieve the desired effect, while minimizing the potential benefit and maximizing the possibility of ADEs (Figure 19.2). With multiple modalities each affecting different aspects of pain processing, including elements of central and peripheral hypersensitization, requirements for each drug are reduced while achieving superior effect and minimizing ADEs. Though difficult to study, there is growing evidence in the veterinary literature that this principle applies in both the acute (Brondani *et al.*, 2009) and chronic (Fritsch *et al.*, 2010) pain setting.

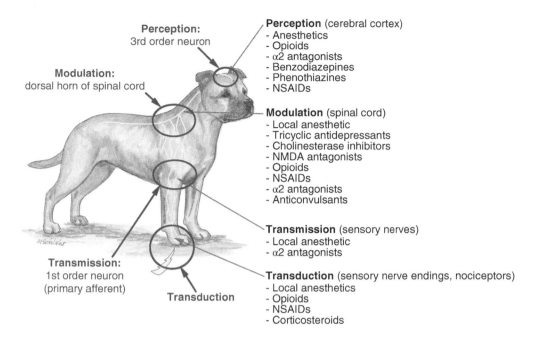

Perception:
3rd order neuron

Modulation:
dorsal horn of spinal cord

Perception (cerebral cortex)
- Anesthetics
- Opioids
- α2 antagonists
- Benzodiazepines
- Phenothiazines
- NSAIDs

Modulation (spinal cord)
- Local anesthetic
- Tricyclic antidepressants
- Cholinesterase inhibitors
- NMDA antagonists
- Opioids
- NSAIDs
- α2 antagonists
- Anticonvulsants

Transmission (sensory nerves)
- Local anesthetic
- α2 antagonists

Transmission:
1st order neuron
(primary afferent)

Transduction

Transduction (sensory nerve endings, nociceptors)
- Local anesthetics
- Opioids
- NSAIDs
- Corticosteroids

Figure 19.2 Multimodal approach to pain management. With multiple modalities each affecting different aspects of pain processing, the requirements for each drug are reduced while achieving superior effect and minimizing adverse drug effects. Source: Illustration by Marcia Schlehr.

Neuropharmacology: the tools in the toolbox

Nonsteroidal anti-inflammatory drugs

Nonsteroidal anti-inflammatory drugs (NSAIDs) are the most commonly used modalities to manage pain, and for good reason: they are highly effective, commonly available, licensed for use in dogs, and safe with proper use. Because inflammation is a prime pain-generating physiological mechanism, NSAIDs are among the most important drugs in the veterinarian's arsenal.

The primary analgesic action of a traditional NSAID results from inhibition of cyclooxygenase 2 (COX2), the membrane enzyme that metabolizes arachadonic acid and results in the production of pro-inflammatory and vasoactive prostaglandins, most specifically prostaglandin E2 (PGE2). NSAIDs also appear to inhibit central perception of pain by modulating multiple gene expression pathways (Wang *et al.*, 2007). Arachadonic acid is also metabolized by lipooxygenase (LOX) to produce leukotrienes, which attract polymorphonuclear neutrophils and promote their adherence to endothelium. The relative roles and molecular dynamics of COX and LOX enzyme variants are still being elucidated, and the optimal LOX- and COX-selective/sparing effect that maximizes effectiveness and limits toxicity remains unclear.

All veterinary NSAID products are effective, although individual patient responses vary. Their main limitation is the potential for adverse effects. COX enzymes are crucial to the production of cytoprotective prostaglandins (COX1 especially in the gastrointestinal (GI) tract and renal tubules, and PGE2 through COX2 in the GI mucosa and renal tubules), so the primary ADEs of NSAIDs include gastroduodenal erosion/ulceration and nephrotoxicity. Additional concerns include rare idiosyncratic hepatotoxicity and effects on tissue healing, and with some but not all NSAIDs, platelet function. There is conflicting evidence whether NSAID ADEs are dependent on longevity of use, in addition to the known risk factors of biological predisposition and (especially) improper use. The single greatest variable in preventing NSAID-related ADEs is the veterinarian and veterinary team, who must be aware of concurrent drug use and patient risk factors, and ensure proper use, patient monitoring, and client education. Seventy five percent of individuals reporting adverse NSAID events to the US Food and Drug Administration (FDA) hotline feel that their veterinarian did not inform them adequately of possible side effects, and/or failed to give the client the drug information sheets (Hampshire *et al.*, 2004).

Tips for use

In the transoperative setting, an edge in efficacy in both human and canine studies goes to presurgical over postsurgical use (Lascelles *et al.*, 1998). Systematic reviews in humans suggest the safety of preoperative NSAID use (Lee *et al.*, 2007), as do studies in healthy dogs, even with moderate intraoperative hypotension (Bostrom *et al.*, 2002). It is axiomatic in veterinary medicine today that patients undergoing general anesthesia should have the benefit of intravenous fluid support and blood pressure monitoring.

New drugs in class

- Grapiprant (Galliprant®) is the first in a new "priprant" class of "non-COX-inhibiting non-steroidal anti-inflammatory" drugs, approved in the United States in 2016 and launched in 2017. Instead of inhibiting COX2, it targets downstream to block the EP4 receptor, one of four "EP" receptors on cell membranes to which PGE2 binds. EP1, EP2, and EP3 are largely (but not exclusively) responsible for GI homeostasis and motility, while EP4 is largely (but not exclusively) responsible for pain and inflammation of osteoarthritis (OA) (Konya *et al.*, 2013). Thus grapiprant is most accurately described as a non-COX-inhibiting, targeted "EP4 receptor antagonist." Its pharmacology suggests anti-inflammatory, analgesic activity in OA while improving upon the adverse event (especially GI) profile so well described with traditional COX-inhibiting NSAIDs. Indeed, it has demonstrated excellent safety in young dogs even at >15× the labeled dose administered daily for 9 months (no GI erosions, ulcers, perforations, or nephrotoxicity observed; Rausch-Derra *et al.*, 2015), and in successful clinical studies of older dogs with OA (Rausch-Derra *et al.*, 2016).

- Robenacoxib (Onsior®) is a unique (coxib class) COX2 selective NSAID now approved for canine and feline perioperative use in the United States for postsurgical pain (Sackett *et al.*, 1996; King *et al.*, 2010). It has an unusually short plasma half-life in both species (<1.7 hours) yet accumulates in inflammatory exudates for over 24 hours (Silber *et al.*, 2010). Safety and toxicity data for this molecule are among the most impressive of the traditional COX2-inhibiting veterinary NSAIDs, being well tolerated in young dogs even at a dose of 20–40× the labeled dose administered daily for 1 month and 5–10× daily for 6 months. In the European Union, canine Onsior® carries a label for OA rather than postsurgical pain.

- Mavacoxib (Trocoxcil®, Europe only) is a sustained-release NSAID approved for chronic pain in dogs. Its pharmacokinetics are established in dogs with OA (Cox *et al.*, 2010) and suggest once-monthly administration. Efficacy and safety appear similar to the daily administration of other veterinary NSAIDs (Walton *et al.*, 2014; Payne-Johnson *et al.*, 2015). However, if an adverse event were to occur, treatment is complicated by the fact that the drug's effects cannot be rapidly withdrawn.

- Nitronaproxen (Naproxcinod®, Europe only for humans) is a cyclooxygenase-inhibiting nitric oxide-donating drug (CINOD) that appears to have the analgesic efficacy of the parent NSAID (Geusens, 2009) but with a greatly reduced incidence of gastropathy (Fritsch *et al.*, 2010).

Acetaminophen

Acetaminophen may elicit some of its antipyretic and analgesic properties by inhibiting one or more centrally acting COX variants (Kuo, 2006), and also appears to have central cannabinoidergic pain-modifying effects (Ghanem *et al.*, 2016). Studies suggest that peripherally it may inhibit COX2-mediated production of PGE2 in cases of mild, but not severe, inflammation (Graham *et al.*, 2013). Its postoperative pain-modifying (and possible anti-inflammatory) effects have been demonstrated clinically in dogs (Mburu *et al.*, 1988), although these studies did not use a validated acute pain clinical measurement instrument, and in a recent limited study acetaminophen did not increase mechanical thresholds (KuKanich, 2016). While the drug has somewhat lower bioavailability in dogs than other species (Nierinckx *et al.*, 2010), interestingly dogs do not produce the *N*-acetyl-*p*-benzoquinoneimine (NAPQI) metabolite responsible for hepatotoxicity in humans. Dogs do, however, produce the *para*-aminophenol metabolite that can cause methemoglobinemia and hemolysis (such as in cats, but without the lack of glucoronidase that substantially exacerbates toxicity) (McConkey *et al.*, 2009). There are no toxicity data to suggest dogs have any unusual level of adverse effects with judicious use of acetaminophen. However, chronic use cannot be advocated in dogs at this time, since long-term safety has not been established.

Tips for use

Acetaminophen can be alternated with NSAIDs, but it is recommended not to exceed 325 mg b.i.d., even for the largest dogs, or for extended use. Acetaminophen can be contraindicated in dogs exposed to methemoglobin-inducing drugs or toxins, and, more controversially, in dogs with liver dysfunction or exposed to hepatotoxic agents.

Opioids

Synthetic opioids are powerful tools to manage pain because receptors for naturally occurring opioids (endorphins, enkephalins) are distributed throughout the body and can be found in both central and peripheral tissues. Several opioid receptor types and subtypes have been isolated, each with a variant effect. The reader is guided to more comprehensive resources regarding opioid neuropharmacology and products (e.g., Epstein, 2015) but a summary follows.

Activation of a mu-opioid receptor inhibits presynaptic release of and postsynaptic response to excitatory neurotransmitters (especially in the dorsal horn of the spinal cord), hyperpolarizing second-order neurons (Barkin *et al.*, 2006). Activation of kappa receptors promotes the release of inhibitory neurotransmitters (predominantly gamma-aminobutyric acid (GABA)).

Pure mu agonists

Morphine remains the prototype opioid and in widest use. It has no ceiling effect on analgesia or respiratory depression, elicits histamine release, and in nonpainful dogs (e.g., as a premedicant) causes vomiting.

Oxymorphone (Numorphan®) and hydromorphone (Dilaudid®) do not elicit histamine release, produce somewhat less nausea, and have a shorter duration of action than morphine.

Methadone may be a parenteral opioid alternative in animals, in part due to its additional effect as an *N*-methyl-D-aspartate (NMDA) antagonist. Some veterinarians favor it as a premedication due to its effectiveness, nice sedation, and low ADE profile (minimal if any nausea, no histamine release) (Ingvast-Larsson *et al.*, 2010).

Fentanyl (Sublimaze®) is a potent short-acting opioid preparation most often used as an intravenous constant rate infusion (CRI). A transdermal patch (Duragesic®) has been used in dogs though a number of studies have demonstrated wide kinetic variability (Kyles *et al.*, 1996). The inherent liability of potential human exposure (purposeful or accidental), especially in children (deaths have occurred), must also be considered.

Oral opioids experience a robust first-pass effect in dogs (KuKanich et al., 2005), but they may not be without utility.

- Codeine: dogs do not convert codeine to morphine as in humans, but do appear to produce significant amounts of another bioactive mu-agonist metabolite, codeine-6-glucuronide. However, oral codeine in this limited study failed to raise mechanical thresholds (KuKanich, 2016).
- Hydrocodone: data in dogs are conflicting, with variable pharmacokinetics reported (some possibly favorable although there is poor conversion to hydromorphone) (KuKanich & Spade, 2013; Benitez *et al.*, 2015a).
- Oxycodone: data are extremely limited in dogs. Rectal suppository opioid formulations may also be prescribed, but appear to provide little advantage in bioavailability over the oral route in dogs (Barnhart *et al.*, 2000).

These drugs are FDA scheduled drugs, and come as separate drugs or combined with acetaminophen. However, in one study of dogs undergoing stifle surgery, oral acetaminophen + hydrocodone given without other analgesics was considered to render inadequate postoperative pain control (as was tramadol in the same study; Benitez et al., 2015b). Therefore acetaminophen + opioid must be considered strictly as an adjunctive analgesic medication to a comprehensive pain management strategy, and not as a stand-alone agent.

Partial mu agonists

Buprenorphine (Buprenex®) has greater affinity than morphine on the mu receptor and it has a ceiling effect. However, it only partially binds to the receptor, meaning it cannot have the analgesic punch of a pure or full mu agonist. Wide variation of onset and duration appears to exist in the dog, even when administered intravenously (Krotscheck et al., 2008), and may be dose-dependent. Compounded sustained-release buprenorphine formulations are available for use in dogs, but they are not FDA-approved products nor are their kinetics well established. Anecdotally, dogs seem to experience significant and prolonged sedation at doses recommended by the compounding pharmacy.

Oral transmucosal (OTM) bioavailability is modest at best in dogs (~40%; Abbo et al., 2008), and the volume required makes OTM administration mostly impractical. Commercial buprenorphine patches (e.g., BuTrans®) have compared favorably in dogs to i.v. buprenorphine in a thermal threshold model (Pieper et al., 2011) and pain scores post-ovariohysterectomy (Moll et al., 2011).

Kappa agonist/mu antagonist

Butorphanol will weakly block the mu-opioid receptor, but its kappa agonism will promote the release of inhibitory neurotransmitters such as GABA. It has a ceiling effect and a very short duration of, and effect on, visceral analgesia in the dog (~30–40 minutes; Sawyer et al., 1991; Grimm et al., 2000). This makes it a poor choice in this species for any kind of significant or protracted pain states. It does have utility in select situations such as when administered in a CRI, and as an adjunct with other medications such as alpha-2 agonists.

Mu antagonist

Naloxone (Narcan®) is a potent mu-opioid receptor antagonist, traditionally used to achieve rapid and complete reversal of opioid overdose or severe ADEs. However, microdoses (as low as 0.01–0.05 µg/kg i.v.) have been used to improve the analgesia provided by buprenorphine (La Vincente et al., 2008) and to minimize adverse effects of i.v. morphine (Cepeda et al., 2004).

New developments in other long-acting opioids including novel formulations and delivery systems may overcome the need for, and limitations of, opioid intravenous CRI, patches, and oral administration. Opioids for all their effectiveness may create clinical challenges as well. In the acute setting, opioid-induced dysphoria, nausea and inappetance, hypothermia, and, in the extreme, hyperalgesia and respiratory depression may be encountered (McNicol & Carr, 2007). Having strategies for recognizing and counteracting these signs will minimize complications. With chronic use in humans, the most commonly reported opioid ADE is constipation. New peripherally acting mu-opioid receptor antagonists (POMORAs) alvimopan (Entereg®) and methylnatrexone (Relistor®, Naloxegol®) permit the central analgesic effect of opioids but block their effect on GI motility (Gevirtz, 2007). These POMORAs have not been clinically evaluated in dogs, and although potentially helpful, their use may be limited due to the generally short duration of opioid use in animals.

Tips for use

Preoperatively, opioids are combined with an anxiolytic (tranquilizer/sedative) to create a profoundly relaxed, stress-free, and anesthetic-sparing state. The choice of opioid, route, dose, and duration of administration is dependent upon clinical preferences and patients' individual needs.

A common postoperative adverse effect of opioid use is nausea and/or inappetance. The preoperative administration of maropitant (Cerenia®) has been shown to speed recovery of appetite in dogs having received hydromorphone

(Hay Krause, 2014), and its use as a premedicant is increasingly routine. There is some evidence, however inconclusive at this time, that maropitant may have a pain-modifying effect as well (Boscan *et al.*, 2011). Treatment strategies for opioid-induced dysphoria include buprenorphine (displaces pure mu agonists from the receptor), butorphanol (antagonizes the mu receptor but activates the kappa receptor), or a microdose of dexmedetomidine; all will diminish dysphoria while maintaining some degree of analgesia.

Oral opioids are recommended for many chronic pain conditions in humans, including OA (American Pain Society, 2002), although it is now accepted that overprescription of strong oral opioids has led to serious problems of dependence and addiction. While to date there are no clinical data supporting the use of oral opioids in dogs, their intermittent, judicious use (+/− combined with acetaminophen) can be considered for dogs experiencing breakthrough pain in acute and chronic pain states, and/or as palliative end of life care.

Locoregional anesthesia

Local anesthetics (LAs) are the principal means used to reduce pain and to provide general anesthesia and concurrent analgesia; they are also used for their anti-inflammatory and antimicrobial activity (Cassuto *et al.*, 2006; Johnson *et al.*, 2008). They are considered quite safe at customary doses. Most techniques are easily mastered, and inexpensive. There no longer exists a rationale against local/regional anesthesia as part of every surgical intervention (Jones, 2008). The 2015 *AAHA/AAFP Pain Management Guidelines* stipulate that insofar as possible, LAs should be utilized with every surgical procedure (Epstein *et al.*, 2015).

LAs bind to a hydrophilic site within sodium channels, thus blockading them; without a Na$^+$ influx, neurons may not depolarize. The effect is complete anesthesia to a site rather than analgesia. Different LAs will have variable onsets, durations of action, and toxicities. A general limitation of LAs is a relatively short duration (hours) of action. This can be overcome in a variety of ways, including the addition of a small amount of opioid (Bazin *et al.*, 1997)

or alpha-2 agonist (Hu *et al.*, 2017) to the LA, and the use of wound diffusion catheters. In 2017, a novel liposome-encapsulated bupivacaine product (Nocita®) was introduced for dogs, labeled for 3 days of postsurgical analgesia.

LA is limited only by the clinician's ability to learn various techniques and anatomic landmarks. Blocks include: local line or paraincisional; subcutaneous infiltrative; intrapleural, intra-abdominal; retrobulbar; intratesticular, intra-articular, carpal ring, epidural, sacrococcygeal, dental (orofacial), brachial plexus, intercostal, paravertebral, and wound diffusion catheters. A rapidly expanding modality is the use of ultrasound and nerve electrolocator devices to enhance precision and dose in perineural delivery for peripheral nerve blockade. Comprehensive discussions of the many techniques are now available (Campoy & Read, 2013; Lerche *et al.*, 2016).

Tips for use

The edge in efficacy goes to preoperative use (Savvas *et al.*, 2008), but infiltration of LAs postincisionally can be effective. To minimize the sting of administration in awake patients, the LA is warmed to body temperature and injected slowly (Hogan *et al.*, 2011); mepivacaine appears to elicit less sting than either lidocaine or bupivacaine. Diluting the LA (with saline to increase the volume for large infiltrative areas) will slow the onset and shorten the duration of action.

Toxicity is most likely to occur when administration occurs at very large doses and/or intravenously (which must be avoided with the potentially cardiotoxic bupivacaine). LAs can result in motor as well as sensory blockade (a special consideration with epidurals). There is little clinical evidence to support the belief that LAs impair wound healing or promote postop infection—in fact LAs are antimicrobial.

To facilitate catheter placement or other minor skin procedures, a transdermal LA formulation, EMLA®, that also comes as a generic, LMX4, may be placed on a shaved area and covered with a bioadhesive dressing or other nonporous wrap (e.g., foil). Although penetration has been reported to be time-dependent (Wahlgren & Quiding, 2000), 20 minutes appears sufficient in canine patients.

Commercial 5% lidocaine patches (Lidoderm®) are labeled for humans with postherpetic neuralgia (shingles), but have been described for postoperative paraincisional analgesia in dogs (Weil *et al.*, 2007), with minimal systemic absorption noted (Weiland *et al.*, 2006). The adhesive patches can be cut to the desired size and shape. One cautionary note is that an entire patch contains 700 mg of lidocaine, a toxic dose if ingested; therefore, adequate precautions must be taken.

Intravenous lidocaine

There is evidence in humans for intravenous lidocaine's (IVL) anesthetic-sparing effect, and its ability to speed the return of bowel function, decrease postoperative pain, minimize opioid consumption, and shorten the hospital stay after abdominal surgery (Groudine *et al.*, 1998). Evidence in dogs is somewhat weaker at this point (MacDougall *et al.*, 2009), although there may be a synergistic effect with other drugs. Formulas for a combination morphine, lidocaine, and ketamine i.v. CRI have been described for dogs (Muir *et al.*, 2003). The combination is profoundly analgesic, fairly sedating, and is superior for the most painful postoperative states. IVL has also been shown to elicit a sustained effect on neuropathic pain in humans (Cahana *et al.*, 1998).

Other drugs in class

• Mexilitine is an oral sodium-channel blocker, often called oral lidocaine and labeled for use as a cardiac antiarrhythmic. It has also been used to treat chemotherapy-induced neuropathic pain states in humans (Egashira *et al.*, 2010). Its utility for chronic pain conditions in dogs is unestablished.

Subanesthetic ketamine constant rate infusion

NMDA receptor antagonism remains a research focus for pain in humans (Fisher *et al.*, 2000). Ketamine is a dissociative anesthetic that binds to a phencyclidine receptor inside the NMDA

receptor (i.e., the calcium channel would already have to be open and active for ketamine to exert its effect). Once bound, it decreases the channel's opening time and frequency, thus reducing Ca^+ ion influx and dampening secondary intracellular signaling cascades. It appears to be protective against hyperalgesia and central hypersensitization in the postoperative setting (Hocking *et al.*, 2007), including in the dog (Slingsby & Waterman-Pearson, 2000), and the evidence in humans is strong for its pain-preventive effects when given intravenously as a CRI at subanesthetic doses. Ideal subanesthetic ketamine plasma concentrations in the dog have been reported at 2–3 µg/mL, which can be achieved by administering ketamine i.v. CRI at 10 µg/kg/min (Boscan *et al.*, 2005). The 2015 *AAHA/AAFP Pain Management Guidelines* state that clinicians should consider the modality as part of a multimodal approach to transoperative pain management, especially in patients at risk for maladaptive pain (Epstein *et al.*, 2015). Such patient populations include, but are not limited to, those with nerve injury (including iatrogenic, e.g., amputation), severe tissue trauma (surgical or otherwise), and with long-standing inflammation (e.g., OA) or pre-existing chronic pain condition.

Tips for use

The recommended intraoperative rate can be accomplished by placing 60 mg (0.6 mL of 100 mg/mL stock) ketamine in 1 L of fluids administered at intraoperative rates of 10 mL/kg/h. Postoperatively, the rate can be reduced to maintenance rates of 2 mL/kg/h, which administers the ketamine CRI at 2 µg/kg/min. A loading dose of 0.25–0.5 mg/kg ketamine i.v. is recommended prior to the initiation of the CRI in order to rapidly achieve plasma levels.

Alpha-2 agonist

Medetomidine and dexmedetomidine bind to opioid-like receptors on C- and A-delta fibers, especially in the central nervous system. Binding presynaptically, norepinephrine production is reduced and sedation occurs; binding postsynaptically, analgesia is produced, and is profoundly synergistic with opioids. It also blocks norepinephrine receptors on blood vessels, resulting in vasoconstriction. The resulting hypertension parasympathetically induces bradycardia, which is extended by a subsequent direct decrease in sympathetic tone. Cardiac index is decreased, although central perfusion is maintained. Many uses are described for the perioperative setting, usually in combination with opioids and at doses much lower than suggested by the manufacturer.

Tips for use

Intravenous microdoses (0.25–1.0 µg/kg)of dexmedetomidine intra- and postoperatively can address rocky anesthetic episodes, postop pain, or dysphoria. This calculates to tiny volumes even in large dogs, and although the effect at these doses may last only 10–15 minutes, it may be re-dosed to effect. CRI doses are also described (Valtolina et al., 2009). In the event a concerning degree of bradycardia arises, anticholinergics (atropine, glycopyrolate) should be avoided as they will increase heart rate, against tremendous vascular resistance, with potentially serious consequences. Instead, atipamezole is used to reverse the bradycardia.

Other drugs in class

- Tizanadine (Zanaflex®, Sirdalud ®) is an oral, centrally acting alpha-2 agonist used in humans primarily as a skeletal muscle relaxant to treat muscle spasticity, and the pain derived from it, in multiple sclerosis and a variety of other painful conditions. Its utility in dogs is unknown.
- Clonidine is a centrally acting alpha-2 agonist that can be administered systemically via oral, i.v., s.c., i.m., transdermal, and epidural routes. Indicated in humans as antihypertensive agent and to treat ADHD, new uses are being found for its antinociceptive effects (Neil, 2011).

Pain-modifying analgesic drugs

Tramadol (Ultram®) is a popular analgesic that in humans breaks down into a highly active mu-agonist opioid (M1) metabolite along with a separate metabolite with serotonin and norepinephrine (inhibitory neurotransmitters) agonism. However, dogs produce very little of the M1 metabolite (Kögel et al., 2014), and what little they make has a very short half-life (1.7 hours) (KuKanich & Papich, 2004). Studies have demonstrated the clinical usefulness of parenteral (i.v., i.m., s.c., epidural) tramadol in dogs (Martins et al., 2010; Seddighi et al., 2009), although presumptively it would not be elicited via mu agonism but rather via the separate metabolite that enhances the inhibitory neurotransmitters serotonin and norepinephrine. Although oral tramadol is a popular adjunct to chronic pain management in humans (Wilder-Smith et al., 2001), its pharmacokinetics in dogs is poor (low plasma levels that decrease to negligible levels after sequential administration over several days) (Malek et al., 2012). There is no strong evidence to suggest any kind of significant pain-modifying effect in dogs. Problems of abuse and diversion in humans have cause the FDA to move tramadol to a Schedule IV status.

Tips for use

Note that adverse drug effects can include GI and extrapyramidal effects.

Other drugs in class

- Tapentadol (Nucytna®) is a centrally acting analgesic with a dual mode of action similar to tramadol: mu-opioid receptor agonism and inhibition of norepinephrine reuptake. It is the parent compound, not a metabolite, that provides both of these effects, and thus it may offer an alternative superior to tramadol in dogs. Unfortunately, recent data reveal low bioavailability in dogs (only 4%) (Young, 2008; Giorgi et al., 2012), and poor performance on a tail-flick analgesia model (Therapeutic Goods Administration, 2011). A more recent study of tapentadol reveals, in contradistinction to tramadol, analgesia in a canine tail-flick model, attributable to an opioid effect of the parent compound otherwise absent with tramadol or its metabolites (Kögel et al., 214). Tapentadol has not been evaluated clinically in dogs.

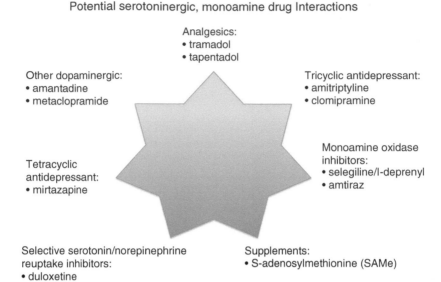

Figure 19.3   Many compounds and chemicals may involve serotoninergic or monoaminergic (especially dopamine) mechanisms, and caution and/or judicious use should be exercised when using them in combination.

See Figure 19.3 for cautions regarding possible serotoninergic drug interactions.

Gabapentin

Gabapentin is labeled as an anticonvulsant drug, yet has become popular in human medicine for many chronic and neuropathic pain conditions (Backonja & Glanzman, 2003). While structurally similar to GABA, it is not a direct agonist; it appears to exert its effect mostly by downregulating voltage-gated calcium channels (Longmire et al., 2006). Its utility in the transoperative setting is supported by a number of systematic reviews (Clivatti et al., 2009; Dauri et al., 2009). Pharmacokinetic studies in dogs reveal that it has a half-life of 3–4 hours (Vollmer et al., 1986), suggesting t.i.d. administration. The primary adverse effect in dogs and humans appears to be somnolescence.

There is no literature to support gabapentin as an adjunctive treatment for OA in dogs or humans, but such literature does exist in rodents. There are a number of case reports describing the successful use of gabapentin in dogs experiencing neuropathic pain (Plessas et al., 2015), and a hypersensitization compo-

nent appears to be present in at least 25% of humans with OA (de Luca et al., 2016). This may explain the increasingly widespread and anecdotally successful use of gabapentin for OA in dogs. Interestingly, a gabapentin analog reduced the development of experimental OA in rodents (Boileau et al., 2005). Gabapentin should be considered for other maladaptive and neuropathic pain states encountered in veterinary medicine.

Tips for use

To avoid drowsiness, a starting dose of 3–5 mg/kg b.i.d. or t.i.d. is recommended for chronic pain. As the patient acclimates, the dose is increased gradually to a target of 10–20 mg/kg b.i.d.. For surgical pain, starting doses are higher (e.g., 10 mg/kg), with one dose administered preoperatively and one to three doses administered in the postoperative period; slight drowsiness does not seem to impede appetite or other daily functions.

Other drugs in class

- Pregabalin (Lyrica®), a gabapentin-like compound, is labeled in humans for pain associated with diabetic neuropathy and postherpetic neuralgia, with a superior kinetic profile to gabapentin (does not require dose escalations). Its utility in dogs remains unknown but it would be expected to have a similar, if not more predictable, effect to gabapentin. A pharmacokinetic-based dose has been proposed for dogs (Salazar *et al.*, 2009). It is an FDA controlled (and rather expensive) drug and a generic version will not be available until after 2018.

- Topiramate (Topamax®) is an anticonvulsant drug in common use for chronic migraine headaches in humans, and with evidence of efficacy for other chronic pain conditions such as lower back pain (Muehlbacher *et al.*, 2006). Studies have established the pharmacokinetics in dogs and one study looked at its use in a canine neuropathic pain disease; improvement was shown but was less effective and had more adverse effects than gabapentin (Plessas *et al.*, 2015).
- Ziconotide (Prialt ®) is a voltage-gated calcium channel blocker that was designed for intrathecal use only. It represents a new class of drug and therapeutic intervention for long-standing severe neuropathic pain in humans (Schmidtko *et al.*, 2010).

Amantadine

Amantadine is an antiviral compound with weak dopaminergic effects, and is reported to exert an analgesic effect through NMDA receptor antagonism (Plumb, 2011). It is the only drug shown to be an effective adjunct to NSAIDs in canine OA, with improved pain scores when the NSAID was combined with amantadine, versus NSAIDs alone (Lascelles *et al.*, 2007). Toxicity and kinetic studies have been performed in humans (Vernier *et al.*, 1969), but not in dogs.

Tips for use

The customary dose in dogs is 3–5 mg/kg s.i.d., but pharmacokinetics suggest a b.i.d. schedule as more rational (Moore, 2016). Agitation, tremors, and diarrhea are adverse effects reported anecdotally.

Other drugs in class

- Orphenadrine, an anti-Parkinson's NMDA-R antagonist blocks voltage-gated sodium channels in the dorsal root ganglion and has demonstrated analgesic action in chronic pain states (Desaphy *et al.*, 2009). Experience in animals is limited.

See Figure 19.3 for cautions regarding possible monoamine drug interactions.

Tricyclic antidepressants

Tricyclic antidepressants (TCAs) exert their analgesic activity by blocking norepinephrine and serotonin (5-HT) reuptake in the dorsal horn, allowing these inhibitory neurotransmitters to exert a prolonged and more pronounced effect. Since clinical depression is also partially mediated through norepinephrine and serotonin, patients may enjoy the benefit of TCAs from these coexisting mechanisms. Additional effects include interaction with NMDA activity and sodium channel blockade. As a class, TCAs are a first-line medication for neuropathic pain in humans (Finnerup *et al.*, 2005). Amitriptyline is the most commonly used TCA in humans, primarily for diabetic neuropathy (Longmire *et al.*, 2006), and is used in animals primarily for chronic feline interstitial cystitis (Chew *et al.*, 1998). The pharmacokinetics of amitryptiline have been evaluated in dogs (Norkus *et al.*, 2015), and there is one published report of its use in a case of neuropathic pain (Cashmore et al., 2009). In humans, despite the efficacy of TCAs in treating neuropathic pain, the adverse effect profile often limits its use. Anecdotally in dogs, suggested doses of up to 3–4 mg/kg b.i.d. seem to be well tolerated (KuKanich, 2013).

Other drugs in class

- Cyclobenzaprine (Flexeril®) is a muscle relaxant with a chemical structure similar to TCAs, and is used in humans for fibromyalgia and pain associated with muscle spasm and myofascial trigger points.

See Figure 19.3 for cautions regarding possible serotoninergic drug interactions.

Selective serotonin reuptake inhibitors and selective serotonin norepinephrine reuptake inhibitors

Serotonin and norepinephrine reuptake inhibitors (SSRIs and SSNRIs, respectively) come in various degrees of selectivity for these inhibitory neurotransmitters. Most are labeled as antidepressants, revealing the shared pathways and well-established comorbidity of depression and chronic pain. Newer SSRIs and SSNRIs such as milnacipran (Savella®) and duloxetine (Cymbalta®) have been developed for chronic neuropathic pain states in humans. Duloxetine's label has expanded from treatment of diabetic neuropathy, postherpetic neuralgia, and fibromyalgia to include OA and low back pain. Pharmacokinetic studies of duloxetine in dogs are conflicting. The European Medicines Agency (2005) found very low bioavailability (Patel *et al.*, 2011; KuKanich, 2013), yet a more recent study suggested a dose-dependent increase of plasma levels equivalent to those found in humans (Baek *et al.*, 2013). Another SNRI, venlafaxine, has demonstrated efficacy in human OA (Sullivan *et al.*, 2009), and in dogs appears to have approximately 50% oral bioavailability (Howell *et al.*, 1994). While no clinical studies exist regarding use of any SNRIs in canine OA, both duloxetine and venlafaxine come as non-controlled generics and may hold possible promise in that area.

Fluoxetine (Prozac®), an SSRI, reveals a less robust impact on chronic pain in humans, suggesting that it is the noradrenergic more than the serotoninergic effect that elicits the most significant pain-modifying effect. Some studies suggest the possible efficacy of fluoxetine for OA in humans (Chappell *et al.*, 2011), and its relative safety margin and low expense may make fluoxetine a consideration in some dogs with OA or other chronic pain states. As veterinarians can neither classify nor diagnose clinical depression in dogs, we cannot know to what degree any clinical response to these drugs might be attributed to improved comfort versus improved state of mind or both.

Other drugs in class

- Trazadone (with many trade names) is an antidepressant serotonin antagonist and reuptake inhibitor (SARI) gaining some utility as an adjunct to SSRIs, opioids, and anticonvulsants for an anxiolytic, tranquilizing, and relaxant effect (Calandre *et al.*, 2011). Its properties as an analgesic are less certain but in humans its off-label use for some neuropathic pain conditions has been reported.

See Figure 19.3 for cautions regarding possible serotoninergic drug interactions.

Anxiolytics

Anxiety contributes directly to the hyperalgesic state through cholecystikinin-mediated nocebo effect (Benedetti *et al.*, 2006). Many studies support the clinical relevance of this in humans, and in animals as well where restraint, social defeat, and rotation (all common veterinary patient experiences) contribute to hyperalgesia (Martenson *et al.*, 2009). The first leg of a strong transoperative pain management protocol involves the use of anxiolytics (i.e., tranquilizers/sedatives). Clinicians may choose between phenothiazines (e.g., acepromazine), benzodiazepines (midazolam or diazepam), or alpha-2 agonists (dex/medetomidine). Additional but significant mindfulness should be granted towards non-pharmacological patient-calming strategies: well-established low-stress and fear-free handling techniques, a patient setting including the use of facial pheromones, the influence of smell and noise, and the benefit of human voice and touch.

Disease-modifying osteoarthritic agents

Disease-modifying osteoarthritic agents (DMOAAs) may not have a primary analgesic mechanism of action, but still have a positive influence on OA in terms of reducing pain and slowing progression of the disease. The only veterinary FDA-approved drug in this category is Adequan®, a polysulfated glycosaminoglycan (PSGAG). PSGAGs inhibit degradative enzymes such as collagenase and metalloproteinases, and reportedly promote the formation of fibrocartilage (Altman *et al.*, 1989; Fujiki *et al.*, 2007), with additional studies that support efficacy. CartrophenVet® is a PSGAG available outside the United States.

Tips for use

The molecule is distantly related to heparin and should be administered cautiously in patients with known bleeding dyscrasias; some clinicians discontinue use prior to surgical procedures. Common off-label applications include chronic use and administration via the subcutaneous route allowing it to be dispensed for administration at home; this improves acceptance by decreasing cost and inconvenience.

Other investigative drugs and targets

- Capsaicin (resiniferatoxin (RTX); Adlea™) is used as a neuroablative in humans with intractable pain conditions (Karai *et al.*, 2004). Some work with this modality has also been done in dogs with osteosarcoma (Brown *et al.*, 2005) and may provide an additional utility in the future.
- Cannabinoid receptor agonists. Centrally located CB2 receptor activity elicits hypoalgesia, and efforts are underway to produce a selective molecule with demonstrable efficacy without psychotropic effect. This modality holds promise in dogs, but it is difficult to recommend despite increasing availability of medicinal and recreational marijuana until more data are available in this species.
- Substance P/neurokinin-1 (NK-1) antagonists. Maripotant (Cerenia®) is an antiemetic approved for use in dogs, and was found to have outcomes equivalent to pre-anesthetic morphine in dogs undergoing ovariohysterectomy (Marquez *et al.*, 2015). However, this molecule failed in human trials as a pain-modifying agent and its true analgesic effect in dogs remains uncertain.
- Glial inhibitors: minocycline, +-nalaxone, and ibudilast have glial inhibitory effects. Glial inhibition may become an essential adjunct to opioid therapy to minimize tolerance, reduce adverse effects, and enhance potency.
- Anti-nerve growth factor (NGF) antibody. NGF contributes to hypersensitization and upregulates in chronic pain. A pilot study using an injectable canine-specific anti-NGF monoclonal antibody product in dogs with

OA revealed improvement for 1 month, similar to that expected with NSAIDs, with no adverse effects (Lascelles *et al.*, 2015).

- Biological therapies (see Chapter 16). Great attention is currently being given to the use of various cell- or other blood-derived preparations, generally for intra-articular injection, but also being explored for use in chronic tendinopathies (Canapp *et al.*, 2016a). The mechanisms of action may be variable and not completely understood, but seem to generally involve the activation of endogenous growth factors and anti-inflammatory cytokines, and the suppression of catabolic and pro-inflammatory cytokines. Evidence so far appears to be generally favorable for each of these preparations, but studies are still relatively few in number and limited by widely variable methodologies of collection, processing, cost, quality control, invasiveness, application, outcome measures, and unknown highest or wisest utility for a given clinical condition. Such biological therapies include:

  ○ Stem cell transplantation: the current technique involves harvesting of autologous adipose tissue and isolation of its mesenchymal stem cells (Vilar *et al.*, 2014) through various commercial systems that vary widely in technique and quality control, then reinjecting the cells into the same patient's joint or tendon. Cells can be banked or cultured for repeat transplantation. A newer technology under investigation uses allogeneic stem cells from a universal canine donor population (Harman et al., 2016).
  ○ Stromal vascular fraction (SVF): the non-cellular portion collected in the process of harvesting and isolating autologous adipose-derived mesenchymal stem cells (Upchurch *et al.*, 2016).
  ○ Platelet-rich plasma (PRP): collected from patients' blood through any of several gravity or centrifugation methods (Fahie *et al.*, 2013), with widely variable characteristics, the ideal of which is not at all known (Franklin *et al.*, 2015). One recent study also suggests a role in possible protective effect in partial canine cruciate injury (Canapp *et al.*, 2016b).

Two different PRP derivative products include: (1) autologous protein solution (APS), which is produced by passing a whole-blood solution over polyacrylamide beads to extract and concentrate therapeutic cytokines; it contains leukocytes (Franklin *et al.*, 2015); and (2) autologous conditioned plasma (ACP), which is leuko-reduced PRP (Franklin & Cook, 2013).

Management of acute pain

There exists a general consensus, supported by best evidence, for the four basic elements that contribute to optimal patient management for the prevention and treatment of postoperative pain. Thereafter, clinicians employ an array of adjunctive pain-modifying pharmacological interventions, each with evidence to make them worthy of clinical consideration.

The basic four elements are:

(1)   Anxiolytics: Pharmacological and non-pharmacological strategies (e.g., low-stress, fear-free environment)
(2)   NSAIDs
(3)   Opioids
(4)   Local anesthetics.

The best of the rest

(1)   Topical dermal/epidermal local anesthetic:
    (a)   Transdermal lidocaine ± prilocain for i.v. catheter placement
    (b)   Lidoderm® patch: applied para-incisionally to especially painful sites for up to 5 days; bandaging is necessary to prevent ingestion.
(2)   Subanesthetic ketamine CRI: Especially in patients at risk for maladaptive pain (nerve injury, significant tissue damage, pre-existing inflammatory conditions, e.g., OA).
(3)   Cold compression: The beneficial effects of cooling damaged tissue should not be underestimated, diminishing inflammation and pain through a variety of proposed mechanisms. Even modest application to injured soft tissue has been shown to reduce pain and speed return to function (Drygas *et al.*, 2011).
(4)   Pain-modifying analgesic drugs: For patients whose procedure may generate more significant pain, or comes to experience unexpected pain:
    (a)   Gabapentin
    (b)   Acetaminophen + hydrocodone or codeine
    (c)   ± Tramadol.

Case Study 19.1   Thoracic limb amputation

Signalment: 4-y.o. M/C 20 kg lab mix undergoing thoracic limb amputation due to ischemic injury.

History:

(1)   Already on NSAID from previous injury; morning dose administered preadmission, along with gabapentin 100 mg p.o.
(2)   Morphine-acepromazine s.c. premedication; catheter i.v. area clipped and topical EMLA® applied
(3)   Intravenous catheter placed; i.v. bolus of ketamine 5 mg and Normosol-R w/ 60 mg/L ketamine administered 200 mL/h
(4)   Propofol induction; isoflurane maintenance
(5)   Brachial plexus block w/ nerve locator: 25 mg of 0.5% bupivacaine (5 mL) + 0.1 mL morphine
(6)   During closure, placement of 5 Fr diffusion catheter s.c., exiting dorsal to incision line; *or:*

layered s.c. application of Nocita® (liposome-encapsulated bupivacaine).

Postoperative management:

(1)   Cold compression applied to incision site
(2)   IVF w/ ketamine CRI 50 mL/h × 24 hours
(3)   If wound diffusion catheter used instead of Nocita®: bupivacaine 0.5% 5 mL + 0.1 mL morphine through diffusion catheter q8h for 32 hours (removed prior to discharge at end of day 1 postop)
(4)   Gabapentin 100 mg p.o. q8h × 3 days
(5)   Therapeutic laser and/or acupuncture if available
(6)   NSAIDs continued for 7 days
(7)   Rehabilitation to facilitate return to function on three legs.

Chronic pain

Osteoarthritis

The most common chronic pain condition recognized in dogs, OA, also presents one of the greatest challenges to treatment because of its progressive pathology and difficulty in early recognition. Indeed, in contradistinction to humans, canine OA is largely conformational in origin, meaning the inflammatory and degenerative process begins at a very early age—as young as puppies. We must begin to conceive of canine OA as a lifetime disease, subtly symptomatic in patients long before they are obviously symptomatic to us, and initiate preventative and therapeutic measures far earlier in life than we are usually accustomed. Furthermore, OA is increasingly recognized as a maladaptive if not abjectly neuropathic pain state (present in 25% of human knee OA patients) (Hochman *et al.*, 2011).

The pain of OA is felt less at the damaged articular surfaces than in the periarticular structures: an inflamed synovium, tension on a fibrotic joint capsule, and exertion on weakened ligaments, tendons, and muscle. OA is a disease of the entire joint organ, and indeed of the entire musculoskeletal system as the patient shifts weight to other limbs, and treatment has to be targeted accordingly.

Given the variable biological nature of OA, paucity of properly designed multimodal treatment studies in dogs, and widely divergent client and veterinarian values, difficulty exists in formulating a standard approach. Yet it is possible to point out where the evidence is strongest and the neurophysiological/pharmacological rationale the most compelling. Note that of the top five modalities from an evidence-based perspective, at least three of them are non-pharmacological in nature. It is not all about drugs!

(1) NSAIDs: An abundance of literature in humans and dogs, as well as two systematic reviews of treatments for canine OA, reveal this class of drug to be, by far, the most predictably effective therapy. The new piprant class of anti-inflammatory, analgesic drugs are included here. The new EP-4 receptor antagonist Galliprant® may be alternatively used.

(2) PSGAGs (Adequan®, CartrophenVet®) and/or nutraceuticals (see Chapter 4).

(3) Weight optimization: This is the primary preventative method to slow the development of OA in dogs (Smith *et al.*, 2006), and is imperative if the patient is already overweight. The role of adipose tissue as a mediator of systemic inflammation, the contribution of central obesity to chronic pain in humans (doubling the risk for it; Ray *et al.*, 2011), and the primacy of weight loss (just 6% in dogs) to diminish OA pain is established (Marshall *et al.*, 2010). With an overweight patient, both the clinician and client are wasting time, energy, and money on other interventions until and unless weight optimization is achieved.

(4) Eicosapentaenoic acid-rich diet (Mehler *et al.*, 2016): These formulations have been demonstrated in several studies to elicit improved gait, mobility, and an NSAID-sparing effect.

(5) Physical rehabilitation, one cornerstone of which is therapeutic exercise. Controlled exercise elicits hypoalgesia through a variety of mechanisms: gate theory (spinal-level blockade of nociceptive signaling in favor of touch, pressure, and proprioception); activation of the endogenous cannabinoid system; increased strength and microstability of joint soft tissue structures; and promoting weight optimization.

(6) Pain-modifying analgesic drugs: One or more of the following:
    (a) Amantadine
    (b) Gabapentin or pregabelin
    (c) ± Tramadol.

(7) New drugs to consider:
    (a) Duloxetine or venlafaxine
    (b) Tapentadol
    (c) Acetaminophen + hydrocodone or codeine (breakthrough pain only)
    (d) Biological therapies (intra-articular PRP, stem cell transplantation, stromal vascular fraction, autologous conditioned serum).

Case Study 19.2 Older patient with mild hip dysplasia and previous surgery for left cranial cruciate ligament deficiency with advancing stifle and hip osteoarthritis

Signalment: 12-y.o. F/S, 40 kg Labrador Retriever w/ BCS 7/9 bilateral hip dysplasia, unilateral stifle injury and clinical signs of mild OA in hips and moderate to severe OA in left stifle.

Management:
First 30 days:

(1) Traditional veterinary NSAID or Galliprant® (non-COX-inhibiting EP4 receptor antagonist)
(2) Weight loss diet/program
(3) Adequan® s.c. (off–label route) induction period: Twice weekly × 4 weeks
(4) Implement at-home therapeutic exercise program
(5) Acupuncture and/or physical modality if available and client consents
(6) Consider intra-articular injection of biological product (e.g., platelet-rich plasma, stem cell transplantation) at least for stifle.

Day 30: Re-evaluate and:

(1) Consider attempting modest (25%) reduction of NSAID or Galliprant® dose (efficacy or utility to minimize ADEs unknown)
(2) Continue with weight loss diet/program
(3) Taper frequency of Adequan® (off-label), targeting once monthly
(4) If patient making inadequate progress, consider addition of:
  (a) Adjunctive pain-modifying analgesic drugs (PMADs): gabapentin (200 mg p.o. b.i.d.) or amantadine (200 mg p.o. s.i.d.)
  (b) Proceed with intra-articular injection of biological agent (stifle at least, hips if possible)
  (c) Referral if available to certified canine rehabilitation therapist (CCRT) or practitioner

(CCRP) for formal rehabilitation/strengthening program
  (d) Oral neutraceuticals (that include avocado soy unsaponifiables (ASU), methylsulfonylmethane (MSM), etc.).

Days 60–90: Re-evaluate and:

(1) If weight optimized, switch to eicosapentaenoic acid (EPA)-rich diet
(2) Can consider attempting another 25% dose reduction of NSAID, or decrease frequency to every other day (efficacy or utility to minimize ADEs unknown)
(3) Further taper Adequan® to frequency based on patient's needs
(4) Continue oral neutraceuticals and adjunctive PMAD medication but dose/schedule adjustments:
  (a) Amantadine: attempt frequency decrease to EOD
  (b) Gabapentin: may need to taper to dose upward to target of 300–600 mg p.o. b.i.d.

Day 90+: If patient has responded well:

(1) Continue EPA-rich diet
(2) Continue Adequan® on lowest-frequency basis:
  (a) Continue oral neutraceuticals and adjunctive PMAD medications but dose/schedule adjustments
  (b) Amantadine: attempt frequency decrease to EOD
  (c) Gabapentin: can attempt dose or frequency reduction
(3) NSAID: Can attempt another dose reduction, or attempt to trial EOD, prn, or withdrawal.

Other non-cancer chronic pain

Many non-OA, non-cancer chronic pain conditions exist in dogs, and most cause, or are likely to cause, neuropathic pain (Mathews, 2008). These include central nervous system lesions of any type (including trauma, intervertebral disc disease, congenital defects, meningoencephalitides); peripheral nerve injury (trauma, amputation, fractures); as well as inflammatory bowel disease and pancreatitis.

As inflammation is a component of the underlying pathology activating nociceptive pathways, NSAIDs can be considered first-line drugs. However, in a neuropathic state, NSAIDs may be expected to contribute a less robust analgesic effect, leaving room for other classes of pain-modifying drugs to occupy a more central treatment role.

Systematic reviews of neuropathic pain in humans (Finnerup *et al.*, 2015) recommend a treatment algorithm, regardless of etiology, that includes as first choice drugs: TCAs, SNRIs, and gabapentin/pregabelin. These papers are drawn mainly from trials involving diabetic neuropathy and post-herpetic neuralgia, leaving the relevance in animals uncertain.

(1) Pain-modifying analgesic drugs:
   (a) Gabapentin or pregabelin
   (b) TCAs, e.g., amitriptyline
   (c) Amantadine
   (d) ± Tramadol
   (e) New drugs to consider:
      (i) duloxetine, venlafaxine
      (ii) tapentadol
   (f) Acetaminophen + hydrocodone or codeine (breakthrough pain only).
(2) NSAIDs
(3) Weight optimization.

Cancer pain

Osteosarcoma, and any cancer metastatic to bone, is one of the most painful chronic pain conditions a dog may encounter. This is due to a combination of unique factors including upregulation of COX enzymes, osteoclast-induced necrosis, lymphatic obstruction, and bioactive, pro-inflammatory cytokines that sustain and enhance the nociceptive pathways in ways distinct from other sorts of chronic inflammatory conditions. When clients have opted for palliative care, it is likely that the patient's pain will be the terminal event. For this reason, it is warranted to access the entire pain-modulating arsenal. The prospect of drug–ADE interaction exists, but since the risk of undermanaging the disease's pain is death (euthanasia), aggressive multimodal polypharmacy pain management is warranted. The International Veterinary Academy of Pain Management (IVAPM) adopted a position/consensus statement supporting the primacy of wise, rational use of pain management medications over the hypothetical fear of ADE in palliative care situations.

A recent review in human literature using a number needed to treat : number needed to harm ratio (NNT:NNH) cited gabapentin, pregabelin, and strong opioids as the most effective and best-tolerated drugs in cancer-related pain, while amitriptyline, tramadol, and NSAIDs elicited more minor effects or an unfavorable safety profile (Tassinari et al., 2011).

(1) NSAIDs: The antineoplastic effects of certain NSAIDs in humans (Gupta & Dubois, 2001) and in dogs (Knapp et al., 1994) have been well established and appear to be mediated through the upregulation of the COX2 enzymes in some neoplasms of these species (Mohammed et al., 2004).

(2) Opioids: Fentanyl (Duragesic®) and buprenorphine (e.g., BuTrans®) patches are labeled precisely for use in cancer breakthrough pain in humans. In dogs one must be mindful that the veterinarian could be liable if a human was exposed to the drug during its use for the canine patient. While the long-term use of oral opioids in animals is currently limited, they would be indicated in this patient population.

(3) Pain-modifying analgesic drugs:
   (a) Gabapentin or pregabelin
   (b) TCAs, e.g., amitriptyline
   (c) Acetaminophen ± hydrocodone or codeine
   (d) Amantadine: though not studied in humans for cancer pain, its NMDA-R antagonist activity makes its consideration worthy
   (e) ± Tramadol
   (f) Additional drugs to consider:
      (i) duloxetine, venlafaxine
      (ii) tapentadol
      (iii) mexilitine—for chemotherapy-induced neuropathic pain.

(4) Bisphosphonates: Compounds that may palliatively alleviate osteosarcoma-related pain by decreasing osteoclast activity, with pamidronate in most common use for dogs (Fan et al., 2005). Intravenous infusions are administered in patients not undergoing amputation and chemotherapy. Anecdotally, 60% of dogs will be responsive within a week, and in about half of those the effect will be durable (i.e., >4 months). It appears to be most effective when administered as part of multimodal therapy (Lorimier, L. P., personal communication). Nephrotoxicosis is reported to be a limiting adverse effect.

(5) Lidoderm® patch: Used with anecdotal success and considered safe due to very little systemic absorption. However, the patch must be secured properly to prevent ingestion.

Webliography

European Medicines Agency. 2005. Document reference: Doc.Ref.:EMEA/590296/2008. http://www.ema.europa.eu/docs/en_GB/document_library/EPAR_-_Scientific_Discussion/human/000572/WC500036776.pdf.

International Veterinary Academy of Pain Management (IVAPM). http://iavpm.org.

Therapeutic Goods Administration. 2011. Australian Public Assessment Report of Tapentadol. Table 1: Minimal efficacious doses in various animal pain models, p9. https://www.tga.gov.au/sites/default/files/auspar-palexia-sr.pdf.

Young, K. 2008. FDA Center for Drug Evaluation and Research: Tapentadol, Application No. 22-304. Section 3.3.5 Metabolism, p60-62. https://www.accessdata.fda.gov/drugsatfda_docs/nda/2008/022304s000_MedR_P1.pdf.

All websites accessed November 2017.

References

Abbo, L. A., Ko, J. C., Maxwell, L. K., Galinsky, R. E., Moody, D. E., Johnson, B. M. & Fang, W. B. 2008. Pharmacokinetics of buprenorphine following intravenous and oral transmucosal administration in dogs. *Vet Ther*, 9, 83–93.

Altman, R. D., Dean, D. D., Muniz, O. E. & Howell, D. S. 1989. Therapeutic treatment of canine osteoarthritis with glycosaminoglycan polysulfuric acid ester. *Arthritis Rheum*, 32, 1300–1307.

AMERICAN PAIN SOCIETY. 2002. *Guideline for the Management of Pain in Osteoarthritis, Rheumatoid Arthritis, and Juvenile Chronic Arthritis*, 2nd edn. Glenview, IL: APS.

Anand, K. J. S. & Hickey, P. R. 1992. Halothane–morphine compared with high-dose sufentanil for anesthesia and postoperative analgesia in neonatal cardiac surgery. *New England Journal of Medicine*, 326, 1–9.

Backonja, M. & Glanzman, R. L. 2003. Gabapentin dosing for neuropathic pain: evidence from randomized, placebo-controlled clinical trials. *Clin Ther*, 25, 81–104.

Baek, I. H., Lee, B. Y., Kang, W. & Kwon, K. I. 2013. Pharmacokinetic analysis of two different doses of duloxetine following oral administration in dogs. *Drug Res (Stuttg)*, 63(8), 404–408.

Barkin, R., Iusco, M. & Barkin, S. 2006. Opioids used in primary care for the management of pain: a pharmacologic, pharmacotherapeutic, and pharmacodynamics overview. In: Boswell, M. V., Cole, B. E. & Weiner, R. S. (eds), *Weiner's Pain Management: A Practical Guide for Clinicians*, 7th edn. Boca Raton, FL: CRC Press/Taylor & Francis, p. 791.

Barnhart, M. D., Hubbell, J. A., Muir, W. W., Sams, R. A. & Bednarski, R. M. 2000. Pharmacokinetics, pharmacodynamics, and analgesic effects of morphine after rectal, intramuscular, and intravenous administration in dogs. *Am J Vet Res*, 61, 24–28.

Bazin, J. E., Massoni, C., Bruelle, P., Fenies, V., Groslier, D. & Schoeffler, P. 1997. The addition of opioids to local anaesthetics in brachial plexus block: the comparative effects of morphine, buprenorphine and sufentanil. *Anaesthesia*, 52, 858–862.

Belshaw, Z., Asher, L. & Dean, R. S. 2016. The attitudes of owners and veterinary professionals in the United Kingdom to the risk of adverse events associated with using non-steroidal anti-inflammatory drugs (NSAIDs) to treat dogs with osteoarthritis. *Prev Vet Med*, 131, 121–126.

Benedetti, F., Amanzio, M., Vighetti, S. & Asteggiano, G. 2006. The biochemical and neuroendocrine bases of the hyperalgesic nocebo effect. *J Neurosci*, 26, 12014–12022.

Benitez, M. E., Roush, J. K., Kukanich, B. & McMurphy, R. 2015a. Pharmacokinetics of hydrocodone and tramadol administered for control of postoperative pain in dogs following tibial plateau leveling osteotomy. *Am J Vet Res*, 76(9), 763–770.

Benitez, M. E., Roush, J. K., McMurphy, R., Kukanich, B. & Legallet, C. 2015b. Clinical efficacy of hydrocodone-acetaminophen and tramadol for control of postoperative pain in dogs following tibial plateau leveling osteotomy. *Am J Vet Res*, 76(9), 755–762.

Boileau, C., Martel-Pelletier, J., Brunet, J., Tardif, G., Schrier, D., Flory, C., *et al.* 2005. Oral treatment with PD-0200347, an alpha2delta ligand, reduces the development of experimental osteoarthritis by inhibiting metalloproteinases and inducible nitric oxide synthase gene expression and synthesis in cartilage chondrocytes. *Arthritis Rheum*, 52, 488–500.

Boscan, P., Pypendop, B. H., Solano, A. M. & Ilkiw, J. E. 2005. Cardiovascular and respiratory effects of ketamine infusions in isoflurane-anesthetized dogs before and during noxious stimulation. *Am J Vet Res*, 66, 2122–2129.

Boscan, P., Monnet, E., Mama, K., Twedt, D. C., Congdon, J. & Steffey, E. P. 2011. Effect of maropitant, a neurokinin 1 receptor antagonist, on anesthetic requirements during noxious visceral stimulation of the ovary in dogs. *Am J Vet Res*, 72, 1576–1579.

Bostrom, I. M., Nyman, G. C., Lord, P. E., Haggstrom, J., Jones, B. E. & Bohlin, H. P. 2002. Effects of carprofen on renal function and results of serum biochemical and hematologic analyses in anesthetized dogs that had low blood pressure during anesthesia. *Am J Vet Res*, 63, 712–721.

Brondani, J. T., Luna, L. S. P., Beier, S. L., Minto, B. W. & Padovani, C. R. 2009. Analgesic efficacy of perioperative use of vedaprofen, tramadol or their combination in cats undergoing ovariohysterectomy. *J Feline Med Surg,* 11, 420–429.

Brown, D. C., Iadarola, M. J., Perkowski, S. Z., Erin, H., Shofer, F., Laszlo, K. J., *et al.* 2005. Physiologic and antinociceptive effects of intrathecal resiniferatoxin in a canine bone cancer model. *Anesthesiology,* 103, 1052–1059.

Cahana, A., Shvelzon, V., Dolberg, O., Magora, F. & Shir, Y. 1998. Intravenous lignocaine for chronic pain: an 18-month experience. *Harefuah,* 134, 692–694, 751, 750.

Calandre, E. P., Morillas-Arques, P., Molina-Barea, R., Rodriguez-Lopez, C. M. & Rico-Villademoros, F. 2011. Trazodone plus pregabalin combination in the treatment of fibromyalgia: a two-phase, 24-week, open-label uncontrolled study. *BMC Musculoskelet Disord,* 12, 95.

Campoy, L. & Read, M. (eds). 2013. *Small Animal Regional Anesthesia and Analgesia.* Ames, IA: John Wiley & Sons, Inc.

Canapp, S. O., Jr, Canapp, D. A., Ibrahim, V., Carr, B. J., Cox, C. & Barrett, J. G. 2016a. The use of adipose-derived progenitor cells and platelet-rich plasma combination for the treatment of supraspinatus tendinopathy in 55 dogs: a retrospective study. *Front Vet Sci,* 3, 61.

Canapp, S. O., Jr., Leasure, C. S., Cox, C., Ibrahim, V. & Carr, B. J. 2016b. Partial cranial cruciate ligament tears treated with stem cell and platelet-rich plasma combination therapy in 36 dogs: a retrospective study. *Front Vet Sci,* 3, 112.

Cashmore, R. G., Harcourt-Brown, T. R., Freeman, P. M., Jeffery, N. D. & Granger, N. 2009. Clinical diagnosis and treatment of suspected neuropathic pain in three dogs. *Aust Vet J,* 87(1), 45–50.

Cassuto, J., Sinclair, R. & Bonderovic, M. 2006. Anti-inflammatory properties of local anesthetics and their present and potential clinical implications. *Acta Anaesthesiol Scand,* 50, 265–282.

Cepeda, M. S., Alvarez, H., Morales, O. & Carr, D. B. 2004. Addition of ultralow dose naloxone to postoperative morphine PCA: unchanged analgesia and opioid requirement but decreased incidence of opioid side effects. *Pain,* 107, 41–46.

Chappell, A. S., Desaiah, D., Liu-SEIFERT, H., Zhang, S., Skljarevski, V., Belenkov, Y. & Brown, J. P. 2011. A double-blind, randomized, placebo-controlled study of the efficacy and safety of duloxetine for the treatment of chronic pain due to osteoarthritis of the knee. *Pain Pract,* 11, 33–41.

Chew, D. J., Buffington, C. A., Kendall, M. S., Dibartola, S. P. & Woodworth, B. E. 1998. Amitriptyline treatment for severe recurrent idiopathic cystitis in cats. *J Am Vet Med Assoc,* 213, 1282–1286.

Clivatti, J., Sakata, R. K. & Issy, A. M. 2009. Review of the use of gabapentin in the control of postoperative pain. *Rev Bras Anestesiol,* 59, 87–98.

Cook, A. K., Niven, C. A. & Downs, M. G. 1999. Assessing the pain of people with cognitive impairment. *Int J Geriatr Psychiatry,* 14, 421–425.

Cox, S. R., Lesman, S. P., Boucher, J. F., Krautmann, M. J., Hummel, B. D., Savides, M., *et al.* 2010. The pharmacokinetics of mavacoxib, a long-acting COX-2 inhibitor, in young adult laboratory dogs. *J Vet Pharmacol Ther,* 33, 461–470.

Dauri, M., Faria, S., Gatti, A., Celidonio, L., Carpenedo, R. & Sabato, A. F. 2009. Gabapentin and pregabalin for the acute post-operative pain management. A systematic-narrative review of the recent clinical evidences. *Curr Drug Targets,* 10, 716–733.

de Luca, K. E., Parkinson, L., Byles, J. E., Lo, T. K., Pollard, H. P. & Blyth, F. M. 2016. The prevalence and cross-sectional associations of neuropathic-like pain among older, community-dwelling women with arthritis. *Pain Med,* epub ahead of print.

Desaphy, J. F., Dipalma, A., De Bellis, M., Costanza, T., Gaudioso, C., Delmas, P., *et al.* 2009. Involvement of voltage-gated sodium channels blockade in the analgesic effects of orphenadrine. *Pain,* 142, 225–235.

Drygas, K. A., McClure, S. R., Goring, R. L., Pozzi, A., Robertson, S. A. & Wang, C. 2011. Effect of cold compression therapy on postoperative pain, swelling, range of motion, and lameness after tibial plateau leveling osteotomy in dogs. *J Am Vet Med Assoc,* 238, 1284–1291.

Egashira, N., Hirakawa, S., Kawashiri, T., Yano, T., Ikesue, H. & Oishi, R. 2010. Mexiletine reverses oxaliplatin-induced neuropathic pain in rats. *J Pharmacol Sci,* 112, 473–476.

Epstein, M. 2015. Opioids. In: Gaynor, J. S. & Muir, W. W. (eds), *Handbook of Veterinary Pain Management,* 3rd edn. St. Louis, MO: Elsevier-Mosby, pp. 161–195.

Epstein, M., Rodan, I., Griffenhagen, G., Kadrlik, J., Petty, M., Robertson, S. & Simpson, W. 2015. AAHA/AAFP pain management guidelines for dogs and cats. *J Am Anim Hosp Assoc,* 51(2), 67–84.

Fahie, M. A., Ortolano, G. A., Guercio, V., Schaffer, J. A., Johnston, G., Au, J., *et al.* 2013. A randomized controlled trial of the efficacy of autologous platelet therapy for the treatment of osteoarthritis in dogs. *J Am Vet Med Assoc,* 243(9), 1291–1297.

Fan, T. M., De Lorimier, L. P., Charney, S. C. & Hintermeister, J. G. 2005. Evaluation of intravenous pamidronate administration in 33 cancer-bearing dogs with primary or secondary bone involvement. *J Vet Intern Med,* 19, 74–80.

Finnerup, N. B., Otto, M., McQuay, H. J., Jensen, T. S. & Sindrup, S. H. 2005. Algorithm for neuropathic pain treatment: an evidence based proposal. *Pain,* 118, 289–305.

Finnerup, N. B., Attal, N., Haroutounian, S., McNicol, E., Baron, R., Dworkin, R. H., *et al.* 2015. Pharmacotherapy for neuropathic pain in adults:

a systematic review and meta-analysis. *Lancet Neurol*, 14(2), 162–173.

Fisher, K., Coderre, T. J. & Hagen, N. A. 2000. Targeting the N-methyl-D-aspartate receptor for chronic pain management. Preclinical animal studies, recent clinical experience and future research directions. *J Pain Symptom Manage*, 20, 358–373.

Franklin, S. P. & Cook, J. L. 2013. Prospective trial of autologous conditioned plasma versus hyaluronan plus corticosteroid for elbow osteoarthritis in dogs. *Can Vet J*, 54(9), 881–884.

Franklin, S. P., Garner, B. C. & Cook, J. L. 2015. Characteristics of canine platelet-rich plasma prepared with five commercially available systems. *Am J Vet Res*, 76(9), 822–827.

Fritsch, D. A., Allen, T. A., Dodd, C. E., Jewell, D. E., Sixby, K. A., Leventhal, P. S., *et al.* 2010. A multicenter study of the effect of dietary supplementation with fish oil omega-3 fatty acids on carprofen dosage in dogs with osteoarthritis. *J Am Vet Med Assoc*, 236, 535–539.

Fujiki, M., Shineha, J., Yamanokuchi, K., Misumi, K. & Sakamoto, H. 2007. Effects of treatment with polysulfated glycosaminoglycan on serum cartilage oligomeric matrix protein and C-reactive protein concentrations, serum matrix metalloproteinase-2 and -9 activities, and lameness in dogs with osteoarthritis. *Am J Vet Res*, 68(8), 827–833.

Geusens, P. 2009. Naproxcinod, a new cyclooxygenase-inhibiting nitric oxide donor (CINOD). *Expert Opin Biol Ther*, 9, 649–657.

Gevirtz, C. 2007. Update on the management of opioid-induced constipation. *Top Pain Manag*, 23, 1–5.

Ghanem, C. I., Pérez, M. J., Manautou, J. E. & Mottino, A. D. 2016. Acetaminophen from liver to brain: new insights into drug pharmacological action and toxicity. *Pharmacol Res*, 109, 119–131.

Giorgi, M., Meizler, A. & Mills, P. C. 2012. Pharmacokinetics of the novel atypical opioid tapentadol following oral and intravenous administration in dogs. *Vet J*, 194(3), 309–313.

Graham, G. G., Davies, M. J., Day, R. O., Mohamudally, A. & Scott, K. F. 2013. The modern pharmacology of paracetamol: therapeutic actions, mechanism of action, metabolism, toxicity and recent pharmacological findings. *Inflammopharmacology*, 21(3), 201–232.

Grimm, K. A., Tranquilli, W. J., Thurmon, J. C. & Benson, G. J. 2000. Duration of nonresponse to noxious stimulation after intramuscular administration of butorphanol, medetomidine, or a butorphanol-medetomidine combination during isoflurane administration in dogs. *Am J Vet Res*, 61, 42–47.

Groudine, S. B., Fisher, H. A., Kaufman, R. P., Jr., Patel, M. K., Wilkins, L. J., Mehta, S. A. & Lumb, P. D. 1998. Intravenous lidocaine speeds the return of bowel function, decreases postoperative pain, and shortens hospital stay in patients undergoing radical retropubic prostatectomy. *Anesth Analg*, 86, 235–239.

Gupta, R. A. & Dubois, R. N. 2001. Colorectal cancer prevention and treatment by inhibition of cyclooxygenase-2. *Nat Rev Cancer*, 1, 11–21.

Hampshire, V. A., Doddy, F. M., Post, L. O., Koogler, T. L., Burgess, T. M., Batten, P. O., *et al.* 2004. Adverse drug event reports at the United States Food And Drug Administration Center for Veterinary Medicine. *J Am Vet Med Assoc*, 225, 533–536.

Harman, R., Carlson, K., Gaynor, J., Gustafson, S., Dhupa, S., Clement, K., *et al.* 2016. A prospective, randomized, masked, and placebo-controlled efficacy study of intraarticular allogeneic adipose stem cells for the treatment of osteoarthritis in dogs. *Front Vet Sci*, 3, 81

Hay Kraus, B. L. 2014. Efficacy of orally administered maropitant citrate in preventing vomiting associated with hydromorphone administration in dogs. *J Am Vet Med Assoc*, 244(10), 1164–1169.

Hochman, J. R., Gagliese, L., Davis, A. M. & Hawker, G. A. 2011. Neuropathic pain symptoms in a community knee OA cohort. *Osteoarthritis Cartilage*, 19, 647–654.

Hocking, G., Visser, E. J., Schug, S. A., Cousins, M. J. & Carr, D. B. 2007. Ketamine: does life begin at 40? *IASP Pain ClinUpdates*, 15(3), 1–6.

Hogan, M. E., Vandervaart, S., Perampaladas, K., Machado, M., Einarson, T. R. & Taddio, A. 2011. Systematic review and meta-analysis of the effect of warming local anesthetics on injection pain. *Ann Emerg Med*, 58, 86–98.

Howell, S. R., Hicks, D. R., Scatina, J. A. & Sisenwine, S. F. 1994. Pharmacokinetics of venlafaxine and O-desmethylvenlafaxine in laboratory animals. *Xenobiotica*, 24(4), 315–327.

Hu, X., Li, J., Zhou, R., Wang, Q., Xia, F., Halaszynski, T. & Xu, X. 2017. Dexmedetomidine added to local anesthetic mixture of lidocaine and ropivacaine enhances onset and prolongs duration of a popliteal approach to sciatic nerve blockade. *Clin Ther*, 39(1), 89–97.

Ingvast-Larsson, C., Holgersson, A., Bondesson, U., Lagerstedt, A. S. & Olsson, K. 2010. Clinical pharmacology of methadone in dogs. *Vet Anaesth Analg*, 37, 48–56.

Johnson, S. M., Saint John, B. E. & Dine, A. P. 2008. Local anesthetics as antimicrobial agents: a review. *Surg Infect*, 9, 205–213.

Jones, R. S. 2008. Combining local and general anaesthesia for better pain relief in dogs and cats. *Vet J*, 178, 161–162.

Karai, L., Brown, D. C., Mannes, A. J., Connelly, S. T., Brown, J., Gandal, M., *et al.* 2004. Deletion of vanilloid receptor 1-expressing primary afferent neurons for pain control. *J Clin Invest*, 113, 1344–1352.

King, J. N., Rudaz, C., Borer, L., Jung, M., Seewald, W. & Lees, P. 2010. In vitro and ex vivo inhibition of canine cyclooxygenase isoforms by robenacoxib: a comparative study. *Res Vet Sci*, 88, 497–506.

Knapp, D. W., Richardson, R. C., Chan, T. C., Bottoms, G. D., Widmer, W. R., Denicola, D. B., *et al.* 1994. Piroxicam therapy in 34 dogs with transitional cell carcinoma of the urinary bladder. *J Vet Intern Med*, 8, 273–278.

KÖGEL, B., Terlinden, R. & Schneider, J. 2014. Characterisation of tramadol, morphine and tapentadol in an acute pain model in Beagle dogs. *Vet Anaesth Analg*, 41(3), 297–304.

Konya, V., Marsche, G., Schuligoi, R. & Heinemann, A. 2013. E-type prostanoid receptor 4 (EP4) in disease and therapy. *Pharmacol Ther*, 138, 485–502

Kreitler, S., Niv, D. & Carr, D. B. 2007. Cognitive impairment in chronic pain. *IASP Pain Clin Updates*, 15(4), 1–4.

Krotscheck, U., Boothe, D. M. & Little, A. A. 2008. Pharmacokinetics of buprenorphine following intravenous administration in dogs. *Am J Vet Res*, 69, 722–727.

Kukanich, B. 2013. Outpatient oral analgesics in dogs and cats beyond nonsteroidal antiinflammatory drugs: an evidence-based approach. *Vet Clin North Am Small Anim Pract*, 43(5), 1109–1125.

Kukanich, B. 2016. Pharmacokinetics and pharmacodynamics of oral acetaminophen in combination with codeine in healthy Greyhound dogs. *J Vet Pharmacol Ther*, 39(5), 514–517.

Kukanich, B. & Papich, M. G. 2004. Pharmacokinetics of tramadol and the metabolite O-desmethyltramadol in dogs. *J Vet Pharmacol Ther*, 27, 239–246.

Kukanich, B. & Spade, J. 2013. Pharmacokinetics of hydrocodone and hydromorphone after oral hydrocodone in healthy Greyhound dogs. *Vet J*, 196(2), 266–268.

Kukanich, B., Lascelles, B. D. & Papich, M. G. 2005. Pharmacokinetics of morphine and plasma concentrations of morphine-6-glucuronide following morphine administration to dogs. *J Vet Pharmacol Ther*, 28, 371–376.

Kuo, G. 2006. Nonsteroidal anti-inflammatory drugs. In: Boswell, M. V., Cole, B. E. & Weiner, R. S. (eds), *Weiner's Pain Management : A Practical Guide For Clinicians*, 7th edn. Boca Raton, FL: CRC Press/ Taylor & Francis, p. 774.

Kyles, A. E., Papich, M. & Hardie, E. M. 1996. Disposition of transdermally administered fentanyl in dogs. *Am J Vet Res*, 57, 715–719.

LA Vincente, S. F., White, J. M., Somogyi, A. A., Bochner, F. & Chapleo, C. B. 2008. Enhanced buprenorphine analgesia with the addition of

ultra-low-dose naloxone in healthy subjects. *Clin Pharmacol Ther*, 83, 144–152.

Lascelles, B. D., Cripps, P. J., Jones, A. & Waterman-Pearson, A. E. 1998. Efficacy and kinetics of carprofen, administered preoperatively or postoperatively, for the prevention of pain in dogs undergoing ovariohysterectomy. *Vet Surg*, 27, 568–582.

Lascelles, B. D. X., Gaynor, J. & Smith, E. S. 2007. Evaluation of amantadine as part of a multimodal analgesic regimen for the alleviation of refractory canine osteoarthritis pain. In: *World Small Animal Veterinary Association World Congress Proceedings*, Sydney, Australia.

Lascelles, B. D., Knazovicky, D., Case, B., Freire, M., Innes, J. F., Drew, A. C. & Gearing, D. P. 2015. A canine-specific anti-nerve growth factor antibody alleviates pain and improves mobility and function in dogs with degenerative joint disease-associated pain. *BMC Vet Res*, 11, 101.

Lee, A., Cooper, M. G., Craig, J. C., Knight, J. F. & Keneally, J. P. 2007. Effects of nonsteroidal anti-inflammatory drugs on postoperative renal function in adults with normal renal function. *Cochrane Database Syst Rev*, 2, CD002765.

Lerche, P., Aarnes, T., Covey-Crump, G. & Taboada, F. M. 2016. *Handbook of Small Animal Regional Anesthesia and Analgesia Techniques*, 1st edn. Chichester: John Wiley & Sons, Ltd.

Longmire, D. R., Jay, G. W. & Boswell, M. V. 2006. Neuropathic pain. In: Boswell, M. V. & Cole, B. E. (eds), *Weiner's Pain Management: A Practical Guide for Clinicians*, 7th edn. Boca Raton, FL: Taylor & Francis, pp. 297–314.

Lovheim, H., Sandman, P. O., Kallin, K., Karlsson, S. & Gustafson, Y. 2006. Poor staff awareness of analgesic treatment jeopardises adequate pain control in the care of older people. *Age Ageing*, 35, 257–261.

MacDougall, L. M., Hethey, J. A., Livingston, A., Clark, C., Shmon, C. L. & Duke-Novakovski, T. 2009. Antinociceptive, cardiopulmonary, and sedative effects of five intravenous infusion rates of lidocaine in conscious dogs. *Vet Anaesth Analg*, 36, 512–522.

Malek, S., Sample, S. J., Schwartz, Z., Nemke, B., Jacobson, P. B., Cozzi, E. M., *et al.* 2012. Effect of analgesic therapy on clinical outcome measures in a randomized controlled trial using client-owned dogs with hip osteoarthritis. *BMC Vet Res*, 8, 185.

Marquez, M., Boscan, P., Weir, H., Vogel, P. & Twedt, D. C. 2015. Comparison of NK-1 receptor antagonist (maropitant) to morphine as a pre-anaesthetic agent for canine ovariohysterectomy. *PLoS One*, 10(10), e0140734.

Marshall, W. G., Hazewinkel, H. A., Mullen, D., DE Meyer, G., Baert, K. & Carmichael, S. 2010. The effect of weight loss on lameness in obese dogs with osteoarthritis. *Vet Res Commun*, 34, 241–253.

Martenson, M. E., Cetas, J. S. & Heinricher, M. M. 2009. A possible neural basis for stress-induced hyperalgesia. *Pain*, 142, 236–244.

Martins, T. L., Kahvegian, M. A., Noel-Morgan, J., Leon-Roman, M. A., Otsuki, D. A. & Fantoni, D. T. 2010. Comparison of the effects of tramadol, codeine, and ketoprofen alone or in combination on postoperative pain and on concentrations of blood glucose, serum cortisol, and serum interleukin-6 in dogs undergoing maxillectomy or mandibulectomy. *Am J Vet Res*, 71, 1019–1026.

Mathews, K. A. 2008. Neuropathic pain in dogs and cats: if only they could tell us if they hurt. *Vet Clin North Am Small Anim Pract*, 38, 1365–1414.

Mathews, K., Kronen, P. W., Lascelles, D., Nolan, A., Robertson, S., Steagall, P. V., *et al.* 2014. Guidelines for recognition, assessment and treatment of pain. *J Small Anim Pract*, 55(6), E10–68.

Mburu, D. N., Mbugua, S. W., Skoglund, L. A. & Lokken, P. 1988. Effects of paracetamol and acetylsalicylic acid on the post-operative course after experimental orthopaedic surgery in dogs. *J Vet Pharmacol Ther*, 11, 163–170.

McConkey, S. E., Grant, D. M. & Cribb, A. E. 2009. The role of para-aminophenol in acetaminophen-induced methemoglobinemia in dogs and cats. *J Vet Pharmacol Ther*, (6), 585–595.

McNicol, E. & Carr, D. B. 2007. Opioid side effects. *IASP Pain Clin Updates*,15(2), 1–6.

Mehler, S. J., May, L. R., King, C., Harris, W. S. & Shah, Z. 2016. A prospective, randomized, double blind, placebo-controlled evaluation of the effects of eicosapentaenoic acid and docosahexaenoic acid on the clinical signs and erythrocyte membrane polyunsaturated fatty acid concentrations in dogs with osteoarthritis. *Prostaglandins Leukot Essent Fatty Acids*, 109, 1–7.

Mohammed, S. I., Khan, K. N., Sellers, R. S., Hayek, M. G., Denicola, D. B., Wu, L., *et al.* 2004. Expression of cyclooxygenase-1 and 2 in naturally-occurring canine cancer. *Prostaglandins Leukot Essent Fatty Acids*, 70, 479–483.

Moore, S. A. 2016. Managing neuropathic pain in dogs. *Front Vet Sci*, 3, 12.

Moll, X., Fresno, L., Garcia, F., Prandi, D. & Andaluz, A. 2011. Comparison of subcutaneous and transdermal administration of buprenorphine for pre-emptive analgesia in dogs undergoing elective ovariohysterectomy. *Vet J*, 187, 124–128.

Muehlbacher, M., Nickel, M. K., Kettler, C., Tritt, K., Lahmann, C., Leiberich, P. K., *et al.* 2006. Topiramate in treatment of patients with chronic low back pain: a randomized, double-blind, placebo-controlled study. *Clin J Pain*, 22, 526–531.

Muir, W. W., 3rd, Wiese, A. J. & March, P. A. 2003. Effects of morphine, lidocaine, ketamine, and morphine-lidocaine-ketamine drug combination on minimum alveolar concentration in dogs anesthetized with isoflurane. *Am J Vet Res*, 64, 1155–1160.

Neil, M. J. 2011. Clonidine: clinical pharmacology and therapeutic use in pain management. *Curr Clin Pharmacol*, 6, 280–287.

Neirinckx, E., Vervaet, C., DE Boever, S., Remon, J. P., Gommeren, K., Daminet, S., *et al.* 2010. Species comparison of oral bioavailability, first-pass metabolism and pharmacokinetics of acetaminophen. *Res Vet Sci*, 89(1), 113–119.

Norkus, C., Rankin, D. & Kukanich, B. 2015. Evaluation of the pharmacokinetics of oral amitriptyline and its active metabolite nortriptyline in fed and fasted Greyhound dogs. *J Vet Pharmacol Ther*, 38(6), 619–622.

Patel, D. S, Deshpande, S. S, Patel, C. G. & Singh, S. 2011. Duloxetine: a dual action antidepressant. *Indo-Glob J Pharml Sci*, 1(1), 63–76.

Payne-Johnson, M., Becskei, C., Chaudhry, Y. & Stegemann, M. R. 2015. Comparative efficacy and safety of mavacoxib and carprofen in the treatment of canine osteoarthritis. *Vet Rec*, 176(11), 284.

Pieper, K., Schuster, T., Levionnois, O., Matis, U. & Bergadano, A. 2011. Antinociceptive efficacy and plasma concentrations of transdermal buprenorphine in dogs. *Vet J*, 187, 335–341.

Plessas, I. N., Volk, H. A., Rusbridge, C., Vanhaesebrouck, A. E. & Jeffery, N. D. 2015. Comparison of gabapentin versus topiramate on clinically affected dogs with Chiari-like malformation and syringomyelia. *Vet Rec*, 177(11), 288.

Plumb, D. C. 2011. *Plumb's Veterinary Drug Handbook*, 7th edn. Stockholm, WI: PharmaVet.

Rausch-Derra, L. C., Huebner, M. & Rhodes, L. 2015. Evaluation of the safety of long-term, daily oral administration of grapiprant, a novel drug for treatment of osteoarthritic pain and inflammation, in healthy dogs. *Am J Vet Res*, 76(10), 853–859.

Rausch-Derra, L., Huebner, M., Wofford, J. & Rhodes, L. 2016. A prospective, randomized, masked, placebo-controlled multisite clinical study of grapiprant, an EP4 prostaglandin receptor antagonist (PRA), in dogs with osteoarthritis. *J Vet Intern Med*, 30(3), 756–763.

Ray, L., Lipton, R. B., Zimmerman, M. E., Katz, M. J. & Derby, C. A. 2011. Mechanisms of association between obesity and chronic pain in the elderly. *Pain*, 152, 53–59.

Sackett, D. L., Rosenberg, W. M., Gray, J. A., Haynes, R. B. & Richardson, W. S. 1996. Evidence based medicine: what it is and what it isn't. *BMJ*, 312, 71–72.

Salazar, V., Dewey, C. W., Schwark, W., Badgley, B. L., Gleed, R. D., Horne, W. & Ludders, J. W. 2009. Pharmacokinetics of single-dose oral pregabalin administration in normal dogs. *Vet Anaesth Analg*, 36(6), 574–580.

Savvas, I., Papazoglou, L. G., Kazakos, G., Anagnostou, T., Tsioli, V. & Raptopoulos, D. 2008. Incisional block with bupivacaine for analgesia after celiotomy in dogs. *J Am Anim Hosp Assoc*, 44, 60–66.

Sawyer, D. C., Rech, R. H., Durham, R. A., Adams, T., Richter, M. A. & Striler, E. L. 1991. Dose response to butorphanol administered subcutaneously to increase visceral nociceptive threshold in dogs. *Am J Vet Res*, 52, 1826–1830.

Schechter, N. L. 1989. The undertreatment of pain in children: an overview. *Pediatr Clin North Am*, 36, 781–794.

Schmidtko, A., Lotsch, J., Freynhagen, R. & Geisslinger, G. 2010. Ziconotide for treatment of severe chronic pain. *Lancet*, 375, 1569–1577.

Seddighi, M. R., Egger, C. M., Rohrbach, B. W., Cox, S. K. & Doherty, T. J. 2009. Effects of tramadol on the minimum alveolar concentration of sevoflurane in dogs. *Vet Anaesth Analg*, 36, 334–340.

Silber, H. E., Burgener, C., Letellier, I. M., Peyrou, M., Jung, M., King, J. N., *et al.* 2010. Population pharmacokinetic analysis of blood and joint synovial fluid concentrations of robenacoxib from healthy dogs and dogs with osteoarthritis. *Pharm Res*, 27(12), 2633–2645.

Slingsby, L. S. & Waterman-Pearson, A. E. 2000. The post-operative analgesic effects of ketamine after canine ovariohysterectomy—a comparison between pre- or post-operative administration. *Res Vet Sci*, 69, 147–152.

Smith, G. K., Paster, E. R., Powers, M. Y., Lawler, D. F., Biery, D. N., Shofer, F. S., *et al.* 2006. Lifelong diet restriction and radiographic evidence of osteoarthritis of the hip joint in dogs. *J Am Vet Med Assoc*, 229(5), 690–693.

Sullivan, M., Bentley, S., Fan, M. Y. & Gardner, G. 2009. A single-blind placebo run-in study of venlafaxine XR for activity-limiting osteoarthritis pain. *Pain Med*, 10(5), 806–812.

Tassinari, D., Drudi, F., Carloni, F., Possenti, C., Santelmo, C. & Castellani, C. 2011. [Neuropathic pain in oncology. Novel evidence for clinical practice]. *Recenti Prog Med*, 102, 220–227.

Upchurch, D. A., Renberg, W. C., Roush, J. K., Milliken, G. A. & Weiss, M. L. 2016. Effects of administration of adipose-derived stromal vascular fraction and platelet-rich plasma to dogs with osteoarthritis of the hip joints. *Am J Vet Res*, 77(9), 940–951.

Valtolina, C., Robben, J. H., Uilenreef, J., Murrell, J. C., Aspegren, J., Mckusick, B. C. & Hellebrekers, L. J. 2009. Clinical evaluation of the efficacy and safety of a constant rate infusion of dexmedetomidine for postoperative pain management in dogs. *Vet Anaesth Analg*, 36, 369–383.

Vernier, V. G., Harmon, J. B., Stump, J. M., Lynes, T. E., Marvel, J. P. & Smith, D. H. 1969. The toxicologic and pharmacologic properties of amantadine hydrochloride. *Toxicol Appl Pharmacol*, 15, 642–665.

Vilar, J. M., Batista, M., Morales, M., Santana, A., Cuervo, B., Rubio, M., *et al.* 2014. Assessment of the effect of intraarticular injection of autologous adipose-derived mesenchymal stem cells in osteoarthritic dogs using a double blinded force platform analysis. *BMC Vet Res*, 10, 143.

Vollmer, K. O., VON Hodenberg, A. & Kolle, E. U. 1986. Pharmacokinetics and metabolism of gabapentin in rat, dog and man. *Arzneimittelforschung*, 36, 830–839.

Wahlgren, C. F. & Quiding, H. 2000. Depth of cutaneous analgesia after application of a eutectic mixture of the local anesthetics lidocaine and prilocaine (EMLA cream). *J Am Acad Dermatol*, 42, 584–588.

Walton, M. B., Cowderoy, E. C., Wustefeld-Janssens, B., Lascelles, B. D. & Innes, J. F. 2014. Mavacoxib and meloxicam for canine osteoarthritis: a randomised clinical comparator trial. *Vet Rec*, 175(11), 280.

Wang, X. M., Wu, T. X., Hamza, M., Ramsay, E. S., Wahl, S. M. & Dionne, R. A. 2007. Rofecoxib modulates multiple gene expression pathways in a clinical model of acute inflammatory pain. *Pain*, 128, 136–147.

Weil, A. B., Ko, J. & Inoue, T. 2007. The use of lidocaine patches. *Compend Contin Educ Vet*, 29, 208–216.

Weiland, L., Croubels, S., Baert, K., Polis, I., DE Backer, P. & Gasthuys, F. 2006. Pharmacokinetics of a lidocaine patch 5% in dogs. *J Vet Med A Physiol Pathol Clin Med*, 53, 34–39.

Wilder-Smith, C. H., Hill, L., Spargo, K. & Kalla, A. 2001. Treatment of severe pain from osteoarthritis with slow-release tramadol or dihydrocodeine in combination with NSAIDs: a randomised study comparing analgesia, antinociception and gastrointestinal effects. *Pain*, 91, 23–31.

20 Imaging in Canine Sports Medicine

Jennifer Brown, DVM, DACVS-LA, DACVSMR, CCRT, CVSMT, and
Kimberly E. Henneman, DVM, DACVSMR, DABT, FAAVA, CVA, CVC

Summary

Diagnostic imaging is an important component of the evaluation of injuries to the musculoskeletal system in the sports medicine and rehabilitation patient. Without a specific diagnosis, it is difficult to design a treatment and rehabilitation plan. While the physical exam is the first step toward diagnosis, appropriate imaging modalities should be used to further determine what may be causing the clinical signs, as well as to determine severity. Imaging techniques can also be used to screen for areas of future concern for an individual, and may help guide conditioning plans and limitations to patients' sporting or work activities. For example, screening radiographs taken in a sound canine athlete may identify mild degenerative changes in a joint that may not be clinically significant at that time. This information can assist both the sports medicine specialist and the client in determining an appropriate exercise and conditioning program to protect those areas from further damage, as well as provide a baseline for monitoring over time, especially if lameness becomes an issue in the future.

The availability of advanced imaging modalities has grown in the past several decades, and they are now widely used beyond research and university settings. With this increased access, a more comprehensive evaluation of bone and soft tissue structures can be performed using multiple diagnostic imaging techniques.

Radiography

Radiography is the foundation of musculoskeletal imaging and should be considered a basic component of a thorough musculoskeletal evaluation after lameness has been localized to a specific region. Typical radiographic images consist of orthogonal views, or the standard two views of the area of interest. These include lateral and dorsal (dorsoventral, dorso-palmar/plantar, craniocaudal) projections. In most circumstances these views will provide significant information. However, when working with performance animals, radiographic abnormalities may be more subtle, and additional views should always be considered.

For a more complete picture of a structure, oblique views are often necessary. These views include the dorso-palmar/plantar medial to lateral oblique (DPMLO) and dorso-palmar/plantar lateral to medial oblique (DPLMO). Since radiography is a 2-D image of a 3-D structure, oblique views will show surfaces obscured by superimposition. For example, in the foot the sesamoid bones are difficult to evaluate in standard lateral and dorso-palmar/plantar views. However, on the oblique views the sesamoids can be viewed more clearly for identification of pathological changes.

Other unique views have been described to fully evaluate specific abnormalities. For example, in the shoulder, a skyline or tangential view will help visualize the intertubercular groove of the humerus and differentiate supraspinatus and biceps tendon mineralization (Flo & Middleton, 1990) (Figure 20.1). Osteochondritis dissecans lesions on the lateral trochlear ridge of the talus are best viewed on the flexed skyline and dorsomedial palmar lateral oblique (DMPLO) images (Gielen et al., 2005).

Joint stressed views can also provide critical information as to the nature of soft tissue injury to the supporting structures of the joint. At rest or in recumbency, sub- or complete luxations may not be visible radiographically, but when stress is applied to the joint, luxations may become apparent. Stressed views can also help determine the degree of instability in the joint, which can be helpful in determining a treatment plan. Often more subtle than luxations, are injuries to the collateral ligaments of the joints. Collateral ligaments exist as medial and lateral supporting structures in almost every joint of the limbs. Medial and lateral stressed views can be very important in determining collateral ligament injury and joint stability.

Stressed views are also useful to evaluate joint angles. These views put the joint of interest in weight-bearing position to determine whether the supporting structures are normal. This is most effectively done by taking the radiograph in standing position, which is common in equine practice. It is more difficult to achieve in small animal practice due to the X-ray tube head being fixed to the radiographic table. When it is not possible to take the radiograph in a standing position, weight bearing can be simulated by putting the limb in stance position with pressure applied to mimic body-weight. Evaluation of carpal hyperextension frequently uses stressed views to determine the joint level of the injury and the subsequent treatment options (Piermattei et al., 2006).

Computed tomography

Computed tomography (CT) is a complex X-ray modality that creates multiplanar 2-D cross-sectional images. (Figure 20.2). This allows for

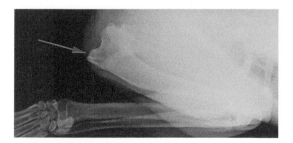

Figure 20.1 Skyline view of the shoulder joint. This view allows better visualization of the bicipital groove and the region of insertion of the supraspinatus tendon on the greater tubercle. Mineralization and remodeling of the greater tubercle of the humerus is present in this image associated with a supraspinatus tendinopathy (arrow).

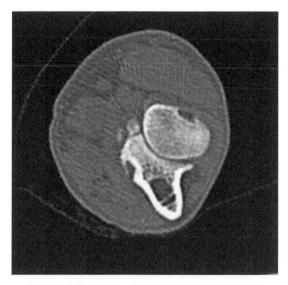

Figure 20.2 CT image of a cross-sectional slice through the elbow joint. The arrow indicates a fragmented coronoid process. Source: Image courtesy of Toby Gemmill, Willows Referral Service, UK.

evaluation of the area of interest in slices and eliminates superimposition of structures that complicate diagnosis in standard radiography. The CT scanner is composed of an X-ray generator and an X-ray detector. The X-ray generator moves around the patient taking thousands of X rays at multiple projection angles that are picked up by the X-ray detector. In a stop-step CT unit, after the projections are acquired, the patient is advanced to obtain the next "slice" along the longitudinal (z) axis. Helical or spiral scanners allow for continuous movement of the patient through the scanner while the X rays are being taken. This allows for a more contiguous scan image and volumetric information for 3-D reconstruction. Images are generated through processing of the attenuation information from the X-ray detectors that is filtered and back-projected to form the digital image. The digital image is then converted to a gray-scale analog image.

Like a radiograph, CT images provide the most detail about bony structures, but CT images are not limited to two planes. This is a significant diagnostic advantage when evaluating for fracture configuration, osteochondral fragmentation, or evaluation of joint incongruity. CT is commonly used in the elbow joint to detect abnormalities associated with elbow dysplasia that can be difficult to assess with standard radiography (Reichle *et al.*, 2000; Gemmill *et al.*, 2006; Moores *et al.*, 2008; Böttcher *et al.*, 2009; Cook & Cook, 2009; Shimizu *et al.*, 2015). In addition to viewing the individual slices for pathology, 3-D rendering can be performed on the entirety of the scan images, reconstructing the area of interest for evaluation (Moores *et al.*, 2008; Dennison *et al.*, 2010) (Figure 20.3).

Although CT is a modality dependent on X-ray attenuation through tissues, making it particularly valuable for osseous injury, it can also be used to evaluate soft tissue lesions and has potential for interventional radiology. CT has a low-contrast resolution setting, and through manipulation of the window and CT number (Houndsfield units), visualization of soft tissue structures can be optimized. It is commonly used for injuries to the spine such as intervertebral disc disease (Newcomb *et al.*, 2012). It has also been used clinically in dogs to evaluate soft tissue abnormalities in the stifle

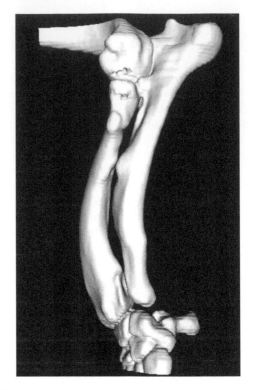

Figure 20.3 Three-dimensional rendering of the radius and ulna including the humeroradial and radiocarpal joints. Source: Image courtesy of Dr. Sherman Canapp.

and iliopsoas (Rossmeisl *et al.*, 2004; Samii *et al.*, 2009). A comprehensive evaluation of the soft tissues using CT or computed tomography angiography (CTA) of the canine shoulder in cadaver dogs showed that this modality may have value in evaluation of the shoulder (Reis Silva *et al.*, 2013). CT may also play a role in both research and clinical settings to evaluate response to rehabilitation therapies by evaluating the CT morphometry of muscle groups in the regions of interest (Cain *et al.*, 2016). Use of CT-guided interventional radiology (IR) procedures for therapeutic purposes in canine patients may be a future application of this imaging modality as well. In one experimental study, CT was used to successfully inject the canine lumbosacral facet joints with methylprednisolone acetate (Liotta *et al.*, 2016).

CT has value in the evaluation of both osseous and soft tissue injuries and may also have future roles in therapeutic IR treatment and outcome measures. Another advantage is that most exams can be done under sedation rather than general anesthesia. It is also much less expensive in most cases than the gold standard modality for soft tissue evaluation, MRI.

Magnetic resonance imaging

Magnetic resonance imaging (MRI) is superior to any other imaging modality for providing exquisite 3-D anatomic detail, especially of soft tissue structures (Figure 20.4). Unlike other modalities, MRI relies on physical and chemical interactions within the tissue to obtain an image. These interactions are primarily exploitation of the physical properties of atomic nuclei throughout the body, in particular the hydrogen atom (Berry, 2002; Gavin & Bagley, 2009). The magnetic resonance (MR) unit produces a signal from changes in hydrogen atoms induced by the application of the magnetic field and radiofrequency pulses. These signals, using Fourier transformation, generate a 3-D image through computer processing. The images are produced in high resolution gray-scale with *increased* signal showing as white and *decreased* signal as black. A higher proportion of hydrogen ions are contained within water and fat, which constitute a large percentage of tissues throughout the body. Most of the signal acquired is from these components.

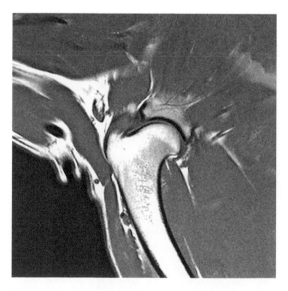

Figure 20.4   Sagittal T1-weighted image of the shoulder joint. T1-weighted images provide excellent anatomic detail. Source: Image courtesy of Dr. Pat Gavin.

When an MRI study is performed, multiple image sequences are obtained. There are standard sequences such as T1-weighted, T2-weighted, T2*-weighted, and STIR, described below. Many more are available and new sequences are being developed. The combinations of sequences selected will depend on the type of MR unit being used (high field vs. low field), the area being studied, and the type of suspected lesion. Some sequences may be more valuable in highlighting a specific lesion or process. T1-weighted, T2-weighted, and STIR are the most common MR sequences (Gavin & Bagley, 2009). In T1-weighted images, fat has an increased or *hyperintense* signal and water a relatively decreased or *hypointense* signal. Anatomic detail is superior in T1-weighted images due to less tissue contrast. In T2-weighted images water has an increased signal and fat a more hypointense signal. T2-weighted images are best for visualizing abnormalities, but have less anatomic definition. In most injuries, increased fluid signal on MRI is a hallmark of tissue damage. This increased signal can stem from any abnormal fluid signal within the tissue such as inflammation, edema, or hemorrhage. STIR and other fat-suppressed sequences suppress the fat signal within tissues and are very good for confirming or identifying pathology in bone characterized by increased signal, as the marrow cavity contains a significant amount of fat. Sclerosis within bone is seen as decreased signal in non-fat-suppressed sequence images.

Gadolinium-based contrast agents can also be used to enhance MR sequences. They are commonly used in human and veterinary medicine in angiography, and when assessing neoplasia or cerebrospinal disease for improved visualization and characterization. Indirect and direct arthrography are considered gold standards for MR evaluation of the joint in human medicine, and have been reported in the hip, knee, ankle, wrist, and shoulder (Applegate *et al.*, 1993; Waldt *et al.*, 2007; Cerezal *et al.*, 2008; Jung *et al.*, 2009; Pozzi *et al.*, 2009; Van Dyck *et al.*, 2009; Rakhra, 2011). Indirect arthrography is performed by intravenous injection of a contrast agent prior to obtaining the desired MRI sequence, whereas direct arthrography is via injection of the contrast agent into the joint. Differences in specificity and sensitivity for lesion detection using direct versus indirect arthrography appear to be slight, with the biggest disadvantage being lack of joint distention using indirect arthrography (Applegate *et al.*, 1993; Waldt *et al.*, 2007; Jung *et al.*, 2009). In dogs, direct MR arthrography has been used for evaluation of the stifle and shoulder joints. In the shoulder, image quality of the soft tissue structures within the joint was found to be enhanced (Vahlensieck *et al.*, 1996). In the stifle, soft tissue structures were also more readily identifiable, and in a group of military working dogs, some pathological changes were only visible after use of direct contrast arthrography (Banfield & Morrison, 2000; Schaefer *et al.*, 2010).

There is significant information in the literature documenting normal anatomy as well as pathological findings of musculoskeletal MRI studies in dogs. While the focus of most MR studies has been on the joints, there is increasing interest in imaging soft tissue injuries and reports include those on the gastrocnemius, supraspinatus, iliopsoas, and long digital extensor tendon (Fitch *et al.*, 1997; Fransson *et al.*, 2005; Murphy *et al.*, 2008; Lafuente *et al.*, 2009; Stahl *et al.*, 2010). MRI can be a very useful diagnostic tool for both soft tissue and bone injury, and MRI should be considered to evaluate any undiagnosed soft tissue or joint injury.

Ultrasonography

Diagnostic ultrasonography generates an image through the use of high-frequency sound waves that are pulsed through the tissue from an ultrasound transducer. The images are a product of wavelength, frequency, and velocity of the sound waves through the tissue (Caine *et al.*, 2009; Drost, 2012; Nyland *et al.*, 2014). These sound waves are reflected back to the transducer as echoes that are converted to an electrical signal to produce a gray-scale image of the tissue being examined. The image produced is a real-time, anatomic picture of the area where the ultrasonography transducer is being applied (Figure 20.5).

Acoustic impedance, determined by the density of the tissue being assessed, is the reflection characteristic of the tissues through which the sound waves travel and produces the echoes. Bone, with high impedance, and air, with low impedance, are perfect reflectors of sound waves, with the components of soft

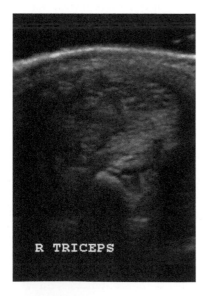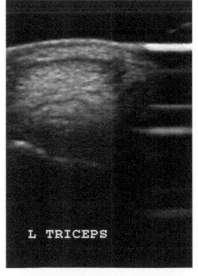

Figure 20.5   Cross-sectional images of the right and left triceps tendon. The left tendon has a normal ultrasonographic appearance. There is significant disruption in the fiber pattern of the right triceps tendon when compared with the left.

tissue falling between the impedance of air and bone. This makes ultrasonography a good diagnostic tool for the evaluation of soft tissues but poor for air-filled structures and pathological changes behind or beneath the surface of bone.

Ultrasonography is becoming more commonly used in diagnosing soft tissue injuries and following tissue healing in canine patients. Appropriate diagnosis with ultrasonography is operator-dependent. Education and experience are vital to develop the skills necessary to use this increasingly requested modality appropriately.

Any muscle, tendon, ligament, or joint suspected of injury could be assessed via ultrasonographic evaluation. There are several studies documenting normal ultrasonographic anatomy in the dog, including most joints and soft tissue structures (Kramer *et al.*, 1997, 1999; Long & Nyland, 1999; Knox *et al.*, 2003; Lamb & Wong, 2005; Liuti *et al.*, 2007; Cannon & Puchalski, 2008; Caine *et al.*, 2009; Turan *et al.*, 2009; Marino & Loughin, 2010; Piórek & Adamiak, 2010; Villamonte-Chevalier *et al.*, 2015). Pathological conditions and their ultrasonographic appearance have also been documented (Kramer *et al.*, 1997, 1999, 2001; Gnudi & Bertoni, 2001; Knox *et al.*, 2003; Mahn *et al.*, 2005; Nielsen & Pluhar, 2005; Vandevelde *et al.*, 2006; Cogar *et al.*, 2008; Arnault *et al.*, 2009; Caine *et al.*, 2009; Cook & Cook, 2009; Seyrek-Intas *et al.*, 2009; Hittmair *et al.*, 2011; Villamonte-Chevalier *et al.*, 2015; Canapp *et al.*, 2016; Cook, 2016). Studies report evaluation of extra-articular soft tissue structures such as the supraspinatus, biceps, abductor pollicis longus, iliopsoas muscle and tendon, menisci, patellar tendons, Achilles tendon, and others (Kramer *et al.*, 1997, 2001; Long & Nyland, 1999; Gnudi & Bertoni, 2001; Mahn *et al.*, 2005; Nielsen & Pluhar, 2005; Vandevelde *et al.*, 2006; Cogar *et al.*, 2008; Arnault *et al.*, 2009; Seyrek-Intas *et al.*, 2009; Turan *et al.*, 2009; Marino & Loughin, 2010; Piórek & Adamiak, 2010; Hittmair *et al.*, 2011; Crema *et al.*, 2015; Villamonte-Chevalier *et al.*, 2015; Canapp *et al.*, 2016; Cook, 2016; Guermazi *et al.*, 2017). Ultrasonography appears to be less useful when evaluating bone and intra-articular structures deep to the bone surfaces such as the cruciate ligaments. However, a recent study suggests that both ultrasonography and MRI, though imperfect, offer clinical usefulness for diagnosing medial meniscal lesions in dogs (Franklin *et al.*, 2017).

Shoulder ultrasonography

The canine shoulder is one of the most common areas for diagnostic ultrasound evaluation due to the lack of radiographic findings and the incidence of tendon and ligament injury in this location, especially in performance dogs. Of primary interest are the supraspinatus and biceps tendons as these structures have been commonly implicated in lameness associated with the shoulder (Fransson *et al.*, 2005; Cogar *et al.*, 2008; Murphy *et al.*, 2008; Lafuente *et al.*, 2009; Van Dyck *et al.*, 2009; Schaefer *et al.*, 2010; Canapp *et al.*, 2016; Cook, 2016).

Ultrasonographic findings in the supraspinatus tendon typically include an increase in size, changes in fiber pattern, and mineralization. When there is an increase in size of the supraspinatus tendon, compression of the adjacent biceps tendon into the biceps groove is often identified due to anatomic proximity (Figure 20.6). The echogenicity of the supraspinatus tendon can vary depending on the degree and chronicity of the tendinopathy. Acute injury, which is less commonly identified, will have a mixed echogenicity with hypoechoic areas indicating more fluid present

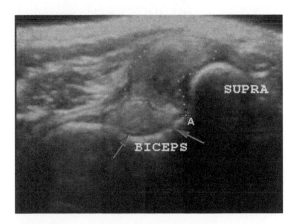

Figure 20.6 Ultrasonographic image of the supraspinatus tendon. The supraspinatus is markedly enlarged and is compressing the biceps tendon into the biceps groove (arrows). The biceps tendon has lost its normal ovoid shape due to the compression.

within the tendon. More commonly, supraspinatus tendon changes are chronic in nature. The echogenicity is also mixed, but the changes will be hyperechoic, indicative of dense fibrous (scar) tissue or potentially dystrophic mineralization. Mineralization is differentiated from fibrous tissue by acoustic shadowing below the lesion (Figure 20.7).

In general, the normal biceps tendon has an increased echogenicity in cross-section and sagittal views compared with the supraspinatus tendon. Biceps tendon abnormalities noted on ultrasound include changes in size and shape, bony reaction along the supraglenoid tubercle due to tearing of fibers from the origin, irregular margins, increased fluid around the biceps tendon, and hypoechoic lesions within the tendon itself. In the craniolateral shoulder, the infraspinatus and teres minor tendons can also be evaluated. Medial shoulder structures are also frequently implicated in shoulder joint lameness, but are difficult to visualize reliably with ultrasound and require special probes and heavy sedation (Cook, 2016).

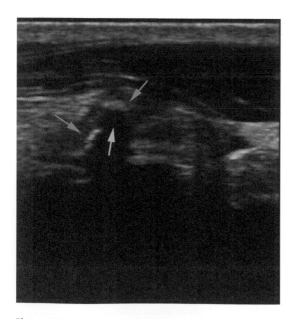

Figure 20.7   Ultrasonographic image of the infraspinatus tendon that has significant disruption and mineralization (blue arrows). Mineralization is hyperechoic with acoustic shadowing present deep to the mineralization (green arrow).

Pelvic limb ultrasonography

Ultrasound evaluation may also prove useful in diagnosis of lesions involving the iliopsoas, stifle, and tarsus.

Iliopsoas

The iliopsoas, from the origin of the psoas major muscle on the cranial lumbar vertebrae to the musculotendinous junction and the tendinous insertion on the lesser trochanter, is subject to both acute and chronic injury. Evaluation of the normal ultrasonographic anatomy has been described (Kramer et al., 1997). Lesions in the muscle belly of the psoas major will have the appearance of either acute or chronic change and may include, depending on severity: irregular boundaries between muscles, increased echodensity indicative of cellular infiltrate, disruption of normal muscle striations, changes in size/thickness, or hypoechoic or anechoic areas within the muscle (Breur & Blevins, 1997). Disruption of the normal linear arrangement of the tendon fibers, changes in echogenicity, and thickening of the tendon are commonly encountered in chronic injuries (Breur & Blevins, 1997; Nielsen & Pluhar, 2005; Cook, 2016).

Stifle

Evaluation of the stifle using ultrasound has mixed results. In two studies looking at the value of ultrasonography to assess for cranial cruciate ligament rupture, it was positively identified in only 19.6% and 15.4% of dogs examined who were definitively diagnosed with rupture at surgery (Gnudi & Bertoni, 2001; Arnault et al., 2009). This low sensitivity is not surprising when understanding the anatomic location of the cruciate ligament as well as the physics of ultrasonography. Bone fragments and osteochondral lesions are also difficult to evaluate for similar reasons. For example, evaluation for fragmented medial coronoid process has been shown to be unreliable due to the anatomic location of the fragments and joint size (Cogar et al., 2008; Cook & Cook, 2009). Evaluation of the meniscus with ultrasound has good sensitivity and specificity for the identification of meniscal injury and may be an important application in evaluation of the stifle joint prior to surgery for cranial cruciate ligament rupture (Kramer et al., 2001; Piórek &

Adamiak, 2010). In addition to the cruciate ligaments, the collateral ligaments, long digital extensor tendon, patellar tendons, and proximal gastrocnemius and fabella can be evaluated with ultrasound.

Tarsus

Evaluation of the tarsus and associated soft tissue structures has been described (Kramer *et al.*, 2001; Nielsen & Pluhar, 2005; Liuti *et al.*, 2007; Caine *et al.*, 2009; Cook, 2016). Ultrasound examination of the components of the Achilles: common calcaneal tendon, gastrocnemius tendon, and superficial digital flexor tendon, to characterize injury and to follow healing post-treatment or surgery is a common clinical application.

Diagnostic ultrasonography can have significant value in evaluating musculoskeletal injuries, despite its limitations. Its image quality is not as good as that of MRI for soft tissue evaluation, but it has some clear advantages:

(1) It can be performed in the awake or lightly sedated patient.
(2) The cost of equipment is significantly less than for MRI or CT, making it more widely accessible to the sports medicine specialist.
(3) Many injuries may be accurately identified using ultrasonography.

Although diagnostic ultrasound is primarily used to assess and identify musculoskeletal injuries, it is also used to follow progression of healing over time, especially when it was diagnosed by other means such as MRI. In these cases, multiple MRI exams to follow healing are impractical, but use of ultrasonography can be quite reasonable for recheck examinations.

Case Study 20.1   Hunting Retriever with waxing and waning thoracic limb lameness

Signalment: 5-y.o. F/I Labrador Retriever. Competes in Hunting Retriever tests. Presented for waxing and waning left thoracic limb lameness.

Physical exam: Sensitive to palpation of left shoulder in flexion and extension, and biceps stretch. Painful on direct palpation of supraspinatus tendon at insertion.

Radiographs: No significant abnormalities (Figure 20.8).

MRI: Reveals tear in the supraspinatus tendon at insertion on greater tubercle and fatty replacement at the myotendinous junction (Figure 20.9). Tendon markedly enlarged, causing compression of the biceps tendon. Following MRI, ultrasonographic exam undertaken to evaluate and document the pathology noted on MRI.

Ultrasonographic findings: Marked enlargement of the supraspinatus tendon with cross-sectional area of 0.92 cm^2 apparently causing compression on the biceps tendon in cross-sectional and longitudinal views. Significant disruption of normal tendon fiber pattern and hypoechoic lesions were present, indicating tear within the tendon (Figure 20.10, red arrow). Multiple hyperechoic areas noted within tendon at dorsomedial aspect, indicating fibrosis or mineralization of tendon in that area (yellow arrow).

Treatment: Patient started in intensive rehabilitation and treatment program with changes in supraspinatus

tendon followed ultrasonographically. Initial improvement observed in the first 8 weeks, with filling of the hypoechoic defect with tendon fibers and a decrease in cross-sectional area of the tendon. By 12 weeks the tendon fibers began to show a more normal and homogenous fiber pattern.

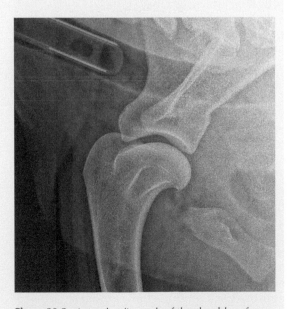

Figure 20.8   Lateral radiograph of the shoulder of a dog diagnosed with a tear of the supraspinatus tendon at the insertion. No significant abnormalities were noted.

(Continued)

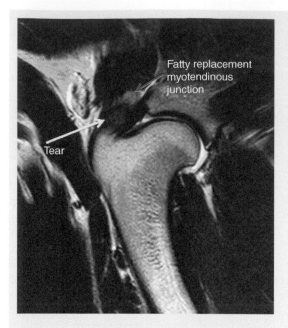

Figure 20.9   T2-weighted sagittal image of the shoulder. The yellow arrow indicates the tear in the supraspinatus tendon at the insertion. The red arrow indicates fatty replacement of the normal tendon at the myotendinous junction. Source: Image courtesy of Dr. Pat Gavin.

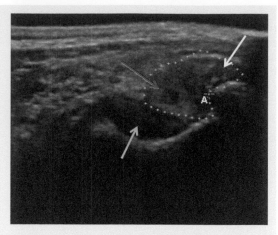

Figure 20.10   Cross-sectional image of the supraspinatus tendon at the insertion on the greater tubercle. The tendon is enlarged at 0.92 cm² in cross-sectional area. Enlargement of the tendon is causing compression of the biceps tendon within the bicipital groove (blue arrow). The hypoechoic tear is indicated by the red arrow. A hyperechoic area of mineralization or fibrosis is indicated by the yellow arrow.

Nuclear scintigraphy

In canine sports medicine and rehabilitation, nuclear scintigraphy may be very useful in localization of lameness attributable to bone lesions that are not apparent on radiographs. Studies have been performed in dogs that highlight this clinical application, including localization of occult lameness, diagnosis of medial coronoid disease, and bone injuries in racing Greyhounds (Tobin *et al.*, 2001; Schwarz *et al.*, 2004; Van Bruggen *et al.*, 2010). In these studies, radiography was inconclusive in identifying the source of the pathological changes in question.

Nuclear scintigraphy is a visual representation of physiological processes rather than an image of an anatomic structure. After intravenous injection of a radiopharmaceutical, technetium-99 m methyl-diphosphonate, labeled to target phosphate in bone, the dog is placed in front of a gamma camera. The gamma

camera uses scintillation material to pick up energy produced by decay of the isotope distributed in the tissues being studied (Driver, 2003). An image is produced from the processing of these gamma-emissions showing the uptake of the radiopharmaceutical. The radiopharmaceutical itself is composed of a radionucleotide and a pharmaceutical. Technetium-99 is the most common isotope used in bone scintigraphy due to its ideal half-life and ability to bind well to diphosphate salts. Diphosphate salts are the primary pharmaceutical used because they localize to bone by binding to hydroxyapatite crystals that are exposed during bone remodeling (Driver, 2003). When increased uptake of the radiopharmaceutical is observed, it reflects increased activity in that area of bone related to blood flow and osteoblastic activity. This increased activity, indicating potential pathology, can be observed before bone changes are apparent radiographically.

Though ubiquitous in equine imaging, the use of bone scintigraphy is not common in small animal practice, likely due in part to the availability of alternative imaging techniques such as CT and MRI. Unlike CT and MRI, scintigraphic exams can be performed in the awake animal under light sedation, and the entire skeleton can be imaged in a short time (Schwarz *et al.*, 2004). Regulations surrounding the use and handling of radiopharmaceuticals and the patient postinjection have made it impractical for many facilities to offer the procedure. Despite these limitations, it is still a viable option for use in canine diagnostic imaging, especially in occult or complex lameness.

Electrodiagnostic testing

Electromyography and nerve conduction studies are used in conjunction with a complete neurological exam to test function of the muscles and nerves. A battery of tests includes: electromyography; peripheral motor and sensory nerve conduction; evaluation of nerve root function with F waves, cord dorsum potential, and H reflex studies; and assessment of the neuromuscular junction with supramaximal repetitive nerve stimulation and stimulated single-fiber electromyography (Cuddon, 2002). Electromyography and motor nerve conduction studies are the most often performed studies in human and veterinary medicine and will be the focus of this section. More information on the additional testing and their indications is available elsewhere (Cuddon, 2002).

Electromyography

Electromyography evaluates the insertional, spontaneous, and voluntary electrical activity of the muscle cell membrane in the motor unit (Chrisman *et al.*, 1972; Brown & Zaki, 1979). By recording the changes in the electrical potential of the muscle cell membrane, electromyography can help differentiate between primary myopathy and neuropathy, identify lesion location, and determine severity of the injury to the nerve (Chrisman *et al.*, 1972; Brown & Zaki, 1979; Cuddon, 2002).

Electrode needles are placed in the muscle unit to be evaluated. These electrodes are connected to an amplifier which enhances the electrical signal from the muscle cell membrane. This electrical activity is shown on an oscilloscope and projected through a speaker providing both visual and auditory evaluation of the signals. There are characteristic visual and auditory signals that are produced by both normally and abnormally functioning motor units (Table 20.1). At rest, muscle is electrically silent. Upon insertion of the electrode needle there is a sharp spike in electrical activity that should return to zero once the insertion is complete and the muscle returns to rest. Incomplete relaxation and voluntary contractions will also produce characteristic electrical activity that also returns to zero upon complete relaxation. Abnormalities are detected with insertion or movement of the electrode needle and observing the produced wave forms and sounds outlined in Table 20.1.

Motor nerve conduction

The focus of motor nerve conduction studies is the function of the peripheral nerves. By calculating the speed of an electrical signal through a muscle innervated by the nerve in question, the integrity of that specific nerve (e.g., radial nerve) can be evaluated. Nerve conduction studies are typically used for differentiating between disuse and dennervation atrophy, as well as the detection of axonal loss in the peripheral nerves. These studies are typically performed in conjunction with electromyography.

Using the same basic equipment as electromyography, and a nerve/muscle stimulator, electrodes are placed proximal and distal on the motor unit to be tested. The compound muscle action potential amplitude, duration, and area are all measured and the velocity of the electrical signal from the anode and cathode are measured after stimulation is applied. The nerve conduction velocity is then calculated from these data using the equation: Nerve conduction velocity = Distance between points/(Proximal conduction latency – Distal conduction latency) (Cuddon, 2002). Normal values for conduction velocity

Table 20.1   Electromyogram potentials and their characteristic oscilloscope wave form and sound of the produced action potential associated with normal and abnormal motor unit responses. Source: Adapted from Brown & Zaki (1979) and Chrisman *et al.* (1972).

Electromyogram potentials	Oscilloscope reading	Auditory signal	Indicates
Insertion	Sharp spike in electrical activity; stops abruptly	Sharp, crisp sound; stops abruptly	Normal response to insertion of the electrode
Minimal contraction potential	Bi- or triphasic action potential; various amplitude	Popping sound with each action potential	Mild normal muscle contraction, incomplete relaxation
Maximal contraction potential	Bi- or triphasic action potentials	Popping sound with each action potential	Significant normal muscle contraction, voluntary withdrawal of the limb
Polyphasic potentials	4+ phase to action potential	Rattling, rasping	Pathology affects motor unit so that summation cannot occur
Positive waves	Primary phase of action potential is downward	Dull thud	Associated with denervation or disease of muscle; neuropathies and myopathies
Fibrillation	Biphasic, low amplitude	Frying eggs	Severe disease of motor unit
Myopathic potentials	Increased number of action potentials for strength of contraction; amplitude and duration are all reduced		Recruitment of additional motor units to compensate for myopathy
Neuropathic potentials	Fewer action potentials during contraction	Motorboat	Loss of motor units firing in neuropathy

have been determined for many of the peripheral nerves (Brown & Zaki, 1979; Cuddon, 2002). Data acquired from the motor nerve conduction study can be compared with normal values or with values on the nonaffected limb. Decreased velocities are indicative of pathology affecting the nerve being tested.

Thermography

Thermal imaging can identify soft tissue changes involved in subtle performance and gait abnormalities, and may be used to monitor rehabilitation progress or to evaluate training stressors before they create injury. Thermography provides a mechanism to capture radiant energy in a clinical setting (Kaplan, 2007; Ring *et al.*, 2004). Interpretation and standardization criteria for the use of thermal imaging have been published (Ring & Ammer, 2012). Current human applications include orthopedic trauma and disease identification (Spalding *et al.*, 2008;

Varju *et al.*, 2004), identification of tissue ischemia (Kulis *et al.*, 2012), response to physical therapy (Cohen & Lee, 2007; Barker *et al.*, 2012), fitness evaluation and identification of soft tissue stress in sports medicine (Ferreira *et al.*, 2008; Castro, 2010; Hildebrandt *et al.*, 2010), infectious disease management (Hidalgo, 2010; Hewlett *et al.*, 2011), and breast cancer detection and surgical management (Brioschi *et al.*, 2010; Wishart *et al.*, 2010; Wang *et al.*, 2011).

Initial use of thermal imaging to detect soft tissue trauma in horses (Purohit & McCoy, 1980; Turner *et al.*, 1986; Turner, 1991) expanded into uses for pregnancy assessment (Bowers *et al.*, 2009), conditioning (Turner, 2006), lesion localization and characterization in neurology (Neimann, 2010), and hoof vascularity (Van hoogmoed & Snyder, 2002). Canine thermal imaging research continues to increase with studies evaluating the use of thermography to identify issues in hips, stifles, elbows, and disc disease (Loughin & Marino, 2007; Infernuso, 2010; Henneman, 2011a; Marino, 2011;

Vainionpää *et al.*, 2012b; Grossbard *et al.*, 2014; McGowan, 2015). Recent papers have reviewed its use in identifying osteoarthritis and hyperthyroidism in cats (Vainionpää *et al.*, 2012a; Waddell *et al.*, 2015). In competitive dogs, thermal imaging is being used to evaluate racing greyhounds before and after racing (Vainionpää *et al.*, 2012c), harness fit in avalanche and sled dogs, foot-fall pattern and thermoregulation in sled dogs wearing booties, and on site at competition (Henneman, 2011b) to quickly localize potential soft tissue causes of lameness for additional exam and diagnostic imaging.

Standardization of the use of thermal imaging in veterinary medicine is now under the guidance of the human medical organization, the American Academy of Thermology. Guidelines for the use of medical thermology in animals were updated in 2016, covering topics such as camera resolution, artifact

---

Case Study 20.2   Thermal imaging of a racing sled dog

Signalment: 5-y.o., M/I, Alaskan Husky. Competes in distance (300–1000 miles) sled dog races. Presented for evaluation of left thoracic limb lameness of 1 day's duration shortly before the start of a race.

History: One day prior to presentation, patient's antebrachium was suddenly entrapped in a loose loop of the gangline (main line connecting dogs to sled) that went suddenly taut as the team took off. Patient had passed a prerace veterinary check with no problems 2 days prior; the distance race was to start the next day. Musher had been treating patient by icing the antebrachium for 10 minutes every 6 hours. When not being iced, arnica cream was placed under neoprene carpal wrap covering the mid-antebrachium to distal border of carpus. Musher withheld any NSAID treatment (not allowed during competition). Patient appeared slightly improved since incident, so musher wanted severity of injury evaluated to decide whether to start patient racing the next day.

Physical exam: 3/5 lameness on rising from rest, becomes 2/5 after warming up. Elbow and shoulder ROM testing (extension and flexion) does not alter lameness; carpal flexion elicits a slight initial guarded response and lameness increased to 3/5. Small area of rope excoriation on mid-dorsal antebrachium, swollen and sensitive to touch. ROM left carpus approximately 25% less than right.

Thermography: Radiology unavailable at race check-in site, so patient had thermal scan of thoracic limbs. Palmar image of left carpal region revealed focal area of increased heat ($\Delta T = 4.8°F$) on medial aspect and smaller area laterally ($\Delta T = 3.4°F$). An area following the tendon sheath of the third digit also warmer ($\Delta T = 3.6°F$) (Figure 20.11). Palpation of toes revealed significantly more sensitivity than at carpus. Extension of toes led to 4/5 lameness.

Outcome: In addition to skin excoriation, patient diagnosed with mild carpitis (normally managed conservatively in distance races, allowing dogs to continue racing) and suspected flexor tendon injury of third digit. Patient was scratched from the race and taken to regular veterinarian for additional imaging and evaluation.

Discussion: When working on-site at a competition where access to traditional diagnostic imaging can be limited, thermal imaging can provide a rapid method to localize a lesion. Toe pathology and trauma is often overlooked in working dogs, and without the thermographic image to draw attention to the thermal asymmetry in the palmar foot of this patient, it might have been allowed to start the race (carpal issues often improve over time in a race as dogs settle into a distance trot). This is a good example of how thermal imaging quickly guided an on-site veterinarian to multiple areas of concern for physical exam, especially in a stoic dog, and assisted in making a decision as to whether the dog should compete.

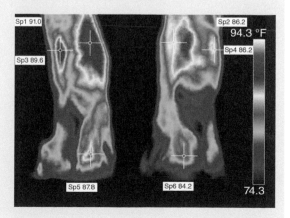

Figure 20.11   Palmar image of the left carpal region revealing a focal area of increased heat on medial aspect and smaller area laterally. An area following the tendon sheath of the third digit was also warmer.

management, patient assessment, and reporting. Veterinarians should be aware that the FLIR ONE camera designed for smart phones and easily available and affordable to clients does not provide sufficient resolution for medical diagnosis.

How thermography works

Thermal imaging is a noninvasive, nonradiating, physiological diagnostic tool (Jiang *et al.*, 2005) that depends on radiant heat from metabolism. Vasoconstriction from increased sympathetic tone decreases regional blood volume and therefore temperature; vasodilation from decreased sympathetic tone or inflammation increases local temperature. By correlating pattern changes in temperature with various diseases, degeneration, or injury processes, thermography may provide a reproducible diagnostic tool (Uematsu *et al.*, 1988; Ring, 2004; Diakides & Bronzino, 2008). Thermal images provide absolute temperatures (aT), and differences in temperatures of similar areas or tissues (ΔT) are noted. A difference of more than 1 °C between areas is considered significant (Turner *et al.*, 1986). Thermal imaging cameras use high-resolution lenses that gather infrared photon energy

packets into high-speed and high spatial resolution focal plane array detectors (Volmer & Mollman, 2010). Images are stored as digital jpeg and video files.

Using thermography

Thermal imaging does not replace, but rather augments, a thorough physical examination, and its use as a physiological imaging tool integrates well with anatomic imaging such as radiography, CT, MRI, and ultrasonography. Though hot spots generally indicate pathological changes, cool areas also can indicate abnormalities (Devereaux *et al.*, 1986) (Figure 20.12).

Environmental factors such as radiant heat sources, lights, and exposure to either direct or indirect sun as well as coats, collars, and harnesses must be controlled during thermal imaging. Fans, breezes, water, topical medication, or uneven hair thickness can create artifacts. Dampness can cause an evaporation artifact for several hours after a bath.

If the environmental temperature is similar to the temperature of the dog, it will be impossible to discern usable heat patterns. In very extreme cold, thermoregulatory vasoconstriction may mask all but the most severe inflammatory changes (Figure 20.13).

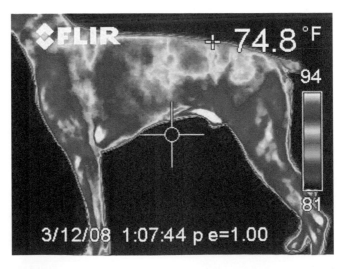

Figure 20.12 Lateral thermal image of an agility Doberman recently involved in a collision with another dog and demonstrating pain to touch in the thoracolumbar region. The range of temperatures read in the scan is shown on the right side of image. The greener areas in the dorsal, lumbar areas were edematous and painful to touch, indicating probable subcutaneous bruising.

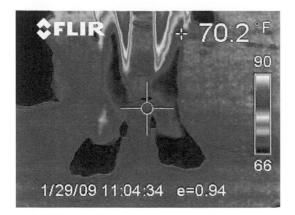

Figure 20.13 Cranial thoracic limbs of an avalanche search-and-rescue dog demonstrating environmental vasoconstriction (thus colder temperatures) of the mid-radius distal to the feet. The lighter blue color of the craniolateral right carpus is in an area that showed discomfort on flexion. A water artifact can also appear similar to this due to evaporative cooling at the skin surface.

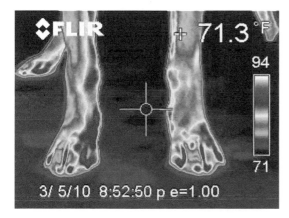

Figure 20.14 Cranial thoracic limbs of a distance sled racing dog during the prerace check-in; the dog was not lame when working. Thermography was used to evaluate the extent of right medial carpal inflammation discovered on physical examination. Inflammation of the right front medial digits and left front lateral digits was also found by thermography and confirmed by palpation. The client opted not to start the dog in the race based on physical and thermographic findings.

Thermal imaging is used to assess for soft tissue injuries including muscle strains, sprains, tendinopathies, and arthritis (Figure 20.14). Thermography may also identify functional fitting problems with both competitive and rehabilitation support or cart harnesses (Figure 20.15).

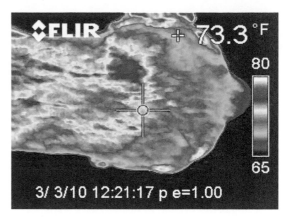

Figure 20.15 Dorsal lumbosacral view of a distance sled racing dog with mild back tenderness (head is to the left). The dog had not been in the harness for over 12 hours. The focal red area in the mid-top of the image was the dog's right ilial crest which showed marked sensitivity on palpation; additionally, the heat pattern along the entire dorsal spine was asymmetrical and a deviation from the normal canine back thermal pattern. The X-back harness pattern can still be seen in addition to possible compensatory heat along the dog's right (top of image) lateral gluteal area.

Webliography

American Academy of Thermology. Guidelines. http://aathermology.org/organization/guidelines/ (accessed October 2017).

References

Applegate, G. R., Flannigan, B. D., Tolin, B. S., Fox, J. M. & Del Pizzo, W. 1993. MR diagnosis of recurrent tears in the knee: value of intraarticular contrast material. *AJR Am J Roentgenol*, 161(4), 821–825.

Arnault, F., Cauvin, E., Viguier, E., Kraft, E., Sonet, J. & Carozzo, C. 2009. Diagnostic value of ultrasonography to assess stifle lesions in dogs after cranial cruciate ligament rupture: 13 cases. *Vet Comp Orthop Traumatol*, 22(6), 479–485.

Banfield, C. M. & Morrison, W. B. 2000. Magnetic resonance arthrography of the canine stifle joint: technique and applications in eleven military dogs. *Vet Radiol Ultrasound*, 41(3), 200–213.

Barker, L. E., Markowski, A. M. & Henneman, K. 2012. Digital infrared thermal imaging following anterior cruciate ligament reconstruction. *J Orthop Sports Phys Ther*, 42(3), 292.

Berry, C. R. 2002. Physical principles of computed tomography and magnetic resonance imaging.

In: Thrall, D. E. (ed.), *Textbook of Diagnostic Veterinary Radiology*, 4th edn. Philadelphia, PA: Saunders, pp. 28–35.

Böttcher, P., Werner, H., Ludewig, E., Grevel, V. & Oechtering, G. 2009. Visual estimation of radioulnar incongruence in dogs using three-dimensional image rendering: an in vitro study based on computed tomographic imaging. *Vet Surg*, 38(2), 161–168.

Bowers, S., Gandy, S., Anderson, B., Ryan, P. & Willard, S. 2009. Assessment of pregnancy in the late-gestation mare using digital infrared thermography. *Theriogenology*, 72(3), 372–377.

Breur, G. J. & Blevins, W. E. 1997. Traumatic injury of the iliopsoas muscle in three dogs. *J Am Vet Med Assoc*, 210(11), 1631–1634.

Brioschi, M. L., Matias, J. E. F., Teixeira, M. J. & Vargas, J. V. 2010. Automated computer diagnosis of IR medical imaging. In: Orlove, G. L. & Brown, D. C. (eds), *InfraMation 2010 Proceedings*, Vol. 11, pp. 115–124.

Brown, N. O. & Zaki, F. A. 1979. Electrodiagnostic testing for evaluation of neuromuscular disorders in dogs and cats. *J Am Vet Med Assoc*, 174(1), 86–90.

Cain, B., Jones, J. C., Holaskova, I., Freeman, L. & Pierce, B. 2016. Feasibility for measuring transverse area ratios and asymmetry of lumbosacral region paraspinal muscles in working dogs using computed tomography. *Front Vet Sci*, 12(3), 34.

Caine, A., Agthe, P., Posch, B. & Herrtage, M. 2009. Sonography of the soft tissue structures of the canine tarsus. *Vet Radiol Ultrasound*, 50(3), 304–308.

Canapp, S. O., Canapp, D. A., Ibrahim, V., Carr, B. J., Cox, C. & Barrett, J. G. 2016. The use of adipose-derived progenitor cells and platelet-rich plasma combination for the treatment of supraspinatus tendinopathy in 55 dogs: a retrospective study. *Front Vet Sci*, 3, 61.

Cannon, M.S. & Puchalski, S.M. 2008. Ultrasonographic evaluation of normal canine iliopsoas muscle. *Vet Radiol Ultrasound*, 49(4), 378–382.

Castro, J. 2010. Thermal imaging and fitness. *In:* Orlove, G. L. & Brown, D.C. (eds), *InfraMation 2010 Proceedings*, Vol. 11, pp. 321–324.

Cerezal, L., Llopis, E., Canga, A. & Rolon, A. 2008. MR arthrography of the ankle: indications and technique. *Radiol Clin North Am*, 46(6), 973–974.

Chrisman, C. L., Burt, J. K., Wood, P. K. & Johnson, E. W. 1972. Electromyography in small animal clinical neurology. *J Am Vet Med Assoc*, 160(3), 311–318.

Cogar, S. M., Cook, C. R., Curry, S. L., Grandis, A. & Cook, J. L. 2008. Prospective evaluation of techniques for differentiating shoulder pathology as a source of forelimb lameness in medium and large breed dogs. *Vet Surg*, 37(2), 132–141.

Cohen, J. M. & Lee, M. H. M. 2007. *Rehabilitation Medicine and Thermography*. Wilsonville, OR: Impress Publications.

Cook, C. R. 2016. Ultrasound imaging of the musculoskeletal system. *Vet Clin North Am Small Anim Pract*, 46(3), 355–371.

Cook, C. R. & Cook, J. L. 2009. Diagnostic imaging of canine elbow dysplasia: a review. *Vet Surg*, 8(2), 144–153.

Crema, M. D., Yamada, A. F., Guermazi, A., Roemer, F. W. & Skaf, A. Y. 2015. Imaging techniques for muscle injury in sports medicine and clinical relevance. *Curr Rev Musculosklet Med*, 8(2), 154–161.

Cuddon, P. A. 2002. Electrophysiology in neuromuscular disease. *Vet Clin North Am Small Anim Pract*, 32(1), 31–62.

Dennison, S. E., Drees, R., Rylander, H., Yandell, B. S., Milovancev, M., Pettigrew, R. & Schwarz, T. 2010. Evaluation of different computed tomography techniques and myelography for the diagnosis of acute canine myelopathy. *Vet Radiol Ultrasound*, 51(3), 254–258.

Devereaux, M. D., Parr, G. R., Lachmann, S. M., Thomas, D. P. & Hazleman, B. L. 1986. Thermographic diagnosis in athletes with patellofemoral arthralgia. *J Bone Joint Surg*, 68(1), 42–44.

Diakides, N. A. & Bronzino, J. D. 2008. *Medical Infrared Imaging*. Boca Raton, FL: CRC Press.

Driver, A. J. 2003. Basic principles of equine scintigraphy. In: Dyson, S. J., Pilsworth, R. C., Twardock, A. R. & Martinelli, M. J. (eds), *Equine Scintigraphy*. Ely: Equine Veterinary Journal.

Drost, W. T. 2012. Physics of ultrasound imaging. In: Thrall, D. E. (ed.), *Textbook of Diagnostic Veterinary Radiology*, 6th edn. Philadelphia, PA: Saunders, pp. 29–39.

Ferreira, J. J., Mendonça, L. C., Nunes, L. A., Andrade FILHO, A. C., Rebelatto, J. R. & Salvini, T. F. 2008. Exercise-associated thermographic changes in young and elderly subjects. *Ann Biomed Eng*, 36(8), 1420–1427.

Fitch, R. B., Wilson, E. R., Hathcock, J. T. & Montgomery, R. D. 1997. Radiographic, computed tomographic and magnetic resonance imaging evaluation of a chronic long digital extensor tendon avulsion in a dog. *Vet Radiol Ultrasound*, 38(3), 177–181.

Flo, G. L. & Middleton, D. 1990. Mineralization of the supraspinatus tendon in dogs. *J Am Vet Med Assoc*, 197(1), 95–97.

Franklin, S. P., Cook, J. L., Cook, C. R., Shaikh, L. S., Clarke, K. M. & Holmes, S. P. 2017. Comparison of ultrasonography and magnetic resonance imaging to arthroscopy for diagnosing medial meniscal lesions in dogs with cranial cruciate ligament deficiency. *J Am Vet Med Assoc*, 251(1), 71–79.

Fransson, B. A., Gavin, P. R. & Lahmers, K. K. 2005. Supraspinatus tendinosis associated with biceps brachii tendon displacement in a dog. *J Am Vet Med Assoc*, 227(9), 1416, 1429–1433.

Gavin, P. R. & Bagley, R. S. 2009. *Practical Small Animal MRI*. Ames, IA: John Wiley & Sons, Inc.

Gemmill, T. J., Hammond, G., Mellor, D., Sullivan, M., Bennett, D. & Carmichael, S. 2006. Use of reconstructed computed tomography for the assessment of joint spaces in the canine elbow. *J Small Anim Pract*, 47(2), 66–74.

Gielen, I., VAN Ryssen, B. & VAN Bree, H. 2005. Computed tomography compared with radiography in the diagnosis of lateral trochlear ridge talar osteochondritis dissecans in dogs. *Vet Comp Orthop Traumatol*, 18(2), 77–82.

Gnudi, G. & Bertoni, G. 2001. Echographic examination of the stifle joint affected by cranial cruciate ligament rupture in the dog. *Vet Radiol Ultrasound*, 42(3), 266–270.

Grossbard, B. P., Loughin, C. A., Marino, D. J. Marino, L. J., Sackman, J., Umbaugh, S. E., *et al.* 2014. Medical infrared imaging (thermography) of type 1 thoracolumbar disk disease in chondrodystrophic dogs. *Vet Sur*, 43(7), 869–876.

Guermazi, A. & Roemer, F. W., Robinson, P., Tol, J. L., Regatte, R. R. & Crema, M. D. 2017. Imaging of muscle injuries in sports medicine: sports imaging series. *Radiology*, 282(3), 646–663.

Henneman, K. 2011a. Thermography in small animals. In: *Ohio State University Annual Thermal Imaging Conference*, Columbus, OH.

Henneman, K. 2011b. Canine thermal imaging: case studies. In: *Ohio State University Annual Thermal Imaging Conference*, Columbus, OH.

Hewlett, A. L., Kalil, A. C., Strum, R. A., Zeger, W. G. & Smith, P. W. 2011. Evaluation of an infrared thermal detection system for fever recognition during the H1N1 influenza pandemic. *Infect Control Hosp Epidemiol*, 32(5), 504–506.

Hidalgo, J. C. 2010. Detecting a H1N1 in Tocumen International Airport in Panama. In: Orlove, G. L. & Brown, D. C. (eds), *InfraMation 2010 Proceedings*, Vol. 11, pp. 361–368.

Hildebrandt, C., Raschner, C. & Ammer, K. 2010. An overview of recent application of medical infrared thermography in sports medicine in austria. *Sensors (Basel)*, 10(5), 4700–4715.

Hittmair, K. M., Groessl, V. & Mayrhofer, E. 2012. Radiographic and ultrasonographic diagnosis of stenosing tenosynovitis of the abductor pollicis longus muscle in dogs. *Vet Radiol Ultrasound*, 53(2), 135–141.

Infernuso, T., Loughin, C.A., Marino, D. J., Umbaugh, S.E. & Solt, P.S. 2010. Thermal imaging of normal and cranial cruciate ligament-deficient stifles in dogs. *Vet Surg*, 39(4), 410–417.

Jiang, L. J., Ng, E. Y., Yeo, A. C., Wu, S., Pan, F., Yau, W. Y., *et al.* 2005. A perspective on medical infrared imaging. *J Med Eng Technol*, 29(6), 257–267.

Jung, J. Y., Yoon, Y. C., Yi, S. K., Yoo, J. & Choe, B. K. 2009. Comparison study of indirect MR arthrography and direct MR arthrography of the shoulder. *Skeletal Radiol*, 38(7), 659–667.

Kaplan, H. 2007. *Practical Applications of Infrared Thermal Sensing and Imaging Equipment*, 3rd edn. Bellingham, WA: SPIE Publications.

Knox, V. W., 4th, Sehgal, C. M. & Wood, A. K. 2003. Correlation of ultrasonographic observations with anatomic features and radiography of the elbow joint in dogs. *Am J Vet Res*, 64(6), 721–726.

Kramer, M., Gerwing, M., Hach, V. & Schimke, E. 1997. Sonography of the musculoskeletal system in dogs and cats. *Vet Radiol Ultrasound*, 38(2), 139–149.

Kramer, M., Stengel, H., Gerwing, M., Schimke, E. & Sheppard, C. 1999. Sonography of the canine stifle. *Vet Radiol Ultrasound*, 40(3), 282–293.

Kramer, M., Gerwing, M., Michele, U., Schimke, E. & Kindler, S. 2001. Ultrasonographic examination of injuries to the Achilles tendon in dogs and cats. *J Small Anim Pract*, 42(11), 531–535.

Kulis, T., Kolaric, D., Karlovic, K., Knezevic, M., Antonini, S. & Kastelan, Z. 2012. Scrotal infrared digital thermography in assessment of varicocele—pilot study to assess diagnostic criteria. *Andrologia*, 44(Suppl. 1), 780–785.

Lafuente, M. P., Fransson, B. A., Lincoln, J. D., Martinez, S. A., Gavin, P. R., Lahmers, K. K. & Gay, J. M. 2009. Surgical treatment of mineralized and nonmineralized supraspinatus tendinopathy in twenty-four dogs. *Vet Surg*, 38(3), 380–387.

Lamb, C. R. & Wong, K. 2005. Ultrasonographic anatomy of the canine elbow. *Vet Radiol Ultrasound*, 46(4), 319–325.

Liotta, A. P., Girod, M., Peeters, D., Sandersen, C., Couvreur, T. & Bolen, G. 2016. Clinical effects of computed tomography-guided lumbosacral facet joint, transforaminal epidural, and translaminar epidural injections of methylprednisolone acetate in healthy dogs. *Am J Vet Res*, 77(10), 1132–1139.

Liuti, T., Saunders, J. H., Gielen, I., DE Rycke, L., Coopman, F. & VAN Bree, H. 2007. Ultrasound approach to the canine distal tibia and trochlear ridges of the talus. *Vet Radiol Ultrasound*, 48(4), 361–367.

Long, C. D. & Nyland, T. G. 1999. Ultrasonographic evaluation of the canine shoulder. *Vet Radiol Ultrasound*, 40(4), 372–379.

Loughin, C.A. & Marino, D.J. 2007. Evaluation of thermographic imaging of the limbs of healthy dogs. *Am J Vet Res*, 68(10), 1064–1069.

Mahn, M. M., Cook, J. L., Cook, C. R. & Balke, M. T. 2005. Arthroscopic verification of ultrasonographic diagnosis of meniscal pathology in dogs. *Vet Surg*, 34(4), 318–323.

Marino, D. J. 2011. Veterinary thermography (medical infrared imaging). In: *Proceedings of North American Veterinary Conference (Small Animal Orthopedics)*.

Marino, D. J. & Loughin, C. A. 2010. Diagnostic imaging of the canine stifle: a review. *Vet Surg*, 39(3), 284–295.

McGowan, L., Loughin C. A., Marino, D. J., Umbaugh, S. E., Liu, P., Amini, M., *et al.* 2015. Medical infrared imaging of normal and dysplastic elbows in dogs. *Vet Surg*, 44(7), 874–882.

Moores, A. P., Benigni, L. & Lamb, C. R. 2008. Computed tomography versus arthroscopy for detection of canine elbow dysplasia lesions. *Vet Surg*, 37(4), 390–398.

Murphy, S. E., Ballegeer, E. A., Forrest, L. J. & Schaefer, S. L. 2008. Magnetic resonance imaging findings in dogs with confirmed shoulder pathology. *Vet Surg*, 37(7), 631–638.

Neimann, N. 2010. Neurology and thermology in the horse. In: *Ohio State University Annual Thermal Imaging Conference*, Columbus, OH.

Newcomb, B., Arble, J., Rochat, M., Pechman, R. & Payton, M. 2012. Comparison of computed tomography and myelography to a reference standard of computed tomographic myelography for evaluation of dogs with intervertebral disc disease. *Vet Surg*, 41(2), 207–214.

Nielsen, C. & Pluhar, G. E. 2005. Diagnosis and treatment of hind limb muscle strain injuries in 22 dogs. *Vet Comp Orthop Traumatol*, 18(4), 247–253.

Mattoon, J. S. & Nyland, T. C. 2014. Fundamentals of diagnostic ultrasound. In: Mattoon, J. S. & Nyland, T. C. (eds), *Small Animal Diagnostic Ultrasound*, 3rd edn. Philadelphia, PA: Saunders, pp. 1–49.

Piermattei, D. L, Flo, G. L. & Decamp, C. E. 2006. *Handbook of Small Animal Orthopedics and Fracture Repair*, 4th edn. Philadelphia, PA: Saunders Elsevier.

Piórek, A. & Adamiak, Z. 2010. Ultrasonography of the canine shoulder joint and its pathological changes. *Pol J Vet Sci*, 13(1), 193–200.

Pozzi, G., Stardiotti, P., Parra, C. G., Zagra, L., Sironi, S. & Zerbi, A. 2009. Femoro-acetabular impingement: can indirect MR arthrography be considered a valid method to detect endoarticular damage? A preliminary study. *Hip Int*, 19(4), 386–391.

Purohit, R. C. & Mccoy, M. D. 1980. Thermography in the diagnosis of inflammatory processes in the horse. *Am J Vet Res*, 41(8), 1167–1174.

Rakhra, K. S. 2011. Magnetic resonance imaging of acetabular labral tears. *J Bone Joint Surg Am*, 93(Suppl. 2), 28–34.

Reichle, J. K., Park, R. D. & Bahr, A. M. 2000. Computed tomographic findings of dogs with cubital joint lameness. *Vet Radiol Ultrasound*, 41(2), 125–130.

Reis Silva, H., Uosyte, R., Clements, D. N., Bergkvist, G. T. & Schwarz, T. 2013. Computed tomography and positive contrast computed tomographic arthrography of the canine shoulder: normal anatomy and effects of limb position on visibility of soft tissue structures. *Vet Radiol Ultrasound*, 54(5), 470–477.

Ring, E. F. 2004. The historical development of thermal imaging in medicine. *Rheumatology (Oxford)*, 43(6), 800–802.

Ring, E. F. J. & Ammer, K. 2012. Infrared thermal imaging in medicine. *Physiol Meas*, 33(3), R33–46.

Ring, E. F. J., Ammer, K., Jung, A., Murawski, P., Wiecek, B., Zuber, J., *et al.* 2004. Standardization of infrared imaging. *Conf Proc IEEE Eng Med Biol Soc*, 2, 1183–1185.

Rossmeisl, J. H., Jr, Rohleder, J. J., Hancock, R. & Lanz, O. I. 2004. Computed tomographic features of suspected traumatic injury to the iliopsoas and pelvic limb musculature of a dog. *Vet Radiol Ultrasound*, 45(5), 388–392.

Samii, V. F., Dyce, J., Pozzi, A., Drost, W. T., Mattoon, J. S., Green, E. M., *et al.* 2009. Computed tomographic arthrography of the stifle for detection of cranial and caudal cruciate ligament and meniscal tears in dogs. *Vet Radiol Ultrasound*, 50(2), 144–150.

Schaefer, S. L., Baumel, C. A., Gerbig, J. R. & Forrest, L. J. 2010. Direct magnetic resonance arthrography of the canine shoulder. *Vet Radiol Ultrasound*, 51(4), 380–385.

Schwarz, T., Johnson, V. S., Voute, L. & Sullivan, M. 2004. Bone scintigraphy in the investigation of occult lameness in the dog. *J Small Anim Pract*, 45, 232–237.

Seyrek-Intas, D., Michele, U., Tacke, S., Kramer, M. & Gerwing, M. 2009. Accuracy of ultrasonography in detecting fragmentation of the medial coronoid process in dogs. *J Am Vet Med Assoc*, 234(4), 480–485.

Shimizu, N., Warren-Smith, C. M., Langley-Hobbs, S. J., Burton, M. H., Kulendra, E., Bradley, K., *et al.* 2015. Inter- and intraobserver agreement in interpretation of CT features of medial coronoid process disease. *J Small Anim Pract*, 56(12), 707–713.

Spalding, S. J., Kwoh, C. K., Boudreau, R., Enama, J., Lunich, J., Huber, D., *et al.* 2008. Three-dimensional and thermal surface imaging produces reliable measures of joint shape and temperature: a potential tool for quantifying arthritis. *Arthritis Res Ther*, 10(1), R10.

Stahl, C., Wacker, C., Weber, U., Forterre, F., Hecht, P., Lang, J. & Gorgas, D. 2010. MRI features of gastrocnemius musculotendinopathy in herding dogs. *Vet Radiol Ultrasound*, 51(4), 380–385.

Tobin, E., Weaver, M., Skelly, C. & McAllister, H. 2001. Bone scintigraphy in racing Greyhounds. Annual Meeting of the European Association of Veterinary Diagnostic Imaging and the European College of Veterinary Diagnostic Imaging, July 18–21, Paris, France. *Vet Radiol Ultrasound*, 42, 393.

Turan, E., Ozsunar, Y. & Yildirim, I. G. 2009. Ultrasonographic examination of the carpal canal in dogs. *J Vet Sci*, 10(1), 77–80.

Turner, T. A. 1991. Thermography as an aid to the clinical lameness evaluation. *Vet Clin North Am Equine Pract*, 7(2), 311–338.

Turner, T. 2006. Observational study of equine swimming for conditioning and physiotherapy at Canterbury Park. In: *Vetel Annual Thermal Imaging Conference*. San Luis Obispo, CA: Vetel Diagnostics.

Turner, T., Purohit, R. C., & Fessler, J. F. 1986. Thermography: a review in equine medicine. *Comp Eq*, 8(11), 855–862.

Uematsu, S., Edwin, D. H., Jankel, W. R., Kozikowski, J. & Trattner, M. 1988. Quantification of thermal asymmetry. Part 1: Normal values and reproducibility. *J Neurosurg*, 69(4), 552–555.

Vahlensieck, M., Peterfy, C. G., Wischer, T., Sommer, T., Lang, P., Schlippert, U., et al. 1996. Indirect MR arthrography: optimization and clinical applications. *Radiology*, 200(1), 249–254.

Vainionpää, M. H., Raekallio, M. R., Junnila, J. J. T., Hielm-Björkman, A. K., Snellman, M. P. & Vainio, O. M. 2012a. A comparison of thermographic imaging, physical examination and modified questionnaire as an instrument to assess painful conditions in cats. *J Feline Med Surg*, 15(2), 124–131.

Vainionpää, M. H., Raekallio, M. R., Tuhkalainen, E., Hänninen, H., Alhopuro, N., Savolainen, M., et al. 2012b. Comparison of three thermal cameras with canine hip area thermographic images. *J Vet Med Sci*, 74(12), 1539–1544.

Vainionpaa, M. H., Tienhaara, E. P., Raekallio, M., Junnila, J., Snellman, M. & Vaiinio, O. 2012c. Thermographic imaging of the superficial temperature in racing greyhounds before and after the race. *Sci Wrld J*, 2012, 182749.

Van Bruggen, L. W., Hazewinkel, H. A., Wolschrijn, C. F., Voorhout, G., Pollak, Y. W. & Barthez, P. Y.

2010. Bone scintigraphy for the diagnosis of an abnormal medial coronoid process in dogs. *Vet Radiol Ultrasound*, 51(3), 344–348.

Van Dyck, P., Gielen, J. L., Veryser, J., Weyler, J., Vanhoenacker, F. M., Van Glabbeek, F., et al. 2009. Tears of the supraspinatus tendon: assessment with indirect magnetic resonance arthrography in 67 patients with arthroscopic correlation. *Acta Radiol*, 50(9), 1057–1063.

Van hoogmoed, L. M. & Snyder, J. R. 2002. Use of infrared thermography to detect injections and palmar digital neurectomy in horses. *Vet J*, 164(2), 129–141.

Vandevelde, B., Van Ryssen, B., Saunders, J. H., Kramer, M. & Van Bree, H. 2006. Comparison of the ultrasonographic appearance of osteochondrosis lesions in the canine shoulder with radiography, arthrography, and arthroscopy. *Vet Radiol Ultrasound*, 47(2), 174–184.

Varju, G., Pieper, C. F., Renner, J. B. & Kraus, V. B. 2004. Assessment of hand osteoarthritis: correlation between thermographic and radiographic methods. *Rheumatology (Oxford)*, 43(7), 915–919.

Villamonte-Chevalier, A. A., Soler, M., Sarria, R., Agut, A., Glelen, I. & Latorre R. 2015. Ultrasonographic and anatomic study of the canine elbow joint. *Vet Surg*, 44(4), 485–493.

Volmer, M. & Mollman, K. P. 2010. *Infrared Thermal Imaging: Fundamentals*, Research and Applications, Weinheim: Wiley-Vch.

Waddell, R. E., Marino, D. J., Loughin, C. A., Tumulty, J. W., Dewey, C. W. & Sackman, J. 2015. Medical infrared thermal imaging of cats with hyperthyroidism. *Am J Vet Res*, 76(1), 53–59.

Waldt, S., Bruegel, M., Mueller, D., Holzapfel, K., Imhoff, A. B., Rummeny, E. J. & Woertler, K. 2007. Rotator cuff tears: assessment with MR arthrography in 275 patients with arthroscopic correlation. *Eur Radiol*, 17(2), 491–498.

Wang, J., Shih, T. T., Yen, R. F., Lu, Y. S., Chen, C. Y., Mao, T. L., et al. 2011. The association of infrared imaging findings of the breast with hormone receptor and human epidermal growth factor receptor 2 status of breast cancer. *Acad Radiol*, 18(2), 212–219.

Wishart, G. C., Campisi, M., Boswell, M., Chapman, D., Shackleton, V., Iddles, S., et al. 2010. The accuracy of digital infrared imaging for breast cancer detection in women undergoing breast biopsy. *Eur J Surg Oncol*, 36(6), 535–540.

21 Conditions and Rehabilitation of the Working Dog

Kimberly E. Henneman, DVM, DACVSMR, DABT, FAAVA, CVA, CVC, and Chris Zink, DVM, PhD, DACVP, DACVSMR, CCRT, CVSMT, CVA

Summary

The last decade has shown increasing veterinary medical awareness of the identification and treatment of orthopedic and particularly soft tissue injuries, especially in the canine athlete. However, most veterinary clinical exposure has been limited to canine athletes participating in competitive endeavors. Increasing global security demands, more awareness and reliance on the incredible abilities of the canine nose, and greater openness towards the role that canine companions play in supporting human physical and mental health is creating ever-growing and diverse noncompetition uses and jobs for dogs.

The use of the term "working dog" can have a variety of meanings, from a specific conformation show category of breeds to dogs trained specifically to assist humans with a variety of tasks. These tasks involve all kinds of aspects from the more traditional protection (military and non-military) and explosives/drug detection to less traditional uses such as health-care support and detection of pests, archeological artifacts, and human diseases. In this chapter, we use the term "working dog" as it relates to dogs that are chosen and trained to work with humans to accomplish very specific tasks. Activities where overlap between competitive sports and noncompetitive jobs (such as mushing, herding, or protection sports) will be touched on briefly; for more in-depth information on the competitive aspect of the canine athlete, the reader is referred to resources listed in Chapter 1.

There is often overlap in the breeds used, training techniques, and physical demands between competitive performance and working dogs. However, there are many unique aspects to the maintenance of health and performance often not recognized by veterinary caregivers (primary medical, surgical, rehabilitation alike), handlers, or trainers. This chapter discusses the unique aspects of working dogs from the perspective of sports medicine injury and rehabilitation.

History of the working dog

The dog was the first animal domesticated by human beings, preceding plants and sedentary agriculture by several thousand years (Larson *et al.*, 2012). It is currently thought that dogs actually domesticated themselves by frequenting human refuse piles for food, but humans evidently figured out very quickly that there were benefits to having these predators as companions. Researchers, however, still cannot agree on when and where geographically this garbage-instigated partnership first happened, much less when humans started using dogs for specific tasks. A recent collaborative effort integrating genetics, paleontology, zooarcheology, advanced morphometrics analysis, and biogeography have now dated domestication to at least 12,000 to 16,000 years ago, with domestication possibly occurring in eastern Eurasia and western Asia simultaneously, rather than just in Asia as previously thought (Larson *et al.*, 2012; Grimm, 2015; Frantz *et al.*, 2016).

Discovering when the first working dog appeared is as problematic as identifying the date of domestication. Taking that next step from using dogs as a food source to more actively manipulating their behaviors to make them hunt, protect, and herd on command obviously happened at some point. The trick is determining when. Much as the equine spine started to show arthritis when humans began to ride, studies on the morphometric differences between ancient wolf and dog skeletons have shown that flattening of the dorsal spinous processes in domesticated dogs developed once they began to be used to carry packs (Grimm, 2015). It is not known exactly when humans first manipulated dogs' prey and pack behavior to assist with hunting wild animals or protecting domesticated hoofstock for food. However, the first documented artifact showing a dog wearing a harness is a 2000-year-old carved knife handle found in Ust'-Polui, Siberia. Nonetheless, the onset of dogs being used to pull sleds is suspected to significantly predate this (Romey, 2016).

The presence of canine working companions at the sides of farmers, hunting in the forests, and marching into war demonstrated that there existed an established relationship by the advent of modern times. Roman, Greek, and Egyptian civilizations have left abundant evidence of dogs used for hunting. Napoleon was known to have posted dogs as sentries in his campaign of Egypt (Lemish, 2008). By the 18th and 19th centuries, the use of carting dogs in Europe (Figures 21.1) was as common as the use of dogs for herding and hunting. In World War I, dogs were used by European forces to perform a variety of specially trained, nonaggressive jobs, from finding and assisting the missing and wounded (mercy dogs) to pulling small artillery and carrying messages through the trenches (Figure 21.2).

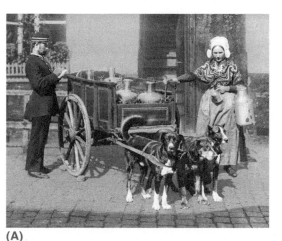
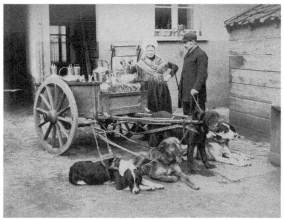

(A)   **(B)**

Figure 21.1   For many centuries, dogs have been used to pull carts such as these dogs delivering milk (**A, B**) and other bottled goods (**B** circa 1880). Source: Public domain—PublicDomainPictures.net.

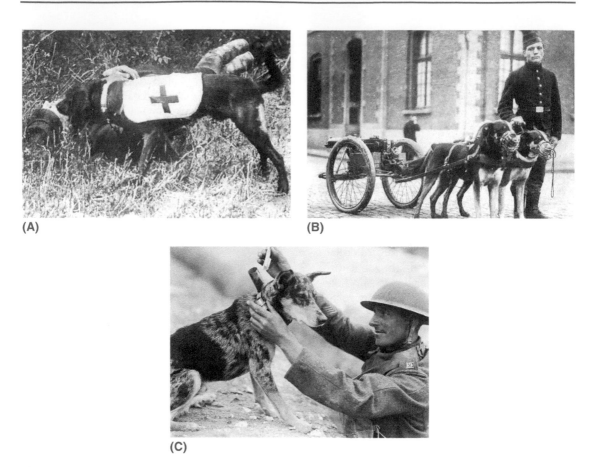

Figure 21.2   World War I saw the first large-scale use of war dogs in military history. **(A)** Ambulance dogs, also known as mercy dogs, wearing saddle bags of medical supplies, sought out the wounded and gave comfort to the dying. Large dogs were used to pull heavy guns **(B)**, and fast medium-sized dogs were used as messengers **(C)**, and these were credited with saving thousands of lives by delivering vital dispatches when phone lines broke down. Source: (A, B) W. E. Mason. (C) The State of Queensland. Public domain—WikimediaCommons.

The United States started using dogs in war during World War II. Interestingly, the first American war dogs were actually sled dogs from Alaska, shipped to Greenland to find lost pilots and to support the 10th Mountain Infantry as pack animals during cold weather operations. These imported American sled dogs probably introduced distemper and rabies into Greenland canine populations, which had been free of these diseases prior to the start of the war. Eventually, a Marine K9 Corps was developed using civilian-donated dogs that were trained to act first as sentries then as scout and messenger dogs (Lemish, 2008). From this humble start, the use of military working dogs (MWDs) progressed to their use in Korea, Vietnam, Afghanistan, and Iraq. MWDs are now used for explosives or drug detection,

sentry duty, tracking, and attack functions, and are even parachuted into hostile areas with their handlers (US War Dogs Association: Types of war dogs). In 1942, during the early stages of World War II, the desire to provide help for soldiers returning home disabled by blindness led to the development of dog guides for the blind—the first modern service dog usage.

Today, in the 21st century, a better scientific understanding of the dog's vast and sensitive olfactory capacity combined with increasing security needs have resulted in a marked increase in the use of detection and service dogs in many different working capacities. Scent-based working dogs are used to detect everything from bed bugs to cancer to drugs to explosives to humans (alive or in various postmortem stages) to endangered animal feces (for location purposes) to forgotten land mines (Critescu *et al.*, 2015; Jezierski *et al.*, 2015; Hackner *et al.*, 2016; Orkin *et al.*, 2016; Prada & Rodriguez, 2016). Dogs accompanying soldiers and police officers for protection, detection, and apprehension is commonly accepted both by the public and by government agencies. Service dogs assisting people with disabilities have expanded beyond those helping the visually impaired to alerting diabetic individuals when their blood sugar is low, notifying those with hearing loss to sounds in their environments, as well as being a comforting presence to humans suffering emotional trauma and shock (emotional assistants, post-traumatic stress disorder dogs); even police dogs have been shown to provide comfort and support to their handlers (Hart *et al.*, 2000). The variety of activities in which working dogs now participate globally presents greater opportunity for musculoskeletal injury and unique challenges for the therapist involved in their care and rehabilitation.

What is a working dog and why are they different?

Working dogs come in all sizes, breeds, and abilities. For the most part, a certain physical type is more desirable for any particular job than a specific breed. There are some instances, however, such as MWDs, for which German Shepherd Dogs, Belgian Malinois, and Dutch Shepherds are the most consistently used breeds for patrol, attack, and detection.

Dogs used for herding tend to be breeds such as Border Collies, Australian Cattle Dogs, and Australian Kelpies, both in working farms or ranches and for competitions. However, one of the authors (KH) has seen a working sheepdog in the Spanish countryside that, despite appearing to be some kind of shaggy terrier, moved the sheep down the road as efficiently as any working Border Collie. Likewise, dogs of clearly mixed heritage can be seen leading sheep and goats on the Navajo and Hopi Indian reservations in Arizona without a human shepherd in sight.

Detection work is based more on ability than any particular selected breed trait. Most of the US Customs and Border Protection (USCBP)/ US Department of Agriculture (USDA) food detection dogs are obtained from pounds and shelters (Figure 21.3). This can create challenges for a veterinary sports medicine or rehabilitation therapist as many of these dogs enter a working career without any physical or behavioral history from their lives before recruitment. Variations in any particular dog's ownership history (physical or emotional abuse), genetics, training, and medical treatments can add unique and sometimes unknown nuances that might play a role in causes of injury as well as in behavioral and physical responses to therapy. Working dogs that originate from a shelter might need to be physically evaluated with particular attention to identify and/or rule out past injuries that could have a significant impact on current ones.

Sometimes there is significant overlap between working dog tasks for which there is a competitive as well as a working aspect, such as sheep herding. In those situations, there might be common injuries and stressors, although it can be impossible for a veterinarian to determine whether work or competition is the cause of any particular injury. Many competitive herding dogs also work cattle and sheep on working farms; many law-enforcement agency dogs may also compete in police-specific contests. While sled dogs in the American lower 48 states are generally used for competitive and recreational functions only, near the Arctic Circle some dogs still perform transportation duties in rural communities. The Russian and Danish military still actively use sled dogs for transportation and patrol in harsh Arctic and Antarctic environments. Dogs function much better and more consistently than machines in subzero cold; the Danish Joint Arctic Command uses their teams for patrol and defense of the Faroe Islands and Greenland. While an American veterinarian is not likely to see a military sled dog, non-racing sled dogs providing winter tours are still popular in many northern latitudes, even in the American lower 48 states. Dry-land racing and tours are growing in popularity in Europe and may eventually find their way to North America, which in turn will expose more veterinarians to the needs of non-competitive, pulling sled dogs.

Why do these dogs do what they do for us, and why should a working dog veterinary therapist care why they do it? The simple answer is

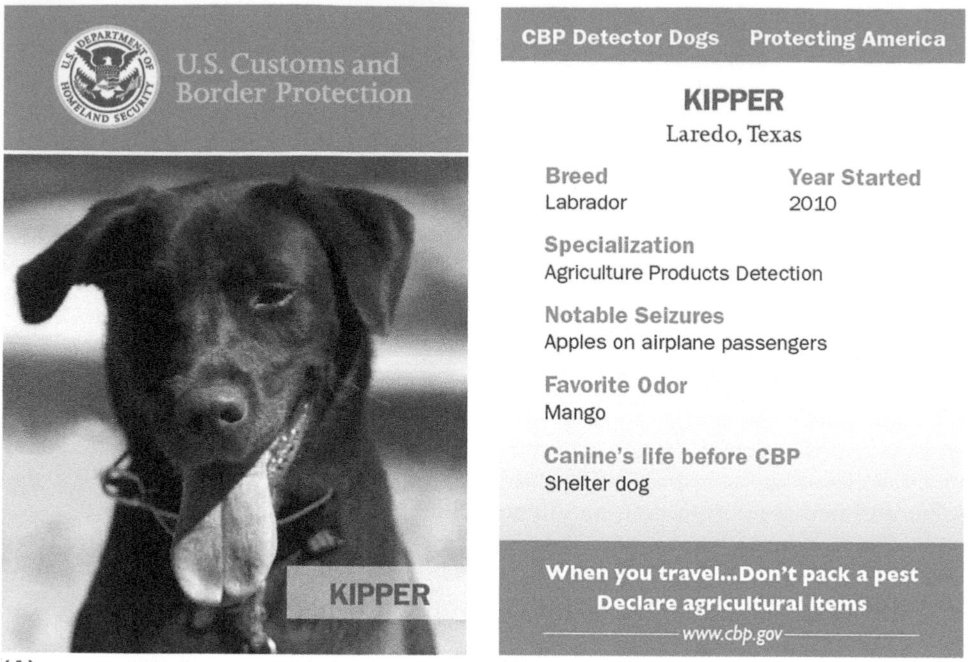

Figure 21.3 US Customs and Border Protection uses food detection dogs, such as Kipper, that are often obtained from shelters. These dogs detect food, plants, and animal products that might endanger US agriculture. Their handlers carry Dog Cards (**A, B**) that contain information about their dogs to give to the public. Source: Card image courtesy of the USCBP.

"drive." Genetically selected drive that is honed through training is the reason that dogs perform the tasks they are trained to do, but also a reason that they can be easy or difficult rehabilitation patients.

Drive is defined as "an innate, biologically determined urge to attain a goal or satisfy a need" (Bryson, 2000; Volhard, 2013) (Box 21.1). This is the instinctive behavior behind environmental stimuli responses in any individual animal. In the dog, certain drives have been selected for and enhanced through years of controlled breeding and training interactions with humans. When the genetic predisposition is then further enhanced with focused training, the dog's drives can be forces to be reckoned with. This is validated by the fact that dogs are still working companions for humans with new uses for dogs being discovered even today. All successful competitive and working dogs will have enhanced drives that are focused above and beyond those of average pet dogs.

These heightened drives create important considerations for the rehabilitation therapist. How an individual dog's drives interact with each other in the face of various stimuli is thought to create temperament in the dog; certain temperaments are desirable and selected for in working dogs (Box 21.2), but might not be appropriate in a pet or even a competitive sport dog. Training a dog to do anything is accomplished by the conditioned manipulation of drives and it can also be affected by the dog's drives. Understanding the basic canine drives is important for any veterinary therapist working with dogs, especially in situations where the animal might be stressed or feel threatened. This cannot be emphasized enough for the therapist who will care for working dogs. Veterinarians and rehabilitation therapists, even those who have personal experience training, working, and/or competing their own dogs, should spend time with and learn specific working dog requirements from experienced dog handlers in the disciplines in which their clients and patients work and/or compete.

High-drive working dogs are usually also accompanied and/or trained by high-drive handlers—another factor that can differ from

---

Box 21.1   Canine working drives.* Source: Adapted from Bryson (2000) and Volhard (2013).

Basic drives

- **Prey** (or **hunt**): hunting, killing, ingesting prey
- **Pack**: emotional contact with other members of a group
- **Defense** (**fight** or **flight**): behaviors associated with survival and self-preservation or preservation of the pack

Subdrives selected for in various working dogs

- **Rank**: a desire to move higher in the pack hierarchy
- **Fight**: attack or aggression towards a perceived threat
- **Guard**: defend territory

- **Protection**: defend individuals of the pack
- **Hunt**: pursue objects even those out of sight
- **Track**: work ground scent
- **Air scent**: work air or windborne scent
- **Retrieve**: instinct to bring an object back to the pack
- **Homing**: return to a specific territory or to the pack
- **Play**: not well understood but play seems to help strengthen pack hierarchy and teach hunting skills among other biological benefits
- **Responsiveness** or **trainability**: desire to obey the pack leader

*These do not include reproduction, urination, defecation and hunger.

Box 21.2   Temperament traits selected for in working dogs. Source: Bryson (2000).

Positive

- **Courage, bravery, hardness:** positive response to stress (thought to be mostly genetic)
- **Confidence**: positive response to stress (conditioned by training)
- **Normal sensory threshold**: lowest level that a stimulus elicits a response

Negative

- **Softness, shyness, aloofness**: negative response to stress
- **Sharpness**: excessively aggressive response to stimuli

---

dealing with pet dogs. While working with high-drive clients can also be true for therapists who work with competitive dogs and their handlers, many working dogs are not owned by individuals but rather by agencies. Each agency has its unique hierarchy of protocols, and goals for their canine "assets" and "property." As a result, there can be many team members, including the veterinarian, trying to resolve the issue of why a dog cannot work. Chains of command can include handlers, budget-watching accountants, and administrators to whom the dog is a tool, not an individual being. Although mindsets and perspectives in some agencies are expanding, there still can be individuals in the team who are unaware of new developments in canine sports medicine or

who still do not perceive dogs as athletes with injuries and treatment needs similar to those in human sports medicine. Sometimes there is more focus on an animal's ability to quickly return to some level of function, rather than the importance of full and stable recovery. This is where a veterinarian knowledgeable in nuances of the sports medicine demands of a particular canine job can communicate and educate those who handle, train, and manage these working canine athletes. And this in the long run can only improve working function and longevity.

Clinical approach to sports medicine and rehabilitation of working dogs

While working dogs share their anatomy, biomechanics, and physiology with pet and competitive dogs, there are unique aspects of veterinary care for working dogs. Instead of the usual partnership between veterinarian and client, working dogs often come with other vested parties. To create a functional team with the goal of restoring the health and function of a working canine athlete, working dog therapists should recognize that there are three elements that must be brought together and balanced. These elements are: (1) the sports medicine and rehabilitation professional's knowledge base and medical perspective; (2) the handler's knowledge base, job, and administrative goals; and (3) the owning or sponsoring agency and its needs and financial constraints. Within each element are factors that the therapist must address to return a patient to a healthy working career.

Element 1: The therapist

Working dog veterinarians and rehabilitation therapists need to understand exactly what is involved with a dog's job. What, exactly, is that dog doing when it is not sitting in the clinic exam room? Obtaining a complete history from the handler is not sufficient to understand the unique needs and stressors of a dog's particular job. Injuries can be from catastrophic single events or from repetitive stresses that ultimately reach the threshold of tissue failure. Knowing the biomechanical demands, harness or clothing, activity frequencies, and other environmental factors (terrain, temperatures, length of time working) that are involved in the dog's training or work is the best way to evaluate the biomechanical causes of any particular injury.

There are many ways that therapists can become familiar with the details of the work done by client handlers and their dogs. It is important to start with an attitude of openness and desire to learn. Asking clients and handlers to share videos and still pictures of a dog in action not only provides insight into what a dog does at training or work, but also creates a bond between handler and therapist that can help with future communication and improve the chances of successful recovery of the dog. Sometimes one video (especially in slow motion) or photo captures that moment in time when an injury could have started (Figures 21.4). Watching animals train, and asking experienced handlers and trainers about their knowledge and techniques, can often provide clues behind vague performance problems that can be otherwise difficult to solve. Even better, attending training sessions and, if possible, accompanying handlers on the job are ideal ways to discover the depths and intensity of a dog's training and physical activities while working.

Understanding total body movement and mechanics is critical for injury diagnosis and therapeutic program design. Focusing on single causes of performance or lameness problems neglects the fact that the body operates as a unit. All animals compensate when there is a part that functions at less than 100%. But the heightened drive characteristics of successful working dogs can mean that it is more difficult to identify when the dog is not fully functioning, especially when subtle problems exist. Loss of function in a muscle, joint, or ligament will lead to compensatory posture and movement alterations that can increase the work and weight load on other structures, which in turn can cause injury and loss of function of those

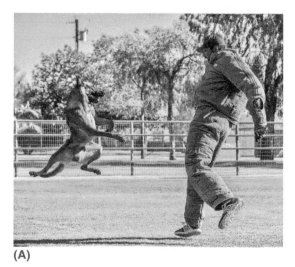
(A)

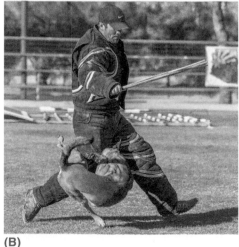
(B)

Figure 21.4 (A, B) A video or photo can reveal actions that could result in injury. Source: Photos by Ro Bastacky.

structures. Eventually, a working dog may become unable to fully perform its duties, with the actual primary cause being difficult to source. Just treating these animals with NSAIDs or rest does not solve the problem until the source musculoskeletal problem(s) can be identified and treated.

Abnormalities in body movement patterns can be understood via two different mechanisms. First, the "Law of Sides" states how lameness compensation patterns tend to progress. Taken from equine gait analysis research, this states that, when there are both primary and compensatory causes of lameness, knowing whether the pattern is contralateral or ipsilateral can help predict which limb has experienced the primary injury.

If the lameness presents as a diagonal pattern (e.g., left thoracic and right pelvic limbs are involved), then there is a significant probability that the primary lameness is present in the thoracic limb. If the lameness presents as an ipsilateral combination (e.g., left thoracic and left pelvic limbs are involved), then there is a significant chance that the primary lameness is in the pelvic limb (Keegan, 2004, 2005a, 2005b; Maliye & Marshall, 2016). While this has not yet been experimentally substantiated in the dog, the authors have found this a useful tool for identifying primary and compensatory injuries in dogs. It is certainly an area open for future research in the canine athlete.

The second way that movement abnormalities can be identified incorporates new work from human fascial research. The common belief that movement is created by compartmentalized and discrete muscle units that act on their own is starting to be transformed as a result of our developing understanding of body-wide muscle and fascial integration (Schleip *et al.*, 2012). Direct morphological continuity of muscular and organized connective tissue in *chains* has been demonstrated in both the human and the horse (Elbrond & Schultz, 2015; Wilke *et al.*, 2016a). These fascial chains transfer tension by regulating changes in stiffness between adjacent myofascial structures (Krause *et al.*, 2016). Stretching and stimulating fascia is a doorway for the therapist into mitigating cellular responses to injury and stress, including the release of resolvins—anti-inflammatory modulators synthesized by polyunsaturated dietary fats (Corey *et al.*, 2012; Berrueta *et al.*, 2016). Stretching of one area along a fascial chain (in this case a pelvic limb) has been demonstrated to improve flexibility in a more remote area such as the neck (Wilke *et al.*, 2016b, 2016c). Understanding the fascial transmission chains can help the veterinary rehabilitation therapist diagnose injury and predict injury propagation.

The presence of these myofascial pathways has not been demonstrated in the dog, but as a quadruped, these chains are postulated to be similar to those in the horse. In addition to their diagnostic and therapeutic value, knowledge of myofascial chain orientations may assist veterinary therapists in designing multifocal rehabilitation protocols for more severe injuries. This interconnectedness means that the little things matter; the foot bone really is connected to the neck bone.

Techniques for identifying dynamic lameness in the dog can include flexion tests similar to those performed in horses by flexing individual joints, holding for 30 seconds, then having the dog trotted or walked off (Figure 21.5). Another lameness assessment technique is to gait the dog on both soft and hard surfaces (e.g., a grass lawn and a cement sidewalk). Clinical observation suggests that a lameness that

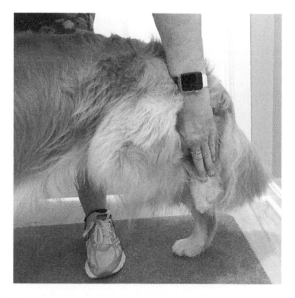

Figure 21.5 Flexing and holding one or more joints then having the dog trot can increase the severity of lameness, thus helping to localize an injury.

worsens on softer terrain usually is associated with a soft tissue injury. A lameness that worsens on a harder surface frequently results from an injury to a bony structure such as a joint articular surface (e.g., osteoarthritis, joint instability, cartilage damage).

Injury therapy end goals can be different for the working dog and handler than those for the average pet and even competitive dog owner. Injury recovery back to basic life functions may be adequate for an animal that is fairly inactive or is competing at focused activities a few days a month, but basic function may not be enough for some working tasks. The physical demands of strenuous physical activity, often combined with the neurological demands on other senses such as scent, vision, and hearing, mean that many working dogs are using maximum body resources in multiple ways while training and working. The presence of lingering pain, weakness, or mechanical dysfunction can affect drive and diminish endurance, scent capacity, and ability to physically negotiate difficult terrain.

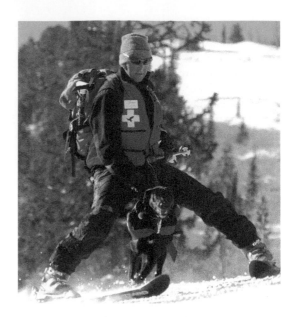

Figure 21.6　Handlers vary in their knowledge of canine anatomy, gait, and health needs. This handler's knowledge helps to keep his dog injury-free under extreme conditions. Source: Photo by Andrea Booher, courtesy of FEMA.

Element 2: The handler

Dogs come with handlers and trainers who have their unique dog knowledge base and their own high determination to succeed at their jobs with their canine partners. Handlers are often the bridge between the therapist and the sponsoring agency, so it is key to have a relationship based on good communication and a common knowledge base (Figure 21.6). Some handlers may be new to dog handling with limited knowledge of anatomy, gait, and the musculoskeletal and neurological demands being placed on their dog, while others may have more experience in specific aspects of dog handling. Some handlers have a sensitive and almost intuitive feel for their dog and others may have a higher threshold before becoming aware that a problem exists.

Most working dog handlers are goal-oriented so their focus may be more on the outcome rather than the process. Taking extra time in the initial consultation with a dog/handler pair can reduce the likelihood of miscommunication later, and helps develop a relationship built on trust and knowledge rather than conflict and misunderstanding. Because of the

goal-intensity of the handler, a veterinary therapist might have to emphasize the importance of rest more than might be necessary with a single-owner dog. Determining a handler's perspective, competence, and even terminology usage are the keys to creating a successful health-care team.

If a veterinarian or therapist is unclear about the terminology that a handler is using, he or she should have no hesitation in asking the handler to explain or clarify. Clear verbal communication and written directions are key so that handlers know what is expected of them, the goals and timeline for rehabilitation, and possible problems that might arise during the rehabilitation period.

An example of terminology confusion between the veterinary medical world and the dog handling world is the use of the word "conditioning." To a veterinary rehabilitation therapist, this term refers to a progressive strengthening program designed to restore a body-wide specific level of musculoskeletal, neurological, and cardiopulmonary function. But to dog trainers, conditioning refers to the process of training a desired behavioral response to a particular stimulus (Department of Defense, 2013). Making sure to clarify terminology is one of the first things that a therapist should do when starting to work with working dog/handler teams, especially those who might be unfamiliar with canine athletic injury management.

Element 3: The controlling agency

Many working dogs are either owned by the military, law enforcement, fire agencies or other sponsoring groups (ski resorts, non-profit organizations, other government bodies). The result is that the decision-making and treatment approval process can be more complex than with animals owned by single clients. Approval for treatment often has to progress through organizational layers, be approved by individuals with no knowledge of canine athlete medical needs, and who might only view the dogs as company or agency assets and tools. Often there are budgetary restrictions, handler time and duty restrictions, and pressure to have the dog "back on the line" by a certain date, regardless of the nature of the injury or whether it is fully healed. It is important for the veterinary rehabilitation community as a whole to continue educating working dog organizations about the importance of rehabilitation after injury diagnosis or surgery, especially for soft tissue musculoskeletal repair.

In many working dog situations, there is a large number of dogs being managed at once, sometimes by the same trainer or administrator, more rarely by the same handler (except in herding and sled dog situations). This can limit not only available funds, but also time that can be dedicated to any single animal. This should not be interpreted by the therapist as an unwillingness to try to do what is best for the individual animal; rather, therapeutic programs should be designed with recognition and respect for the limitations presented.

Each organization has its own techniques, protocols, and regimens for training its dogs. Becoming familiar with training regimens, including the presence of rest periods, is important for the veterinary therapist. Normal physical conditioning and training has been shown to create physiological stress changes—changes that are tolerable and create adaptive changes

in the body (Bruchim *et al.*, 2014; Diverio *et al.*, 2015). However, strenuous training or working in environmental extremes can lead to nonadaptive stress and injury. Chronic or severe stress can also affect the body's ability to heal from injury (Baker & Miller, 2013).

The key is for the therapist to listen to the handler, be aware of restrictions, and design a plan that works within those boundaries. Designing flexible plans that do not necessarily require the use of an underwater treadmill, for example, and that can be undertaken during a handler's breaks in their duties, or in the environment of the organization's kennel is important for success. While a therapist might be faced with a situation that is less than ideal, some rehabilitation is usually preferable to none. Maintaining a flexible attitude can go a long way in negotiating treatment compromises.

Rehabilitation concerns

Specific exercises for various injuries and fitness goals are covered in Chapter 8. The rehabilitation plan for any particular injury or problem involves the same body mechanics for a working dog as for an active pet or competitive dog. Nonetheless, understanding and keeping in mind the unique considerations of working dog rehabilitation can be just as important to success as the specific exercises themselves.

Drive

Working dogs, no matter their job, are selected for temperaments that involve heightened drive or behavior characteristics (such as prey, hunt, nondistractibility, aggression, etc.), which can either help during therapy tasks or hinder. A veterinary rehabilitation therapist who is used to handling more social pet and competition dogs might not initially understand the drives of a working dog or know how to use them to advantage. The ability to identify which drives are particularly strong (drive intensity) in any given patient, as well as how those drives interact, can assist the therapist (and the handler) to safely examine and handle a working dog during diagnosis and rehabilitation, and to improve the likelihood of a successful outcome.

Individual animals will naturally have different thresholds wherein an external stimulus will change a particular response. A rehabilitation therapist caring for working dogs should be very familiar with canine behavioral theory. Understanding working dog temperaments and reading an animal's responses quickly allows for appropriate adaptation of goals during rehabilitation sessions. For example, if a responsive, high-drive, low-threshold dog (especially one suffering from a fairly fresh injury or that is new to rehabilitation) starts to become overwhelmed by therapy tasks, the therapist should know when to reduce the pressure on the dog, letting the dog take a break or even cutting the session short. Maintaining a rigid schedule in which therapy is forced on an animal that is shutting down will almost guarantee a more difficult patient at the next therapy session. It might even create a situation in which the dog experiences significant musculoskeletal and neural fatigue/degeneration.

A good therapist is aware that any individual dog might have variations in its responsiveness to therapy in any given session. Sometimes a dog can lack energy during a particular stage of the healing process. The ability to listen to a handler's observations, evaluate the willingness and ability for a high-drive dog to complete therapeutic tasks on a given day, and to have the flexibility to admit (despite a busy schedule) that perhaps an individual animal just is not ready for an intense rehabilitation session, is a sign of a caring and successful working dog therapist.

It is the authors' experience that many high-drive, responsive dogs, especially those in patrol, apprehension, protection, and guarding disciplines have high pain tolerances and do not like to be touched—two aspects that can make evaluation of patient responses difficult. Additionally, the need to use a muzzle can compromise the ability to work in water or perform other rehabilitation exercises. For example, working dogs with high pain thresholds may not quit when musculoskeletal structures start to hurt from overuse; they might just adaptively change their gait. There is a joke with marathon sled dogs that "if a dog has his leg fall off in a race, he'll just pick it up on the way back and tell you that he is fine." This is descriptive of an attitude that carries across many disciplines besides racing sled dogs. For the working dog therapist, this means that strict attention must be paid to minute clues of posture, gait, and muscle tension to determine whether a healing tissue boundary has been exceeded, since typically high-drive working dogs will not stop working until an injury is very advanced.

Other factors

It is critical to obtain a thorough job-orientated history to understand a working dog's stressors, especially as the dog begins to resume work. If a dog wears a harness, vest, or booties, the therapist should request that the handler bring the equipment to an appointment, and watch the handler place the equipment on the dog. Uneven packing of supplies in search and rescue dog harness pockets or poorly designed harnesses that are restrictive or create areas of increased pressure can block full return to function and even lead to continuing injury (Figure 21.7). Harnesses, vests, and booties should be observed for all activities in which a dog participates because some design problems only manifest in certain conditions (Figure 21.8). As therapy progresses, the dog should wear its working equipment during rehabilitation sessions so that fit can be evaluated and progressive conditioning can take place in a manner similar to that which the dog encounters on the job. A thoughtful approach to the ergonomics of canine clothing and equipment design should be taken, and changes made as needed.

Additionally, veterinary rehabilitation therapists should try to determine whether there are other environmental factors that a dog faces at work, and rehabilitation protocols should be adapted appropriately. If a dog is required to work outside in heat and humidity, then having therapy sessions occur only in an air-conditioned

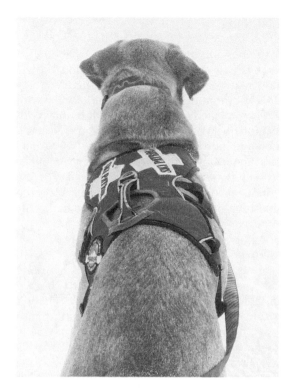

Figure 21.7 Poorly designed or fitting harnesses such as this one can restrict a dog's movement and/or create areas of increased pressure that can lead to injuries.

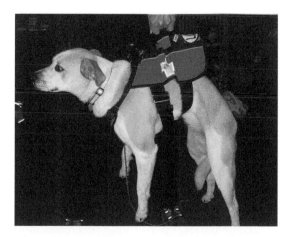

Figure 21.8 This harness is not appropriately designed to support a dog's body when being air-lifted.

clinic might not fully prepare the dog for its work. If a dog has to climb over suitcases or rubble, or has to make sudden starts, stops, or turns, the therapist should design and

incorporate exercises that attempt to mimic these environments and thus appropriately condition muscle fitness and neurological proprioceptive responses.

The therapist should also be aware of whether the dog could come into contact with toxic materials. Being lower to the ground, dogs are closer to spilled chemicals than their human counterparts and are often sent to search damaged buildings, exterior areas, and cars, or to apprehend individuals in environments that might contain illegal drugs. As a result, they might drink or ingest contaminated substances or fluids on the ground (Figure 21.9). Exposures can occur via skin (usually the feet), the gastrointestinal tract (direct ingestion or by licking the feet), and/or the respiratory tract (inhalation). Past exposures could affect the dog's pulmonary response to therapeutic exercise (including the underwater treadmill and pool), and exposure while healing from an injury (e.g., if the dog is deployed prior to complete recovery) could interfere with physiological mechanisms important for tissue healing and immunity. Nearly a third of dogs used after the Oklahoma City bombing displayed negative health effects (including irritation from cement lime and fiberglass) and 60% of dogs working the World Trade Center after the 9/11 attack displayed some type of respiratory problem (Duhaime *et al.*, 1998; Fox *et al.*, 2008).

When dealing with a MWD or a detection dog that has been deployed to other areas of the

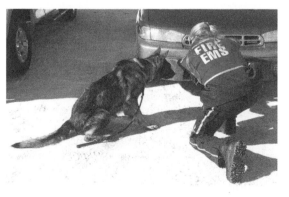

Figure 21.9 Working dogs are often in contact with toxic materials on the ground, such as spills from vehicles.
Source: Photo by Andrea Booher, courtesy of FEMA.

country or other parts of the world, it is advisable to verify that the dog has been checked for blood-borne and gastrointestinal parasitic diseases that may be common in the region of deployment (Toffoli & Rolfe, 2006). Many areas of Europe are prone to *Borrellia* species not commonly found in the United States (Alho *et al.*, 2016), which could create underlying musculoskeletal and joint inflammatory abnormalities.

Nutrition

Many working dogs are trained and used for more than one job purpose. While herding dogs only herd and sled dogs only pull, most law enforcement and military working dogs are trained to be dual purpose—patrol and apprehension, or patrol and detection (explosives or drugs). Search and rescue (SAR) dogs (wildland, urban, avalanche) must multitask by maintaining scent focus while also scrambling over difficult terrain; this creates a great demand of energy for scenting, neurological, and muscular functions. Returning to these functions after an injury layoff can be fatiguing. Handlers need to be cautioned to watch for a dog shutting down and adjust work and food as needed.

It is outside of the scope of this chapter to discuss working dog nutrition in detail, but it bears repeating that it is important to maintain these dogs in proper body condition. In this vein, providing appropriate sources of energy and protein for tissue repair is critical during rehabilitation (see Chapter 4). Borrowing from the marathon sled dog world and from clinical use with wildland SAR dogs, post-loading the body with a source of readily absorbed glucose after a rehabilitation session may speed body recovery and minimize fatigue. It can be beneficial to feed a small carbohydrate meal of simple sugars (honey, berries, rice-based glucose polymers) within 30 minutes of a strenuous rehabilitation session (whether in or outside the clinic), especially if the dog seems mentally and/or physically fatigued (Reynolds *et al.*, 1997; Wakshlag *et al.*, 2002; Reynolds, 2014). Handlers report that dogs seem to recover faster from rehabilitation exercises with this treatment, and many successfully continue the practice of glycogen post-loading after training and exercise, even after the dog is completely healed.

Handling

Working dog compliance with rehabilitation exercises can sometimes be challenging due to a dog's drive, intensity, and sensitivity. Being able to communicate well with the dog is a critical key to successful recovery. More than with pet, competitive, or service dogs, many detection and patrol/apprehension dogs are trained to respond to commands in another language to keep personnel who are not involved in law enforcement from trying to confuse or delay an attacking dog with conflicting commands. The most common command languages in patrol/apprehension and protection dogs are English, German, Dutch, and French.

Improved compliance with many working dogs can be achieved if the handler is allowed and encouraged to participate in the rehabilitation exercises. The therapist should also learn from the handler how the dog is usually rewarded and adapt that reward system to clinical therapeutic protocols. Working dogs can be rewarded either by praise, play, or food.

Creative protocols

Flexibility and creativity are important keys to developing successful therapeutic plans for working dogs. With many working disciplines, there are time and budgetary limitations on the parts of the client or agency. Some service dog organizations have contractually fixed protocols for how certain diagnosed conditions must be handled, thus restricting these clients to obtain approval from the agency and its medical staff. Frequently a sponsoring agency will pay for surgical repair, but will not cover rehabilitation. In these situations, the handler might personally take on the responsibility and cost of rehabilitation, performing exercises and manual therapies in-between or after other duties.

There can be additional restrictions and limitations that make a therapist modify a patient's physical rehabilitation program. The veterinary rehabilitation therapist should have the ability and confidence to modify and adapt the plan to fit the given circumstances. Often, the need for modification leads to the discovery of new and different methods to assist with optimal musculoskeletal and neurological recovery.

Rehabilitation equipment can be constructed from just about anything as long as the therapist has the right mindset and a touch of creativity. If no underwater treadmill is available in the winter, soft snow of various heights for walking and trotting exercises can be used. Smaller dogs can use in-home bathtubs (or in one case, the bathtub in a fire station). The slanted roof of an old dog house at a sled dog kennel was used as a replacement for a physioball and a disc. A racing sled with gangline and empty harnesses attached can be used instead of cavaletti. Wobble boards can be made from dowels or PVC and small pieces of plywood. The key to creative equipment design is to make sure that materials are free from splinters, sharp components, and toxic coatings. Terrain should be inspected to ensure that the footing is appropriate and free of embedded hazards.

Working disciplines

This is a brief overview of some of the working dog disciplines, organizations, and agencies in the United States at the time of writing. Sometimes there is overlap between disciplines as many dogs are trained to be *dual* or *multipurpose*.

Detection

Detection dogs are specially trained to detect and indicate the presence and position of specified substances. There are already many types of detection dogs and the list continues to grow; many are used by federal, regional, and local law enforcement agencies. The USDA obtains dogs from regional rescues and shelters. Other agencies purchase dogs from local and/or international sources. Detection dogs work by bracketing odor gradients, both ground and airborne (each dog is different), and must be able to do so in various types of terrain and environments (Figure 21.10). Most regional detection dogs are trained to Police Officer Standardization Training (POST) certification standards.

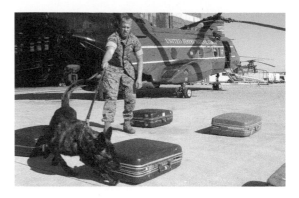

Figure 21.10 Detection dogs are trained to detect and indicate the presence of specified substances. They work by bracketing odor gradients and must be able to function in a variety of environments. Source: Photo public domain—USMC.

Detected scents and common federal agencies

- Drugs: Drug Enforcement Agency (DEA)
- Currency: Treasury, Customs and Border Protection (CBP)
- Concealed humans: CBP, Transportation Security Agency (TSA)
- Explosives (standard, vapor wake): TSA's National Explosives Detection Canine Training Program (NEDCTP), Bureau of Alcohol, Tobacco and Firearms (ATF)
- Plant protection and quarantine (PPQ): US Department of Agriculture (USDA), US Border Patrol (USBP), Animal and Plant Health Inspection Service (APHIS), US Customs and Border Protection Office of Field Operations (USCBP OFO), National Detector Dog Training Center (USDA, 2017)
- Wildlife: US Fish and Wildlife Service (USFWS)—wildlife and exotic animal smuggling, location of wildlife in wilderness (Cristescu *et al.*, 2015; Orkin *et al.*, 2016)
- Forensics: firearms, weapons, articles
- Arson: accelerants
- Search and rescue: technically SAR dogs are detection dogs since they are specifically seeking human scent (alive or dead). However, due to the unique environmental nature of the work, they are covered here as a separate type of working dog
- Cancer (Hackner *et al.*, 2016; Jezierski *et al.*, 2015)
- Medical: seizures, diabetes

- Pests: bed bugs, moles/ground hogs/mice/rats, invasive species
- Human remains: crime scene, blood, clandestine graves, cadaver (Institute of Canine Forensics, 2015)
- Antiquities, historic and archeological (Baxter & Hargrave, 2013).

Potential issues

- Mental fatigue: nose shut-down
- Exposure to toxic chemicals
- Medications prescribed to dogs that might affect ability to detect odor
- Diet: fat amounts and types in the diet of detection dogs have been shown to have an effect on scent discrimination (Altom et al., 2003; Angle et al., 2014), with diets higher in polyunsaturated fatty acids (linoleic) showing some mild enhancement of scent detection
- Environment: heat, humidity, terrain.

Military

Military working dogs are used in many aspects of defense, detection, and scouting. The majority of breeds used are Belgian Malinois, Labrador Retrievers, and German Shepherd Dogs, with some Dutch Shepherds and the occasional sporting or herding breed. Dogs are now allowed to be adopted by civilian law enforcement agencies, previous military handlers, and private individuals after they have completed service (US War Dogs Association: Working dog adoptions), so rehabilitation therapists may end up seeing these dogs as retired or geriatric patients.

Specific tasks

Most dogs are considered dual purpose:

- Detection: human, explosives, drugs
- Patrol: protection, pursuit, apprehension, tracking/trailing.

Potential issues

- Fatigue: nasal, musculoskeletal
- Heat stroke: extreme environments, equipment and protection vests, booties (Toffoli & Rolfe, 2006; Baker & Miller, 2013)

- Shoulder joint and soft tissue injuries from poorly fitting, imbalanced, and/or restrictive protection and equipment vests
- Infectious disease exposures from foreign postings (Toffoli & Rolfe, 2006; Alho et al., 2016)
- Trauma: gunshot wounds, explosives (Baker et al., 2009; Bruchim et al., 2014)
- Repetitive stress wear and tear: feet issues; early osteoarthritis in shoulder, elbow, hips, stifles; chronic soft tissue injuries leading to structural and gait changes; spondylosis; intervertebral disc disease (IVDD); lumbosacral stenosis (Evans et al., 2007; Linn et al., 2003; Moore et al., 2001)
- Cancer: studies of MWDs (German Shepherd and Belgian Malinois) show a cancer incidence higher than in the general canine population. Overseas deployments with potentially increased carcinogen exposure may play a role (Peterson et al., 2000).

Police and federal agencies (excluding military)

Since September 11, 2001, increased security needs in the United States and internationally have led to a marked increase by civilian law enforcement agencies in the purchase and use of working dogs (Figure 21.11). Dogs are acquired by adoption of retired MWDs, purchase through private agents (domestic and international), and direct purchase from kennels.

Specific tasks

These dogs are often dual purpose:

- Detection: explosives, drugs
- Patrol: protection, pursuit, apprehension, tracking/trailing.

Potential issues

These are similar to those of MWDs and detection and miscellaneous protection dogs. However, unlike in the MWD, and related to a more focused, urban, law-enforcement

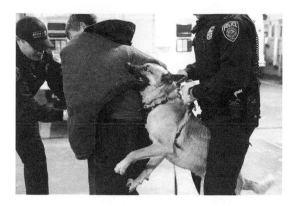

Figure 21.11   Police and law enforcement agencies throughout the United States are dramatically increasing the use of working canines for patrol, apprehension, and detection. Shortly before going to publication, this Salt Lake Unified Police dog, Dingo, was killed in the line of duty while apprehending a wanted Federal fugitive. Source: Photo courtesy of Lt. Chad Reyes and Salt Lake Unified Police.

setting, the three leading causes of death for police dogs are: being struck by a vehicle, heat stroke, and gunshot trauma. While exertional hyperthermia is certainly an issue with working police dogs, sadly the highest incidence of fatal hyperthermia comes from animals being left unattended in vehicles (Stojsih *et al.*, 2014).

Protection (miscellaneous)

These are dogs used for protection, law enforcement, and MWD-like work in many other civilian and personal protection situations.

Specific tasks

- Secret Service (Goodavage, 2017)
- FBI Hostage Rescue Team
- Prisons
- Personal protection
- Ring sports: used as training for personal protection dogs and breeding stock (Schutzhund, Mondio Ring, French Ring)
- Private security.

Potential issues

- Repetitive stress injuries: often unaddressed or unrecognized until significant symptomatic threshold is crossed; by then multiple areas of trauma are often involved
- Conditioning: physical fitness
- Cervical spinal trauma: cervical whiplash, IVDD (from repetitive bite work training)
- Lumbar spinal trauma: iliopsoas and other hypaxial muscles, ventral longitudinal ligament (from rotational hyperextension of spine during repetitive apprehension and bite training)
- Fatigue: nasal and musculoskeletal
- Trauma: musculoskeletal.

Case Study 21.1   Supraspinatus insertionopathy

Signalment: 2-y/o M/I Border Collie, working sheep-ranch dog, presented twice for post-trauma evaluations.

First presentation: Patient worked sheep at ranches throughout the United States and Canada as client traveled presenting clinics and competing. Four months before first presentation patient became distracted and fell into a small ditch while working sheep, hitting the opposite side with his chest. Patient cried out, was NWB on left thoracic limb for 5-10 minutes then seemed to move and work normally. Because of patient's talent and athletic ability, client wanted a thorough examination to rule out residual issues.

Physical examination: No obvious gait abnormalities. Physical and musculoskeletal examination unremarkable except for a small palpable defect in left supraspinatus at level of acromion process, and slight sensitivity to palpation.

Thermal imaging: Thermal images taken from cranial chest and left and right laterals demonstrate a significant asymmetrical pattern between right and left shoulders with a focus of heat in the area of left supraspinatus tendon (Figure 21.12).

Ultrasonography: Ultrasonographic exam of supraspinatus muscles demonstrated mild hyperechogenicity in the left distal supraspinatus (possibly displaying bruising or muscle trauma) with repeatable muscle hypoechoic core lesion just distal to this (Figure 21.13).

Treatment: As patient was traveling for the next month with other dogs competing in sheepdog trials, client was advised not to train or work the patient, allowing only strict leash walking for 3–4 weeks.

(Continued)

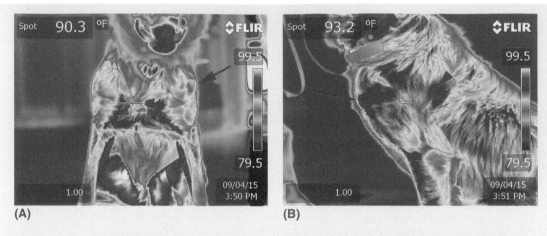

Figure 21.12 **(A)** Thermal image of the cranial chest demonstrating an asymmetrical pattern between the right and left shoulders with a focus of heat in the area of the left supraspinatus tendon (arrow). **(B)** Left lateral view showing the same pinpoint area of heat in the area of the distal supraspinatus (pink arrow). This heat signature radiates caudally and dorsally along the proximal supraspinatus and proximal deltoideus. There is another strong heat signature just caudal to the scapula (pink arrowhead) which is consistent with increased blood supply to the teres major.

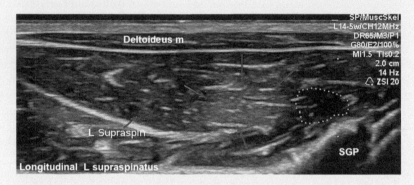

Figure 21.13 Ultrasonographic exam of the supraspinatus muscle demonstrating mild hyperechogenicity in the distal supraspinatus muscle (arrows) possibly displaying bruising or muscle trauma, with a repeatable muscle hypoechoic core lesion distally (dashed circle).

Client given instruction on PROM exercises, and manual and cryo/thermal therapies. Client advised to seek professional canine rehabilitation therapy including laser and acupuncture if symptoms worsened while traveling or upon arriving home.

Second presentation: One year later, patient presented for re-evaluation of left shoulder and right pelvic limb. Patient had been successfully working larger flocks and bigger areas, and had competed in several small, novice-level herding competitions. Eight months previously, he had displayed a mild, undiagnosed lameness of right pelvic limb that had improved gradually over the next few months. No problems had been reported until 3 weeks prior to the second presentation. Patient disappeared from

Client's view while moving sheep behind a barn, reappearing with a significant lameness of right pelvic limb.

Physical examination: Patient shows slight (1/5) gait abnormality of right pelvic limb at trot with shortened posterior stance phase and jerky, spastic lift into swing phase. Patient crabs slightly to right with a loss of normal reach to midline (right pelvic limb places directly under hip and left pelvic limb moves toward midline). Patient appears to have wider stance on thoracic limbs and to use front end to pull himself forward. Left shoulder has no loss of ROM in extension, but slight initial resistance to flexion before moving into full flexion. No obvious abnormalities in neutral postural position, visual gait movement, or muscle development. No sensitivities or

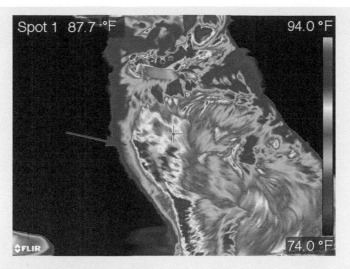

Figure 21.14   Thermal image of the lateral left shoulder demonstrating a small but definite focus of heat at the insertion of the left supraspinatus tendon a year after initial diagnosis.

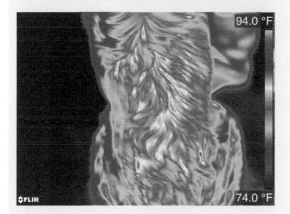

Figure 21.15   Dorsal lumbar spine thermal image (cranial is at the top of the image). An increased heat signature can be seen along the right cranial ribcage and lumbar epaxial musculature and over the left sacroiliac area.

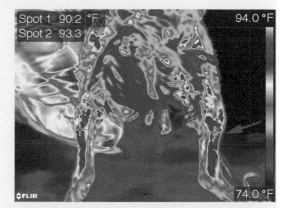

Figure 21.16   Thermal image of the caudal aspect of the pelvic limbs. The right pelvic limb demonstrates a significant focal heat pattern at the proximal caudal aspect of the right lateral tibia (arrow).

muscle defects on palpation of either right or left supraspinatus muscles. Slight resistance to full extension of the right pelvic limb, especially if digits also placed into flexion. Slight sensitivity and thickening palpable on right lateral proximal tibia. No medial buttress or joint laxity in either stifle joint. Slight sensitivity and muscle hypertonicity over right mid-lumbar spine with mild loss of lateral spinal flexibility.

Thermal imaging: Lateral chest image shows mild increase in heat present on cranial aspect of left shoulder at supraspinatus insertion (Figure 21.14). Patient shows asymmetrical heat pattern over lum-

bar spine, with greater heat present over right epaxial muscles (Figure 21.15), possibly representing increased blood flow from increased muscle demand compensating for right pelvic limb lameness (holding the leg up to minimize weight bearing) or chronic overuse from left shoulder (chronic stretching and tearing of epaxial muscle fibers). Right tibial image shows significantly elevated temperature in area of proximal caudolateral tibia (Figure 21.16).

(Continued)

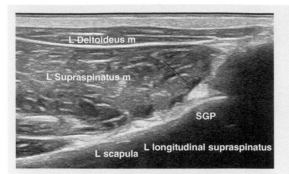

Figure 21.17 Longitudinal ultrasound of the left supraspinatus. A circular area of hyperechogenicity is visible just dorsal to the supraglenoid process in the same area as the defect imaged a year prior.

Ultrasonography: Ultrasound of left shoulder demonstrates no abnormal echo pattern of supraspinatus muscle belly. A triangular hyperechoic area of suspected fibrosis is well delineated in same area as previous core lesion (Figure 21.17). Ultrasound of right caudolateral tibia demonstrates significant disruption of normal muscular structure of long digital extensor (Figure 21.18). Patient shows slight discomfort with pressure of ultrasound probe on year-old left shoulder and acute right tibial injuries.

Treatment: Cryotherapy initiated on right pelvic limb injury, followed by manual therapy, gentle PROM, and low-level laser therapy (LLLT). Field and pen work discontinued. Once patient fully weight bearing at stance with no lameness visible at walk, exercises, PROM, and manual therapy for the chronic left thoracic limb supraspinatus muscle injury initiated. Client advised to gradually increase appropriate loading and movement exercises as patient could tolerate for next 16 weeks.

Discussion: This case illustrates several important aspects of managing complex working dog cases that can involve both chronic and acute issues.

Thermal imaging demonstrated increased blood supply demand (warmer temperatures) in muscles that could be compensating for a slight gait abnormality and structural asymmetry (triceps, teres minor, epaxials). A biomechanical compensatory link

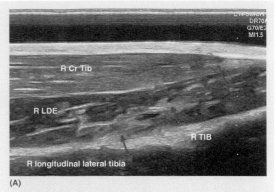

(A)

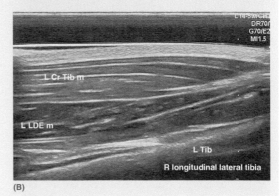

(B)

Figure 21.18 (A) Longitudinal ultrasound of the right proximal caudolateral tibia showing marked disruption of the architecture of the long digital extensor muscle. The cranial tibial muscle appears unaffected. (B) Longitudinal ultrasound of the left proximal caudolateral tibia for comparison.

between thoracic and pelvic limbs can be demonstrated with the presence of hypertonicity and increased blood flow of the lumbar epaxial muscles.

While the left pelvic limb injury could perhaps be a discrete event, there is a high probability that the diagonal pattern of left thoracic limb and right pelvic limb injuries are related. A thorough practitioner needs to consider and rule out the possibility that the left thoracic limb injury has not fully healed or has affected gait mechanics to the point that extra mechanical load has been placed on the right pelvic limb, thus contributing to the failure of muscle or tendinous structure.

Herding

While herding as a competitive sport is common through the United States and the United Kingdom, many ranches and farms actively use dogs in day-to-day herding operations with

sheep and cattle (Figure 21.19). Herding can be broken down to two distinct activities: either gathering and moving animals in and around a property, or guarding sheep or cattle (mostly sheep) from predators such as coyotes, feral dogs, and wolves. Dogs performing the latter

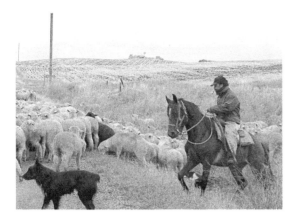

Figure 21.19   Working dogs on a ranch in Idaho.

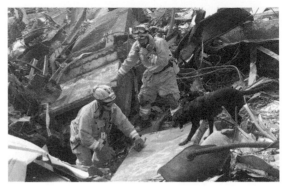

Figure 21.20   Search and rescue dogs need to be able to work on various terrains including rubble, rock scree, and hot desert sand. Source: Photo by Andrea Booher, FEMA, World Trade Center.

activity are often referred to as livestock guardian dogs. Commonly used breeds for movement herding include the Border Collie, Australian Cattle Dog, Australian Shepherd, and Australian Kelpie. Commonly used breeds for guarding livestock include Anatolian Shepherds, Great Pyrenees, Meremma, and Akbash Dogs. The herding ability of many Border Collies has also been effectively channeled around airports and golf courses to chase off waterfowl.

Specific tasks

- Farm and ranch work
- Herding sheep/goats/cattle
- Geese police (golf courses/airports).

Potential issues

- Repetitive musculoskeletal stress from sudden stopping/starting with sudden changes in direction
- Insufficient conditioning
- Blunt trauma from livestock
- Stereotypical behavior from inappropriate management or environment (occurs in both movement herding and guardian dogs)
- Border Collie collapse syndrome (exercise intolerance disorder): affected breeds may include Border Collies, Australian Cattle dogs, Australian Kelpies, Australian Shepherds, Whippets, Shetland sheepdogs, Bearded collies, Belgian Malinois, and Belgian Tervuren.

Search and rescue

The use of search and rescue dogs has grown throughout the world as their value in urban settings such as the rescue or recovery of earthquake victims has gained in international attention (American Rescue Dog Association, 2002). In the United States, many ski resorts have owned and used dogs specifically for avalanche rescue for decades. Avalanche dogs are usually very specifically trained for work in snow only. In regions of human–wilderness interface, there are usually volunteer or law-enforcement-associated groups who regularly practice scent training and urban or wilderness rescue training to stay ready for deployment at a moment's notice. Dogs can be specifically trained for either live-find or cadaver recovery (including searching for bodies underwater) or can be trained for any scent (Judah, 2014). Dogs need to be fit to handle various terrains such as building rubble, avalanche conditions, mountain rock scree, and hot desert sand/exposure (Bulanda, 2010) (Figure 21.20).

Specific tasks/sites

- Wilderness
- Urban
- Avalanche
- Rescue versus recovery
- Victims dead for over 10 years, cadaver, and other decomposed tissue.

Potential issues (Duhaime *et al.*, 1998; Slensky *et al.*, 2004)

- Fatigue: extreme environments such as rubble, steep slopes, elevation changes, heavy vegetation, heat, uneven firmness, and texture of footing
- Restrictive vests affecting shoulder, neck, and back movement
- Hyperthermia
- Gastrointestinal issues: diarrhea, vomiting, diminished appetite
- Foot problems: worn pads, foreign bodies, flexor tendon injuries, carpal tunnel inflammation and injury, carpal hyperextension
- Hypoglycemia, electrolyte imbalances, dehydration
- Encounters with wildlife
- Injuries from inhaling or walking through toxins in demolished buildings
- Injuries from working on rough, exposed surfaces of destroyed buildings.

Water rescue

The use of dogs for water rescue is not common in North America, except as a training exercise for Newfoundlands, Portuguese Water Dogs and other breeds with water rescue as a component of their heritage. However, actively working Newfoundlands (and some Labradors and Golden Retrievers) can be found working with water-rescue units in the United Kingdom (Royal Navy Reserve) and Italy (Coast Guard, Scuola Italiana Cani Salvataggio (Italian School of Water Rescue Dogs)) (Figure 21.21).

Potential issues

- Heli-deployment: water impact trauma, ear infections
- Conditioning
- Pneumonia, upper respiratory tract infection from water inhalation.

Sled dogs

The use of dogs to pull sleds and sledges may be one of the oldest documented uses of dogs working for humans. Today in the continental

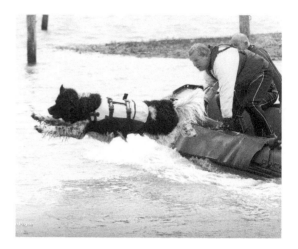

Figure 21.21 In many parts of the world, dogs are trained for water rescue. Here a Newfoundland in the United Kingdom practices water rescue skills.
Source: Photo by Cheryl and Phil Payne.

United States, sled dogs are mostly used for competitive sport. However, in parts of Alaska and northern Canada (e.g., Nunavut), dogs are still used as an important form of transportation of humans, mail, and cargo, both in the interior, and along the western and northern coasts. The US Post Office discontinued regular mail service by sled dog in 1963 when the last sled dog mail driver on the Bering Sea retired. While many villagers in Alaska rely more on airplanes and snowmobiles for transportation, many Native families still keep small sled dog teams for short transportation and competitive sport. The Russian and Danish militaries still use working sled dogs as transportation in remote areas. The most common breeds used are Siberian Huskies, Alaskan Huskies, and Malamutes. Working sled dogs would be expected to have the same type of health issues as racing sled dogs; much of the research done solving sled dog health issues has been applied to sports medicine issues with other competitive and working canine athletes.

Potential issues (Lee *et al.*, 2014)

- Gastric ulcers
- Maintenance of weight
- Aspiration pneumonia
- Musculoskeletal: shoulders, triceps, carpi, feet, hamstrings

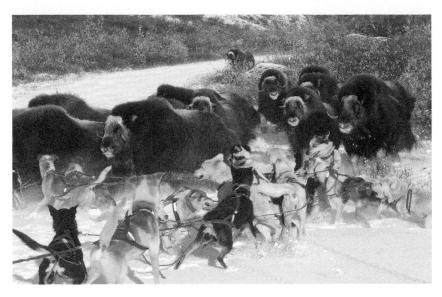

Figure 21.22 Working dogs can be faced with many different and unexpected situations, such as this sled dog team that met a herd of musk oxen on the trail. Source: Photo by Heather Williams.

- Hyperthermia
- Poorly fitting harnesses
- Encounters with wildlife (especially moose, muskox, caribou) (Figure 21.22)
- Cardiac arrhythmias: genetic, electrolyte imbalance, hyperkalemia from exertional myopathy
- Exertional myopathy.

Service dogs

There is a wide variety of roles that service dogs play. Effective March 15, 2011, under the Americans with Disabilities Act (ADA), a Service Animal is defined as any dog that is individually trained to do work or perform tasks for the benefit of an individual with a disability, including a physical, sensory, psychiatric, intellectual, or other mental disability. Other species of animals, whether wild or domestic, trained or untrained, are not service animals for the purposes of this definition. The work or tasks performed by a service animal must be directly related to the individual's disability. There are many different tasks that service dogs perform; some dogs perform more than one role.

Examples of the work that these dogs might perform include assisting individuals who are blind or have low vision with navigation and other tasks, alerting individuals who are deaf or hard of hearing to the presence of people or sounds, providing nonviolent protection or rescue work, pulling a wheelchair, assisting an individual during a seizure, alerting individuals to the presence of allergens, retrieving items such as medicine or the telephone, providing physical support and assistance with balance and stability to individuals with mobility disabilities, and helping persons with psychiatric and neurological disabilities by preventing or interrupting impulsive or destructive behaviors. The crime deterrent effects of an animal's presence and the provision of emotional support, well-being, comfort, or companionship do not constitute work or tasks for the purposes of this definition.

It is not known how many working dogs there are in the United States or other countries. For example, Guide Dogs for the Blind reports having trained 14,000 total teams since their inception in 1942; they currently claim 2200 active dog guides. There probably are 10,000 dog guides working across the United States when one considers dogs trained by all guide dog schools.

According to the University of Arizona, in 2014 0.9% of persons with disabilities were partnered with service dogs (see the Service Dog Central website). In 1990, Congress found that there were 43 million Americans with disabilities, suggesting there are probably more than 387,000 service dogs across the United States. However, this figure probably includes emotional support animals, which are sometimes grouped with service animals, such as under the Fair Housing Act or Air Carrier Access Act. A more reasonable estimate of the number of public access (task-trained) service dogs in the United States might be 100,000 to 200,000.

Service dog categories

- Diabetic alert dogs
- Severe allergy alert dogs
- Visual assistance dogs
- Hearing assistance dogs
- Wheelchair assistance dogs
- Psychiatric service dogs
- Mobility assistance dogs
- Medical alert dogs
- Seizure alert dogs
- Seizure response dogs
- Autism assistance dogs.

Potential issues

- Poor conditioning
- Working with subtle, unrecognized injuries
- Poorly fitting harnesses
- Chemical or environmental exposures due to increased exposure potential (travel)
- Fatigue (nose).

Webliography

Americans with Disabilities Act. 2011. https://www.ada.gov/archive/adastat91.htm#Anchor-33869.
Baxter, C. & Hargrave, M. 2015. Guidance on the use of historic human remains detection dogs for locating unmarked cemeteries. http://www.dtic.mil/docs/citations/AD1001858.
Guide Dogs for the Blind. FAQ. https://www.guidedogs.com/explore-resources/faq.
Institute of Canine Forensics. 2015. *In the news*. http://www.hhrdd.org.
ITALIAN SCHOOL of WATER RESCUE DOGS. http://www.waterrescuedogs.com.
Romey, K. 2016. Sled dogs have been pulling us for millenia, archeology shows. *National Geographic*. http://news.nationalgeographic.

com/2016/03/20160318-ancient-sled-dogs-archaeology-Iditarod-Arctic-Siberia/.
Service Dog Central. http://www.servicedogcentral.org/content/.
United States Department of Agriculture. 2017. *National Detector Dog Manual*. USDA/Animal Plant Health Inspection Service. https://www.aphis.usda.gov/import_export/plants/manuals/ports/downloads/detector_dog.pdf.
United States War Dogs Association. 0000a Types of war dogs. http://www.uswardogs.org/war-dog-history/types-war-dogs/.
United States War Dogs Association. 0000b Working dog adoptions. http://www.uswardogs.org.
Volhard, W. 2013. A Personality Profile for your Dog. http://www.volhard.com/pages/canine-personality-profile.php.
WikimediaCommons. File: The Battle of Frontiers, August-September 1914. https://commons.wikimedia.org/wiki/File:The_Battle_of_Frontiers,_August-september_1914_Q70232.jpg.
All websites accessed October 2017.

References

Alho, A. M., Pita, J., Amaro, A., Amaro, F., Schnyder, M., Grimm, F., *et al.* 2016. Seroprevalence of vector-borne pathogens and molecular detection of *Borrelia afzelli* in military dogs from Portugal. *Parasites Vectors*, 9(1), 225.
Altom, E. K., Davenport, G. M., Myers, L. J. & Cummins, K. A. 2003. Effect of dietary fat source and exercise on odorant-detecting ability of canine athletes. *Res Vet Sci*, 75, 149–155.
American Rescue Dog Association. 2002. *Search and Rescue Dogs: Training the K-9 Hero*, 2nd edn. Hoboken, NJ: John Wiley & Sons, Inc.
Angle, T., Wakshlag, J. J., Gillette, R. L., Steury, T., Haney, P., Barrett, J. & Fisher, T. 2014. The effects of exercise and diet on olfactory capability in detection dogs. *J Nutr Science*, 13(3), e44.
Baker, J. & Miller, L. 2013. The effects of environmental extremes on working dogs: a collaborative initiative. *US Army Med Dept J*, 22–27.
Baker, J., Truesdale, C. A. & Schlanser, J. R. 2009. Overview of combat trauma in military working dogs in Iraq and Afghanistan. *US Army Med Dept J*, 33–37.
Berrueta, L., Muskai, I., Olenich, S., Butler, T., Badger, G. J., Colas, R. A., *et al.* 2016. Stretching impacts inflammation resolution in connective tissue. *J Cell Physiol*, 231(7), 1621–1627.
Bruchim, Y., Aroch, I., Eliav, A., Abbas, A., Frank, I., Kelmer, E., *et al.* 2014. Two years of combined high-intensity physical training and heat acclimatization

affect lymphocyte and serum HSP70 in purebred military working dogs. *J Appl Physiol*, 117, 112–118.

Bryson, S. 2000. *Police Dog Tactics*. Calgary, AB: Detselig Enterprises Ltd.

Bulanda, S. 2010. *Ready! Training the Search and Rescue Dog*, 2nd edn. Irvine, CA: i-5 Publishing.

Cristescu, R. H., Foley, E., Markula, A., Jackson, G., Jones, D. & FrÈRe, C. 2015. Accuracy and efficiency of detection dogs: a powerful new tool for koala conservation and management. *Sci Rep*, 5, 8349.

Corey, S. M., Vizzard, M. A., Bouffard, N. A., Badger, G. J. & Langevin, H. M. 2012. Stretching of the back improves the gait, mechanical sensitivity and connective tissue inflammation in a rodent model. *PLoS One*, 7(1), e29831.

DEPARTMENT of DEFENSE. 2013. *US Military Working Dog Training Handbook*. Guilford, CT: Lyons Press.

Diverio, S., Guelfi, G., Barbato, O., Di Mari, W., Egidi, M. G. & Santoro, M. M. 2015. Non-invasive assessment of animal exercise stress: real-time PCR of GLUT4, COX1, SOD1 and HSP70 in avalanche military dog saliva. *Animal*, 9(1), 104–109.

Duhaime, R.A., Norden, D., Corso, B., Mallonee, S. & Salman, M. D. 1998. Injuries and illnesses in working dogs during the disaster response after the bombing in Oklahoma City. *J Am Vet Med Assoc*, 212(8), 1202–1207.

Elbrond, V. S. & Schultz, R. M. 2015. Myofascia—the unexplored tissue: myofascial kinetic lines in horses, a model for describing locomotion using comparative dissection derived from human lines. *Med Res Arch*, 3, 1–22.

Evans, R. I., Herbold, J. R., Bradshaw, B. S. & Moore, G. E. 2007. Causes for discharge of military working dogs from service: 268 cases (2000–2004). *J Am Vet Med Assoc*, 231(8), 1215–1220.

Fox, P. R., Puschner, B. & Ebel, J. G. 2008. Assessment of acute injuries, exposure to environmental toxin, and five-year health surveillance of New York Police Department working dogs following the September 11, 2001 World Trade Center terrorist attack. *J Am Vet Med Assoc*, 233(1), 48–59.

Frantz, L., Mullin, V., Pionnier-Capitan, M., Lebrasseur, O., Ollivier, M., Perri, A., et al. 2016. Genomic and archaeological evidence suggests a dual origin of domestic dogs. *Science*, 352(6290), 1228–1231.

Goodavage, M. 2017. *Secret Service Dogs: The Heroes Who Protect the President of the United States*, 1st edn. New York: Dutton.

Grimm, D. 2015. Dawn of the dog. *Science*, 348(6232), 274–279.

Hackner, K., Errhalt, P., Mueller, M., Speiser, M., Marzluf, B. A., Schulheim, A., et al. 2016. Canine scent detection for the diagnosis of lung cancer in a screening situation. *J Breath Res*, 10(4), 046003.

Hart, L. A., Zasloff, R. L., Bryson, S. & Christensen, S. L. 2000. The role of police dogs as companions and working partners. *Psychol Rep*, 86(1), 190–202.

Jezierski, T., Walczak, M., Ligor, T., Rudnicka, J. & Buszewski, B. 2015. Study of the art: canine olfaction used for cancer detection on the basis of breath odour. Perspectives and limitations. *J Breath Res*, 9(2), 027001.

Judah, C. 2014. *Training a Search and Rescue Dog for Wilderness Air Scent Detection*, 1st edn. Holden Beach, NC: Coastal Books.

Keegan, K. 2004. How to evaluate head and pelvic movement to determine lameness. *AAEP Proc*, 50, 206–211.

Keegan, K. 2005a. Head movement patterns in horses with forelimb and hindlimb lameness. *AAEP Proc*, 51, 114–120.

Keegan, K. 2005b. Pelvic movement pattern in horses with hindlimb and forelimb lameness. *AAEP Proc*, 51, 121–127.

Krause, F., Wilke, J., Vogt, L. & Banzer, W. 2016. Intermuscular force transmission along myofascial chains: a systemic review. *J Anat*, 228(6), 910–918.

Larson, G., Karlsson, E. K., Perri, A., Webster, M. T., Ho, S. Y., Peters, J., et al. 2012. Rethinking dog domestication by integrating genetics, archeology and biogeography. *Proc Natl Acad Sci USA*, 109(23), 8878–8883.

Lee, J., VON Pfeil, D., Thompson, S. & Hinchcliff, K. 2014. *The Musher and Veterinary Handbook*, 3rd edn. Marlboro, VT: International Sled Dog Veterinary Medical Association.

Lemish, M. 2008. *War Dogs: A History of Loyalty and Heroism*. Washington, DC: Potomac Books.

Linn, L. L., Bartels, K. E., Rochat, M. C., Payton, M. E. & Moore, G. E. 2003. Lumbosacral stenosis in 29 military working dogs: epidemiologic findings and outcome after surgical intervention (1990–1999). *Vet Surg*, 32, 21–29.

Maliye, S. & Marshall, J. 2016. Objective assessment of the compensatory effect of clinical hind limb lameness in horses: 37 cases (2011–2014). *J Am Vet Med Assoc*, 249(8), 940–944.

Moore, G. E., Burkman, K. D., Carter, M. N. & Peterson, M. R. 2001. Causes of death or reasons for euthanasia in military working dogs: 927 cases (1993–1996). *J Am Vet Med Assoc*, 219(2), 209–214.

Orkin, J. D., Yang, Y., Yang, C., Yu, D. W. & Jiang, X. 2016. Cost-effective scat-detection dogs: unleashing a powerful new tool for international mammalian conservation biology. *Sci Rep*, 6, 34758.

Peterson, M., Fommelt, A. & Dunn, G. 2000. A study of the lifetime occurrence of neoplasia and breed differences in a cohort of German Shepherd dogs and Belgian Malinois military working dogs that died in 1992. *J Vet Intern Med*, 14(2), 140–145.

Prada, P. A. & Rodriguez, M. 2016. Demining dogs in Colombia—a review of operational challenges, chemical perspectives, and practical implications. *Sci Justice*, 56(4), 269–277.

Reynolds, A. 2014. The role of glucose polymers in recovery from exercise in sled dogs. In: Lee, J., von Pfeil, D., Thompson, S. & Hinchcliff, K. (eds), *The Musher and Veterinary Handbook*, 3rd edn. Marlboro, VT: International Sled Dog Veterinary Medical Association, pp. 48–50.

Reynolds, A. J., Carey, D. P., Reinhart, G. A., Swenson, R. A. & Kallfelz, F. A. 1997. Effect of postexercise carbohydrate supplementation on muscle glycogen repletion in trained sled dogs. *Am J Vet Res*, 58(11), 1252–1256.

Schleip, R., Findlay, T., Chaitow, L. & Huijing, P. 2012. *Fascia: The Tensional Network of the Human Body: The Science and Clinical Applications in Manual and Movement Therapy*, 1st edn. Edinburgh: Churchill Livingstone.

Slensky, K. A., Drobratz, K. J., Downend, A. B. & Otto, C. M. 2004. Deployment morbidity among search-and-rescue dogs used after the September 11, 2001 terrorist attack. *J Am Vet Med Assoc*, 225(6), 868–873.

Stojsih, S. E., Baker, J. L., Les, C. M. & Bir, C. A. 2014. Canine deaths while in service in civilian law enforcement (2002–2012). *J Spec Ops Med*, 14(4), 86–91.

Toffoli, C. A. & Rolfe, D. S. 2006. Challenges to military working dog management and care in the Kuwait theater of operation. *Military Med*, 171(10), 1002–1005.

Wakshlag, J. J., Snedden, K. A., Otis, A. M., Kennedy, C. A., Kennett, T. P., Scarlett, J. M., *et al.* 2002. Effects of post-exercise supplements on glycogen repletion in skeletal muscle. *Vet Ther*, 3(3), 226–234.

Wilke, J., Krause, F., Vogt, L. & Banzer, W. 2016a. What is evidence-based about myofascial chains: a systemic review. *Arch Phys Med Rehabil*, 97(3), 454.

Wilke, J., Niederer, D., Vogt, L. & Banzer, W. 2016b. Remote effects of lower limb stretching: preliminary evidence for myofascial connectivity? *J Sports Sci*, 34(22), 2145–2148.

Wilke, J., Vogt, L., Niederer, D. & Banzer, W. 2016c. Is remote stretching based on myofascial chains as effective as local exercise? A randomized-controlled trial. *J Sports Sci*, 7, 1–7.

22 The Role of Acupuncture and Manipulative Therapy in Canine Rehabilitation

Carolina Medina, DVM, DACVSMR, CVA, CVCH, CCRT, Christine Jurek, DVM, CCRT, CVA, CVC, and Rosemary J. LoGiudice, DVM, DACVSMR, CCRT, CVA, CVSMT, FCoAC

Summary

Reducing pain, providing the best possible quality of life for patients, and restoring and maintaining normal form and function is the focus of veterinary rehabilitation therapy. Acupuncture is the insertion of thin, sterile needles into specific points, based on anatomic structures, which leads to physiological responses. These physiological responses are due to stimulation of the nervous system, and lead to a release of endogenous substances such as beta-endorphins, dynorphins, enkephalins, serotonin, epinephrine, gamma-aminobutyric acid (GABA), cortisol, and various hormones. Approximately 360 acupuncture points have been described, having various impacts on pain relief and on organ systems. Acupuncture points can be stimulated via dry needle, electroacupuncture, aquapuncture, acupressure, laser acupuncture, moxibustion, hemoacupuncture, pneumoacupuncture, and gold implantation. The selection of acupuncture points is critical to the success of treatment, and is based upon the clinical condition, patient temperament, and treatment goals. Acupuncture has clinical applications in rehabilitation and sports medicine including pain relief, performance and endurance enhancement, and nerve regeneration.

Veterinary manipulative therapy, also referred to as veterinary spinal manipulative therapy and animal chiropractic, is a valuable manual, neurological receptor-based somatic therapy. It is a potent modality for maintaining overall health and mobility, focusing on restoration of function as well as relief and management of pain. The American College of Veterinary Sports Medicine and Rehabilitation (ACVSMR) recognizes chiropractic as an integrative veterinary therapy related to veterinary sports medicine and rehabilitation.

This chapter describes the evidence basis for acupuncture and chiropractic and discusses the precautions, contraindications, and limitations for the use of these integrative modalities.

Canine Sports Medicine and Rehabilitation, Second Edition. Edited by Chris Zink and Janet B. Van Dyke.
© 2018 John Wiley & Sons, Inc. Published 2018 by John Wiley & Sons, Inc.

Acupuncture overview

Acupuncture is the insertion of fine, sterile needles into specific acupuncture points to create a physiological response. These physiological responses are due to stimulation of both the central and peripheral nervous systems. Acupuncture stimulation releases endogenous substances such as beta-endorphins, dynorphins, enkephalins, serotonin, epinephrine, GABA, cortisol and various hormones (Soligo et al., 2013). The earliest scientific studies done on acupuncture focused on its analgesic effects. In the late 1970s researchers discovered that acupuncture stimulation led to an increased concentration of endogenous opioids in the serum and cerebral spinal fluid (Pan et al., 1984; He, 1987). Additional studies showed that naloxone, an opioid antagonist, blocked the effects of acupuncture and decreased the pain threshold in acupuncture subjects (Mayer et al., 1977). These were the first studies showing that endogenous opioids played a role in the mechanism of action of acupuncture analgesia.

Acupuncture stimulation increases the blood concentration of the serotonin precursor free tryptophan (Costa et al., 1982). Others have shown an increase in serotonin in the central nervous system (CNS) after acupuncture stimulation (Zhong, 1989). Beta-endorphins stimulate serotonergic nerves within the descending tract to release serotonin (He, 1987). It is speculated that acupuncture analgesia involves serotonergic neurons since acupuncture releases beta-endorphins, which in turn releases serotonin.

Acupuncture analgesia may be related to one or more of the four phases of pain perception: insult from a noxious stimulus, transduction of the painful stimulus via electrical signals, transmission of the painful stimulus into the spinal cord, and perception of pain by the higher brain centers and somatosensory cortex. One hypothesis proposes that acupuncture stimulation can block perception of pain before it reaches the CNS. This is based on Wall and Melzack's gate control theory of pain perception (Melzack & Wall, 1965; DeLeo, 2006). Acupuncture stimulates A-beta and A-delta fibers to rapidly carry information to the spinal cord, synapsing with inhibitory interneurons to close the gate before ascending pain impulses arrive from the C fibers. This prevents pain impulses from reaching the higher brain centers and blocks conscious perception of pain. Regional acupuncture analgesia is also speculated as A-delta fibers are transmitted cranially and caudally within spinal segments before entering the dorsal horn gray matter (Steiss, 2001). Acupuncture also activates the descending pain control pathway modulating nociceptive signals at the level of the brain and spinal cord (Murotani et al., 2010; Silva et al., 2011). Acupuncture has also been shown to alleviate inflammatory pain in rats and human models, thereby reducing inflammatory mediators such as lipopolysaccharides, interleukin 6 (IL-6), IL-1β, and tumor necrosis factor alpha (TNF-α) (Jeong et al., 2003; Yim et al., 2007; Zhang et al., 2012).

Acupuncture points

Dogs have approximately 360 acupuncture points located throughout the body. There are four types of points depending on their associated neural structures: Type I motor points, Type II midline points, Type III nerve or nerve plexus points, and Type IV muscle–tendon junction points. Motor points make up 67% of all points, and are located in areas where nerves penetrate a muscle. SI-9 is located at the junction of the deltoideus and the long head of the triceps brachii, where the axillary and radial nerves emerge. Type II points are located on the superficial nerves on dorsal and ventral midlines. Bai-hui lies in the depression between the spinous processes of the 7th lumbar and the 1st sacral vertebrae on the dorsal midline and it is supplied by the dorsal branch of the 7th lumbar nerve. Type III points are located at high-density loci of superficial nerves and nerve plexuses. GB-34 is the point where the common peroneal nerve divides into the deep and superficial branches. Type IV points are located at muscle–tendon junctions where Golgi tendon organs exist. BL-57 is located at the junction of the gastrocnemius muscle and the common calcanean tendon (Gunn et al., 1976; Gunn, 1977).

Most acupuncture points are located in areas of low electrical resistance and high electrical conductance (Brown et al., 1974; Reichmanis et al., 1975; Urano & Ogasawara, 1978). Histological studies reveal that acupuncture points are located in areas where there are free nerve endings, arterioles, lymphatic vessels, and an aggregation of mast cells (Pan *et al.*, 1986). Due to their anatomic location, there are many local effects that occur with acupuncture point stimulation. These local effects include an increase in local blood flow and circulation; release of Hageman's factor XII which activates the clotting cascade, complement cascade, and release of plasminogens and kinins; mast cell degranulation which releases histamine, heparin, and proteases; release of bradykinin which leads to vasodilation; and production of local prostaglandins which leads to smooth muscle relaxation (Kendall, 1989a; Omura, 1975). The vasoactive effects that occur with acupuncture stimulation follow a specific sequence. There is an initial short vasoconstriction phase (lasting 15–30 seconds), followed by a quasi-control state (lasting 10 seconds to 2 minutes), and a final vasodilation phase (lasting 2 minutes to 2 weeks) (Omura, 1975). This results in an enhanced local tissue immune status, improved local tissue perfusion, and muscle and tissue relaxation. Pain relief occurs as a result of improved perfusion and muscle spasm relief caused by local effects of acupuncture stimulation and somatovisceral reflexes (Steiss, 2001).

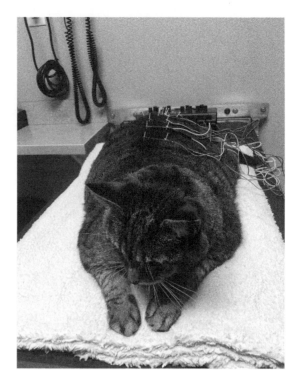

Figure 22.1 Thirteen-year-old domestic shorthaired cat receiving electroacupuncture for the treatment of osteoarthritis. As demonstrated here, animals frequently find this treatment very relaxing.

Methods of acupuncture point stimulation

There are nine ways to stimulate acupuncture points: dry needle, electroacupuncture, aquapuncture, acupressure, laser acupuncture, moxibustion, hemoacupuncture, pneumoacupuncture, and gold implantation (Xie & Preast, 2007). Dry needle is defined as the insertion of acupuncture needles into acupuncture points. These needles vary in length (0.25, 0.5, 1, 1.5, and 2 inches) and gauge (28, 30, 32, 34, and 36 gauge), and they are typically left in place for approximately 20 minutes. Dry needle is the most commonly used acupuncture technique in dogs.

Electroacupuncture is the attachment of electrical leads to dry needles and connection to an electroacupuncture unit (Figure 22.1). The unit can be set to a variety of frequencies and each frequency stimulates a different pathway in the nervous system. Low-frequency (1–20 Hertz) electroacupuncture predominantly stimulates A-delta fibers and releases beta-endorphins,

enkephalins, and orphanins. High-frequency (80–100 Hertz) electroacupuncture predominantly stimulates C fibers which releases dynorphins, and serotonergic fibers which releases serotonin and norepinephrine (Melzack & Wall, 1965; Kendall, 1989b; Fry *et al.*, 2014). Lower frequencies provide longer lasting and more cumulative analgesia (Han, 2003). Canine patients are frequently treated with a combination of dry needle and electroacupuncture (Figure 22.2).

Aquapuncture is the injection of a sterile liquid directly into acupuncture points. The pressure of the liquid induces stimulation of acupuncture points until it is absorbed. The most commonly used injectable liquids include saline, vitamin B12, and lidocaine.

Acupressure is the application of manual pressure on acupuncture points for a period of 1–5 minutes per point. This is a safe and easy technique to demonstrate and instruct clients to perform at home.

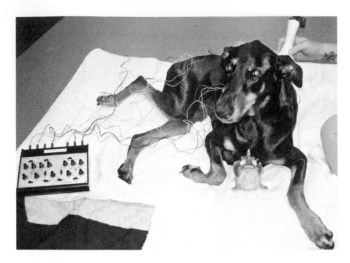

Figure 22.2   Doberman receiving a combination of electroacupuncture and dry acupuncture.

Low-level laser therapy can be applied directly on acupuncture points to induce stimulation of the points. Treatment can be done with either a class 3B or class 4 therapeutic laser at routine settings for the individual body region.

Moxibustion is performed using the dried herb *Artemisia* rolled into a cigar shape and burned 1.5 cm over the acupuncture point without touching the skin. This stimulates acupuncture points through a warming technique and is typically used on patients with chronic arthritis that is worse in cold weather.

Hemoacupuncture has two forms of stimulation. The first form is the withdrawal of a small amount of blood from acupuncture points located directly on blood vessels. For example, *Tai-yang* is located on the transverse facial vein just lateral to the lateral canthus of the eye. This technique is primarily used for febrile diseases. The second form is the injection of the patient's blood into acupuncture points. This technique is used for autoimmune diseases.

Pneumoacupuncture is the injection of air into the subcutaneous space in areas where there is muscle atrophy. The theory behind this technique is that the air puts pressure on the acupuncture points and stimulates them until the air is absorbed.

Gold therapy is the injection of sterile gold, in the form of a small wire or bead, directly into acupuncture points. The gold creates an ionic change in the tissues that stimulates the points for a prolonged period of time.

Acupuncture point selection

Local points are those located directly in the area to be treated, and they are selected largely to treat pain. ST-36 is a local point for the stifle as it is located just distal to the tibial plateau in the cranial tibial muscle. Distal points are located either distal or caudal to the area to be treated, and they are selected for the patient that finds it too painful at the local site and/or to draw edema or swelling from the local site. LIV-3 is located between the 2nd and 3rd metatarsals proximal to the metatarsophalangeal joint, so quite distal to the stifle, and is commonly used to treat stifle pain. Another option is to select points proximal/cranial and distal/caudal. A patient with intervertebral disc disease at T13–L1 can be treated with BL-20 (lateral to the caudal border of the dorsal spinous process of T12) and BL-23 (lateral to the caudal border of the dorsal spinous process of L2).It is important to know the anatomic location and clinical indication of acupuncture points to make an appropriate therapeutic point selection. Since there are approximately 360 acupuncture points there are many options for point selection for individual conditions. Points that are most commonly used in veterinary medicine are selected for their ease of anatomic location and acceptance by animal patients. Points along the neck, back, hips, and shoulders are commonly used in dogs as they are well tolerated due to their location in large

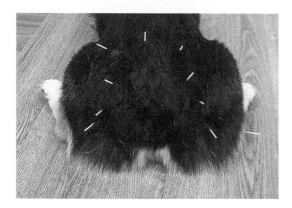

Figure 22.3   Acupuncture points along the back and hips, as shown here, and in other large muscle groups are well tolerated.

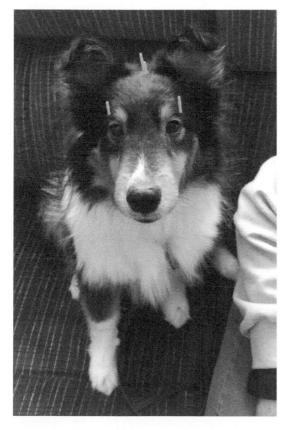

Figure 22.4   Dog tolerating acupuncture in the very sensitive, highly innervated areas adjacent to the eyes.

muscle groups (Figure 22.3). Points located in areas with smaller muscles, such as the elbows, feet, and face are less well tolerated by the canine patient (Figure 22.4). Most veterinary acupuncturists select the commonly used

Table 22.1   Acupuncture points for specific conditions

Clinical condition	Acupuncture point selection
General pain	LIV-3, GB-34, BL-60, SI-9
Hip pain	BL-54, GB-29, GB-30, *Jian-jiao*, BL-40, BL-23, LIV-3
Stifle pain	ST-36, GB-33, GB-34, SP-9, SP-10, BL-40, LIV-3
Hock pain	BL-60, KID-3, ST-41, KID-6, LIV-3
Shoulder pain	LI-15, TH-14, SI-9, LU-1
Elbow pain	LI-10, LI-11, LU-5, HT-3, PC-3
Carpal pain	HT-7, LU-7, LU-9, TH-4, PC-7
Intervertebral disc disease (IVDD)	Local, cranial, and caudal BL points to the site of IVDD, KID-1, *Liu-feng*
Wobbler's syndrome	*Jing-jia-ji*, LI-4, SI-16, SI-3
Degenerative myelopathy	ST-36, LI-10, BL-23, *Bai-hui*, BL-54, BL-40, KID-1, *Liu-feng*
Vestibular disease	GB-20, GB-21, GV-20, TH-21, SI-19, GB-2, *An-shen*
Urinary incontinence	BL-39, KID-3, KID-6, SP-6, CV-1
Fecal incontinence	GV-1, BL-25, ST-36, ST-37, LI-10
Appetite stimulation	BL-20, BL-21, *Shan-gen, Jian-wei*

Source: Xie & Preast (2007)

acupuncture points for individual conditions (Table 22.1) as these points are easy to locate (Table 22.2) and are well tolerated by animal patients (Xie & Preast, 2007).

Integrating acupuncture into sports medicine and rehabilitation therapy

Acupuncture has many applications in sports medicine practice including its use for performance and endurance enhancement, as well as treating conditions to which canine athletes are prone such as muscle spasms, trigger points, osteoarthritis, intervertebral disc disease, and nerve damage. Acupuncture improves endurance and physical performance, and helps to regulate heart rate and blood pressure (Ehrlich & Haber, 1992). Treatment is typically performed

Table 22.2   Anatomic locations of acupuncture points

Acupuncture point	Anatomic location
BL-20	Lateral to caudal border of dorsal spinous process of T12
BL-21	Lateral to caudal border of dorsal spinous process of T13
BL-23	Lateral to caudal border of dorsal spinous process of L2
BL-24	Lateral to caudal border of dorsal spinous process of L4
BL-25	Lateral to caudal border of dorsal spinous process of L5
BL-26	Lateral to caudal border of dorsal spinous process of L6
BL-27	Lateral to caudal border of dorsal spinous process of L7
BL-28	Lateral to caudal border of dorsal spinous process of S1
BL-39	Lateral to popliteal crease on medial border of biceps femoris tendon
BL-40	Center of popliteal crease
BL-52	Lateral to caudal border of dorsal spinous process of L2 and lateral to BL-23
BL-54	Dorsal to greater trochanter
BL-67	At nail bed of lateral aspect of fifth digit of pelvic limb
CV-1	Between external genitalia and anus
CV-2	Ventral midline at cranial border of pubis
CV-3	Ventral midline 3/4 distance from umbilicus to pubis
CV-4	Ventral midline 2/3 distance from umbilicus to pubis
CV-5	Ventral midline 1/3 distance from umbilicus to pubis
CV-6	Ventral midline 1/4 distance from umbilicus to pubis
GB-2	Ventral to tragus
GB-20	Caudal and lateral to occipital protuberance
GB-21	Groove cranial to scapula halfway between C7–T1 junction and acromion
GB-29	Cranial to greater trochanter
GB-30	Caudal to greater trochanter
GB-33	On lateral side of pelvic limb, proximal to lateral femoral epicondyle
GB-34	Cranial and distal to head of fibula
GV-1	Between tail base and anus
GV-17	On dorsal midline of head at level of caudal rim of ears
GV-20	On dorsal midline of head at level of ear canals
GV-21	On dorsal midline of head at level of cranial rim of ears
HT-3	Cranial to medial epicondyle of humerus
HT-7	On transverse crease of carpal joint lateral to flexor carpi ulnaris tendon
KID-1	Under central pad of pelvic limbs
KID-3	Proximal to medial malleolus
KID-6	Distal and plantar to medial malleolus
LI-4	Between 2nd and 3rd metacarpals proximal to metacarpophalangeal joint
LI-10	1/6 of distance between elbow and carpus between extensor carpi radialis and common digital extensor

Table 22.2   (*Continued*)

Acupuncture point	Anatomic location
LI-11	Between biceps tendon and lateral epicondyle of humerus
LI-15	Cranial and distal to acromion
LIV-3	Between 2nd and 3rd metatarsals proximal to metatarsophalangeal joint
LU-1	In superficial pectoral muscle medial to greater tubercle of humerus
LU-5	In cubital crease lateral to biceps tendon
LU-7	Proximal to styloid process of radius
LU-9	Distal to styloid process of radius
PC-3	In cubital crease medial to biceps tendon
PC-7	Proximal and medial to accessory carpal pad
SI-3	Proximal and lateral to metacarpophalangeal joint
SI-9	Between deltoid and triceps at level of shoulder joint
SI-16	Dorsal border of brachiocephalicus at level of C2–C3
SI-19	Rostral to the tragus
SP-6	Medial and caudal aspect of tibia and distal to saphenous vein
SP-9	On medial side of pelvic limb, distal to medial condyle of tibia
SP-10	On medial side of pelvic limb, proximal to medial femoral condyle between two bellies of sartorius
ST-36	Just distal to tibial plateau in cranial tibialis muscle
ST-37	Distal to ST-36 in cranial tibialis
ST-41	Cranial aspect of tarsus
TH-4	At radiocarpal joint cranial to common digital extensor tendon
TH-14	Caudal and distal to acromion
TH-21	Dorsal to tragus
An-shen	Large depression behind ears
Jian-jiao	Dorsolateral aspect of hip in depression ventral to cranial dorsal iliac spine
Jian-wei	1/3 down lateral neck between jugular groove and lateral process of cervical vertebrae
Jing-jia-ji	Dorsal and ventral to lateral processes of each cervical vertebrae (28 points)
Liu-feng	Dorsal to metatarsophalangeal and metacarpophalangeal joints between digits 2–3, 3–4, and 4–5 (total of 12 points)
Shan-gen	Dorsal midline of nose between haired and non-haired junction
Yan-chi	Dorsolateral caudal lumbar region

Source: Xie & Preast (2007)

2–5 days before a competition. Acupuncture is also useful after a competition to alleviate pain or stress on the musculoskeletal system. It is important for the athlete to be cooled down and relaxed before doing an acupuncture treatment. Generally, acupuncture is done approximately 2–4 hours after performance. However, it is still effective if initiated the day after a competition. Acupuncture points used for performance enhancement include ST-36, LI-10, CV-4, CV-6, BL-24, BL-26, LI-4, and LIV-3.

Acupuncture is a useful modality to integrate into a rehabilitation program due to its analgesic properties and nerve stimulation effects. Many patients that receive rehabilitation therapy have pain that might hinder their ability to perform physical activity. By decreasing or eliminating pain, acupuncture allows more aggressive rehabilitation treatments to be instituted. Acupuncture can be administered as the final step in the rehabilitation protocol. A patient with cranial cruciate ligament rupture might receive laser therapy, massage, underwater treadmill, and exercises such as sit-to-stands. This patient would benefit from acupuncture therapy at the end of the exercises once they have cooled off. For these patients, acupuncture therapy can be given once or twice per week. A patient with intervertebral disc disease would likely receive a rehabilitation protocol of physioball work, isometric contractions, assisted walking with slings, toe pinches, ear scratches, neuromuscular electrical stimulation, and underwater treadmill. Because acupuncture can promote nerve regeneration (La et al., 2005) it is indicated for these patients, and it is commonly used 1–5 days per week depending on the grade of disc disease. Acupuncture is not only beneficial for pain management and nerve regeneration but it also has calming/sedating effects that are useful for patients that need to be cage-rested (Kim et al., 2006). Acupuncture points used for their calming/sedating effects include GV-17, GV-20, GV-21, An-shen, and HT-7.

Case Study 22.1   Acupuncture to treat a Greyhound with decreased mobility

Signalment: 8 y.o. F/S Greyhound.

History: Patient has decreased activity, difficulty getting onto bed, and right pelvic limb lameness after activity for past few months.

Physical examination: On presentation patient is bright, alert, and responsive. Body condition score 6/9, weight 70.8 pounds. Mild muscle atrophy of right pelvic limb (47.5 cm) compared to left (48 cm). Exhibits pain (4/10) on lumbosacral junction and slow conscious proprioception on right pelvic limb, but patellar reflexes and withdrawal normal. Patient on Cosequin® and fish oil for over a year.

Treatment plan: Continue Cosequin® and fish oil, start gabapentin at 10 mg/kg p.o. t.i.d., and weekly laser therapy and acupuncture for 4 weeks. Clients instructed to not allow patient to jump onto bed while undergoing therapy.

Initial treatment:
Laser therapy: Wavelength 905 nm, power 1.2 Watts, frequency 292 Hz, dose 4 J/cm², 229.624 J along lumbosacral spine and paraspinal muscles.
  Acupuncture:

● Dry needle: Bai-hui, LIV-3, BL-60, KID-3, BL-35, BL-36, GB-29, GB-30
● Electroacupuncture: Shen-shu, Shen-peng, Shen-jiao, BL-54 + Jian-jiao, BL-23 @ 20 Hz × 20 minutes.

Follow-up treatment (1 week later):
Update: Patient more comfortable and more active at home.

Laser therapy: Repeated as above.
Acupuncture:

● Dry needle: Bai-hui, LIV-3, BL-60, KID-3, BL-35, BL-36, GB-29, GB-30
● Electroacupuncture: Shen-shu, Shen-peng, Shen-jiao, BL-54 + Jian-jiao, BL-23 @ 20 Hz × 20 minutes.

Follow-up treatment (1 week later):
Update: Patient is doing well, although she jumped on the bed and yelped.
  Laser therapy: Repeated as above.
  Acupuncture:

● Dry needle: Bai-hui, LIV-3, BL-60, KID-3, BL-35, BL-36, GB-29, GB-30
● Electroacupuncture: Shen-shu, Shen-peng, Shen-jiao, BL-54 + Jian-jiao, BL-23 @ 20 Hz × 20 minutes.

Follow-up treatment (1 week later):
Update: Patient is doing very well at home and clients are lifting her on and off bed to prevent jumping.
  Laser therapy: Repeated as above.
  Acupuncture:

● Dry needle: Bai-hui, LIV-3, BL-60, KID-3, BL-35, BL-36, GB-29, GB-30
● Electro-acupuncture: Shen-shu, Shen-peng, Shen-jiao, BL-54 + Jian-jiao, BL-23 @ 20 Hz × 20 minutes.

Outcome: On the last visit, patient has no evidence of lumbosacral pain or right pelvic limb lameness. Patient able to return to activities she used to enjoy, and has not required any follow-up treatments to date.

Cautions and contraindications

There are numerous acupuncture points located around the eyes, which should be used with caution so as not to puncture the globe. Points located along the lateral thorax and abdomen should be inserted at an oblique angle to avoid entering the pleural or abdominal cavities. It is imperative to note that electroacupuncture is contraindicated in patients with a history of seizures, epilepsy, cardiac arrhythmias, and those that have a pacemaker; and it should be used with caution in patients with neoplasia and congestive heart failure (Altman, 1994). Acupuncture should never be performed directly into or around a tumor, into open wounds or scar tissue, or directly into skin that has severe dermatitis. There are certain acupuncture points that cause uterine contraction and induce parturition, therefore these points are contraindicated in pregnancy that is not at term. Points contraindicated in pregnancy include LI-4, SP-6, BL-23, BL-24, BL-25, BL-26, BL-27, BL-28, BL-40, BL-52, BL-60, BL-67, ST-36, CV-2, CV-3, CV-4, CV-5, CV-6, and *Yan-chi* (Xie & Preast, 2007).

Training and certification

In most states, only licensed veterinarians can perform acupuncture. Before engaging in the practice of acupuncture, successful completion of a certified veterinary acupuncture training program is required. Institutions that offer veterinary acupuncture training programs in the United States include the Chi Institute of Chinese Medicine, the International Veterinary Acupuncture Society, and Medical Acupuncture for Veterinarians. In addition, there is a unique opportunity to receive a Master's Degree in Traditional Chinese Veterinary Medicine (TCVM) through China's Southwest University. This is a chance for veterinarians certified in basic acupuncture to pursue a greater understanding of veterinary acupuncture and Chinese herbal medicine.

What is manipulative therapy/ chiropractic?

Spinal manipulation or chiropractic focuses on the relationship between structure (primarily the spine) and function (as coordinated by the nervous system) and how that relationship affects the preservation and restoration of health (see the Association of Chiropractic Colleges website). The basis of chiropractic is to improve the mobility of hypomobile joints (all joints, not just vertebral), which, in turn, improves appropriate afferent and efferent neurological function. Appropriate neurological function is necessary for maintaining all bodily functions, including proper muscle action.

The word chiropractic was coined in American English from *chiro* (hand) and *praktikos* (practical), which loosely means *done by hand* (Etymology Dictionary). Chiropractic is the study of the relationship between structure (primarily of the spine) and function (primarily of the nervous system), and how that relationship affects the restoration and preservation of overall health and mobility (Gatterman, 2005).

Modern-day chiropractic, credited to Dr. Daniel David Palmer, who performed the first adjustment in September 1895, started by adjusting a patient's vertebral mobility. A traditional adjustment is a precise, high-velocity, low-amplitude (HVLA) thrust, similar to a Maitland Grade V thrust manipulation (see Chapter 6). The difference between joint mobilization and joint manipulation (adjustment) is that during mobilization a joint is manually brought from its normal range of motion into its passive range of motion, but during a manipulation the joint that has been brought into its end passive range of motion is then brought into its paraphysiological space/range of motion without exceeding the boundaries of its anatomic integrity (Vernon & Mrozek, 2005).

To perform manipulative therapy/animal chiropractic appropriately, one needs to have keenly honed palpation skills, appropriate training in adjustment techniques, and the ability to integrate biomechanics, anatomy, neurology, and physiology to determine the patient's differential diagnoses and the potential results of an adjustment.

An anatomic abnormality requiring adjustment has traditionally been referred to as a *subluxation* (Gatterman, 2005). This term meets with significant controversy as subluxations have not been scientifically proven to exist and there is no agreement as to a specific definition of the term. Some medical sources require

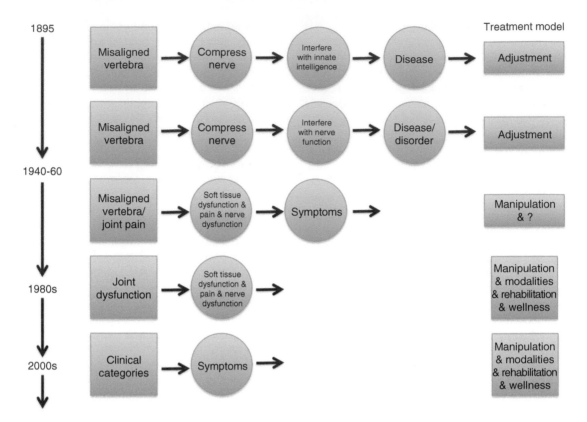

Figure 22.5 Evolution of subluxation theory. Subluxation theory has grown and developed since the early days of chiropractic, reflecting a more thorough understanding of complexity in both pathophysiology and treatment. Source: Vernon (2010).

radiographic evidence for a joint to qualify as having a subluxation (Gatterman, 2005). Current chiropractic practitioners often use the term subluxation for articular abnormalities that cannot be visualized on radiographs, but respond to appropriate adjustments. For example, *sacroiliac subluxation* implies that ligamentous stretching has been sufficient to permit the ilium to slip on the sacrum. An irregular prominence on one articular surface becomes wedged upon a prominence of the other articular surface, the ligaments are taut, reflex muscle spasm is intense, and pain is severe and continuous until a reduction is effected. The displacement is so slight that it cannot be recognized in radiographs. The pain of subluxation is often relieved dramatically and suddenly by manipulation (Turek, 1977).

Another definition for subluxation is, "A motion segment in which alignment, move-ment integrity, and/or physiologic function are altered although contact between joint surfaces remains intact" (World Health Organization, 2005). A motion segment is defined as "a functional unit made up of two adjacent articulating surfaces and the connecting tissues binding them to each other" (Gatterman, 2005). The subluxation theory continues to evolve (Figure 22.5).

A subluxation is believed to result in decreased joint range of motion, which results in a vicious cycle of decreased afferent and efferent nervous system signals, decreased joint health, and pain. With joint immobilization, cartilage degeneration and joint capsule contracture, especially of the flexor side of the joint capsule, occurs (Millis & Levine, 2014). The goal of manipulative therapy or chiropractic is to help improve the joint range of motion and restore function.

Chiropractic/manipulative therapy is a receptor-based therapy. A functional knowledge of neurology is required for the appropriate use of manipulative therapy. Every manual adjustment affects the nervous system in some manner, and the manipulative therapist should understand the neurological impact that an adjustment might have on the patient.

Anatomy and function

Many patients that present to rehabilitation therapists are experiencing changes in gait and/or mobility. Training in neuroanatomy and neural function as well as honing palpation and manual skills are critical components of training in manipulative therapy/chiropractic. These skills can be tremendously beneficial in helping to determine the longitudinal level of a neurological lesion with which a rehabilitation patient presents (Beck, 2011; Lorenz *et al.*, 2011).

Knowledge of the anatomy and function of the nervous system is necessary to appropriately diagnose musculoskeletal problems encountered in rehabilitation patients and to determine when and how to prescribe and apply chiropractic and manipulative therapies. A working knowledge of spinal cord anatomy and function, including locations of motor and sensory tract pathways and how afferent information is processed and affected by chiropractic adjustments, can help to improve rehabilitation diagnosis and subsequent treatments.

The joints formed by the articular facets of the spine are true synovial (diarthrodial) joints referred to as zygapophyseal joints, or Z joints for short. The joint capsules of the Z joints have a tremendous concentration of sensory innervation, including mechanoreceptors and nerve endings containing substance P for nociception (Giles & Taylor, 1987; Yamashita et al, 1996; Cramer & Darby, 2014). Gapping or separating of the Z joints and breakdown of intra-articular adhesions between Z joints have been hypothesized as a beneficial effect of spinal adjusting (Cramer *et al.*, 2002). Research has demonstrated that vertebral hypomobility results in degenerative changes of the Z joints, including adhesions in the Z joints themselves, the amount and severity of which are time-dependent (Cramer, *et al.*, 2004, 2010).

The anatomic components of a joint, including the joint capsules and ligaments, are rich in mechanoreceptors that provide abundant afferent information to the CNS about joint position and proprioception. Sensory information (received from both the external environment and from within the body) is processed and integrated by the CNS to produce appropriate output (Zimny, 1988). An adjustment of a joint provides sensory input through the motion imparted on the motion segment.

The intervertebral foramen (IVF) forms a bony–ligamentous boundary and provides protection between the central and peripheral nervous systems. Intervertebral foramina are found from the 2nd cervical vertebrae to the sacrum. The structures that pass through the IVF are the dorsal root ganglia, spinal nerve, cerebrospinal fluid (CSF), recurrent meningeal nerve, dura, veins, arteries, lymphatics, transforaminal ligaments, and adipose tissue.

Because discs receive direct nociceptive innervation, an injury to the disc can be a sole cause of back pain. In addition, an inflamed disc can compress or entrap a dorsal root exiting the IVF, and the histamine-like substances that leak from injured intervertebral discs have been found to irritate exiting dorsal roots. Both of these situations cause sharp, stabbing pain known as radicular pain (Cramer & Darby, 2014).

When performing an adjustment, the goal of the animal chiropractor/manipulative therapist is not to return a vertebra or joint back to a specific position, but to activate or initiate the homeostatic mechanisms of vertebral or articular kinesthetics. An adjustment concentrates on one specific motion segment at a time. Effects of a local change may have widespread physiological effects, so the properly trained manipulative therapist will have performed a comprehensive evaluation and established a list of differential diagnoses for the patient before any adjustments or treatments are undertaken.

Functional neurology and manipulative therapy

The nervous system, composed of the central and peripheral nervous systems, is a complex and highly organized system that, when functioning properly, gathers sensory information from both outside and inside the body and processes this information to signal and activate body systems in a coordinated manner. The function of the nervous system can be assessed through the response of the autonomic nervous system (such as through heart rate, pupillary light reflex, sweating, and blood pressure) and somatic system (muscle function).

Knowledge of the origin of cranial nerves can assist the rehabilitation veterinarian in determining the approximate location of a suspected brain lesion in a patient. Likewise, knowledge of the innervation of skeletal muscles assists the rehabilitation therapist in further localizing the longitudinal level of a suspected spinal cord lesion. This can be especially beneficial when referring a patient for MRI.

Manipulative and rehabilitation therapists must be familiar with the innervation of skeletal muscles and of cutaneous regions (dermatomal pattern), and from which spinal cord segments the nerves emerge. Especially important are the brachial and lumbar plexi, because most of the muscles of the thoracic and pelvic limbs are innervated from these associated nerves (Lorenz *et al.*, 2011).

Musculoskeletal biomechanics

The manipulative therapist should understand how the bones, joints, and muscles move in concert with one another and how the nervous system signals the muscles to contract. The three dimensions of vertebral motion, in the X, Y, and Z axes (Figure 22.6) allow for coordinated motion in flexion/extension, lateral bending, and axial rotation, respectively (see Chapter 17), as well as with *coupled motion*—vertebral movement around one axis (e.g., X axis) that is associated with movement around a different axis (e.g., Y axis) (Figure 22.7).

While each vertebra has the ability to move in each of the axes, the structure and articulation of the articular facets (Z joints) contribute to increased motion in certain directions. The angulation of the articular facets of the quadruped cervical vertebrae is approximately 45 degrees caudal to cranial, dorsal to ventral, and lateral to medial.

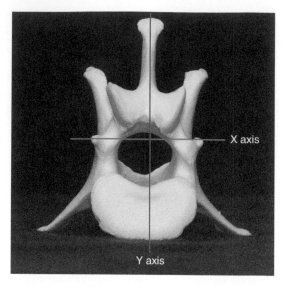

Figure 22.6   Axis of motion. End on view of a lumbar vertebra with schematic of x and y axes. The x-axis is horizontal, the y-axis is perpendicular to the ground, and the z-axis is planar (parallel to the vertebral bodies of the lumbosacral spine).

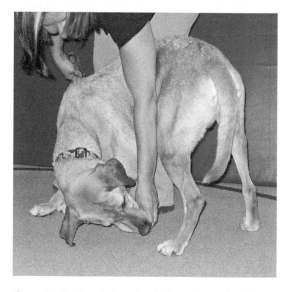

Figure 22.7   Coupled motion in the spine. A dog does a cookie reach to the rear toes, exhibiting flexion, lateral bend, and rotation.

The angulation of the articular facets of the quadruped thoracic vertebrae cranial to the anticlinal vertebrae (T11 in the canine) is such that the primary movement of the thoracic spine cranial to the anticlinal vertebrae is lateral flexion or side bending, with a small amount of axial rotation.

The angulation of the articular facets of the quadruped thoracic vertebrae caudal to the anticlinal vertebrae is such that the motion of the thoracic spine caudal to the anticlinal vertebrae and of the lumbar vertebrae is primarily dorsoventral flexion and extension.

Pelvis and sacrum

The canine sacrum is composed of three fused sacral vertebrae. The angle of the canine L7–S1 articular facets is approximately 45 degrees from each of the sagittal, transverse, and coronal axes. The angle of the canine sacroiliac articulation varies among dogs and is a topic of research through the American Kennel Club Canine Health Foundation (AKC-CHF) and North Carolina State University, the goal of which is to determine variations within and among breeds and the relationship of the canine sacroiliac joint angle to the lumbosacral, pelvic, and stifle joint angles.

Extremities

In addition to palpation and evaluation of vertebral motion segments, the manipulative therapist evaluates the motion quality of the motion segments of the extremities, performing appropriate motion palpation to challenge the mobility of each motion segment in the direction of normal mobility. If hypomobility or restriction of normal motion is detected, the manipulative therapist determines whether to perform a manual adjustment to help restore function and/or modulate pain.

Case Study 22.2   Sporting dog with thoracolumbar heat, left thoracic limb short stride, and paraspinal muscle sensitivity

Signalment: 9-y.o. M/N English Cocker Spaniel. Active in upland hunting, barn hunt, dock jumping, and family pet.

History: Several-day history of mild palpable heat over the thoracolumbar spine. No lameness noted. Patient normally runs and works at least 30 minutes daily.

Examination: BCS 4.5/9. Posture square at down, sit, stand. No appreciable weight shift. Active spinal ROM (cookie stretches) good in all directions (extension, flexion, lateral bend, coupled rotation). Gait fluid and even on clinical evaluation, but when viewed in slow motion video, at the trot, slight short stride of the left thoracic limb noted. No pain on palpation of the limbs. Slight muscular sensitivity and fasciculation elicited upon palpation of paraspinal muscles in the area of T13–L2. Slight tenderness at stretch of left iliopsoas muscle. Slight resistance to full extension of left thoracic limb. No restriction of PROM of coxofemoral joints. No instability palpated in shoulder or stifle joints.

Muscle girth symmetrical (using a Gulick girthometer) at proximal and mid-femur measurements, and at mid-tibia, and distal humerus measurements.

VSMT (veterinary spinal manipulative therapy) exam: Tenderness at T13–L2. Restricted motion at left temporomandibular joint (TMJ). The following restrictions/hypomobilities were found on motion palpation: ADR (atlas dorsal right), C6BL (6th cervical vertebral body left), T13PL (13th thoracic vertebrae posterior (dorsal) left), L4PL (4th lumbar vertebrae posterior (dorsal) left), left T9 rib dorsal.

Assessment: Several areas of hypomobility or restrictions in the caudal thoracic and cranial lumbar spine. Left 9th rib restricted dorsally—discomfort associated with this rib restriction could affect thoracic limb extension as upon extension the dorsal–caudal angle of the scapula normally glides caudal–ventral along the dorsal arches of the adjacent ribs. Patient may resist full extension of the thoracic limb to prevent this scapular motion. In addition, the brachial plexus originates from the last three cervical and first two thoracic nerves, so any vertebral restrictions in this area could alter nerve activity, potentially leading to increased nociception, decreased mobility, and diminished activity. Because of the slight discomfort elicited by the iliopsoas stretch test, iliopsoas muscle strain cannot be ruled out. The sensitivity to palpation at T13–L2 correlates to iliopsoas origin (last thoracic and first 4–5 lumbar vertebrae). Restriction of L4 correlates with emergence of one nerve root of the femoral nerve, which innervates the iliopsoas muscle.

(Continued)

Treatment: VSMT adjustments performed to address VSMT hypomobilities/restrictions: left TMJ and TMJ traction, atlas (C1) dorsal and right, 6th cervical vertebra body left, 13th thoracic vertebra dorsal and left, 4th lumbar vertebra dorsal and left, left 9th rib dorsal. Additional treatment of the iliopsoas and left shoulder muscles, such as laser, massage therapy, and therapeutic exercises indicated if discomfort not resolved post-VSMT.

Results: Restriction in scapular extension, tenderness on iliopsoas stretch, and paraspinal muscle palpation were resolved following VSMT adjustments.

Plan: Avoid rigorous activity for 2 days before returning to closely monitored training. Discontinue activity if symptoms, including gait changes, return. Recheck recommended 1 week later. If symptoms do not resolve or if they return, recommend additional diagnostics, including possible vertebral radiographs and ultrasound examination of the iliopsoas muscle.

Follow-up: Patient returned to normal activity 3 days following the VSMT adjustments. A video revealed that the patient's gait was normal. One week later, a follow-up chiropractic/VSMT exam was performed and no major restrictions were found. The patient has maintained problem-free activity, and receives VSMT therapy every 4–6 weeks.

Comment: Appropriate VSMT evaluation of canine athletes can detect hypomobilities before they lead to clinical abnormality and/or lameness, and thereby help an animal to maintain its best functional potential.

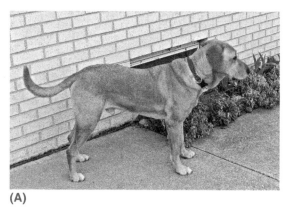
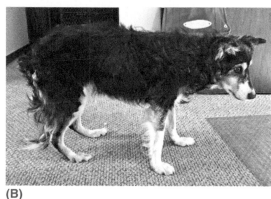

(A)   (B)

Figure 22.8 (A) Normal posture. Note the squarely placed limbs, level topline, and smooth muscle outlines in this dog. (B) Abnormal posture. This geriatric canine has pelvic limbs held forward under her body and a slightly kyphotic topline. There is also some loss of the secondary curvature in the lower cervical spine, resulting in low head carriage.

Chiropractic evaluation and treatment

As with any examination, a thorough history, including the physical activities of the patient and the client's goals should be taken. Observing the patient's posture and stance (Figure 22.8), and watching the patient move and transition between positions (e.g., between sitting and standing) gives the therapist important clues as to the mobility of the patient and potential difficulties and compensations. Video recordings of the patient in motion (such as during a sporting event or while the patient moves around the home), viewed in slow motion may reveal subtle gait and body position changes that would otherwise go undetected.

A thorough hands-on evaluation of the patient follows. The manipulative therapist uses two types of palpation skills, static palpation and motion palpation. In static palpation, the soft tissue and bony structures are manually assessed for texture, quality, alignment, heat, swelling, tenderness, and symmetry. Motion palpation, performed after static palpation, assesses the movement of each motion segment for quality of motion and symmetry (Gatterman, 2005) (Figure 22.9). Motion palpation is performed on the entire patient unless severe pain or discomfort is revealed, prompting the therapist to seek additional diagnostics.

The therapist should understand normal joint biomechanics to properly perform motion

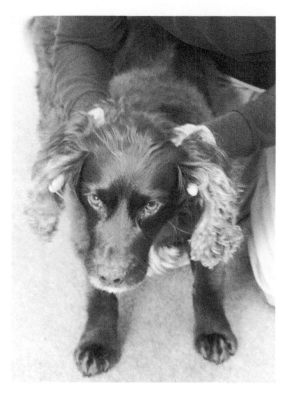

Figure 22.9 Motion palpation to evaluate symmetry at the occipito-atlantal joints.

palpation, challenging each motion segment in its correct line of motion to determine whether normal joint motion is present. Hypomobile joints are assessed to determine the quality and direction of the restriction and whether manual therapy, and possibly manipulative therapy/ chiropractic, would be appropriate. An unstable or hypermobile joint is not a candidate for adjustment. If adjustment is indicated, the manipulative therapist performs the adjustment in the correct direction to reduce the restriction and restore more appropriate joint motion (Figure 22.10).

Information gathered during the neurological evaluation, including motor, muscular strength, reflexes, and sensory responses, helps to localize a suspected neurological impairment. Upon formulation of a list of differential diagnoses, an appropriate rehabilitation therapy plan that might include manipulative therapy/chiropractic can be prescribed.

Clinical uses of manipulative therapy

Spinal manipulation is commonly used to treat low back pain in humans (National Institutes

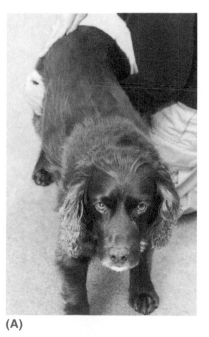
(A)

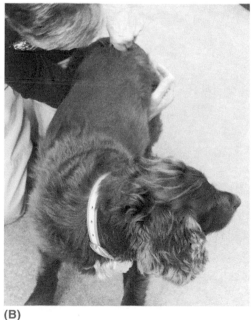
(B)

Figure 22.10 **(A, B)** The therapist performs the adjustment in the correct direction to reduce the restriction and restore more appropriate joint motion.

of Health, 2013). One report states that for treatment of low back pain "some people benefit from chiropractic therapy or acupuncture" (Goodman *et al.*, 2013). Another report summarized evidence regarding the effectiveness of spinal manipulation/mobilization in human adults for managing a variety of both musculoskeletal and non-musculoskeletal conditions, finding that spinal manipulation/mobilization was effective for treating or managing low back pain that is acute, subacute, and chronic in nature, migraine headache, cervicogenic headache, and dizziness (Bronfort *et al.*, 2010). Thoracic manipulation/mobilization was shown to be effective for acute and subacute neck pain. In addition, it was reported that manipulation/mobiliza-

tion was effective for several extremity joint conditions (Bronfort *et al.*, 2010).

Spinal manipulative therapy/animal chiropractic is used to help treat conditions such as lameness, paresis, pain, sports injuries, temporomandibular joint (TMJ) problems, and incontinence.

As discussed in Chapter 18, incontinence can be a primary reason for euthanasia of geriatric dogs (American Humane Association, 2016). One of the top five reasons for inappropriate fecal elimination and house soiling in geriatric patients is an underlying orthopedic condition that may prevent the dog from posturing correctly, or causes pain when the dog tries to defecate (Rudinsky, 2016). Manipulative therapy can be used to help improve mobility and

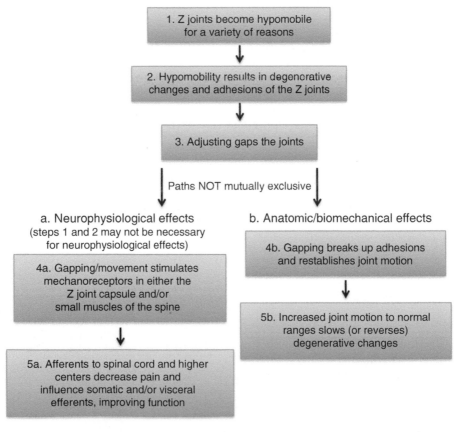

Figure 22.11   Manipulative therapy can be used to control or dampen pain via the neurophysiological effects of an adjustment stimulating mechanoreceptors in the joint capsule and small muscles of the spine thus sending afferent signals to the spinal cord and higher centers.

reduce pain, and thereby may possibly help improve continence.

Manipulative therapy can remove vertebral Z-joint adhesions that cause degenerative changes developing from hypomobility. Periodic manipulative therapy, then, can help maintain the best possible spinal and overall patient mobility (Cramer & Darby, 2014). Chiropractic manipulation has been documented to treat debilitating chronic sacroiliac joint syndrome in humans with good results (Cramer & Darby, 2014).

Pain management

In addition to improving function and mobility, manipulative therapy can be used to control or dampen pain (Figure 22.11). In a 1-year study of 148 human patients with low back pain and leg pain due to disc herniation treated with chiropractic therapy, all patients experienced significant improvement (Leemann *et. al.*, 2014). Managing pain is important in canine rehabilitation practice, allowing the patient to move and respond appropriately to rehabilitation therapies. Stimulation of large-diameter afferent nerve fibers by a high velocity, low amplitude thrust influences the pain gate modulation as hypothesized by Wall and Melzack (Melzack & Wall, 1965; Potter *et al.*, 2005).

Safety and contraindications

Manipulative therapy (chiropractic), is safe when performed properly. The incidence of adverse events as a result of manual therapy (including chiropractic adjustments) was found to be lower than that experienced from taking medication, and with no more risk than that inherent in other health interventions (Cassidy *et al.*, 2008; Carnes *et al.*, 2010; Church *et al.*, 2016).

Animal chiropractic should not be performed in areas with neoplasia, fracture, or other hypermobility, or hemorrhage.

Because it helps to improve and maintain appropriate nervous system and musculoskeletal health, manipulative therapy can be a beneficial part of a rehabilitation, general health, or sports medicine program.

Webliography

American Association of Rehabilitation Veterinarians (AARV). http://rehabvets.org.

American College of Veterinary Sports Medicine and Rehabilitation (ACVSMR). http://www.vsmr.org.

American Humane Association (AHA). 2016. Euthanasia: making the decision. 2016 fact sheet. http://www.americanhumane.org/fact-sheet/euthanasia-making-the-decision/.

American Kennel Club Canine Health Foundation (AKC-CHF). http://www.akcchf.org/research/participate-in-research/The-Canine-Sacroiliac-Joint-Angle-Breed-Variations-and-Relationship-to-Lumbosacral-Pelvic-and-Stifle-Angles.html.

Association of Chiropractic Colleges. http://www.chirocolleges.org/resources/chiropractic-paradigm-scope-practice/.

Chi Institute of Traditional Chinese Veterinary Medicine. www.tcvm.com.

Chi Institute of Traditional Chinese Veterinary Medicine. Traditional Chinese Veterinary Medicine Master's Program. http://www.tcvm.com/MastersDegree.aspx.

Etymology Dictionary. Chiropractic. http://www.etymonline.com/search?q=chiropractic.

Goodman, D., Burke, A. & Livingston, E. Low back pain. JAMA Patient Page April 24, 2013; 309(16), 1738. http://jamanetwork.com/journals/jama/fullarticle/1681414.

International Veterinary Acupuncture Society (IVAS). www.ivas.org.

National Institutes of Health (NIH). 2013. Spinal manipulation for low-back pain. NIH: National Center for Complementary and Integrative Health, NCCIH Pub No. D409, April 2013. https://nccih.nih.gov/health/pain/spinemanipulation.htm.

Rudinsky, A., 2016. Top 5 reasons for fecal house soiling in senior pets. Veterinary Team Brief, September 2016. www.veterinaryteambrief.com/article/top-5-reasons-fecal-house-soiling-senior-pets.

World Health Organization (WHO). 2005. *WHO Guidelines on Basic Training and Safety in Chiropactic*. http://www.who.int/medicines/areas/traditional/Chiro-Guidelines.pdf.

All websites accessed November 2017.

References

Altman, S. 1994. Techniques and Instrumentation. In: Schoen, A. M. (ed.), *Veterinary Acupuncture: Ancient Art to Modern Medicine*. St. Louis, MO: Mosby, pp. 86–97.

Beck, R. W. 2011. *Functional Neurology for Practitioners of Manual Medicine*, 2nd edn. Edinburgh: Churchill Livingstone Elsevier.

Bronfort, G., Haas, M., Evans, R., Leininger, B. & Triano, J. 2010. Effectiveness of manual therapies: the UK evidence report. *Chiropr Osteopat*, 18, 3.

Brown, M. L., Ulett, G. A. & Stern, J. A. 1974. Acupuncture loci: techniques for location. *Am J Chin Med*, 2, 67–74.

Carnes, D., Mars, T. S., Mullinger, G., Froud, R. & Underwood, M. 2010. Adverse events and manual therapy: a systematic review. *Man Ther*, 15(4), 355–363.

Cassidy, J. D., Boyle, E., Cote, P., He, Y., Hogg-Johnson, S., Silver, F. L. & Bondy, S. J. 2008. Risk of vertebrobasilar stroke and chiropractic care. *Spine*, 33(4S), S176–S183.

Church, E. W., Sieg, E. P., Zalatimo, O., Hussain, N. S., Glantz, M. & Harbaugh, R. E. 2016. Systematic review and meta-analysis of chiropractic care and cervical artery dissection: no evidence for causation. *Cureus*, 8(2), e498.

Costa, C., Ceccherelli, F., Ambrosio, F., Baron, P., De Antoni, A., Vanzan, S., *et al*. 1982. The influence of acupuncture on blood serum levels of tryptophan in healthy volunteers subjected to ketamine anesthesia. *Acupunct Electrother Res*, 7, 123–132.

Cramer, G. D. & Darby, S. A. 2014. *Clinical Anatomy of the Spine, Spinal Cord, and ANS*, 3rd edn. St. Louis: MO: Elsevier Mosby.

Cramer, G. D., Gregerson, G. M., Knudsen, J. T., Hubbard, B. B., Ustas, L. M. & Cantu, J. A. 2002. The effects of side-posture positioning and spinal adjusting on the lumbar z joints. *Spine*, 27(22), 2459–2466.

Cramer, G. D., Fournier, J. T., Henderson, D. N. R. & Wolcott, C. C. 2004. Degenerative changes following spinal fixation in a small animal model. *J Manipulative Physiol Ther*, 27(3), 141–154.

Cramer, G. D, Henderson, C. N. R., Little, J. W., Daley, C. & Grieve, T. J. 2010. Zygapophysial joint adhesions following induced hypomobility. *J Manipulative Physiol Ther*, 33, 508–518.

DeLeo, J. A. 2006. Basic science of pain. *J Bone Joint Surg Am*, 88(Suppl. 2):58–62.

Ehrlich, D. & Haber, P. 1992. Influence of acupuncture on physical performance capacity and haemodynamic parameters. *Int J Sports Med*, 13, 486–491.

Fry, L. M., Neary, S. M., Sharrock, J. & Rychel, J. K. 2014. Acupuncture for analgesia in veterinary medicine. *Top Compan Anim Med*, 29, 35–42.

Gatterman, M. I. 2005. *Foundations of Chiropractic*, 2nd edn. St. Louis, MO: Elsevier Mosby.

Giles, L. G, Taylor, J. R. 1987. Human zygapophyseal joint capsule and synovial fold innervation. *Br J Rheumatol*, 26, 93–98.

Gunn, C. C. 1977. Type IV acupuncture points. *Am J Acupunct*, 5, 51–52.

Gunn, C. C., Ditchburn, F. G., King, M. H. & Renwick, G. J. 1976. Acupuncture loci: a proposal for their classification according to their relationship to known neural structures. *Am J Chin Med*, 4, 183–195.

Han, J. S. 2003. Acupuncture: neuropeptide release produced by electrical stimulation of different frequencies. *Trends Neurosci*, 26, 17–22.

He, L. F. 1987. Involvement of endogenoius opiod peptides in acupuncture analgesia. *Pain*, 31(1), 99–121.

Jeong, H. J., Hong, S. H., Nam, Y. C., Yang, H. S., Lyu, Y. S., Baek, S. H., *et al*. 2003. The effect of acupuncture on pro-inflammatory cytokine production in patients with chronic headache: a preliminary report. *Am J Chin Med*, 31, 945–954.

Kendall, D. E. 1989a. Part I: A scientific model of acupuncture. *Am J Acupunct*, 17, 251–268.

Kendall, D. E. 1989b. Part II: A scientific model of acupuncture. *Am J Acupunct*, 17, 343–360.

Kim, M. S., Soh, K. S., Nam, T. C., Seo, K. M. & Litscher, G. 2006. Evaluation of sedation on electroencephalographic spectral edge frequency in 95 dogs sedated by acupuncture at GV20 or Yingtang and sedative combination. *Acupunct Electrother Res*, 31, 201–12.

La, J. L., Jalali, S. & Shami, S. A. 2005. Morphological studies on crushed sciatic nerve of rabbits with electroacupuncture or diclofenac sodium treatment. *Am J Chin Med*, 33, 663–669.

Leemann, S., Peterson, C. K., Schmid, C., Anklin, B. & Humphreys, B. K. 2014. Outcomes of acute and chronic patients with magnetic resonance imaging-confirmed symptomatic lumbar disc herniations receiving high-velocity, low-amplitude, spinal manipulative therapy: a prospective observational cohort study with one-year follow-up. *J Manipulative Physiol Ther*, 37(3), 155–163.

Lorenz, M. D., Coates, J. R. & Kent, M. 2011. *Handbook of Veterinary Neurology*, 5th edn. St. Louis, MO: Elsevier Saunders.

Mayer, D. J., Price, D. D. & Rafii, A. 1977. Antagonism of acupuncture analgesia in man by the narcotic antagonist naloxone. *Brain Res*, 121, 368–372.

Melzack, R. & Wall, P. D. 1965. Pain mechanisms: a new theory. *Science*, 150, 971–979.

Millis, D. L. & Levine, D. 2014. *Canine Rehabilitation and Physical Therapy*, 2nd edn. St. Louis, MO: Elsevier Saunders.

Murotani, T., Ishizuka, T. & Nakazawa, H. 2010. Possible involvement of histamine, dopamine, and noradrenaline in the periaqueductal gray in electroacupuncture pain relief. *Brain Res*, 1306, 62–68.

Omura, Y. 1975. Pathophysiology of acupuncture treatment; effects of acupuncture on cardiovascular and nervous systems. *Acupunct Electrotherap Res*, 1, 51–140.

Pan, C., Zhao, A. & Zhang, X. 1986. *Research on Acupuncture, Moxibustion and Acupuncture Anesthesia*. New York, NY: Springer-Verlag.

Pan, X. P., Zhang, B. H., Wang, D. L., Gao, H., Du, G. Z., Chen, B. Y. & Zheng, L. F. 1984. Electroacupuncture analgesia and analgesic action of Naga. *J Trad Chin Med*, 4, 273–278.

Potter, L., McCarthy, C. & Oldham, J. 2005. Physiological effects of spinal manipulation: a review of proposed theories. *Phys Ther Rev*, 10, 163–170.

Reichmanis, M., Marino, A. A. & Becker, R. O. 1975. Electrical correlates of acupuncture points. *IEEE Trans Biomed Eng*, 22, 533–535.

Silva, J. R., Silva, M. L. & Prado, W. A. 2011. Analgesia induced by 2 or 100 Hz electroacupuncture in the rat tail-flick test depends on the activation of different descending pain inhibitory mechanisms. *J Pain*, 12, 51–60.

Soligo, M., Nori, S. L., Protto, V., Florenzano, F. & Manni, L. 2013. Acupuncture and neurotrophin modulation. *Int Rev Neurobiol*, 111, 91–124.

Steiss, J. E. 2001. The neurophysiologic basis of acupuncture. In: Schoen, A. M. (ed.), *Veterinary Acupuncture Ancient Art to Modern Medicine*, 2nd edn. St. Louis, MO: Mosby, pp. 27–46.

Turek, S. L. 1977. *Orthopaedics Principles and their Application*, 3rd edn. Philadelphia, PA: Lippincott.

Urano, K. & Ogasawara, S. 1978. A fundamental study on acupuncture points phenomena of dog body. *Kitasato Arch Exp Med*, 51, 95–109.

Vernon, H. 2010. Historical overview and update on subluxation therories. *J Chiropr Humanit*, 17, 22–32.

Vernon, H. & Mrozek, J. 2005. A revised definition of manipulation. *J Manipulative Physiol Ther*, 28(1), 68–72.

Xie, H. & Preast, V. 2007. *Xie's Veterinary Acupuncture*. Ames, IA: John Wiley & Sons, Inc.

Yamashita, T., Minaki, Y., Ozaktay, A. C., Cavanaugh, J. M. & King, A. I. 1996. A morphological study of the fibrous capsule of the human lumbar facet joint. *Spine*, 21, 538–543.

Yim, Y. K., Lee, H., Hong, K. E., Kim, Y. I., Lee, B. R., Son, C. G. & Kim, J. E. 2007. Electro-acupuncture at acupoint ST-36 reduces inflammation and regulates immune activity in collagen-induced arthritic mice. *Evid Based Complement Altern Med*, 4, 51–57.

Zhang, Z. J., Wang, X. M. & Mcalonan, G. M. 2012. Neural acupuncture unit: a new concept for interpreting effects and mechanisms of acupuncture. *Evid Based Complement Altern Med*, 2012,429412.

Zhong, X. H. 1989. Correlation between endogenous opioid-like peptides and serotonin in laserpuncture analgesia. *Am J Acupunct*, 17, 39–43.

Zimny, M. L. 1988. Mechanoreceptors in articular tissues. *Am J Anat*, 182(1), 16–32.

23 The Business of Canine Rehabilitation

Amy Kramer, PT, DPT, CCRT

Summary

The American Society for the Prevention of Cruelty to Animals estimates that 78 million dogs are owned in the United States. Approximately 68% of all households in the United States have a dog. Pet spending is easily at an all-time high—Americans were expected to spend more than $60 billion on their pets in 2017 (Manning, 2016). With the internet being so readily available, people who are interested in options and alternative treatments for their pet will search for the best source. With a little advanced preparation, that best source could be you. When starting a canine rehabilitation business, there are many factors to consider. Knowing some of your options in advance can help a start-up canine rehabilitation business become successful and profitable. This chapter is designed to provide foundational information and to present some of the important decisions and options to consider when initiating a new rehabilitation business or reshaping an existing one.

Canine rehabilitation business scenarios

There are two initial options to consider when a therapist is considering building a canine rehabilitation business. The business can consist of a department in an existing veterinary hospital/clinic or a stand-alone rehabilitation practice. Each scenario has advantages and disadvantages. Several factors come into play when trying to decide between the two, including finances, space, and location.

Free-standing rehabilitation practice

Advantages
- The entire space can be designed for optimal rehabilitation practice
- Referrals are more easily obtained as there is no perceived competition with area general practices
- All services are unique and offered as a specialty.

Disadvantages

- All services must be marketed to the veterinary community and public to generate business
- All costs of doing business must be covered by the income generated from rehabilitation
- There may be spaces that are required but not always used, resulting in inefficiency (e.g., kennels).

Rehabilitation department within a veterinary hospital

Advantages

- Existing reception staff, waiting areas, and kennels can be shared with other services
- Potential in-house referral system is in place
- In-patient rehabilitation can be offered
- Rehabilitation can be started immediately postoperatively, prior to discharge of the patient
- Rehabilitation sessions can be built into the cost of surgery.

Disadvantages

- Outside referrals may be more difficult to obtain
- Patients may be fearful due to previous experiences, smells, and other animals crying/barking in this facility
- May have insufficient space for rehabilitation treatment areas and large equipment such as an underwater treadmill, and may need to renovate flooring/electrical system to accommodate
- Rehabilitation services must be promoted throughout the hospital to assure a culture of in-house referral
- Hospital renovations may result in downsizing of rehabilitation department if income does not meet expectations.

Business structure

How the business is structured financially is the next factor to consider. The business's financial structure is based upon details such as whether there are partners, tax benefits that might be available, and the risks and liabilities that would be assumed based on the type of structure. A good small business attorney and accountant can help with choosing the best financial structure. There are many websites that provide excellent information on how to structure a business, including Entrepreneur.com, Incorporate.com, SBA.gov, and IRS.gov. Helpful book titles include *Legal Guide for Starting and Running a Small Business* (Steingold, 2017) and *The Small Business Start-Up Kit* (Pakroo, 2003).

Sole proprietorship

A sole proprietorship is an unincorporated business with no partners. There are several reasons a therapist might choose this structure. One is that it is the least expensive and easiest to form and organize. The sole proprietor has complete control. All income generated is the proprietor's to reinvest or keep, and, if need be, a sole proprietorship is simple to dissolve. However, with a sole proprietorship the owner is responsible for all debts of the business and is personally liable, putting their own assets at risk. It can be difficult to raise funds when there are no shares of the business to sell or with which to attract long-term employees.

Limited liability corporation (LLC)

This business structure is often used to limit the owner's personal liability risk. There is less organizational paperwork required to set up an LLC as compared with a corporation. Further, there is the benefit of pass-through taxes, in which profits from the business flow directly through the owner's personal tax returns; the business does not file a completely separate tax return. Earnings in an LLC are usually subject to self-employment tax. Those choosing to create an LLC must make sure to check state laws for limits in the life of an LLC. For example, in some states, the LLC has to be dissolved if a member leaves the LLC. An LLC may be challenging to sell unless converted to a corporation, which can be difficult.

Corporations

A corporation is a group of people or a company acting as a single entity. There are several different types of corporations depending on whether they issue stock and whether they are for-profit or not. If the corporation is set up to issue stock, shareholders use money to purchase stock/shares in the company. The cost to purchase stock/shares is based on the valuation of the business as determined by an accountant assessing several variables. There is significantly more paperwork required to start a corporation than an LLC or partnership. There are two types of corporations, S and C, with the differences listed below.

C-Corporation

In general, all corporations are automatically classified as C-corporations unless the corporation elects instead to be an S-corporation. The C-corporation offers great tax planning flexibility and can shield shareholders from direct tax liability because the corporation is taxed separately from its owners. There is no limit on the number of shareholders allowed.

S-Corporation

An S-corporation is considered a pass-through corporation based on how it is taxed. An S-corporation requires the shareholders to have *reasonable compensation* but it allows them to consider all earnings profits as *distributions*, and to pass them through their personal tax returns. This avoids *double taxation*. It also provides the same protection from personal liability as a C-corporation. S-corporations are limited to 100 shareholders, and can have only one class of stock.

Business start-up team

Legal

Having a good corporate attorney is essential when choosing the right business structure, setting up the corporate binder, issuing stock certificates, and assuring that all documents are in order. The attorney can also help to write partnership/shareholder and employment agreements, job descriptions, and employee handbooks. Having good legal representation from the beginning will help minimize legal issues in the long run.

Accountant

An accountant helps to determine the tax implications associated with each type of business entity. The accountant should have experience with small to mid-sized businesses, and can help to minimize tax liability. An accountant can oversee and generate reports, projections, and profit and loss statements and business valuations. They can help with decisions regarding new equipment lease/finance/purchase, accounts receivables, and cash flows.

Business plan

A good business plan is essential to starting a business. It will explain the structure of the business, and can assist when pursuing funding from a bank/lender. Books such as *How to Write a Great Business Plan* (Sahlman, 2008) and *How to Write a Business Plan* (McKeever, 2017) are helpful. Useful websites include GoBusinessPlans.com, Business.com, and BizPlanEasy.com. These resources offer detailed information on proper layout and what to include in each section of the plan, and also provide templates for business plans. The business plan should include the following information, the purpose of which is to show the feasibility of business success.

Executive summary

This is the most important part of the business plan, and some suggest writing it last as it is a summary to highlight what has been written elsewhere in the plan. An individual reading this short summary will continue reading if their interest has been piqued. If not, they will discard it. Make it stand out!

Business description/products/services

This section describes what products/services the business offers. Rather than specifically discussing costs, this section should describe how the product/service meets the needs of customers or fills a gap that exists in the market.

Market analysis summary

This section reveals the market needs, trends, and growths that should make this business marketable. Key customers, future markets, and any existing competition are described here. Advantages of the proposed business and what makes it different from competitors are spelled out.

Strategy and implementation summary

Sales, marketing plans, and how customers are to be drawn to the business location are explained here. Location, equipment, technology, and key metrics that will be tracked to ensure the business is headed in the right direction are listed.

Company and management summary

The management team and the organization of the business are described here. This should include the company owners/officers/directors along with a summary of the value they bring to the organization and the role(s) each will play. It should also include the date of incorporation.

Financial plan

The financial plan details projected profits and loss as well as a sales forecast. This will give a potential lender/shareholder an idea of anticipated revenue.

Business funding

Knowing how much funding the business will require to get started is key. Finding ways to attain funding is another issue. There are several ways to secure funding for a sports medicine/rehabilitation business.

Traditional bank loans

These can be challenging in certain financial times. However, a cogent business plan that shows substantial financial projections is helpful. Having good credit history is also important.

Investment partners

It is possible to find an investor to provide start-up funds. Investors are especially helpful if they have invested in similar small businesses before, as their insight and experiences can be invaluable.

Shareholders

If the business is set up as a corporation, shares of the company can be sold. Shareholders will then own a portion of the business and will have a proportionate say in overall business operations such as equipment purchases and corporate structure. Having shareholders requires establishing the *value* of a business that may not even be running yet, which can be difficult.

Small business administration

Often the federal government's Small Business Administration (US SBA) will offer financial assistance and loan options to small businesses especially if they are women- or minority-owned.

Naming/branding the practice

Special consideration should be given to the name of the practice because it can help *brand* the business for its lifetime. It is never easy to change a business name, so taking time to assure an excellent name at the start will be key in marketing success. The practice will also need a logo, and some owners elect to add a tagline. Resources that can help with business branding include www.TheGuardian.com and www. Entrepreneur.com.

The first step in branding a business is knowing the business's *persona*. This involves understanding the needs, goals and behaviors of potential clients. Determining a company's persona can be accomplished using a free tool found at sites such as www.MakeMyPersona. com. Once the consumer/client has been identified, the next step in the branding process, naming, can be pursued.

Name

The name should be short and catchy or even be a pneumonic to help shorten a longer business name. A business name like "Joe's Canine Rehabilitation Clinic" might not be easy for potential clients to remember, and also might not present the desired image of professionalism. "Noah's ARC" (Noah's Animal Rehab Center) might be something that people will remember because it is easy to pronounce and everyone has heard of Noah's Ark!

Logo

A logo is a significant part of branding. It will be featured on the building, door, uniforms, letterhead, brochures, and business cards of the practice. The logo should stand out, be simple and easily recognized, yet different from logos of existing rehabilitation centers. In addition, it should provide an indication of what the business specializes in or at least pique the curiosity of the viewer. If the brochure is on a rack in a veterinary practice along with many others, will it stand out? Will people reach for it to read more information? There are many ways to develop logos, including hiring a graphic artist or visiting websites such as Designmantic.com, Logoworks.com, or 99designs.com, which are easy to use and can provide great ideas just by providing the business name and industry.

Taglines

Taglines are not essential but can be included in branding, and may be the catchy phrase that people will remember. Taglines should be short

and should provide an indication of what the business does. Examples include *Sit, Stay, Heal, Healing one paw at a time*, and *Giving your pet a longer leash on life*.

Rehabilitation team

The ideal team for canine rehabilitation combines the expertise and knowledge of both veterinarians and physical therapists. Individuals from both disciplines should be certified in canine rehabilitation (see Chapter 5). Veterinarians and physical therapists with the CCRT (certified canine rehabilitation therapist) or CCRP (certified canine rehabilitation practitioner) credentials have advanced education in the field of canine rehabilitation. Veterinary technicians can receive CCRP or CCRA (certified canine rehabilitation assistant) credentials. The veterinarian and the physical therapist working together bring significant value to improve patient outcomes beyond what either can accomplish alone.

Veterinarians

Veterinarians have the knowledge and experience in animal medicine to help guide rehabilitation in the areas of nutrition, supplements (see Chapter 4), medications, pain management (see Chapter 19), and overall wellness of the patient. They can also be certified in acupuncture and chiropractic (see Chapter 22), which can be beneficial to the rehabilitation process.

Physical therapists

Physical therapists have years of experience in the appropriate use of modalities (see Chapter 7) as well as manual therapy skills (see Chapter 6), which are key to improving range of motion. They are also experts in therapeutic exercise (see Chapter 8) and designing exercise programs to achieve the goals desired in rehabilitation.

Technicians/rehabilitation assistants

Rehabilitation-certified technicians are key to any rehabilitation setting as they can help guide patients through exercise programs, assist in hydrotherapy (underwater treadmill or pool) and modalities, hold a patient during acupuncture or therapy sessions, address client education, and manage the service's equipment. This frees up the veterinarian and the physical therapist to do patient evaluations, design treatment plans, and manage the practice.

Location/space needs

If the rehabilitation practice is a department in an existing veterinary practice, the location is already determined. The department will be located where the practice owners have allotted space. Opening a stand-alone practice will require careful consideration of possible facility locations.

Location

The ideal location has minimal competition, so that it can be "the only game in town." This tactic will help to attract clients from a greater radius. Consideration should be given to population density and proximity to veterinary hospitals that can be a source of referrals.

Lease/buy

The decision to lease or buy will be determined by finances, as purchase costs and financing fees must be covered in addition to the other costs involved in opening a new rehabilitation facility. Leasing requires finding a landlord that will allow an animal practice, and will allow the planned improvements/renovations. Both leasing and buying require that city ordinances permit an animal business in the area, and allow overnight boarding if that is a planned service.

Parking

There must be sufficient parking not only for customers but for staff as well. Many clients will be bringing pets that are large and unable to walk. They will be hesitant to bring their pet to the practice if parking is inconvenient. Considerations of space for staff parking should include the possibility that the number of staff will grow as the practice does and the resultant need for additional parking should not reduce the availability of client parking.

Space requirements

If the rehabilitation service is a component of an existing practice, some creativity will be required to make the most of the space allotted. For example, the underwater treadmill (UWTM) may need to be in the room where treatments take place. This may limit the number of patients that can be seen at one time. Another consideration is that the distance between the kennels and the rehabilitation area can impact profitability because time is spent moving dogs, especially large nonambulatory patients.

A free-standing facility will require a detailed layout that demonstrates how the services being offered will be accommodated. Ideally, the area for exercise should be large enough that two or more dogs can be treated simultaneously without the animals being forced to interact. Acupuncture or manual therapy treatments are best done in a private room, so the plans should consider how many such rooms are needed. Hydrotherapy equipment (pools and UWTMs) require significant specialized space, and this also needs to be taken into consideration. The reception and waiting area must be large enough that dogs do not have to be close to one another during check in/check out. Kennels are necessary, whether offering overnight boarding or not, especially for patients with clients that prefer to drop their dogs off for treatments and pick them up at the end of the workday. Additional space must be allotted for office, charting desks, staff break room, office manager space, bathrooms (addressing requirements for mens'/womens'/unisex and ADA (see later in this chapter)), laundry room, and meeting room/conference space for staff meetings or educational classes.

Construction considerations

Build out requirements are determined by the services to be offered. Each service has its own space and equipment needs that require specific considerations in terms of construction. An individual starting a rehabilitation business must think like an owner in terms of profitability. Fancy art and chairs will not generate a return on investment, although indirectly they might make a client more comfortable, which might translate into personal recommendations and thus increased business. However, in general, the emphasis should be on equipment, supplies that can be sold, and services.

Therapy room/gym

This room will need to have space to set up cavaletti poles and cones, wobble boards, peanuts, and a land treadmill (Figures 23.1 and 23.2). Flooring in this room is important since many patients will have a compromised gait and will need extra traction to help them walk/stand.

Acupuncture

This service requires a calming, quiet area away from other animals where the patient is not tempted to get up in the middle of treatment. Here, comfortable flooring or a soft mat, quiet music, dimmable lighting, and windows in the door to avoid unnecessary interruptions are all suggested (Figure 23.3).

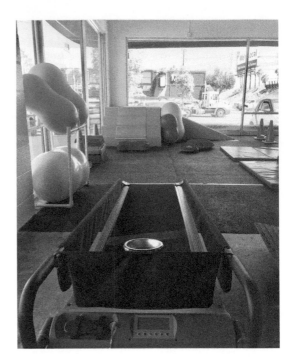

Figure 23.2   Gym equipment including land treadmill, cavaletti poles and cones, and physio rolls. Source: Image courtesy of the Beach Animal Rehabilitation Center.

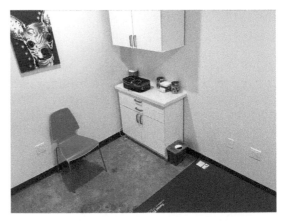

Figure 23.3   Acupuncture room with mat rather than exam table. Source: Image courtesy of the Beach Animal Rehabilitation Center.

Pool

The space for this will depend on the dimensions of the pool. There are requirements in terms of drains, equipment, and power needs that will vary depending on whether the pool is

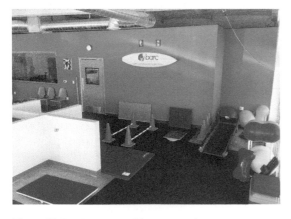

Figure 23.1   Gym area with treatment bays, demonstrating large space with natural light and good nonslip flooring. Source: Image courtesy of the Beach Animal Rehabilitation Center.

in-ground or above-ground and also on local codes. Nonslip flooring is critical in this room to prevent slipping on wet surfaces.

Underwater treadmill

Treadmill manufacturers have very specific space and power requirements for their machines. One important feature to consider when building is that the door to the room that will house the underwater treadmill is large enough to allow the equipment to be added after construction, and to be removed if that ever becomes necessary. It is wise to have the floor sloped toward a central drain in case of accidental overflow. A nonskid flooring surface here is advisable as well (Figure 23.4). Locker room flooring such as Dri-Dek® is a good choice as it allows the water to flow through while keeping the traction surface dry.

Evaluation room

A larger room always helps with analyzing a dog's stance and in preventing the patient from feeling crowded or threatened. Often there are several family members that stay for the initial evaluation, so having a larger area makes everyone feel more comfortable.

Reception/waiting area

This area needs to be large enough to allow patients plenty of space (Figure 23.5). If possible, having separate check-in and check-out areas improves traffic flow. The waiting area is not an area that makes money directly. It should be sufficiently comfortable for someone waiting for their dog, but its luxury should not compromise the purchase of equipment, which is more directly profitable.

Cats and exotics

If the service will treat cats/rabbits/pigs or any other small animal, an additional smaller, quieter space may be required.

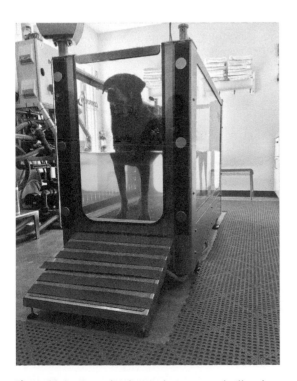

Figure 23.4 Example of an underwater treadmill and nonslip flooring. Source: Image courtesy of the Beach Animal Rehabilitation Center.

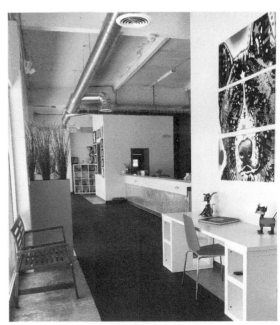

Figure 23.5 Open reception area with nonslip flooring. Source: Image courtesy of the Beach Animal Rehabilitation Center.

Kennels

Researching the type of kennels, including size, material, and drainage is essential prior to beginning construction (Figure 23.6). Kennels on the ground (using a concrete floor) must have drains cut into the floor that are connected to the main drain. This can be costly. Another option is to elevate the floor of the kennel room so that drains from the cages direct fluids into one central drain. Cameras can be installed to allow staff and the client to monitor the pet in the kennel.

Storage

Dedicated space is required for items that will be stocked and sold in the rehabilitation practice. Common retail items include slings/harnesses, booties, cold/heat packs, treats/food, supplements, and fitness equipment.

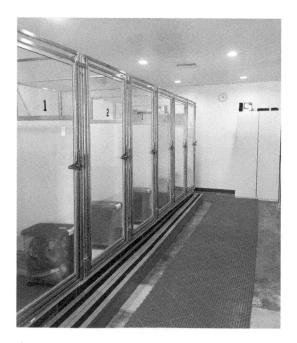

Figure 23.6   Kennels appropriately sized for medium to large dogs and good traction flooring. Source: Image courtesy of the Beach Animal Rehabilitation Center.

General construction concepts

Insulation

Insulation helps modulate temperature changes and reduces noise. The need for sufficient insulation becomes apparent when dogs in the kennels are barking while the therapist is working on a nervous patient in the acupuncture room.

Heat/air conditioning

Heating, ventilation, and air conditioning (HVAC) is especially important if the practice has hydrotherapy equipment, which creates substantial humidity. This should be discussed with the contractor well in advance, because special accommodations are often required. Thermostat units that connect to the internet are very helpful, allowing the staff to control them remotely.

Lighting/natural light

Good lighting is essential to improve employee performance, health, and safety (Dianat *et al.*, 2013). When possible, windows and or skylights should be used, because they help reduce electricity usage. Dimmable lights are beneficial in an acupuncture room.

Flooring

The flooring in a rehabilitation department/facility is extremely important. Most patients are compromised in some way, and having a floor with good traction throughout the facility will help them ambulate and gives the clients more confidence in the practice. There are many excellent options including rubber flooring, yoga mat runners, and rough concrete; different surfaces might be used in different areas of the facility. It is also helpful to have large, movable, waterproof floor mats in the evaluation and treatment rooms. Flooring products should be nonporous, easy to clean, provide good traction, and if possible (though less important), should be esthetically pleasing.

ADA (Americans with Disabilities Act) requirements

This part of the construction phase can be challenging. Research is important, and one should not expect the contractor, architect, or subcontractors to know the ADA requirements for this specific type of facility. It is advisable to consult with an ADA specialist known as a CASp (Certified Access Specialist) instead of learning during a building inspection that a component of the construction does not meet ADA requirements. ADA requirements are for exterior (entrances and access to public right of way) as well as interior (bathrooms, hallways, doorways) components of the building.

Electrical requirements

Some pieces of equipment require dedicated electrical circuits or specific types of outlets (dryer, underwater treadmill). It is best to have these details established during the building phase, rather than having the electrician make modifications after construction. LED lights and lights that are on a solenoid or timer can save energy costs. It is generally easier to install extra outlets during construction than it is to add them later.

Low voltage/phones/computers

Today's world revolves around computers, so it is important to have enough telephones and computers to start the business, enough CAT 5e or 6 cable (category of cable used for computer wiring with Cat 6 preferred due to increased upload/download speeds), and telephone outlets, and the ability to add telephone lines to expand as the business grows. A strong Wi-Fi signal throughout the facility is suggested. Repeaters or boosters can be helpful to extend the range of a Wi-Fi signal from the router.

Rehabilitation equipment

Equipment for rehabilitation can include large expensive items such as an underwater treadmill or laser as well as small inexpensive items

such as goniometers and Gulick tape measures. It is important to consider what is truly *needed* versus *wanted*. Some large ticket items, such as an underwater treadmill, are not essential to get started and can be purchased later when finances improve.

Evaluation equipment

- Goniometer: Used to measure joint range of motion. Multiple sizes are needed
- Gulick girthometer: Used to measure muscle and joint girth
- Reflex hammer: Used to test reflexes
- Penlight flashlight: To test pupillary light reflex and illuminate lesions.

Treatment equipment (inexpensive)

Available at markets/pharmacies

- Ice/heat packs
- Hair bands
- Air mattress.

Available online through canine rehabilitation suppliers

- Rocker/wobble boards: Nonslip surface with interchangeable components allowing unidirectional or multidirectional movement
- Physioballs or peanuts: Available in multiple sizes and shapes; a stabilizing rack can be built of PVC pipe
- Therapy band or therapy tubing: Available in different resistances; can be to cut to size
- Cavaletti systems: Cones and PVC poles with holes marked at 4 cm intervals
- Neuromuscular electrical stimulation (NMES or e-stim): Carbon fiber electrodes seem to work better than adhesive pads that lose adhesive quality due to fur.

Treatment equipment (expensive)

- Laser: Class 3b or 4. Many come with interchangeable heads and all come with protective glasses
- Therapeutic ultrasound: Can have large or small interchangeable heads

- Underwater treadmill: This is a great treatment tool but certainly not appropriate for all cases. There are several different manufacturers of treadmills with varying features. Space, plumbing, electrical, and HVAC requirements must be addressed before installation
- Swimming/therapy pool: Can be quite expensive, so the costs of purchase, installation, maintenance, and water supply must be weighed against potential income. Pools can be in-ground, above-ground, or all-in-one units with resistance jets as well as built-in ramps and decks
- Gait analysis system to analyze gait, providing objective measures including pressure, stride length, force, acceleration, and stance times (see Chapter 2 for details on the pros and cons of different systems).

Software: scheduling/documentation

Software

Of the many veterinary practice software programs available, many offer a free trial period prior to purchase. Beneficial features include employee timeclock, appointment scheduler, and the ability to create note templates. Many enable the practice to contact clients through the program via text and email, manage appointment reminders and inventory, and integrate online home exercise programs and accounting programs such as QuickBooks®.

Scheduling

Practice software programs often include an appointment scheduler that allows for varied appointment times for different treatment sessions, such as evaluations, rechecks, underwater treadmill sessions, or acupuncture visits. Often the treatments can be color coded for easy visual cues.

File storage

Becoming a more cloud-based practice saves time and paper cost, and reduces the risk of losing documentation that is necessary to keep available. Another great benefit is the opportunity to access records remotely, allowing for charting to be completed while off site.

Fee schedule

Determining the costs of services is based on time and service provided. Initial evaluation/assessment takes longer than an acupuncture or hydrotherapy therapy session, and the staff required is different. It is important to make sure that the fee charged covers more than the cost of providing the service. Aside from the cost of the staff participating in the patient's care there are overhead costs (electricity, space, equipment wear/tear, materials used) that need to be built into fees. For example, an acupuncture session fee must include the costs of the veterinarian to insert the needles, the technician holding the pet, the needles used, the electricity for lights, music, electro-unit, and the space in which the treatment takes place. Each session must make more than it costs to make it a profitable treatment.

Some practices charge based on time, others charge based on treatment type (acupuncture, hydrotherapy, physical therapy), and some charge based on modality (laser, ultrasound, massage). Still others use combinations of the above options.

Marketing

Marketing is essential for the success of any business. The public needs to be informed that the practice has opened, where it is located, the services offered, the qualifications of the staff, the hours of operation, and, very importantly, the benefits of rehabilitation.

Website

Every rehabilitation practice should have a searchable website that contains all the pertinent information that both the public and referring veterinarians will be interested in finding, especially how to schedule an appointment. Websites should include: hours of operation, services provided, contact information, location, staff (including their qualifications and areas of special interest), and testimonials. Hiring someone who specializes in search engine optimization is helpful to assure that the right keywords are used to achieve a high rank on search engines. As many people access webpages via mobile devices, the web designer should create a responsive website that will adjust to the size of the screen on which it is being viewed.

Printed materials

It is helpful to have printed materials such as brochures/rack cards and business cards that can be placed at referring veterinary hospitals, dog parks, pet stores, and other places frequented by clients. Printed materials should be eye catching with great photos and pertinent information so that potential clients can make contact.

Lunch 'n' learns

It is important to schedule opportunities to speak to potential referring veterinarians about the services provided at the rehabilitation practice and how this can help their patients and clients. As rehabilitation is still in the growing stages, not all veterinarians know what constitutes rehabilitation therapy and how rehabilitation can benefit their patients and improve their outcomes. Bringing lunch to a potential referring veterinary clinic, and presenting material using either a PowerPoint® presentation or a demonstration using dogs can help these potential referral sources to better understand the services offered. These presentations should make it clear that the rehabilitation practice has an ethical referral policy in place to prevent clients from leaving their referring hospital to receive routine care at the new facility.

Advertising

Print, television, and radio advertisements are great ways to get a new business name in front of many potential clients. Television and radio spots can recruit large numbers of clients but can be difficult to produce. A "feel-good" pet story can lure in a news team from the local television station, newspaper, or magazines in the region of the facility. The rehabilitation team can offer to write a pet-related column in a local paper or in a highly subscribed national magazine to encourage new business. Providing sponsorship to a local youth sports team or community event where the business logo is seen on team jerseys or banners can be very effective.

Social media

It is recommended to have a presence on social media, including Instagram, Facebook, and Twitter. Giving potential clients a glimpse into what is going on inside the facility can pique an interest in the services offered. Existing clients enjoy seeing their own pet on a social media page, and may repost the original post, thus increasing the business's visibility. Google and Yelp have business reviews that allow potential clients to read reviews by existing clients of the business. A customer review survey in 2016 by BrightLocal, a Search Engine Optimization company that helps companies get their business found on the internet, showed that word of mouth is still the most popular (68%) way for people to recommend a local business (Bonelli, 2016). The survey also showed that 84% of people trust online reviews as much as a personal recommendation. Staying up to date on social media pages with at least weekly new postings as well as continued reviews from existing clients on sites like Yelp, Facebook, and Google can help to bring in more customers.

Conclusion

Opening a rehabilitation practice/department takes a lot of forethought and energy. Making it successful and profitable requires hard work and patience. This chapter was designed to provide basic insight as to how to build a rehabilitation facility. It is wise to consider consulting with others in the field who have been successful to gain insight. Visit existing practices to learn what has worked well and what the owners would do differently the next time, and, no matter what, enjoy the process.

Webliography

Business structure

Entrepreneur Staff. 2010. Business structure basics. In: *Start Your Own Business, The Only Start-Up Book You Will Ever Need*, 5th edn, pp. 124–142. www.entrepreneur.com/start-your-own-business.

Internal Revenue Service. Business structures. https://www.irs.gov/businesses/small-businesses-self-employed/business-structures.

United States Small Business Administration. Choose a business structure. www.SBA.gov.

Business plan

Boachie, P. 2017. 7 must-have ingredients of a successful business plan. www.Business.com.

Duvald'Adrian, S. 2017. Do you really need a business plan? www.Business.com.

Go Business Plans Business Plan Consultant Group: www.GoBusinessPlans.com.

Naming/branding the practice

Campbell, H. 2015. The 7 Tenets of Branding. www.Entrepreneur.com.

Jafri, S. 2016. What's in a Name? In Branding, Pretty Much Everything. www.Salmajafri.com.

Scrimgeour, H. 2015. A guide to branding your small business. www.TheGuardian.com.

Logos

- Designmantic: www.Designmantic.com
- Logoworks: www.LogoWorks.com
- 99 Designs: www.99Designs.com.

Social media statistics

Bonelli, S. 2016. Local consumer review survey. www.BrightLocal.com.

Rehabilitation equipment

- Balanced Canine Products: www.BalancedCanineProducts.com
- Balls n Bands: www.BallsnBands.com

- Canine Rehab Products: www.CanineRehabProducts.com
- Canine Rehab Systems: www.CanineRehabSystems.com
- FitPAWS: www.FitpawsUSA.com
- TotoFit: www.totofit.com
- Wizard of Paws: www.WizardofPaws.net.

Cloud-based veterinary practice software

- Cure Pet: www.CurePet.com
- Evet Practice: www.EvetPractice.com
- Ezyvet: www.ezyVet.com
- Hippo: www.HippoManager.com
- Onward Vet: www.OnwardVet.com
- Provet: www.ProVet.info
- Vetter: www.VetterSoftware.com.

Online home exercise programs

- Canine Exercise Solutions: www.CanineExercise.com (integrates with several software programs).

References

Dianat, I., Sedghi, A., Bagherzade, J., Jafarabadi, M. A. & Stedmon, A. W. 2013. Objective and subjective assessments of lighting in a hospital setting: implications for health, safety and performance. *Ergonomics*, 56(10), 1535–1545.

Manning, S. 2016. Americans spent just over $60 billion on their pets last year, a record fueled by a big jump in what owners shelled out for services like grooming, boarding and training. https://www.usnews.com/news/business/articles/2016-03-17/americans-pony-up-record-60b-keeping-pets-healthy-happy (accessed November 2017).

Mckeever, M. 2017. *How to Write a Business Plan*, 13th edn. USA: Nolo.

Pakroo, P. 2003. *The Small Business Start-Up Kit*, 9th edn. USA: Nolo.

Sahlman, W. 2008. *How to Write a Great Business Plan*. Boston, MA: Harvard Business School Publishing.

Steingold, F. S. 2017. *Legal Guide for Starting and Running a Small Business*, 15th edn. USA: Nolo.

Index

Locators in *italic* refer to figure; those in **bold** to tables

Canine Sports Medicine and Rehabilitation, Second Edition. Edited by Chris Zink and Janet B. Van Dyke.
© 2018 John Wiley & Sons, Inc. Published 2018 by John Wiley & Sons, Inc.